# Modern Antenatal Care of the Fetus

# Modern Antenatal Care of the Fetus

EDITED BY
Geoffrey Chamberlain
MD, FRCS, FRCOG
*Professor of Obstetrics and Gynaecology*
*St George's Hospital Medical School*
*London*

BLACKWELL SCIENTIFIC PUBLICATIONS
OXFORD LONDON
EDINBURGH BOSTON MELBOURNE

Editorial Offices:
Osney Mead, Oxford OX2 0EL
25 John Street, London WC1N 2BL
23 Ainslie Place, Edinburgh EH3 6AJ
3 Cambridge Center, Suite 208
Cambridge, Massachusetts 02142, USA
107 Barry Street, Carlton
Victoria 3053, Australia



First published 1990

Set by Best-set Typesetter Ltd, Hong Kong
Printed and bound in Great Britain by William Clowes Limited, Beccles and London

DISTRIBUTORS
Marston Book Services Ltd
PO Box 87
Oxford OX2 0DT
(*Orders:* Tel: 0865 791155
Fax: 0865 791927
Telex: 837515)

USA
Year Book Medical Publishers
200 North LaSalle Street
Chicago, Illinois 60601
(*Orders*: Tel: (312) 726-9733)

Canada
The C.V. Mosby Company
5240 Finch Avenue East
Scarborough, Ontario
(*Orders:* Tel: (416) 298-1588)

Australia
Blackwell Scientific Publications
(Australia) Pty Ltd
107 Barry Street
Carlton, Victoria 3053
(*Orders*: Tel: (03) 347-0300)

British Library
Cataloguing in Publication Data

Modern antenatal care of the fetus.
1. Man. Fetuses. Disease
I. Chamberlain, Geoffrey, *1930–*
618.3′2

ISBN 0–632–02703–7

# Contents

# List of contributors

LINDSEY D. ALLAN MD, FRCP, *Senior Lecturer in Paediatric Cardiology, Guy's Hospital Medical School, St Thomas's Street, London SE1*

GEOFFREY CHAMBERLAIN MD, FRCS, FRCOG, *Professor of Obstetrics and Gynaecology, St George's Hospital Medical School, Cranmer Terrace, London SW17 0RE*

DEMETRIOS L. ECONOMIDES MB, MRCS, MRCOG, *Research Fellow, Harris Birthright Research Centre for Fetal Medicine, Department of Obstetrics and Gynaecology, Kings' College Hospital, Denmark Hill, London SE5 9RS*

NICHOLAS M. FISK MBBS, FRACOG, MRCOG, DDU, *Lecturer and Honorary Senior Registrar, Fetal Medicine Unit, Institute of Obstetrics and Gynaecology, Royal Postgraduate Medical School, Queen Charlotte's and Chelsea Hospital's, Goldhawk Road, London W6 0XG*

HAROLD FOX MD, FRCPath, FRCOG, *Professor of Reproductive Pathology, Department of Pathology, University of Manchester, Stopford Buildings, Oxford Road, Manchester M13 9PT*

DAVID R. GRIFFIN MB, MRCOG, *Consultant Obstetrician and Gynaecologist, Watford General Hospital, Vicarage Road, Watford WO3 8HB*

J. GEDIS GRUDZINSKAS MD, FRCOG, *Professor of Obstetrics and Gynaecology, 4th Floor, Holland Wing, The London Hospital, and St Bartholomew's Hospital Medical College, London E1 1BB*

HOWARD M.L. JENKINS DM, MRCOG, *Consultant Obstetrician and Gynaecologist, Derby City Hospital, Uttoxeter Road, Derby DE3 3NE*

FRANK D. JOHNSTONE MD, FRCOG, *Department of Obstetrics and Gynaecology, Centre for Reproductive Biology, University of Edinburgh, 37 Chalmers Street, Edinburgh EH3 9EW*

K. MICHAEL LAURENCE MA, DSc, FRCP, FRCPath, *Professor of Paediatric Research, Institute of Medical Genetics, University of Wales College of Medicine, Heath Park, Cardiff CF4 4XN*

RICHARD J. LILFORD PhD, MRCOG, MRCP, *Professor of Obstetrics and Gynaecology, St James's University Hospital, Leeds LE9 7TF*

LIST OF CONTRIBUTORS

STUART LOGAN MB, ChB, MSc, MRCP, *Senior Lecturer in Paediatric Epidemiology, Institute of Child Health, London WC1*

PETER J. McPARLAND MRCOG, MRCPI, *Senior Registrar, Hammersmith Hospital, Du Cane Road, London W12 0HS*

ELIZABETH MILLER BSc, MB, *Consultant Epidemiologist, PHLS Communicable Disease Surveillance Centre, 61 Colindale Avenue, London NW9 5EQ*

JACQUELINE MOK MD, FRCP, *Consultant Paediatrician, Community Child Health, Lothian Health Board, 15–17 Carlton Terrace, Edinburgh EH7 5DG*

JAMES P. NEILSON BSc, MD, MRCOG, *Senior Lecturer, Department of Obstetrics and Gynaecology, Centre for Reproductive Biology, University of Edinburgh, 37 Chalmers Street, Edinburgh EH3 9EW*

KYPRIANOS H. NICOLAIDES MB, BSc, *Research Fellow, Harris Birthright Research Centre for Fetal Medicine, Department of Obstetrics and Gynaecology, Kings' College Hospital, Denmark Hill, London SE5 9RS*

J. MALCOLM PEARCE MD, FRCS, MRCOG, *Senior Lecturer, Fetal Welfare Laboratory, St George's Hospital, Cranmer Terrace, London SW17 0RE*

GEOFFREY L. RIDGWAY MD, BSc, FRCPath, *Consultant Medical Microbiologist, University College Hospital, Grafton Way, London WC1E 6AU*

CHARLES H. RODECK MB, BSc, FRCOG, *Professor and Honorary Consultant, Royal Postgraduate Medical School, Institute of Obstetrics and Gynaecology, Queen Charlotte's and Chelsea Hospital, Goldhawk Road, London W6 0XG*

GURLEEN SHARLAND BSc, MBBS, MRCP, *Registrar, Perinatal Cardiology, Guy's Hospital Medical School, St Thomas's Street, London SE1*

JOHN A.D. SPENCER BSc, MB, MRCOG, *Senior Lecturer and Consultant, Institute of Obstetrics and Gynaecology, Royal Postgraduate Medical School, Queen Charlotte's and Chelsea Hospital, Goldhawk Road, London W6 0XG*

PHILIP J. STEER BSc, MD, MRCOG, *Professor of Obstetrics and Gynaecology, Charing Cross and Westminster Medical School, West London Hospital, Hammersmith Road, London W6 7DQ*

RICHARD WARREN MB, DCH, MRCOG, *Consultant Obstetrician and Gynaecologist, Norfolk and Norwich Hospital, Brunswick Road, Norwich, Norfolk NR1 3SR*

# Preface

Modern antenatal care of the fetus includes that part of antenatal care which concentrates on the fetus. The mother and her unborn child are one unit, but for the ease of discussion some aspects of care relate more to the mother, others to the fetus and a large number to both. In this volume we consider some facets of antenatal care as it concentrates on the fetal diagnosis and treatment. A group of British authors has been selected, all of whom have contributed recently to this subject, many performing original research in it. Their reviews have been produced in the winter of 1988/89 and we have married them together to give us an updated account of an expanding subject.

Geoffrey Chamberlain
*St George's Hospital*
*London*

# 1: What is modern antenatal care of the fetus?

GEOFFREY CHAMBERLAIN



Antenatal fetal care has been an integral part of antenatal medicine since it started in Edinburgh at the turn of the century. The antenatal diagnosis of monsters was one of the three stated aims of the Ballentyne and Haig-Ferguson group, the acknowledged founders of antenatal clinics (see Table 1.1).

The next major advance was led by Janet Campbell in the 1920s when she organized antenatal clinics as we know them now (Campbell, 1927). Working from the Ministry of Health, Dr Campbell derived a uniform structure of antenatal care for women throughout the country. A pattern of examinations was proposed for all visits. After 16 weeks, at each visit the uterine height would be checked, the fetal heart listened for, the mother's blood pressure taken and the urine tested. The first examination and those at 32 and 36 weeks would be done by a general practitioner or clinic medical officer and at the other visits performed by a midwife. This pattern of four-weekly visits to 32 weeks, fortnightly to 36 weeks and weekly thereafter has entered the collective obstetricians' subconscious and has rarely been challenged until the last 15 years. Dame Janet Campbell, as she was later to be, was a pioneer of women's health but modern fetal care probably started after the Second World War. By

**Table 1.1** The aims of promaternity care. From Ballantyne (1901)

| | |
|---|---|
| **1** | The antenatal diagnosis of monsters |
| **2** | The treatment of medical diseases |
| **3** | The avoidance of fits |

then, maternal mortality rates had been reduced by a combination of better training of midwives and doctors looking after women (either consultant or general practitioner obstetricians), the wider use of antibiotics in the treatment of puerperal infections and the availability of blood following systematic organization of the Regional Transfusion Services. Obstetricians coming back from the Second World War faced a different scene from the one which they had left; now they could concentrate more on improving perinatal mortality and morbidity. Among the pioneers of this major change in the philosophy of obstetrics was Dugald Baird of Aberdeen. This scientist examined perinatal deaths in detail and from his studies derived a system of analyses which stood the test of time. From this pathological base, Dugald Baird was able to develop a management procedure to be used for the care of the fetus and the newborn.

Following the epidemiological work of Dugald Baird, we needed a system of measurement of the individual fetus that could be used to assess any therapeutic efforts made to improve well-being. This came when Ian Donald opened a window on the uterus by using ultrasound scanning in the human. For the first time, safe, precise and non-invasive measurements could be made reproducibly; this allowed serial readings to be made on the same fetus and permitted longitudinal records of growth to be constructed. Biophysical measurements of fetal movements, respiratory movements and cardiovascular activities soon followed. Some led to a more precise measurement of variations in fetal growth and function; others like cardiotocography, while clinically popular, has not been shown scientifically to be of proven benefit to the fetus. The use of cardiotocography in labour has been well assessed in a large randomized controlled trial in Dublin (O'Donnell 1986). In pregnancy, the general impression is that an abnormal tracing relates closely to poor fetal outcome (Solum *et al.* 1981) but that a normal tracing cannot be used absolutely for reassurance. Lumley *et al.* (1983) in a randomized controlled trial confirmed the lack of precision in antenatal cardiotocography amongst women at higher risk.

From measures like this, fetal therapy could be directed more precisely; it could be used directly as in helping the surgeon to navigate intrauterine surgical interventions or indirectly by monitoring pharmacological therapy performed through the mother. Both styles of treatment are now expanding but they needed longitudinal fetal monitoring as provided by biophysics.

Historically, biochemical measures preceded the biophysical ones. At first, laboratory ranges of results were wide; soon more sophisticated biochemical techniques led to a greater precision in measuring the chemistry of the sample provided. However, distribution curves of even the more precise results covered so wide a range that the boundary between normal and abnormal was imprecise. Of necessity the relevance of these results was only indirect, for we could not perform assays on the biochemical levels of fetal intracellular fluid or even, until very recently, the fetal extracellular bathing fluids such as blood. We had to depend on the transfer of catabolites back across the placenta and measure them after the passage into the mother's blood, which represents the fetal milieu exterieur. In consequence, the range of variation of fetal products in maternal body fluids were wide in both normality and abnormality. Often the levels in patients with and without the biochemical alteration overlapped, so the tests did not allow precision in the prediction or outcome. They have mostly disappeared as diagnostic agents from the late pregnancy scene but are being actively explored in very early pregnancy (see Chapter 4).

Biological measurements of the fetus had to await invasive harvesting methods in order to investigate cells derived from the fetus directly. Fritz Fuchs from Copenhagen reported the determination of the sex of the future baby by examining cells derived by amniocentesis in 1956; chorionic villus biopsy came in the early 1970s. From these cells, cultures could be made and the karyometric optical analysis of chromosomes performed. The subject has advanced to use improved DNA technology, allowing the diagnosis of an increasing number of major fetal diseases.

All this new science is woven into modern fetal antenatal care which acts as a screening service to detect fetal problems early enough to allow action to the taken. Such action at present is the nihilistic use of abortion; this reflects the inability of fetal therapy to keep up with fetal diagnosis, a well-known problem in medicine generally. However, the capacity to diagnose problems must precede the ability to treat them; without specific

**Table 1.2** When did modern fetal antenatal care start? The reader is invited to make his own judgement; the author considers the era began with Ian Donald and his pioneering of the use of ultrasound

| | | |
|---|---|---|
| Promaternity care formulated | Haig-Ferguson<br>Ballentyne | 1899 |
| Systematic antenatal clinics | Campbell | 1927 |
| Perinatal death analyses | Dugald Baird | 1952 |
| Placental function biochemistry | Brown<br>Klopper | 1955 |
| Amniocentesis for chromosome studies | Fuchs | 1956 |
| Static diagnostic ultrasound | Donald | 1961 |
| Continuous fetal heart rate monitoring | Hammacher | 1962 |
| Chorionic villus sampling | Hahnemann | 1968 |
| Percutaneous fetal blood sampling | Hobbins<br>Mahoney | 1974 |
| Alpha-fetoprotein levels | Brock | 1977 |
| Realtime ultrasound | Manning | 1984 |
| Doppler blood flow studies | Trudinger | 1985 |
| Recombinant DNA diagnosis | McDonald | 1986 |

diagnoses, the group of fetuses needing treatment cannot be delineated. Advances in DNA technology are currently so rapid that treatment may well be available in the next few years for many conditions we can only diagnose at the moment and for which we at present can only offer termination of pregnancy. The speed of advance can be gauged by the current resistance of many gynaecologists to offer permanent sterilization to couples with certain hereditary states for they feel a cure may be available just around the corner.

When did modern fetal antenatal care begin? A gradual process of increased diagnostic ability to measure the fetus has accelerated exponentially (Table 1.2). If any point has to be set as the beginning, it is probably Ian Donald and the revelations he showed with the ultrasound scanner, an instrument he played as delicately as a viola.

## The perinatal period

Since the 1820s, data have been collected about stillbirths and from a little later about neonatal deaths. The former related to babies who were born dead after the 28th week of pregnancy while the latter included all those who died in the first four weeks of life. In the 1920s, a new term was phrased — perinatal mortality. Seventy years ago this was intended to bring together those babies whose deaths might relate to obstetrical events so as to correlate attributability. Thus all stillbirths and all first week neonatal deaths were included among perinatal deaths. It was considered that after the first seven days, neonatal deaths were due to paediatric problems and not obstetrical ones.

This concept is obviously a dated one. We have now moved far enough to drop these old definitions in western countries. The problems with the definition of the perinatal period are at the beginning and the end. At the beginning, the 28th week of pregnancy is not a very well defined gestational zone for many women; without the help of ultrasound it is probably incorrect in one-third of a literate population and two-thirds where literacy and numeracy are uncommon. Further, many babies are now surviving in modern western neonatal units at gestational ages of 25 and even 24 weeks. Hence the beginning of the zone needs to be rethought.

The later boundary of the seventh day of extrauterine life is too restrictive. More babies are now surviving in the western countries because of neonatal intensive care; it would be wise to take the later time limit to four weeks again. Many babies who die in the second, third and fourth weeks of life with conditions such as necrotizing enteritis and respiratory immaturity are delivered early because of obstetrical conditions. The deaths of these immature newborns relate as much to obstetrics as deaths in the first week do.

There is another fundamental philosophical problem with the perinatal span. Whilst it may be acceptable, with a change in limits of the time zone, it is not a good adjective to describe a subject. No one doctor has the skills to cover the whole perinatal period from 28 weeks to the end of the first week of life. The former time is covered by the obstetrician, the latter by the neonatal paediatrician. Although in some parts of the world liaison is good between two groups, they are not the same people. The doctor who can make a correct diagnosis and treat intrauterine growth retardation or perform a Kjelland's forceps delivery in labour is not the same person who can look after the complexities of modern neonatal care in the intensive care unit. The term perinatal has become debased. In America and with American-derived educational systems, the word perinatal equals neonatal, ignoring the obstetrical component. The term perinatal therefore would seem to have had a useful life in describing the timing of events around birth but now may have outlived its usefulness and possibly should be laid to rest. There are no firm rules about the use of English but words slip in and out of usage as decades pass. Perhaps we should let perinatal drop in the future, referring to events in the intrauterine and neonatal periods as fetal and neonatal incidents.

### The concept of higher risk

Many consider that one of the major functions of modern antenatal care is to detect those mothers who are *at higher risk*. These women are then so categorized and they are expected to have more intensive antenatal care. There are however two important questions to ask here.

The first is: *At higher risk for what?* There may be a familial problem in the family so that a future baby might be at higher risk for haemophilia or Duchenne's muscular dystrophy. They are thus at higher risk for these conditions but not of necessity for any other problem such as intrauterine growth retardation. Most women, however, are just labelled *at high risk* because of some perceived risk factor such as heavy cigarette smoking or a raised blood pressure. The observers must decide for which fetal hazards the mother is at higher risk; the increased relative risks to a given fetus vary according to the measure of outcome examined.

The three major hazardous outcomes to a fetus are: (i) low birth weight; (ii) hypoxia; and (iii) congenital abnormalities. Each of these outcomes may require maternal, fetal or neonatal treatment depending on the degree of effect. The factors leading to each of these three measures of higher risk overlap but will vary in importance according to which measure of outcome is used. For example, a mother who is a heavy cigarette smoker will have a much greater relative risk of producing a low birth weight baby. The risks to this fetus of hypoxia in labour are not so great and those of congenital abnormalities are probably low. The concept of indiscriminate higher risk labelling of mothers at the booking antenatal clinic is not a wise one. It labels the woman without being specific as to what the risk is. Further, if she sees her notes with this phrase written on them, the mother is greatly worried.

The second question in the concept of risk is: *What is the degree of risk to the individual fetus?* Generally speaking, the screening tests at the antenatal clinic are performed to decide which women are in the various groups of higher risk categories for these conditions. These should aim at providing an actuarial measure of higher risk, placing the mother into a mathematical category of degree of increased risk. It is then for the thinking obstetrician to examine the individual woman and assess her fetus by investigations to check if there is any fetal deficit or alteration of function. This allows one to move from an actuarial higher risk group to the real or actual risk to the individual fetus itself in any given pregnancy.

The real risk may be perceived to be so great that labour should be avoided and an elective Caesarean section performed before the woman goes into labour. A lesser degree of actual risk to that fetus might permit the obstetrician to allow a labour at a given time, i.e. an induction is performed followed by careful monitoring during the labour. A lower still risk level may allow the woman to proceed to labour at the time nature and the fetus decide with full monitoring in labour. The fourth category will be those considered at lowest risk who would be allowed to pass into labour when the fetus decides and who require the minimum of monitoring during labour itself. Modern antenatal care of the fetus should divide women by screening into those groups who seem to be at an actuarial higher risk for low birth weight, hypoxia or congenital abnormalities, and then testing those women individually to see if their fetuses are at real or actual risk for these conditions. This subject is well pursued by James and Stirrat (1988) who have published a first rate account of this aspect of antenatal care.

## The pattern of modern antenatal care

The functions of modern antenatal care may be considered under six headings:

**1** The screening and prevention of maternal problems.
**2** The screening and prevention of fetal problems.
**3** The management of maternal symptomatic problems.
**4** The management of fetal symptomatic problems.
**5** The preparation of the couple for childbirth.
**6** The preparation of the couple for child rearing.

All these features are interlinked but in this volume, items 2 and 4 will be considered in more detail.

Modern antenatal care is not a uniform practice; it is carried out by a range of professionals including the midwife, the general practitioner, junior hospital doctors and, occasionally, the consultant obstetrician. The latter is usually involved when there are major problems of the mother or fetus such as maternal diabetes or heart disease, or intrauterine growth retardation of the fetus. For the rest of the time in the UK, the consultant will be in charge of a team and is there to be consulted on real problems. The junior hospital doctor probably carries out much of the hospital antenatal care. Such juniors vary enormously in their experience and the enthusiasm with which they perform their duties. The general practitioner in the UK now performs an increasing proportion of normal antenatal care ranging up to 70% of the total load in some districts. The midwives' contribution to antenatal care is also an increasing one. In the 1970s, she was an obstetrical aide in many places, but now midwives perform their own antenatal clinics in many centres; these are sited in the community, usually away from the main hospital and are very popular for waiting times are often less and care seems more personal.

The frequency and number of visits women pay to antenatal clinics is very variable. There is no firm association between increased numbers of visits and reduced perinatal mortality; the women at highest risk may have the most visits for obvious reasons. In the UK, most women have about ten visits during pregnancy; other European countries like Switzerland and Luxembourg report as few as five visits (mean) whilst in Holland and Finland, 14 visits are the average. Probably the number of visits depends more upon the traditional pattern laid down by Campbell in 1926 than upon any reasoned thought. Chamberlain (1978) suggested that one could reduce the number of visits in mid-trimester for little seemed to happen in that time but he met resistance from three groups of users of antenatal clinics — the senior obstetricians, the midwives and the women having babies. All these groups had been conditioned to consider the Campbell pattern to be sent from Mount Sinai on pillars of stone. Now, shared care between the hospital centre and GPO (general practitioner obstetrician) or midwives' clinics in the community is the nearest one gets to a rational programme of antenatal care for the pregnant woman.

There are few objective measures of the effectiveness of antenatal visits for the measures of outcome have been hard to delineate. Hall *et al.*

**Table 1.3** Minimum care for normal primigravidae. Modified from Hall (1989) with permission

| Gestation in weeks | Main purposes of visit* |
|---|---|
| 12 | History and examination, clarification of uncertain gestation, identification of risk factors for antenatal care and confinement. Advice on diet, drugs, work and exercise |
| 16 | Alpha-fetoprotein screening and ultrasonic scan |
| 22 | Fundal height, baseline weight |
| 26 | Blood pressure, urinalysis, discussion of delivery and feeding, etc. |
| 30 | Fundal height, weight gain: identification of high risk for intrauterine growth retardation and pre-eclampsia |
| 34 | Blood pressure, urinalysis, discussion of delivery and feeding, etc. |
| 36 | Fundal height, weight gain, identification of malpresentation |
| 38 | Blood pressure, urinalysis, discussion of delivery and feeding, etc. |
| 40 | Assessment of need for induction |
| 41 | Blood pressure, urinalysis, discussion of delivery and feeding |

* Blood pressure and urinalysis performed at every visit.

**Table 1.4** Minimum care for normal multigravidae. Modified from Hall (1989) with permission

| Gestation in weeks | Main purposes of visit* |
|---|---|
| 12 | History and examination, clarification of uncertain gestation, identification of risk factors for antenatal care and confinement. Advice on diet, drugs, work and exercise |
| 16 | Alpha-fetoprotein screening and ultrasonic scan |
| 22 | Fundal height, baseline weight |
| 30 | Fundal height, weight gain: identification of high risk for intrauterine growth retardation and pre-eclampsia |
| 36 | Fundal height, weight gain, identification of malpresentation |
| 40 | Assessment of need for induction |

* Blood pressure and urinalysis at every visit.

(1980) suggested a concept of productivity, examining the proportion of routine visits which resulted in an identification of the first time of any major problem. These workers took pre-eclampsia and malpresentation as their marker problems. From this Hall (1989) derived logical schemes of minimum care for a normal primigravida and minimum care for a normal multigravida (Tables 1.3 and 1.4).

On top of the clinical regime, modern fetal antenatal care has accepted a whole series of complex tests, many of which are dealt with in this book. These too have correct times for application but we must be careful to use the most useful tests, being prepared to put to one side the tests that are less helpful in predicting fetal compromise so that we can concentrate on the more useful ones.

## Prepregnancy care

In practice, modern antenatal fetal care should start at the prepregnancy clinic. Here aspects of the woman's past life and her past obstetrical career can be assessed along with those of her partner; they are potential guides to the various aspects of the fetal well-being. This is a helpful step, for once pregnancy starts the couple only have two options — to continue the pregnancy or to abort it. Prepregnancy consultation widens the spectrum of choice; while in some cases it may allow time for the correction of any problems detected such as susceptibility to rubella infection.

## The first antenatal visit

When pregnancy starts, the woman attends for a booking visit where a full history is taken; events that have occurred already in the present pregnancy are assessed, particularly those that might be teratogenic (exposure to drugs or X-rays).

### Menses

The menstrual cycle should be assessed and the last menstrual period demarcated as precisely as possible for it is hard to expect the woman to remember details in later months when some precision might be important.

### Medical history

The past medical history should be established with particular reference to specific illnesses such as lupus erythematosus or diabetes.

### Family history

A family history may contain elements indicating features of increased fetal risk such as early hypertension, early diabetes or twinning.

### Sociobiological background

The woman's age relates to problems of genetic origin whilst her ethnic group may relate to variations in diet and upbringing. Smoking has an effect on fetal growth and neonatal development, while alcohol and other addictive drugs are also noxious agents to the fetus. The social class of the woman can be derived from the occupation of herself or her partner, flagging a mixed group of factors such as nutrition in youth, diseases in youth, education and attitudes to medical care. It is also a guide to the woman's height; since the baby's likely birth weight is strongly correlated with maternal height, then social class relates to birth weight. Maternal weight is important for fetal growth and relates strongly to nutrition in early pregnancy which bears some relation to weight.

### Past obstetrical events

The past obstetrical history needs detailed scrutiny for it is one of the best predictors of the woman's and her fetus's behaviour in pregnancy and labour. Details should be sought of the previous pregnancies, any complications that occurred, the timing and method of delivery and the birth weight of the child. Conditions such as preterm labour or intrauterine growth retardation are often recurrent and a relative risk of problems in this pregnancy can be assessed from the past obstetrical history, using also the other factors that may be co-variables in this.

### Examination

Physical examination at this stage may reveal a raised blood pressure or a uterus inconsistent in size with gestational dates. Some abnormality of the uterus such as fibroids or, if relevant, a wider than normal cervical os may also be found. These can affect fetal health and should be noted and dealt with.

### Investigations

Investigations include those on the blood where ABO and rhesus groupings are performed. Hepatitis antibodies and serological tests for syphilis may be helpful as may the rubella antibody titres. Some units test for HIV in at-risk populations. Electrophoresis should be performed on the haemoglobin of a woman who comes from a relevant part of the world or who has a past history relating to this. Alpha-fetoprotein testing for open neural tube abnormalities is done in most hospitals; in some it is conjoined with other biochemical tests such as plasma oestrogen and plasma hCG to screen younger women who may have a baby with Down's syndrome. A specimen of urine is checked for bacilluria and glycosuria.

Commonly, an ultrasound scan of the fetus is performed, not necessarily at the booking visit but at about 18 weeks of gestation, to assess fetal size and in many clinics to look for any abnormality. Scanning at this time is usually done to estimate the fetal biparietal diameter; it is possible to train radiographers, midwives and doctors to do this fairly simple test reproducibly in a short time. The ultrasound screen shows a clear image of the fetal head and, with modern cursors, the diameter can be detected precisely. These same observers, however, are not necessarily the right people to screen for congenital abnormalities. Whilst anencephaly is relatively easy to detect at this stage, spina bifida is not. Most fetal heart problems cannot be resolved at 18 weeks and neither can abnormalities of gut or renal tract. In consequence, it would be ideal to measure the fetus for the biparietal diameter fairly early in pregnancy (16 weeks), to provide the first point on a chart to assess growth. Later on (22–24 weeks), there should be a second check for fetal abnormalities by more skilled ultrasonographers than are usually provided in most district hospitals for routine measurement work. This double testing is hard to perform in practice and in many centres has been conjoined into a single visit at 18 weeks as a compromise.

As well as this very practical point, enthusiasts should remember that many of the ultrasound tests have been developed in teaching units where there is a larger proportion of staff available who are interested in the subject and are more skilled in detecting variations in the ultrasound image. The 18 week ultrasound visit is a compromise between these two ideals in order to make the best use of man and woman power.

## Subsequent antenatal clinic visits

The history of events since the last visit should be assessed as they may contain symptoms which need treatment under item 4 of the list of aims of antenatal care on p. 6, the management of fetal symptomatic problems. For example, there may be a sudden increase in maternal girth indicating polyhydramnios or a diminution of fetal movements indicating fetal compromise. Maternal health is also considered, for infections acquired by the mother in pregnancy can pass readily to the fetus. Some of these involve routine screening, others depend on the identification of higher risk groups (e.g. animal workers are at higher risk of cytomegalic virus infections) while a few conditions relate to maternal symptomatic infection (see Chapters 11–14).

The woman's weight is commonly measured at each antenatal visit and changes at subsequent visits are assessed but it is not a very specific indicator of fetal well-being. More useful is the measurement of blood pressure which can be compared with previous readings; if it has risen, this may be associated with pre-eclampisa, particularly if proteinuria has also occurred. The urine is also checked for glycosuria as an indication of diabetes or carbohydrate intolerance.

The fetal presentation will be established and its size is assessed in relation to the amount of amniotic fluid. Many units do a second ultrasound reading of fetal size at 32 weeks, hoping by this means to rule out those with intrauterine growth retardation. The efficacy of this is considered in Chapter 5.

Of those women shown to be at higher risk from one of the problems, further ultrasound tests can be performed on abnormalities, placental site and function. These are arranged specifically for the women who have fetuses with these problems. Antenatal cardiotocography (CTG) is performed as a screening test although its precise value is difficult to ascertain (Chapter 9). If CTG indicates some degree of fetal compromise, a fetal biophysical profile screening may be performed (Manning *et al.* 1987).

Doppler ultrasound is now being assessed to measure various components of blood flow in the placental bed and umbilical vessels (Chapter 6). This is a logical measure to try to assess; the flow of maternal blood to the placental bed and the flow of fetal blood from it are the major components in the provision of nutrients and oxygen to maintain normal fetal growth and oxygenation.

More invasively, the assessment of the fetus through the fetoscope has almost ceased in the UK. Occasionally one may wish to use it to guide fetal blood sampling in mid-trimester but bed navigation for this can be done by good high resolution ultrasound. The use of blood samples to assess the biochemical and acid base status, or to obtain fetal cells for swift karyometric analysis has increased. This procedure is discussed in Chapter 7.

A whole new science of fetal electrocardiography (FECG) is starting. At present this relates more to labour but research is advancing on assessing the various electrical aspects of the fetal cardiac cycle in pregnancy (Chapter 10).

## Conclusions

Antenatal care started to prevent fits, prevent malformations and to treat any medical condition of the mother. There was a phase before the Second World War when the emphasis was on trying to prevent maternal mortality or morbidity. After the Second World War, antenatal care turned to the reduction of perinatal mortality. Now, much of antenatal care is fine tuning in order to produce a better product. With lower birth rates and smaller family size, parents expect each child to be perfect and are upset when this is not so. Obstetricians and their co-workers can assist this process by the early detection and correction of fetal problems. No fetal tests are yet perfect and many have been introduced without full assessment. It is by a more rigid scientific scrutiny of the new tests at their early phase with randomized controlled trials that we might determine which of the tests are more valuable. Then we can introduce these more widely and exclude the tests which are not worthwhile.

## References

Ballantyne J.W. (1901) A plea for a pro-maternity hospital. *British Medical Journal*, **1**, 413–14.

Campbell J. (1927) *Protection of Motherhood*. HMSO, London.

Chamberlain G. (1978) A re-examination of antenatal care. *Journal of the Royal Society of Medicine*, **71**, 662–8.

James D.K. & Stirrat J.M. (1988) *Pregnancy and Risk*. Wiley, Chichester.

Hall M.J. (1989) A critique of antenatal care. In *Obstetrics*, (Ed. by A. Turnbull & G. Chamberlain), p. 230. Churchill Livingstone, London.

Hall M.J., Chang P.K. & MacGillivray I. (1980) Is routine antenatal care worthwhile? *Lancet*, **ii**, 78–80.

Lumley J., Lester A., Anderson I., Renou P. & Wood C. (1983) A randomised trial of weekly cardiotocography in high risk obstetrical patients. *British Journal of Obstetrics and Gynaecology*, **90**, 101–8.

Manning F.A., Morrison I. & Harman C.R. (1987) Fetal assessment based on fetal biophysical profile scoring. *American Journal of Obstetrics and Gynecology*, **157**, 880–4.

Solum T., Ingemarsson I. & Nygren A. (1981) The accuracy of ultrasonic fetal cardiotocography. *Journal of Perinatal Medicine*, **9**, 54–62.

# 2: Decision analysis in obstetrics

RICHARD J. LILFORD



Doctors usually make clinical decisions on the basis of intuition; informed intuition, but nevertheless intuition. Every clinical decision can lead to a number of possible outcomes; the decision options and their possible consequences can therefore be shown in a decision diagram. The use of decision theory will be illustrated with a clinical example with which all gynaecologists will be familiar: the management of microscopic invasive cancer of the cervix.

Imagine two women, each with cancer invasion to 2 mm below the basement membrane and each with lymph channel involvement. One of these women is 20 years old and about to get married, the other is a 40-year-old mother who has been sterilized. In each case let us assume that the diagnosis has been made by a cone biopsy with a wide excision of normal tissue around the disease. The main treatment options lie between no further therapy, simple hysterectomy and extended hysterectomy with lymphadenectomy. The outcomes are death from cancer, death from surgery, major surgical morbidity, infertile survival following hysterectomy or fertile survival following no treatment. This decision is shown on a decision tree in Figure 2.1.

Clearly the decision should depend on the operative mortalities of surgical treatments, the likelihood that the disease has spread to pelvic lymph nodes and the chance of cure by surgery if it has done so. The best possible assessment of these probabilities can be obtained by detailed

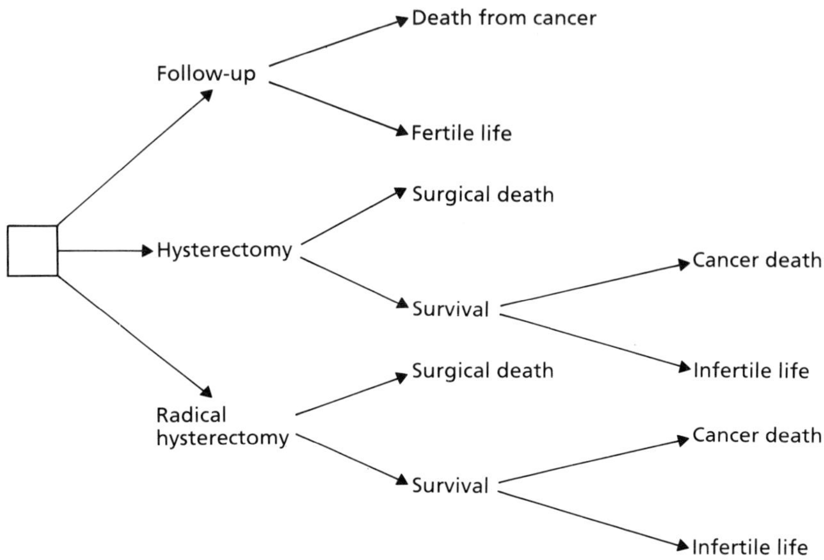


**Fig. 2.1** Decision tree for management of a patient with microscopic cervical cancer, invading to a depth of 2 mm and with lymph vascular channel involvement, where the lesion is excised with a wide margin of normal tissue. If (i) operative mortality is 0.05 per cent for hysterectomy and 0.5 per cent for radical hysterectomy, (ii) the chance of lymph-node spread is 2 per cent and (iii) the chance of cure of such spread by radical surgery is 50 per cent, then the mortality of conservative therapy (2 per cent) exceeds that of radical treatment 0.5 per cent + (2 per cent × 0.5) = 1.5 per cent. Simple hysterectomy will always have a slightly worse mortality.

review of the literature. This would show that the operative mortality of simple hysterectomy is 0.5 per thousand rising to 5 per thousand for radical hysterectomy (Shingleton & Orr 1983). Further extensive literature review shows the chance that the cancer has spread beyond the cervix, given the above histological features, is 2 per cent and the chance of cure by radical surgery, if spread is present, is about 50 per cent (Johnson *et al.* 1989).

If all we are concerned about is increasing the chances of survival, we can calculate the probability of survival and death with each method of management. The chance of death from cancer with no further surgery is 2 per cent, whereas the chance of death with radical surgery is the operative mortality plus the risk of dying from cancer despite surgery. This can be calculated as shown in the legend to Figure 2.1. Survival rates are improved most by radical surgery and least with simple hysterectomy. This does not necessarily mean that all patients should be treated by radical surgery. Firstly, the young patient who wishes to have a family may be prepared to surrender an improved chance of survival in order to retain her fertility. Secondly, patients may have relative preference for cancer death compared to surgical death or vice versa. Lastly, morbidity of radical surgery has not been taken into account.

If we knew how a patient valued these outcomes, relative to each other, then we could calculate the best treatment for that patient. This best treatment is referred to as the treatment with the highest expected utility. It is the treatment that will improve the outcome most for that patient, taking into account the probabilities of the various outcomes and their relative values. Once these values have been ranked on a scale from 1 (the best outcome) to 0 (the worst outcome), the expected utility of each treatment option can be calculated by a technique similar to that used to determine the probabilities of survival with each method of treatment (Figure 2.1), except that we now use the product of the probability of each outcome and the value of that outcome in place of these probabilities alone. The problem, of course, is to determine these relative values.

Before returning to this problem, we will discuss, in more detail, the use of decision theory where we are not concerned with values, but merely with improving a particular outcome, e.g. survival. We may wish to do this as a prelude to a more sophisticated analysis incorporating value estimates or in situations where values are not really important, i.e. where everyone's values are the same and either 0 (death) or 1 (survival). These are situations of *probabilistic dominance*; an example would be the best management of suspected tubal pregnancy or appendicitis. Broadly speaking all patients would prefer the treatment which most improves the chances of survival and the disadvantages of certain treatment options, such as the pain of surgery, are so small relative to the two main outcomes of death or survival, as to make no appreciable difference to the decision.

## Probabilities and decision theory

There are few decisions in obstetrics more controversial than the management of the low-risk, term breech presentation. Some clinicians recommend Caesarean section for all cases, while others favour a trial of labour. When the author and Dr Bingham began to analyse this problem, we had imagined that the decision would involve a trade-off between the safest course of action for the baby (Caesarean section) and the safest treatment for the mother (vaginal delivery). Proper structure of the decision has shown that this is not necessarily so and that the decision may be one of virtual probabilistic dominance.

### Establishing a framework for the decision

In the past, retrospective series of breech presentation have compared fetal outcome following vaginal delivery and Caesarean section, as shown in Figure 2.2a. This, however, is not the decision with which the clinician is confronted; in Figure 2.2b we show that the decision which the obstetrician faces is between trial of vaginal delivery and elective Caesarean section. This correct structuring of the decision immediately shows that mortality and morbidity, both fetal and maternal, resulting

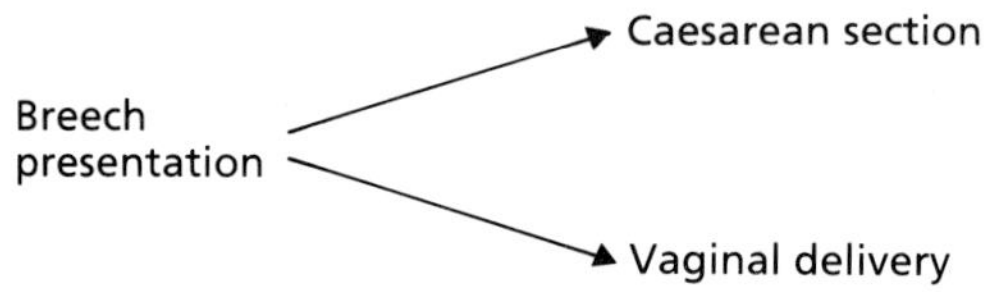


(a)

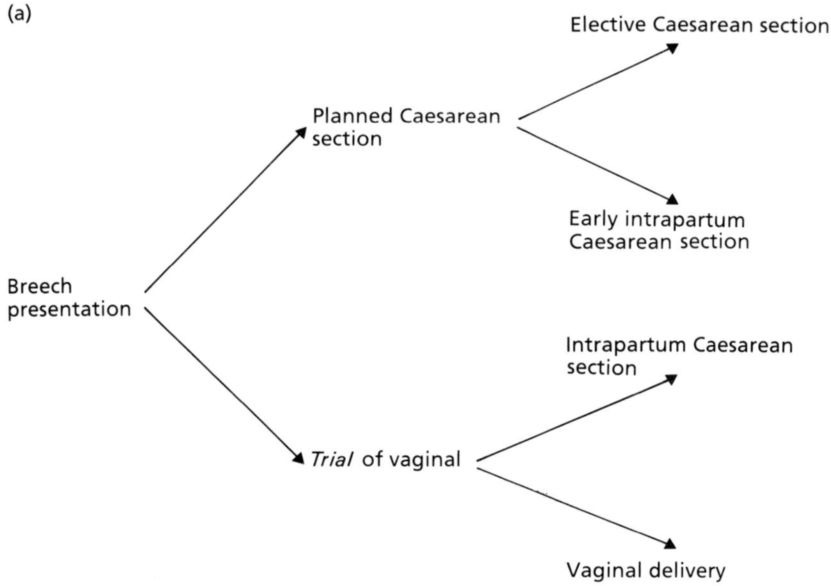


(b)

**Fig. 2.2** (a) The incorrect construction of the breech presentation controversy and (b) a construction which comes much closer to reality.

from emergency intrapartum Caesarean section is actually attributable to the decision to recommend a trial of vaginal delivery.

## Quantifying the outcomes

Having determined the outcomes which may result from alternative methods of management, the next step is to quantify the probabilities of these outcomes. In the case of vaginal breech delivery, the only randomized trial comparing elective Caesarean section with trial of vaginal delivery for properly selected cases (Collea *et al.* 1980) was much too small to produce estimates of the relative risks of major fetal mortality and morbidity.

Bingham & Lilford (1987) have examined the entire literature from the last twenty years and concluded that the additional risk of fetal death or permanent brain damage, attributable to trial of vaginal breech delivery, is between 1 in a 100 and 1 in 200. Examination of the correctly constructed decision tree (Figure 2.2b) shows that maternal risks are not necessarily greater with elective section. Since there is a higher maternal morbidity and mortality after intrapartum Caesarean section than elective operation, the maternal risk of elective surgery may be less than that of trial of vaginal delivery. Trials of vaginal breech delivery fail in between 20 and 50 per cent of all cases where this is attempted (Bingham & Lilford 1987; Songane *et al.* 1987).

The techniques outlined can be used to calculate the safest course of action for the mother, taking into account the probability that a trial of vaginal delivery will fail and the relative risks of vaginal delivery, elective Caesarean section and intrapartum Caesarean section. Intrapartum Caesarean section is about three times as dangerous as elective Caesarean section which, in turn, has a 5-fold increased risk of death over vaginal delivery (Bingham & Lilford 1987).

## Calculating the safest treatment

From these figures it can be calculated that trial of vaginal delivery is actually the more dangerous option for the mother when the probability that this will succeed drops to under 70 per cent. Major and minor morbidity is also at least three times more likely following intrapartum Caesarean section than elective surgery. Thus, a mother with a breech presentation, or any other condition which predisposes to failed trial of vaginal delivery (such as previous Caesarean section for poor progress) has little to gain, in terms of mortality and morbidity, from trial of vaginal delivery. In the case of breech delivery the relevant trade-off is between a small additional fetal and maternal risk with trial of vaginal delivery versus maternal inconvenience, psychological upset and effects on future pregnancies with elective surgical delivery.

Since the preservation of fetal brain function and the maintenance of maternal health are the most important considerations for most people, this decision is used as an example of virtual probabilistic dominance. There may, of course, be some women who would be prepared to sacrifice a modicum of fetal safety in order to avoid the psychological disadvantages of Caesarean section and we will return to this issue under the discussion of measurement of human values.

## Dealing with uncertain probability estimates

Up to this point we have discussed probabilities obtained from review of the literature — preferably from randomized trials or alternatively from observational studies, using judgement to modify these estimates according to local circumstances. It is as wrong to ignore probabilities in the literature as it is to accept and extrapolate these to different populations at different times without appropriate, albeit subjective, modification. In some cases, however, there may be no published data whatsoever. Under these circumstances, probabilities must be almost or entirely subjective and can be obtained from experts or by concensus from teams of experts, by the Delphi technique (Weinstein & Fineberg 1980).

## Measurement of values

In the example of microinvasive carcinoma of the cervix, the expected utilities of each method of treatment could not be calculated because the values attributable to the various outcomes, such as infertility or death from cancer, were unknown. Even in the second example, which we present as one of almost complete probabilistic dominance, the case for planned Caesarean section cannot be established firmly without the consideration of values, e.g. psychological factors relating to the desire to deliver naturally. Statisticians coming from other disciplines are often surprised at the poor quality of probabilistic medical data. This results from the huge diversity of human biology with its many untidy groups, leading in turn to imprecision and bias in many comparative studies. The measurement of human values is even more difficult (Tversky & Kahnemann 1974). However, it is these values that determine most clinical decisions and the study of human value assessment is therefore essential to an analysis of medical decisions (Pauker & Kassirer 1987).

Most work on value measurement in our speciality has been carried out in the field of prenatal diagnosis (Pauker & Pauker 1987; Thornton *et al.* 1988). This is not surprising, as the importance of values is very obvious in this subject; decisions in prenatal diagnosis clearly hinge on the values which people attach to outcomes such as termination of pregnancy, accidental abortion, mental handicap, etc. and the concept of non-directive counselling is therefore best developed in this field. Most of the work discussed, therefore, relates to prenatal diagnosis, but the much smaller number of value studies related to later pregnancy management is considered also. How, then, may we obtain values between 1 (the best health state) and 0 (a person's least preferred health state).

### Ranking

Ranking consists of determining the worst and best outcomes and those in between in the order chosen by the ranker.

### Visual analogue scales

This is an extension of the ranking method in which the relative preferences of the ranked outcomes are indicated on an unmarked scale. This method does not give reliable results as it provides falsely pessimistic impressions of intermediate outcomes, i.e. those in the middle of the ranking scale (Torrance 1986). Many decisions in late pregnancy depend on the relative values associated with the outcomes of surgical versus vaginal delivery.

Measurement of the relevant values was attempted by Silver & Minogue (1987) but their work was flawed because the authors used a linear analogue scale (0 = full health, 1 = maternal death) to elicit values from eight perinatologists. Hysterectomy, a possible outcome, was valued at 62 which would imply that the subject would run a risk of death of up to 38 per cent in preference to being rendered infertile by hysterectomy (Thornton 1988). The perinatologist assessors would not have given this value if they had understood the implications in terms of the precise trade-off implied and the consequences for decision making. Similarly, the discomfort of labour was valued at 6, implying that a woman would choose a 1 : 20 risk of death to avoid it. These results thus confirm that analogue scales tend to result in a bunching of values towards the middle of the scale.

### Individual lottery

This method is based on game theory and originated from the work of von Neumann & Morgenstern (1947). It has been widely used in economics and more recently, in medicine. Value scores are obtained by asking patients or subjects to take part in a series of lotteries. The subject is asked to specify her best, worst and intermediate health states or outcome. In each lottery she is asked to choose between the certainty of an intermediate health state and a gamble between her best and worst health outcome.

Returning to our problem of microscopic cervical cancer, let us imagine that a subject would regard death from cervical cancer as her worst health state, infertility following radical hysterectomy as her intermediate health state and intact survival as the best possible outcome. In this situation, the patient would be offered a choice between the intermediate health state (infertile life) and a gamble between the other two (intact survival, death from cervical cancer). The relative likelihood of the two extreme states (intact survival, cancer death) is then varied and the point observed where the patient is unable to make a decision between the certain health state and the gamble. Once values are obtained in this way (they will come out between 0 and 1) they can be multiplied by the probability of that outcome to obtain the product of the value of the outcome and the probability that it will happen. This can then be combined with the probabilities and the values of other outcomes, in order to choose the method of treatment with the best overall expected utility, by the standard method shown in Figure 2.3.

This is called a certainty equivalence method for determining values. An alternative lottery, the probability equivalence method, uses choices nearer to those actually faced by patients in conventional clinical practice. The different treatments available are described to the subject, along with the probabilities of the various outcomes, e.g. no specific therapy versus radical hysterectomy for our patient with microscopic cervical cancer. The patient is then asked to choose the treatment she prefers. The probabilities are varied and again the point determined where she finds it impossible to select between two treatment options. Again, a point of indifference is reached. Information is presented in the same way as it is in non-directive clinical counselling.

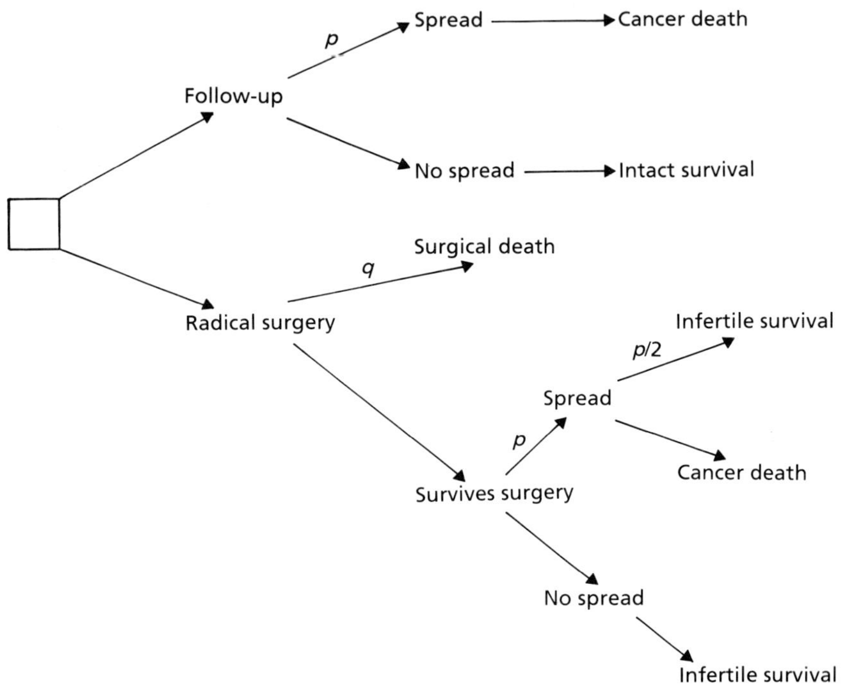


**Fig. 2.3** Calculating the management with the greatest expected utility: $U(c)$ = Expected utility follow-up; $U(s)$ = Expected utility radical surgery.

$U(c) = p \times U(cD) + (1 - P) \times U(L)$

and

$U(s) = q \times U(sD) + (1 - q) \times (1 - P) \times U(I) + (1 - q) \times P/2 \times U(I) + (1 - q) \times P/2 \times U(cD)$

where $P$ = chance of spread = 0.02 (2 per cent); $q$ = probability surgical death = 0.005 (0.5 per cent); $U(L)$ = utility of intact survival = 1; $U(I)$ = utility of infertile survival, say 0.95; $U(cD)$ = utility of cancer death, say 0.05; $U(sD)$ = utility of surgical death, say 0, i.e. this person will run a 5 per cent chance of death to retain fertility and slightly prefers death from cancer to sudden death from surgery

$U(c) = (0.02 \times 0.05) + (0.98 \times 1) = 0.981$

$U(s) = 0 + (0.995 \times 0.98 \times 0.95) + (0.995 \times 0.01 \times 0.98) + (0.995 \times 0.01 \times 0.05) = 0.936,$

i.e. conservative management is best for this patient.

## Values and the prenatal diagnosis of Down's syndrome

I will discuss these methods within the context of prenatal diagnosis for Down's syndrome. Amniocentesis is usually performed to diagnose and allow selective termination of Down's syndrome fetuses but it may lead to accidental abortion of a normal pregnancy. The risk of trisomy 21 varies with certain biochemical markers and with the mother's age. The risk of procedure-related abortion is somewhere between 0.5 and 1 per cent (Tabor *et al.* 1986). Pauker & Pauker (1977) were the first to perform a quantitative approach to this problem and they performed certainty equivalence lotteries to obtain the utilities of loss of normal pregnancy, birth of a Down's syndrome baby, termination of a Down's syndrome pregnancy, normal delivery and spontaneous abortion at about 20 weeks. They obtained value assessments of these outcomes and then used them in directive genetic counselling. They found this useful as a method to help patients understand the decisions which they were making.

Our group (Thornton & Lilford 1988) extended the work of Pauker using the probability equivalence method in which choices are given in the same way as they are in conventional clinical practice. We compared womens' perception of the relative risks of chorion biopsy, amniocentesis and the risk of having a baby with Down's syndrome.

We carried out three multiple gambles among 73 women. The first choice, having given the women background information about procedure-related abortions with amniocentesis (which we put at 1 : 100), was the choice between amniocentesis and nothing at various risks of Down's syndrome. These risks were presented from opposite ends of the scale, from 1 : 10 to 1 : 20 000, in order to avoid any anchoring to the midpoint of the scale. The next gamble was between amniocentesis and chorion villus biopsy (CVS), at a risk of Down's syndrome of 1 : 100, but differing risks of miscarriage with CVS. The third gamble was between CVS and nothing, with a fixed miscarriage risk from CVS (1 : 25) and different risks of Down's syndrome; the third gamble was to measure coherence.

## Coherence

Coherence implies the ability of subjects to make internally consistent choices. Broadly speaking, subjects should be able to make their gambles in such a way that the answer to the third gamble should be very similar to that which would be predicted on the basis of the first two. Such a patient would be internally consistent or coherent. This coherence measure, according to some authorities, can be faulted, because it implies that values are independent of probability; in other words that a 1 : 100 risk of spontaneous abortion is seen to be twice as bad as a 1 : 200 risk. This is referred to as the constant proportion risk attitude and people frequently do not conform with this. Nevertheless, a subject who understands what is going on, should be able to make a choice on the third gamble within reasonable limits of that predicted from the first two.

Our findings were as follows:

**1** Ten per cent of women would not want amniocentesis, even at a 1 : 10 risk of Down's syndrome. Similarly, 20 per cent of women would want this test, even if the risk of Down's was as low as 1 : 2000. The median point of indifference was a risk of 1 : 800, i.e. half of women would want to have amniocentesis, despite a 1 per cent miscarriage risk, down to a Down's risk of 1 : 800. Aversion to Down's syndrome, compared to accidental loss of a normal pregnancy, was slightly greater than that found by Pauker & Pauker (1977) but slightly less than that found by

Tabor and colleagues (1986) when making real offers of this test to unselected women of all ages.

**2** Half of all women, with a 1 : 100 Down's risk, would accept a doubling of the miscarriage risk associated with amniocentesis in order to get the advantage of early diagnosis by CVS.

These results were independent of social class or whether the patient was a doctor, para-medical worker or a non-medical person.

**3** A little over half of subjects were coherent in that their answer to the third gamble was within a halving or doubling of that which would have been expected from their first two answers. Thus, an important implication of this decision analysis is that many people are not able to fully internalize and understand the trade-offs which they are prepared to make. Only coherent choices can be said to reflect a true value system. It is therefore desirable in decision theory to incorporate a measure of coherence, so that the analysis can be confirmed among subjects who understand the choices which they are making. In the case of the experiment described the trade-off choices made among coherent subjects were not significantly different from those made by incoherent subjects. Coherence was (statistically) significantly greater in medical than non-medical people, but this difference was small.

## Interpretation of results

### Structuring the decision for the average patient

In our original decision paradigm of the treatment of two women with microinvasive cancer, we obtained the probabilities of the various outcomes. We can now present women with choices in which we simply vary these probabilities (probability equivalence multiple gambles). Alternatively, we can do a full decision analysis. For this we use the values attributable to the various possible outcomes (infertility, cancer death, etc.), obtained by the certainty equivalence multiple gamble method. Typical results when this experiment was carried out were:

| | |
|---|---|
| intact survival, young woman | 1 |
| infertile life, young woman | 0.95 |
| cancer death | 0.05 |
| surgical death | 0 |

This patient would run a 5% risk of death to preserve her fertility and has a marginal preference for cancer death over immediate surgical death. (Most patients have a preference for late death over early death because of the greater value of the years immediately ahead.) In Figure 2.3 these results are combined with the probabilities of the various outcomes and the calculation of expected utilities is demonstrated. We can now choose the optimum treatment for a particular woman or for someone whose values are those of the average younger or older person and who has microinvasive cancer with the histological features described in the first section.

### Sensitivity analysis

We can now examine how the decision might change for a woman with different values or a doctor who has formed different conclusions about the probabilities of certain outcomes. This is a sensitivity analysis. It turns out that this decision is very sensitive to the value of infertility. Even a value for infertility of 0.98 (which implies that the subject will run a risk of death from cancer of up to 1 : 50 in order to preserve fertility) favours the decision to use conservative treatment, although this will not maximize most the chances of survival. However, relative preference for cancer or surgical death makes little difference to the preferred method of treatment and our older patients, or any women who do not wish to preserve fertility, should be treated by extended hysterectomy if the chance of lymphatic spread is 2 per cent.

The ability to perform this sensitivity analysis is one of the attractive features of decision analysis, because it enables us to vary the probabilities and values of various outcomes and (i) individualize decisions; and (ii) determine the factors that have greatest influence on the decision.

Thus, for a surgeon claiming a lower operative mortality rate, different probability estimates can be fed into the model and the effect of this on the best treatment determined. Similarly, for individual patients who place higher or lower importance on preserving fertility, or on cancer death relative to surgical death, an individualized expected utility can be calculated for the different treatment options.

## Other examples of decision theory in obstetrics and gynaecology

In the example of management of the mature breech delivery, we saw that this was not quite a decision of probabilistic dominance. A choice must be made between greater fetal safety with planned surgical delivery and less pain, disappointment and difficulty in subsequent pregnancies with vaginal delivery. As maternal risks are about equal with planned surgery and vaginal delivery, Thornton and Lilford asked women to make trade-offs between fetal safety and the above disadvantages of planned Caesarean section (Thornton & Lilford 1987; Thornton 1988; Thornton & Lilford 1989). Multiple gambles were administered in which alternatively low and high fetal risks were offered in a series of lotteries of fetal safety versus the psychological disadvantages of Caesarean section. All subjects ($n = 123$) would opt for Caesarean section if the risk of fetal death or brain damage was 1 : 50. Most subjects were prepared to run a risk of 1 : 10 000 of fetal death or brain damage to avoid surgery, although a small number would actually prefer Caesarean section to vaginal delivery even if there was no fetal or maternal advantage. The median point of indifference, i.e. the risk half the women were prepared to run, was 1 : 4000. These values, even allowing for sampling error, cannot be taken totally at face value because:

**1** Coherence was not measured in this study, so we do not know how well subjects understood and internalized the information.
**2** A large proportion (30 per cent) of subjects were women on postnatal wards who might be especially biased towards the fetus.
**3** The way the trade-offs were formulated may have made subjects feel that they were being selfish if they did not put a very high premium on fetal safety and the questionnaire is being repeated by computer with an in-built test for coherence.

In the mean time, these results, even if they are biased towards fetal safety, nevertheless show that women are prepared to run much lower fetal risks than might otherwise have been expected. Two further interesting findings have come from this study:
**1** Obstetricians and husbands place a lower premium on fetal safety and a higher premium on maternal well-being than mothers themselves.
**2** Analysis of results from a subset of women who had had or had wished to have home delivery showed a lower premium on fetal safety and the mean fetal risk they would accept in order to avoid surgery was 1 : 100 ($n = 14$). Whether this was because these women understood the trade-off information better (and would have been more coherent if tested) or because they genuinely have different values, cannot be stated with certainty. It should be noted, however, that a 1 : 100 risk is a similar fetal risk to that attributable to mature selected vaginal breech delivery and these results confirm that this decision can be regarded as one of virtual probabilistic dominance. In addition, the small fetal risks that women are prepared to run can be used as evidence that small improvements in fetal outcome are worthwhile, even if planned Caesarean section is required, but we do not yet know how these trade-offs would change in cases where the chances that trial of vaginal delivery will result in vaginal delivery are high and where maternal danger is therefore greater with planned abdominal delivery. These trade-offs are very difficult to make because the possible outcomes are not only fetal versus maternal death, but also fetal brain damage or serious maternal morbidity (e.g. hysterectomy). This is an area of almost impossible difficulty. P. Bingham (pers. comm.) was able to get subjects to rank these outcomes, but believable trade-off functions for this range of outcomes were almost impossible to obtain and we have seen that analogue scales produce completely meaningless results. As many perinatal decisions involve precisely these trade-offs, this is a serious limiting factor on the use of formal decision theory in obstetrics.

Decision theory can be used to model the decision and clarify difficult issues such as prophylactic treatment of pulmonary thromboembolism (Klein & Pauker 1981; Klein & Pauker 1988). Recognizing the difficulties, these authors did not bother to obtain precise value estimates for possible outcomes (e.g. maternal death, fetal damage, fetal death), but merely used a range of plausible estimates in a number of sensitivity analyses. Clinicians can refer to these and see how their own best estimates of various probabilities affect the decision. Also, the clinician can determine the effect of any individual patient's values on the decision.

A certain patient may have a particular fear of drug-induced fetal damage, while another, the mother of three children, might be concerned almost exclusively with minimizing her risk of death. In other words, there is a half-way house between complete reliance on decision analysis and the completely unstructured, largely intuitive methods generally used. The difficulties of obtaining precise value trade-offs for the range of fetal and maternal risks in obstetrics are such that the main place of decision theory is not to produce conclusions, but to structure decisions appropriately before applying the intuition and judgement which can never be dispensed with.

Decision analysis has been used to examine the role of elective repeat Caesarean section (Shy *et al.* 1981), radiotherapy in advanced cervical cancer (Twiggs & Potish 1984), management of genital herpes in pregnancy (Binkin *et al.* 1984), whether to treat recurrent ovarian cancer (one of the best examples of this subject (Simes 1985)) and hormone replacement therapy (Holzman *et al.* 1984; Elstein *et al.* 1986). Similar logical processes are used in cost utility studies designed to determine where resources will do the most good (Williams 1985). Within our speciality this methodology has been used to consider the economic advantages and disadvantages of routine hormone replacement therapy (Weinstein & Schiff 1983), screening for neural-tube defects (Tyrrell *et al.* 1988), tocolytic therapy (Korenbrot *et al.* 1984) and screening for Down's syndrome (Hagard & Carter 1976). In these studies the most favourable outcome for communities rather than individuals is determined and again, the dialectic — the argument — is more important than the conclusions reached.

## What is the role of decision analysis?

It can be seen that there are many problems with decision analysis and that the beauty of the technique *resides in its logic,* not in the numbers it produces. The latter should not be used to imply certainty or finality. Breaking the decision into numbers is merely a way of disciplining the mind and the dialectic. The first problem is that it is often difficult to get good probability estimates in medicine. Secondly, it is difficult to obtain entirely believable and coherent values from individuals; different methods give different results and many subjects will be incoherent because they make choices almost at random. Thirdly, there is a philosophical argument based on the observation that peoples' values are not entirely independent of probability (Hershey & Schoemaker 1985).

Some argue that this lack of independence is irrational and arises from a limitation of human cognition (a faulty heuristic) which can be corrected by determining absolute values by the certainty equivalence method. Others claim that this method is over-rigorous and remote from real decisions which should be allowed to reflect human irrationality.

Despite these difficulties, decision analysis is an extremely useful and powerful tool for the following reasons.

**1** It allows us to structure the decision properly and avoid the facile analysis of decisions which is sometimes encountered, i.e. that amniocentesis should be offered when the risk of Down's syndrome is greater than the risk of miscarriage from the procedure; that radical surgery should be carried out for microinvasive cancer when the risk of metastasis to lymph nodes equals the operative mortality of the operation; that one should always try for vaginal delivery just because it may succeed.

**2** By structuring the decision carefully, the precise origins of controversy can be identified and instead of instinctive arguments, based on simplistic slogans, precise areas of disagreement can be pinpointed. Clinical discussion and argument therefore becomes much more productive and areas where the most urgent research effort is needed are identified.

**3** Many intelligent patients appreciate decision analysis and Pauker & Pauker (1977) found that this technique increased satisfaction of their patients with genetic counselling.

**4** The subject is fun and trains and disciplines and mind.

**5** Decision analysis always involves review of the literature. However, it is a much more pointed tool than simple review articles, since it inevitably places results of published studies in the context of the framework for clinical decisions. It shows the reader how published results affect clinical decisions.

We present two further novel uses of decision theory.

**6** Decision analysis is not only a very powerful method for determining the likely benefits that can be realistically anticipated from new treatment but it is useful for determining the size of benefit which would make the treatment worthwhile, taking into account known and postulated side-effects. Decision analysis is therefore a very suitable technique for determining the sample sizes for envisaged randomized trials. The size of these trials depends on the magnitude of the treatment effect which the trial will detect, along with the designated power and precision of the trial. Clinicians should not be asked to place patients in trials unless these have a reasonable probability of demonstrating treatment effects which will actually alter clinical practice. De Bono *et al.* (1989) have used this method to determine the sample size for a test of fetal well-being. The alpha and beta errors of all clinical trials should be set to be equal and the relative disadvantages or potential dangers of alternative treatments should be reflected purely in the magnitude of treatment effect the trial is designed to detect. The trial should be sufficiently large to detect the size of difference which would influence clinical practice and this can be determined by decision theory.

**7** Value assessments are useful in studying the values of the population pertaining to ethical problems and this has been used for surrogate parenthood (Bromham *et al.* 1988) and the degrees of equipoise necessary for randomized trials (Johnson & Lilford 1989).

These population value trade-offs are ethometrics. Gaudee & Puka (1988) have also used decision theory to enhance expected utility in difficult ethical choices. The argument that the utilitarian approach ignores intrinsic morality (deontological/Kantian principles) can be countered with the notion that subjects will include these moral imperatives in their utility value judgements.

## Conclusion

Formal decision analysis is an enjoyable and powerful tool for considering clinical decisions. The important role of values in determining clinical actions is demonstrated by this technique. As the world becomes more confusing and complex and as slogans and simplistic solutions are presented to us, so the importance of the formal study of clinical problems will grow. Decision analysis in obstetrics and gynaecology represents an attempt to bring logic to bear on the numerous and complex decisions in our diverse and rich speciality. However, like the study of medical ethics, it should not be taken too seriously. The greatest disservice to decision theory is done by those who imply that the numerical conclusions are correct and binding. Decision theory, especially in obstetrics, is a tool; an adjunct to clinical judgement and not a means to replace it. Many of the criticisms of decision theory disappear if it is regarded in this spirit.

## Acknowledgements

I would like to acknowledge Drs P. Bingham, N. Johnson and J. Thornton who have worked with me on this subject and who have done most of the field-work.

## References

Bingham P. & Lilford R.J. (1987) Management of the term breech presentation: assessment of the risks of selected vaginal delivery versus cesarean section for all cases. *Obstetrics and Gynecology*, **69**, 965–78.

Binkin N.J., Koplan J.P. & Cates W. (1984) Preventing neonatal herpes: the value of weekly viral cultures in pregnant women with recurrent genital herpes. *Journal of the American Medical Association*, **251**, 2816–21.

de Bono M., Fawdry R. & Lilford R.J. (1989) Decision analysis to determine size of a trial to evaluate tests of fetal well-being. *Journal of Perinatology* (in press).

Bromham D.R., Bryce F.C. & Savage J. (1988) The ethics of surrogacy — IVF. The opinion of selected informed groups. In *Philosophical Ethics in Reproductive Medicine*, (Ed. by M. Dalton & D.R. Bromham). University of Leeds.

Caudee D. & Puka B. (1988) An analytical approach to resolving problems in medical ethics. In *Professional Judgement*, (Ed. by J. Dowie & A. Elstein), pp. 474–91. Cambridge University Press.

Collea J.V., Chein C. & Quilligan E.J. (1980) The randomised management of the term frank breech presentation: A study of 208 cases. *American Journal of Obstetrics and Gynecology*, **137**, 235.

Elstein A.S., Holzman G.B., Ravitch M.M., Metheny W.A., Holmes M.M., Hoppe R.B., Rothert M.L. & Rovner D.R. (1986) Comparison of physicians' decisions regarding estrogen replacement therapy for menopausal women and decisions derived from a decision analytic model. *American Journal of Obstetrics and Gynecology*, **80**, 246–58.

Hagard S. & Carter F.A. (1976) Preventing the birth of infants with Down's syndrome: a cost benefit analysis. *British Medical Journal* March, **1**, 753–6.

Hershey J.C. & Schoemaker P.J.H. (1985) Probability versus certainty equivalence methods in utility measurement: are they equivalent? *Management Science*, **31**, 1213–31.

Holzman G.B., Ravitch M.M., Metheny W., Rothert M., Holmes M. & Hoppe R.B. (1984) Physicians' judgements about estrogen replacement therapy for menopausal women. *Obstetrics and Gynecology*, **63**, 303–11.

Johnson N. & Lilford R.J. (1989) Collective equipoise and the ethics of randomised trials. (Submitted).

Johnson N., Appleby L., Jones S., Songane F. & Lilford R.J. (1989) A decision analysis on microscopic lesions of the ectocervix. (Submitted).

Klein K. & Pauker S.G. (1981) Recurrent deep venous thrombosis in pregnancy: analysis of the risks and benefits of anticoagulation. *Medical Decision Making*, **1**, 181–202.

Klein K. & Pauker S.G. (1988) Recurrent deep venous thrombosis in pregnancy: analysis of the risks and benefits of anti-coagulation. In *Professional Judgement*, (Ed. by J. Dowie & A. Elstein), pp. 277–97. Cambridge University Press.

Korenbrot C.C., Aalto L.H. & Laros R.K. (1984) The cost-effectiveness of stopping preterm labour with beta-adrenergic treatment. *New England Journal of Medicine*, **310**, 691–6.

Pauker S.G. & Kassirer J.P. (1987) Decision analysis. *New England Journal of Medicine*, **316**, 250–8.

Pauker S.P. & Pauker S.G. (1977) Prenatal diagnosis: a directive approach to genetic counselling using decision analysis. *Yale Journal of Biology and Medicine*, **50**, 275–89.

Pauker S.P. & Pauker S.G. (1987) The amniocentesis decision: ten years of decision analytic experience. In *Genetic Risk, Risk Perception and Decision Making*, Vol. 23(2) (Ed. by G. Evers-Kiebooms, J. Cassiman, H. Van den Berghe & G. d'Ydewalle), pp. 151–69. Alan R. Liss, New York.

Shingleton H. & Orr J.W. (Eds) (1983) Cancer of the cervix. Current review. In *Obstetrics and Gynaecology*, pp. 329–82. Churchill Livingstone, Edinburgh.

Shy K.K., Logerfo J.P. & Karp L.E. (1981) Evaluation of elective repeat cesarean section as a standard of care: an application of decision analysis. *American Journal of Obstetrics and Gynecology*, **139**, 123–9.

Silver R.K. & Minogue J. (1987) When does a statistical fact become an ethical imperative? *American Journal of Obstetrics and Gynecology*, **157**, 229–33.

Simes R.J. (1985) Treatment selection for cancer patients: application of statistical decision theory to the treatment of advanced ovarian cancer. *Journal of Chronic Diseases*, **38**, 171–86.

Songane F.F., Thobani S., Malik H., Bingham P. & Lilford R.J. (1987) Balancing the risks of planned caesarean section and trial of vaginal delivery for the mature, selected, singleton breech presentation. *Journal of Perinatal Medicine*, **15**, 531–43.

Tabor A., Madsen M., Obel E.B., Philip J., Bang J. & Norgaard-Pedersen B. (1986) Randomised controlled trial of genetic amniocentesis in 4606 low-risk women. *Lancet*, **i**, 1287–93.

Thornton J.G. (1988) Measuring patients' values in reproductive medicine. *Contemporary Reviews in Obstetrics and Gynaecology*, **1**, 5–12.

Thornton J.G. & Lilford R.J. (1987) When a woman asks for a caesarean section. *British Medical Journal*, **294**, 703.

Thornton J.G. & Lilford R.J. (1988) Value assessments applied to the prenatal diagnosis of Down's syndrome by chorionic villus biopsy or amniocentesis. *Medical decision Making* (in press).

Thornton J.G. & Lilford R.J. (1989) The Caesarean section decision: patients' choices are not determined by their immediate emotional reactions. *Journal of Obstetrics and Gynaecology*, **9**, 283–8.

Torrance G.W. (1986) Measurement of health state utilities for economic appraisal. A review. *Journal of Health Economics*, **5**, 1–30.

Tversky A. & Kahnemann D. (1974) Judgement under uncertainty: heuristics and biases. *Science*, **185**, 1124–31.

Twiggs L.B. & Potish R.A. (1984) Decision theory: analysis of the enteric morbidity and surgical staging in the treatment of advanced cervical cancer. *American Journal of Obstetrics and Gynecology*, **148**, 134–40.

Tyrrell S., Howel D., Bark M., Allibone E. & Lilford R.J. (1988) Should maternal alpha-fetoprotein estimation be carried out in centers where ultrasound screening is routine? *American Journal of Obstetrics and Gynecology*, **158**, 1092–9.

Von Neumann J. & Morgenstern O. (1947) *Theory of Games and Economic Behaviour*, 2nd edn. Princeton University Press, Princeton.

Weinstein M.C. & Fineberg H.V. (1980) *Clinical Decision Analysis*. W.B. Saunders Philadelphia.

Weinstein M.C. & Schiff I. (1983) Cost-effectiveness of hormone replacement therapy in the menopause. *Obstetrical and Gynecological Survey*, **38**, 445–54.

Williams A. (1985) Economics of coronary artery bypass grafting. *British Medical Journal*, **291**, 326–30.

# 3: Placental structure in health and disease

HAROLD FOX



## The placenta

The placenta, as expelled from the uterus, appears to be a complete organ: this, the fetal placenta, is not however the total structure for there is also a maternal component of the placenta which comprises the placental bed and the uteroplacental vessels.

### Development of the fetal placenta

The fertilized ovum enters the uterine cavity as a morula which rapidly converts into a blastocyst and loses its surrounding zona pellucida. The outer cell layer of the blastocyst proliferates to form the primary trophoblastic cell mass from which cells infiltrate between those of the endometrial epithelium at implantation. The endometrium degenerates and the trophoblast thus comes into contact with the endometrial stroma, implantation being complete by the 10th or 11th post-ovulatory day. In the seven-day ovum the trophoblast forms a peripheral circumferential plaque which rapidly differentiates into two layers, an inner layer of large, mononuclear cytotrophoblastic cells with well-defined limiting membranes and an outer layer of multinucleated syncytiotrophoblast, this latter being a true syncytium. It is now well established that the syncytiotrophoblast is derived from the cytotrophoblast, not only at this early stage but throughout gestation, for even when trophoblast is growing rapidly DNA synthesis and mitotic activity occurs only in the nuclei of the cytotrophoblastic cells, the syncytiotrophoblast being a post-mitotic, terminally differentiated, tissue (Richart 1961; Galton 1962). The syncytiotrophoblast appears to be formed by breaking down the limiting membrane of the cytotrophoblastic cells for although no true intercellular membranes are present in the syncytial layer, remnants of such membranes can occasionally be found on electron microscopy (Enders 1965). Cells with a cytoplasmic complexity and nuclear structure intermediate between those of the trophoblastic layers can also be identified on electron microscopy and these intermediate-type cytotrophoblastic cells appear to be ones which are beginning to differentiate into syncytiotrophoblast but have not yet lost their limiting membranes.

Between the 10th and 13th post-ovulatory days a series of intercommunicating clefts, or lacunae, appear in the rapidly enlarging trophoblastic cell mass (Figure 3.1): these are probably formed as a result of engulfment within the trophoblast of endometrial capillaries. The lacunae soon become confluent to form the precursor of the intervillous space and, as maternal vessels are progressively eroded, this becomes filled with maternal blood. At this stage the lacunae are incompletely separated from each other by trabecular columns of syncytiotrophoblast which, between the 14th and 21st post-ovulatory days, tend to become orientated radially (Figure 3.2) and come to possess a central cellular core that is produced by proliferation of the cytotrophoblastic cells at the chorionic base. These trabeculae are not true villi but serve as the framework from which the villous tree will later develop, the placenta at this time being a labyrinthine rather than a villous structure and the trabeculae being best known as primary villous stems (Boyd & Hamilton 1970). Continued growth of the cytotrophoblast leads to its distal extension into the region of decidual attachment (Figure 3.3) whilst, at the same time, a mesenchymal core appears within the villous stems, this being formed by

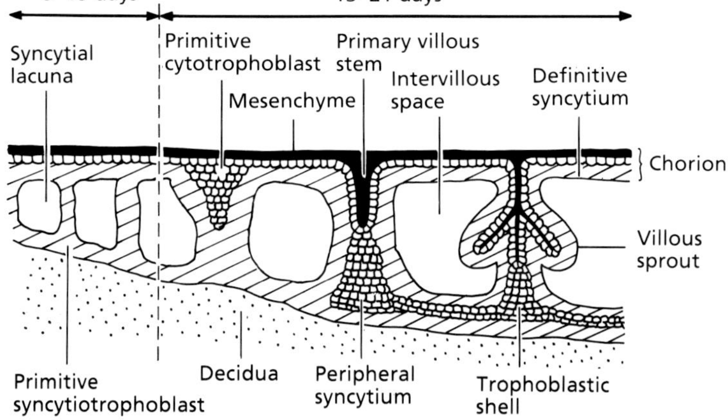


**Fig. 3.1** Diagrammatic representation of the early development of the placenta. (Reproduced with permission from Fox 1978.)

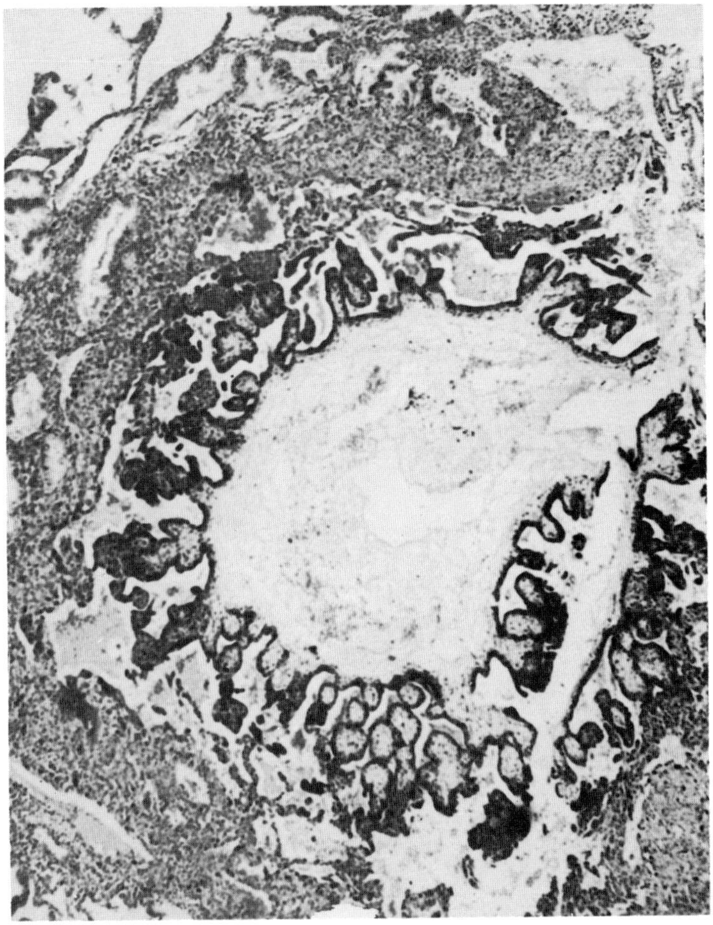

**Fig. 3.2** A developing conceptus approximately 14 days after conception. Trabecular primary villous stems are arranged radially and divide the precursor of the intervillous space into a labyrinth. H & E × 24. (Reproduced with permission from Fox 1978.)

a distal extension of the extra-embryonic mesenchyme. Later, the villous stems become vascularized, the vessels developing from mesenchyme within the core and establishing, in due course, functional continuity with others differentiating in the body stalk and inner chorionic mesenchyme.

The distal part of the villous stems is now formed almost entirely by cytotrophoblastic cells which form columns anchored to the decidua of the basal plate. The cells in these *cytotrophoblastic cell columns* proliferate and spread laterally to form a continuous cytotrophoblastic shell which splits the syncytiotrophoblast into two layers, the definitive syncytium on the fetal aspect of the shell and the peripheral syncytium on the maternal side. The definitive syncytium persists as the lining of the intervillous space but the peripheral syncytium eventually degenerates and is replaced by fibrinoid material (Nitabuch's layer). The establishment of the cytotrophoblastic shell is a mechanism to allow for rapid circumferential growth of the developing placenta and this leads to an expan-

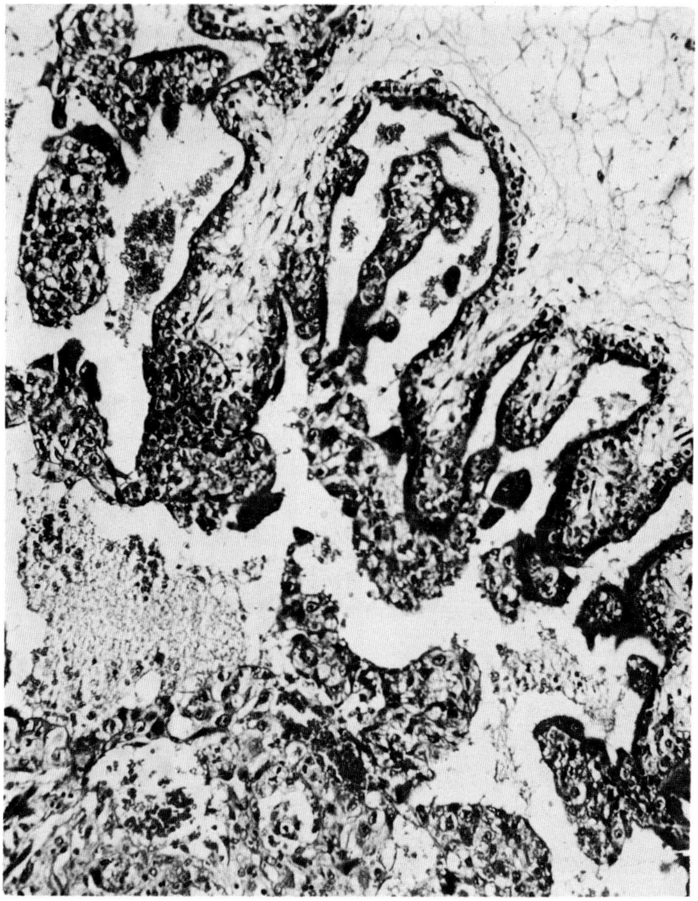

**Fig. 3.3** Detail of primary villous stem in a 14-day-old conceptus. The stems have a mesenchymal core and the growing tip of each is formed by a mass of proliferating cytotrophoblastic cells. H & E × 68. (Reproduced with permission from Fox 1978.)

sion of the intervillous space into which sprouts extend from the primary villous stems. These offshoots consist initially only of syncytiotrophoblast but as they enlarge they pass through the stages previously seen during the development of the primary villous stems, i.e. intrusion of cytotrophoblast, formation of a mesenchymal core and eventual vascularization. These sprouts are the primary stem villi and, as they are true villous structures, the placenta is by the 21st post-ovulatory day a vascularized villous organ. The primary stem villi later grow and divide to form secondary and tertiary stem villi and these latter eventually break up into the terminal villous tree.

Between the 21st post-ovulatory day and the end of the fourth month of gestation there is not only continuing growth but also considerable remodelling of the placenta. The villi orientated towards the uterine cavity degenerate and form the chorion laeve whilst the thin rim of decidua covering this area gradually disappears to allow the chorion laeve to come into contact with the parietal decidua of the opposite wall of the uterus. The villi on the side of the chorion orientated towards the decidual plate proliferate and progressively arborize to form the chorion frondosum which develops into the definitive fetal placenta. During this period there is some regression of the cytotrophoblastic elements in the chorionic plate and in the trophoblastic shell whilst the cytotrophoblastic cell columns largely degenerate and are replaced by fibrinoid material (Rohr's layer): clumps of cells persist, however, as the *cytotrophoblastic cell islands*.

The placental septa appear during the third month of gestation: they protrude into the intervillous space from the basal plate and divide the maternal surface of the placenta into 15–20 lobes. These septa are simply folds of the basal plate, being formed partly as a result of regional variability in placental growth and partly by the pulling up of the basal plate by the anchoring columns which have a poor growth rate (Boyd & Hamilton 1970). As the basal plate is formed principally by the remnants of the trophoblastic shell embedded in fibrinoid material it follows that the septa are similarly constituted, though some decidual cells may also be carried up into the folds. The septa are an incidental by-product of the architectural remodelling of the placenta and have no physiological or morphological role to play.

By the end of the fourth month of gestation the fetal placenta has achieved its definitive form and undergoes no further anatomical modification. Growth continues, however, until term and is due principally to continuing branching of the villous tree and formation of fresh villi.

## Development of the maternal placenta

During the early weeks of gestation cytotrophoblastic cells stream out from the tips of the anchoring villi, penetrate the trophoblastic shell and extensively colonize the decidua and adjacent myometrium of the placental bed, these cells being known as the *interstitial extravillous cytotrophoblast*: in addition, trophoblastic cells stream into the lumens of the intradecidual portions of the spiral arteries of the placental bed where they form intraluminal plugs and constitute the *intravascular extravillous cytotrophoblast*. These endovascular trophoblastic cells destroy and replace the endothelium of the maternal vessels and then invade the media with resulting destruction of the medial elastic and muscular tissue (Brosens *et al.* 1967): the arterial wall becomes replaced by fibrinoid material which appears to be derived partly from fibrin in the maternal blood and partly from proteins secreted by the invading trophoblastic cells (de Wolf *et al.* 1973). This process is complete by the end of the first trimester, at which time these physiological changes within the spiral arteries of the placental bed extend to the myometrio-decidual junction. There then appears to be a rest phase in this process but between the 14th and 16th week of gestation there is a resurgence of endovascular trophoblastic migration with a second wave of cells moving down into the intramyometrial segments of the spiral arteries, these cells extending as far as the origin of these vessels from the radial arteries. Within the intramyometrial portion

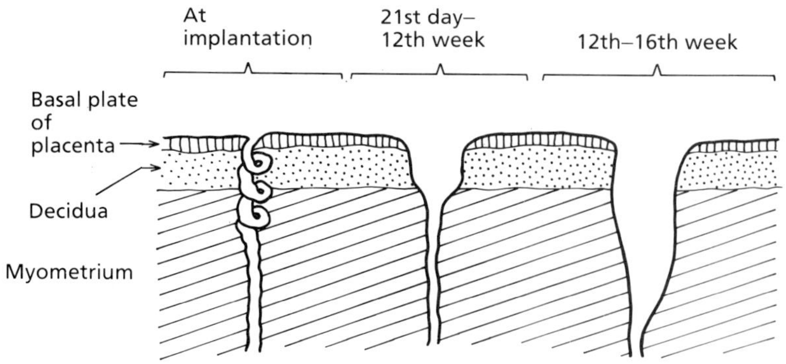


**Fig. 3.4** Diagrammatic representation of conversion of spiral arteries into uteroplacental vessels. (Reproduced with permission from Fox 1986.)

of the spiral arteries the same process as occurs in their intradecidual portion is repeated, i.e. replacement of the endothelium, invasion and destruction of the medial musculo-elastic tissue and fibrinoid change in the vessel wall. The end result of this trophoblastic invasion of, and attack on, the vessels is that the thick-walled muscular spiral arteries are converted into flaccid, sac-like uteroplacental vessels (Figure 3.4) which can passively dilate in order to accommodate the greatly augmented blood flow through this vascular system which is required as pregnancy progresses.

It will be apparent that the extravillous intravascular population of trophoblastic cells plays a key role in placentation and that via these cells the placenta establishes its own low pressure, high conductance, vascular system, thus ensuring an adequate maternal blood flow to itself and an ample supply of oxygen and nutrients to the fetus.

Whilst the function of the intravascular population of extravillous trophoblastic cells appears clear that of the interstitial extravillous trophoblastic cells is obscure. The number of these cells has, in the past, been seriously underestimated for it is now known that they are a major component of the placental bed (Pijnenborg *et al.* 1981). The interstitial trophoblastic cells tend to aggregate around the spiral arteries and it has been suggested that they prime these vessels to allow them to react to their eventual invasion by endovascular trophoblast (Pijnenborg *et al.* 1983): if this is indeed the function of these cells then their mode of action on the vessels is unknown.

The extravillous trophoblastic cells differ, as a whole, from villous trophoblast in their ability to express Class 1 major histocompatibility antigens (Redman *et al.* 1984) and in the fact that their principal synthetic product is human placental lactogen (hPL) rather than human chorionic gonadotrophin (hCG) (Gosseye & Fox 1984; Kurman *et al.* 1984). Studies with monoclonal antibodies have, however, shown that the apparently morphologically homogeneous extravillous trophoblastic cells are actually constituted by a number of antigenically heterogeneous populations (Bulmer & Johnson 1985).

## Anatomy of the fetal placenta

The fetal placenta is made up of a number of subunits which are now generally known as *lobules*. The injection studies of Wilkin (1965) have shown that the primary stem villi break up just below the chorial plate into a number of secondary stem villi which, after running for a short distance parallel to the chorionic plate, divide into a series of tertiary stem villi. The lobules are derived from these tertiary stem villi which sweep down through the intervillous space to anchor on to the basal plate: during the course through the intervillous space they give off multiple branches which ramify into the terminal villous network. As the tertiary stem villi pass down towards the basal plate they are arranged in a circular fashion around the periphery of an empty cylindrical space; the lobule thus forms a hollow globule (Figure 3.5) with the bulk of the terminal villi being mainly in the outer shell of this globular structure and the centre of the lobule being relatively empty and free of villi. The lobules are separated from each other by interlobular areas which are in continuity with the subchorial space.

There has been considerable confusion as to the meaning of the term *cotyledon* when applied to the human placenta. This name should not be used to describe the lobes seen on the maternal surface for these are merely the areas lying between the septa and lack any other morphological significance. The term cotyledon should be restricted to the functional unit of the placental villous tree and this is best defined as that part of the

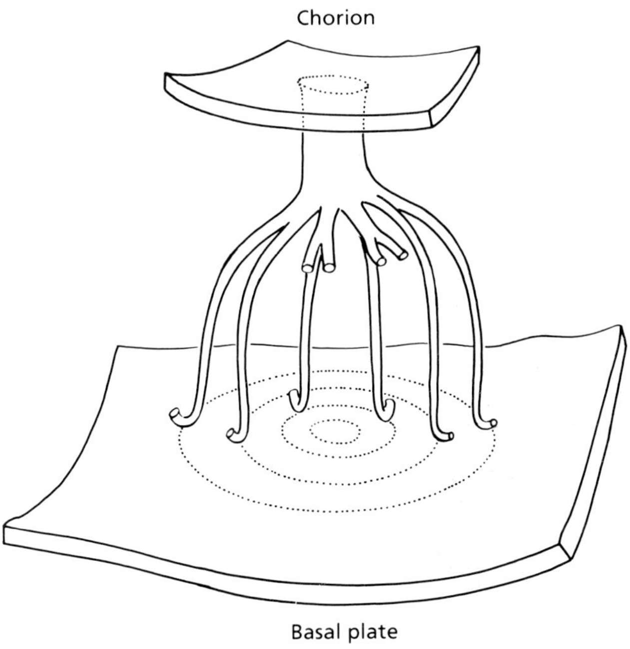


**Fig. 3.5** Diagrammatic representation of a fetal lobule. The stem villi are arranged in a circular fashion around a central hollow core. (Reproduced with permission from Fox 1978.)

villous tree that is derived from a single primary stem villus (Ramsey 1959). A primary stem villus can, however, give rise to a varying number of secondary stem villi and thus to a differing number of lobules, there being no fixed relationship between cotyledons and lobules. Thus centrally placed cotyledons may contain as many as five lobules whilst those situated laterally may have only one or two lobules. The situation has, however, been made unduly complicated by the fact that some have applied the term cotyledon to the maternal surface lobes and others have also used this name to describe the lobule: the human placenta is not really a cotyledonary structure and there is much to be said for the suggestion that the word cotyledon be abandoned when referring to human and primate placentas (Ramsey 1975).

### **The maternal uteroplacental circulatory system** (Figure 3.6)

Maternal blood enters the intervillous space via arterial inlets in the basal plate and is then driven by the head of maternal pressure towards the chorionic plate as a funnel-shaped stream (Ramsey & Donner 1980). The driving head of maternal pressure is gradually dissipated, a process aided by the baffling effect of the villi, and lateral dispersion of the blood occurs. This forces the blood already present in the intervillous space out through basally sited wide venous outlets into the endometrial venous network. Indian ink injection studies originally suggested that the maternal blood entered the intervillous space as a jet or spurt but cineangiography has shown that these terms give an undue impression of both speed and intermittency, the maternal blood entering the space 'much as water from an actively flowing brook penetrates a reed-filled marsh' (Ramsey 1965).

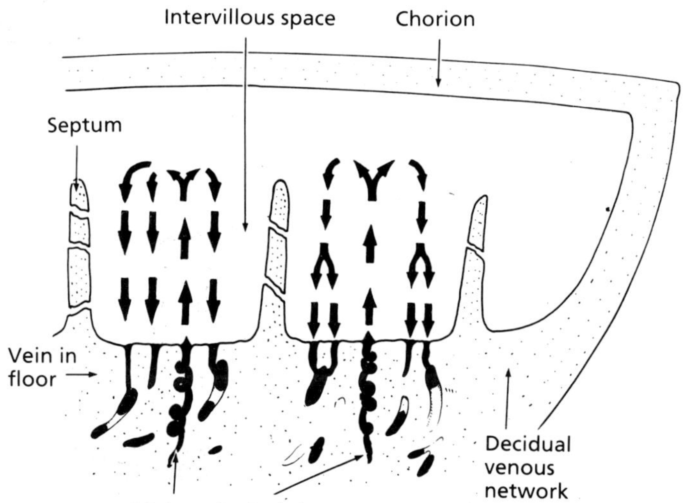


**Fig. 3.6** Diagrammatic representation of the maternal circulation through the placenta. (Reproduced with permission from Fox 1978.)

The physiological basis for this circulatory system is a series of pressure differentials, the pressure in the maternal arterioles being higher than the mean intervillous space pressure which, in turn, exceeds that in the maternal veins during a myometrial diastole. This entire system is, however, a low pressure one for whereas in most organs there is a progressive decrease in the diameter of the arteries as they approach their target tissues, the reverse is true for the placenta, the uteroplacental vessels assuming an increasing diameter as they approach their entry into the intervillous space. There is, therefore, a considerable drop in pressure from the proximal to the distal portion of these vessels and the full arterial pressure is not transmitted to the intervillous space. The placenta itself offers little flow resistance to maternal blood and has a high vascular conductance: there is thus very little fall in pressure across the intervillous space and the main factor governing the rate of maternal blood flow in a normal pregnancy is the vascular resistance within the radial arteries (Moll *et al.* 1975; Moll 1981). Despite the fact that the pressure difference between arterial and venous sides of the intervillous space is small, it is apparently sufficient to drive arterial blood towards the chorionic plate, to stop short-cutting of the stream into adjacent venous outlets and to prevent mixing of neighbouring arterial inflows.

Cineangiography has shown that the individual uteroplacental arteries act independently of each other and are not all patent and discharging blood simultaneously into the intervillous space. Furthermore, during myometrial contractions the afferent blood flow through the intervillous space may be markedly reduced or can even cease. This is probably due to compression and occlusion of the veins draining the intervillous space (Adamson & Myers 1975) but ultrasonic studies have shown that during a myometrial contraction the intervillous space distends (Bleker *et al.* 1975) and thus the fetus is not severely deprived of an oxygen supply during myometrial systole.

## Relationship of maternal circulatory system to fetal lobule

The haemodynamic system originally proposed by Ramsey (1965) postulated that the maternal blood flow into the intervillous space was through randomly situated arterial inlets but it has since become clear that this is not the case and that a definite relationship exists between the maternal vessels and the fetal lobules: this is not coincidental for it is probable that the lobules tend to develop preferentially around the flow from eroded maternal vessels (Reynolds 1966). The exact nature of this relationship is still not fully determined and two contrasting schemes have been proposed. Thus, Freese (1966) and Wigglesworth (1967) thought that arterial inlets into the intervillous space are so situated that the inflow from each uteroplacental vessel is into the central villous-free space of a fetal lobule and that the maternal blood then flows laterally through the lobule into the interlobular area from which it is drained by basal venous outlets (Figure 3.7). Others (Lemtis 1970; Gruenwald 1973; Schumann 1981)

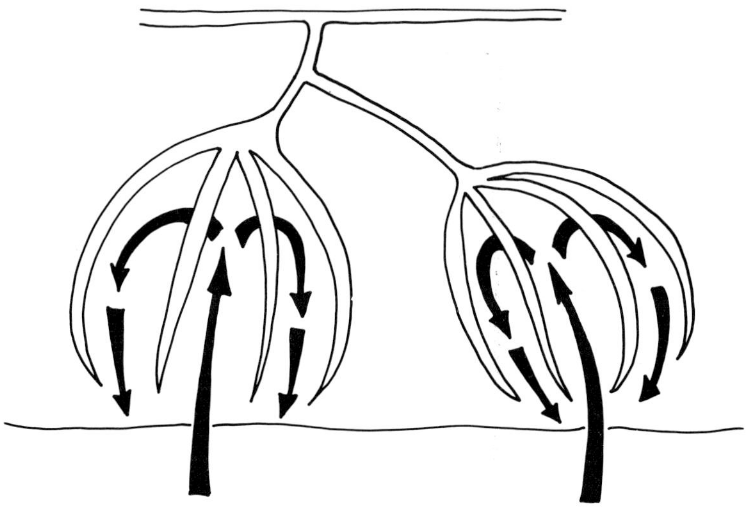

**Fig. 3.7** Diagram of the relationship between maternal uteroplacental blood flow and the fetal lobule as envisaged by Freese and Wigglesworth. (Reproduced with permission from Fox 1986.)

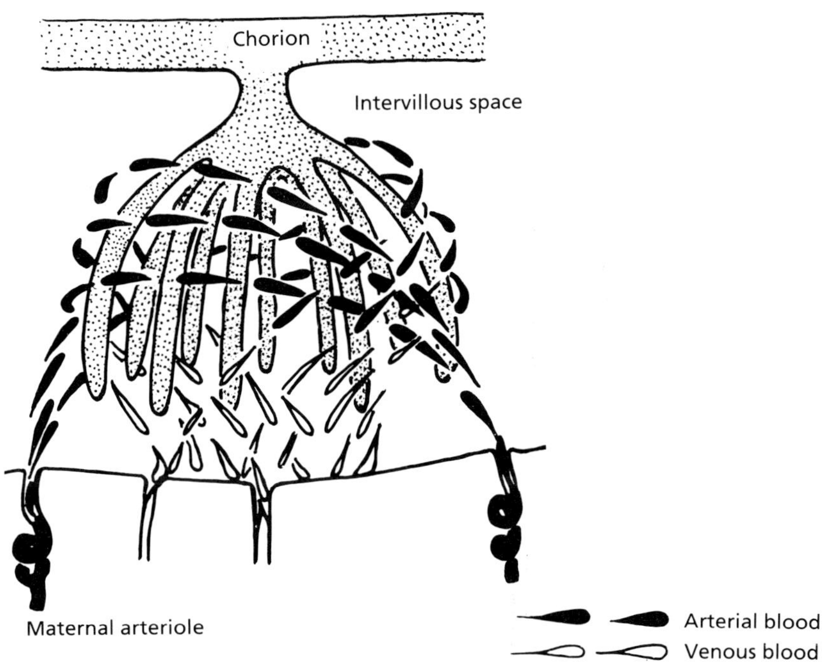


**Fig. 3.8** Diagram of the relationship between maternal uteroplacental blood flow and the fetal lobule as envisaged by Gruenwald and Lemtis. (Reproduced with permission from Fox 1978.)

consider that the maternal vessels open, not into the central space of a lobule, but into the interlobular spaces and that the maternal blood then encircles the lobule in streams to form a shell around them, entering and leaving the lobule whilst doing this and before draining through the basal outlets (Figure 3.8).

Whichever of these two concepts is correct it is clear that maternofetal exchange takes place principally in those villi that form the shell of the lobule and that it is only here that a true functional intervillous space, which is probably only of capillary calibre, exists; elsewhere, in the subchorial lake, the interlobular spaces and the central intralobular spaces villi are either sparse or absent and these areas in functional terms are physiological dead spaces.

## Histology of the placental villi

In the first 2 months of pregnancy the villi are relatively few in number, have a homogeneous pattern and measure approximately 170 μm in diameter (Figure 3.9). Their outer surface is covered by a trophoblastic mantle which is two layered, an outer layer of syncytiotrophoblast and an inner layer of cytotrophoblastic cells (Langhans' cells). The latter, which form a complete layer, are cuboid, polyhedral or ovoid and have well marked cell borders. No cell boundaries are visible between the nuclei of the syncytiotrophoblast and, indeed, microinjection studies have shown that substances flow freely through this layer and can pass from one villus to another, this indicating that there is a continuous common cytoplasm over the entire surface of the placental villi (Gaunt & Ockleford 1986). The syncytiotrophoblast is of uniform thickness whilst the syncytial nuclei are regularly spaced and are smaller and more densely staining than those of the cytotrophoblast.

A delicate brush border is often discernible on the outer surface of the syncytium and this corresponds with the microvilli that are seen on electron microscopy: these probably have no absorptive function but may well play a role in pinocytotic vesicle formation and could also serve to increase the density of specific surface receptor sites (Dearden & Ockleford 1983). It is worth noting that the syncytiotrophoblast lines the intervillous space and thus acts as an endothelium: the structure of the syncytiotrophoblast is quite unlike that of an endothelial cell and hence its ability

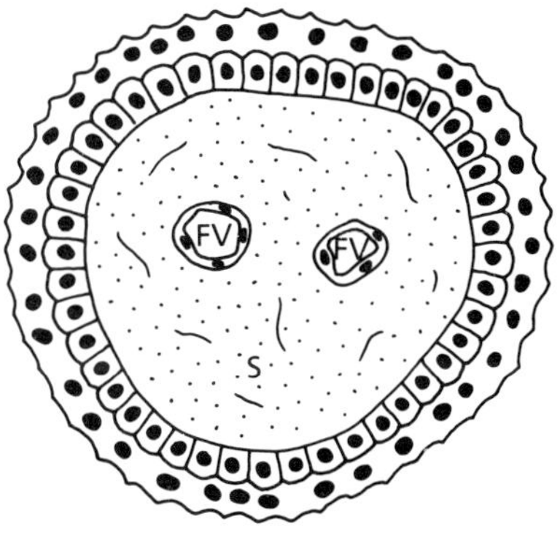


**Fig. 3.9** Diagrammatic representation of the histological appearances of a typical first trimester villus. (Reproduced with permission from Fox 1986.) FV = fetal vessels; S = villous stroma.

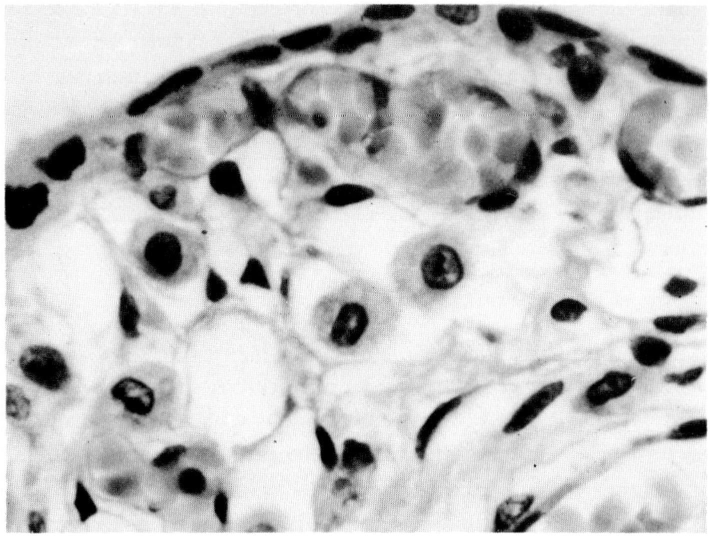

**Fig. 3.10** Several typical Hofbauer cells in the stroma of a placental villus. H & E × 990. (Reproduced with permission from Fox 1967.)

to function in this manner is somewhat of a mystery. It is possible, however, that some of the many placental proteins secreted by the syncytiotrophoblast act to prevent coagulation whilst studies with monoclonal antibodies have shown that, despite their structural dissimilarity, syncytiotrophoblast and endothelial cells do appear to share otherwise specific antigens (Voland *et al.* 1986).

The villous stroma is, at this stage, formed by loose mesenchymal tissue: by the end of the second month of gestation small centrally placed vessels, lined by large immature endothelial cells, are present. Hofbauer cells are a prominent feature of the villous stroma: these cells may be round, ovoid or reniform, measure about 25 μm in diameter and have an eccentrically placed nucleus (Figure 3.10). There is now overwhelming evidence that the Hofbauer cells are fetal tissue macrophages (Fox & Kharkongor 1969; Moskalewski *et al.* 1975; Castellucci *et al.* 1980; Demir & Erbengi 1984): their origin is, however, obscure for they are present in the villi before they are vascularized by fetal vessels and before haematopoiesis begins in the fetus. It has, however, recently been suggested that there are several populations of Hofbauer cells, those in early pregnancy developing from chorionic mesenchyme but being later supplemented by cells derived either from the fetal liver or bone marrow (Castellucci *et al.* 1987). The Hofbauer cells probably play a number of roles, some related to transport mechanisms and others to immunological protection of the fetus; in this latter respect their ability to trap maternal antibodies crossing over into the placental tissues is almost certainly of considerable importance.

Between the 8th and 30th weeks of gestation the villi become more numerous and most villi have an average diameter of about 40 $\mu$m (Figure 3.11). In these villi the cytotrophoblastic cells are less prominent

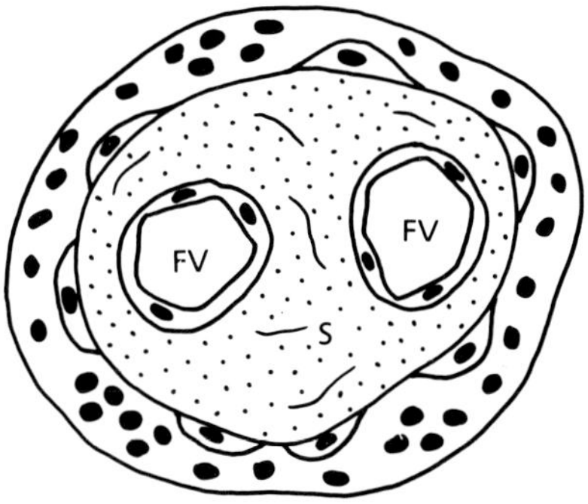


**Fig. 3.11** Diagrammatic representation of the histological appearances of a typical second trimester villus. (Reproduced with permission from Fox 1986.) FV = fetal vessels; S = villous stroma.

whilst the syncytiotrophoblast is thinner and somewhat irregular: the syncytial nuclei are less evenly distributed than in the first trimester and often show a degree of clustering. A distinct, but thin, trophoblastic basement membrane is present, separating the trophoblast from the stroma. The stroma is more compact than is the case in the villi of early gestation and contains a variable number of fibroblasts, myofibroblasts and delicate collagen fibres. Hofbauer cells are seen in the stromal interfibrillary spaces but appear less numerous than in the villi of the early placenta. The villous fetal capillaries are quite prominent, tend to lie more towards the villous periphery and are linked by flattened, fully mature endothelial cells.

From about the 30th week of gestation small terminal villi, measuring about 40 μm in diameter, begin to appear and these are the predominant form of villi seen in the term placenta (Figure 3.12). Their trophoblastic covering layer is irregularly thinned whilst cytotrophoblastic cells are few and inconspicuous.

In terminal villi the syncytial nuclei are irregularly distributed and are often aggregated to form multinucleated protrusions into the intervillous space (Fox 1978). It has been claimed that many, even most, of these knots are histological artefacts due to tangential sectioning of the

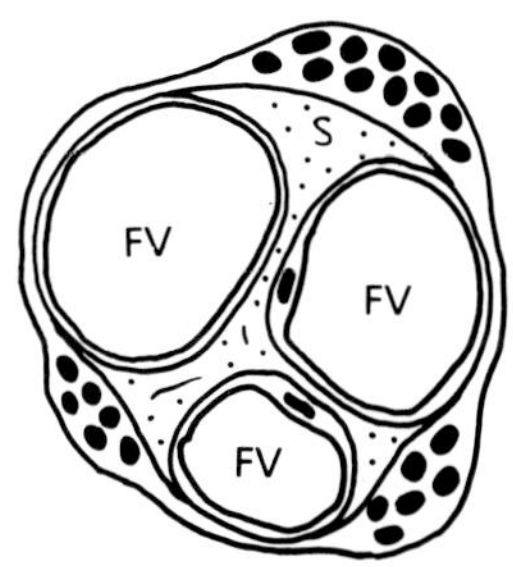


**Fig. 3.12** Diagrammatic representation of a terminal villus, the predominant type of villus in the term placenta. (Reproduced with permission from Fox 1986.) FV = fetal vessels; S = villous stroma.

villi (Küsterman 1981; Cantle *et al.* 1987) but nevertheless the nuclei within these knots differ considerably from those in the rest of the villous syncytiotrophoblast and show all the ultrastructural features of senescence: it appears therefore that syncytial knots are formed of aged nuclei which become sequestrated away from the functional areas of the syncytium, their loss being made up for by the formation of fresh syncytial nuclei from the cytotrophoblast (Jones & Fox 1977).

In many terminal villi the syncytiotrophoblast is focally attenuated and anuclear (Figure 3.13): these thinned areas commonly overlie a dilated fetal capillary vessel and form the *vasculo-syncytial membranes* (Getzowa & Sadowsky 1950). These membranous areas of the syncytiotrophoblast differ markedly from the non-thinned areas of the syncytium in their content of histochemically detectable enzymes (Amstutz 1960), in their ultrastructure (Burgos & Rodriguez 1966) and in their surface characteristics (Fox & Agrofojo-Blanco 1974) and it is almost certain that they are specialized zones for the facilitation of gas transfer across the placenta.

The trophoblastic basement membrane of the terminal villi is well defined whilst the villous stromal tissue is reduced to a thin layer between the sinusoidally dilated villous capillaries. Hofbauer cells are present in the stroma but are difficult to recognize because of their compression by vessels and collagen fibres.

In the terminal villi there are usually between two and six fetal capillary vessels which are characteristically situated towards the villous periphery in close approximation to the covering trophoblast. These vessels are commonly sinusoidally dilated and occupy most of the cross-sectional area of the villus. Aherne (1975) thought that the dilatation of the fetal villous vessels was a mechanism for crowding flow lines, and hence increasing concentration gradients, for substances crossing from maternal

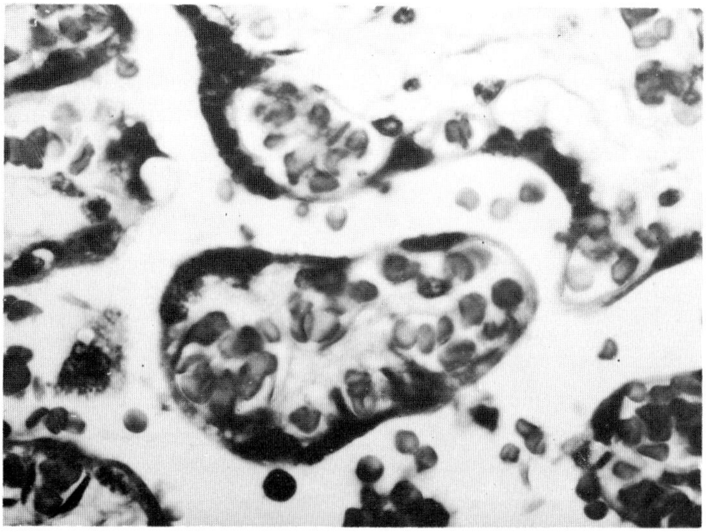

**Fig. 3.13** A terminal villus with a vasculo-syncytial membrane (on the right). H & E × 850. (Reproduced with permission from Fox 1985.)

to fetal blood and was thus a mechanism for augmenting the efficiency of placental transfer mechanisms. By contrast, Kaufmann *et al.* (1985) considered that the sinusoidal dilatation of these vessels was a means of decreasing blood flow resistance, for allowing an evenness of blood flow throughout the placenta and for facilitating fetal placental perfusion.

## Placental pathology

It is not proposed to give in this section a detailed account of the placental abnormalities seen in every complication of pregnancy but rather to consider the general pattern of placental pathology: in particular the concept of *placental insufficiency* will be considered.

### Developmental abnormalities

The only common developmental abnormality of the placenta is extrachorial placentation, in which the chorionic plate of the placenta, from which the villi arise, is smaller than the basal plate, the transition from villous to non-villous chorion taking place not at the placental margin but at some distance within the circumference of the fetal surface of the placenta. If this transition is marked by a flattened ring of membranes the placenta is classed as circummarginate, whereas if this ring has a raised, rolled edge, the placenta is circumvallate.

The clinical significance of this anomaly has been much debated but it is now clear that the circummarginate form is devoid of clinical importance, and that although circumvallate placentation is associated unduly frequently with a rather small baby, and possibly with a slight excess of congenital malformation (Ladermacher *et al.* 1981), it does not appear to be associated with an increased perinatal mortality (Fox & Sen 1972). Other aberrant forms of placentation are either of no functional significance (e.g. bilobate placenta, accessory lobe) or so rare that they can, in practical terms, be ignored (e.g. placenta membranacea, girdle placenta).

There have been claims that marginal or velamentous insertion of the cord is related to a high perinatal mortality rate but modern studies have agreed that the site of cord insertion is unrelated to the incidence of premature labour, low birth weight, or fetal hypoxia (Uyanwah-Akpom & Fox 1977; Wood & Malan 1978). Velamentous insertion does, of course, present a small risk because of the danger of traumatic damage to, and bleeding from, the unprotected vessels running through the membranes.

### Gross lesions of the placenta

Few, if any, of the various plaques, thrombi, or cysts seen on cutting the placenta are of any importance (Fox 1978); macroscopically visible calcification, however marked, is also a banal finding, devoid of clinical significance. This unimportance of gross lesions applies equally to those, such as perivillous fibrin deposition and fetal artery thrombosis, that functionally inactivate, and thus exclude from playing any role in materno-fetal transfer, a proportion of the villous population. Indeed, the loss in this manner of a third of the villous parenchyma is without any effect on fetal development, growth, or viability and this bears eloquent witness to the considerable functional reserve capacity of the placenta.

This, however, leaves unexplained the apparently paradoxical finding that extensive infarction, e.g. necrosis of more than 10 per cent of the villous parenchyma, is associated with a very high incidence of fetal hypoxia, growth retardation, and death. Extensive infarction is, however, caused by widespread thrombosis of maternal uteroplacental vessels. This is a process that one would not expect to occur in a healthy vascular tree and it is, therefore, no coincidence that extensive infarction is virtually confined to placentas from women with pre-eclampsia, a condition in which an acute *atherosis* is found in the uteroplacental vessels and which predisposes to thrombosis. Far more importantly, however, there is in pre-eclamptic women, whether thrombosis occurs or not, a severely restricted blood flow to the placenta (the reasons for this are discussed later). Extensive infarction, therefore, occurs only against a backcloth of a severely compromised uteroplacental circulation, and its true significance is that it is the visible hallmark of a markedly abnormal maternal vasculature and a reduced maternal placental blood flow, these being the real causes of the apparent effects of infarction on fetal nutrition and oxygenation. It is true that the situation is further worsened in these cases by infarction superimposed on a placenta, the functional reserve of which has been already dissipated by uteroplacental ischaemia, but the infarction, *per se*, is not the primary cause of the fetal complications and would be of little importance if it occurred in placentas with a normal blood supply.

## Placental weight

It is difficult, and in routine practice virtually impossible, to obtain a true estimate of placental mass and, indeed, a knowledge of placental weight is, by itself, of little value. Placental/fetal weight ratios are more useful but it would not be an undue oversimplification to suggest that the only conclusion that can be drawn from the many studies of this ratio is that small babies usually have small placentas whereas big babies have large placentas. It then becomes almost an article of faith as to whether one believes that the baby is small because the placenta is small or that the placenta is small because the baby is small. Several findings suggest, however, that placental mass is unlikely to be a limiting factor for fetal growth. First, if fetal weight was narrowly limited by placental mass, this would imply that the term placenta has no functional reserve capacity. As already remarked, simple pathologic findings indicate that this is not the case and experimental studies involving either surgical reduction of placental mass (Robinson *et al.* 1979) or artificially increased fetal oxygen consumption (Lorijn & Longo 1980) have confirmed the striking functional reserve capacity of the placenta. Second, the placenta also has a normally unrealized potential for further incremental growth as evidenced by the large placentas encountered in such conditions as pregnancy at high altitude, severe maternal anaemia, and decompensated maternal heart disease.

This ability of the placenta to show a compensatory increment of growth in the face of an unfavourable maternal milieu is further evidence against limitation of fetal weight by placental mass and it must therefore be concluded that the placenta is usually small because the baby is small, the placenta sharing in the generally reduced growth of the fetal organs and its small size not acting as a contributory factor to fetal growth retardation.

## Histological abnormalities of the placental villi

Most of the changes observed in the placental villi are either a manifestation of villous maturation and trophoblastic differentiation or reflect a response to alterations in one or other of the two circulatory systems of the placenta.

The characteristic response of the villi to a reduced maternal blood flow is a proliferation of villous cytotrophoblast and an accompanying thickening of the trophoblastic basement membrane (Fox 1978). The villous cytotrophoblastic elements are, throughout pregnancy, the stem cells of the trophoblast, DNA synthesis and mitotic activity being confined to these cells. During the course of a normal pregnancy, however, the cytotrophoblastic elements diminish in number and prominence as gestation proceeds, presumably because in the late stages of pregnancy there is little need for fresh growth of trophoblast. Therefore the cytotrophoblast can, at this stage, be regarded as a largely quiescent germinative zone. In conditions of placental ischaemia, however, this germinative zone is reactivated, for the cytotrophoblastic elements become more numerous and unduly prominent and often show mitotic activity, all changes indicating a resurgence of proliferative activity. It is almost certain that this activation of the germinative zone represents a repair and hyperplasia phenomenon in which cytotrophoblast proliferates, in an attempt to replace and repair ischaemically damaged syncytiotrophoblast. It is true that syncytial damage is not apparent on light microscopy of placentas subjected to ischaemia but electron microscopy shows small focal areas of syncytial necrosis in such cases, usually of only very slight extent and detectable only after prolonged search (Jones & Fox 1980). The basement membrane thickening seen in ischaemic placental villi is probably only an incidental by-product of the cytotrophoblastic hyperplasia, for basement membrane protein is almost certainly secreted, in part at least, by the cytotrophoblast, and an unusual degree of proliferation of these cells is therefore accompanied by an excessive production of basement membrane material.

It is clear, therefore, that the essential response of the placenta to ischaemia is a highly efficient reparative one, a phenomenon that does not suggest severe functional damage to the organ. It is true that at the ultrastructural level the ischaemic villi show decreased pinocytotic activity and a reduced number of secretory droplets, but whether these indices of diminished transfer and synthetic activity are caused simply by oxygen lack or are indicative of placental damage is a moot point. Certainly, however, the unimpaired replicative and regenerative capacity of the placenta and the slight, but definite, evidence of compensatory mechanisms in the placenta subjected to ischaemia suggest that the trophoblast is not insufficient in these circumstances but is fulfilling as adequately as possible its physiologic role in the face of an unfavourable maternal environment.

The placental villi have a dual blood supply but are in no way dependent upon fetal blood for their supply of nutrients or oxygen. The morphologic effects of decreased villous blood flow are stromal fibrosis and an increased number of syncytial knots. The reasons why a reduced fetal villous perfusion should result in these morphologic changes is obscure but there is no evidence that they are associated with any decline in placental function.

## Ageing of the placenta

It is widely believed that the placenta ages as pregnancy progresses and that the term organ is in, or on the verge of, a decline into morphologic and functional senescence. The villi of the term placenta are often described as showing all the morphologic hallmarks of senescence, but this view is based almost entirely upon a misinterpretation of the normal processes of maturation of the villous tree and of trophoblastic differentiation. There are in fact no morphologic features of the term placenta, at either light or electron microscopic level, that can be considered as a manifestation of ageing (Fox 1979). Claims that lipofuscin, or ageing, pigment is present in the term placenta have recently been refuted (Haigh & Fox 1984). Further adduced as evidence of placental ageing is the cessation of DNA synthesis and of placental growth that has been claimed to occur at the 36th week of gestation. More recent studies have, however, indicated that total placental DNA levels continue to rise in a linear fashion until, and beyond, the 40th week of gestation (Sands & Dobbing 1985), and this would be in accord with histologic evidence of fresh villous growth and the autoradiographic demonstration of continuing DNA synthesis in the term placenta (Geier *et al.* 1975).

Placental growth does, therefore, appear to continue to term though there is no doubt that there is a decrease in the growth rate during the later stages of pregnancy. This decrease is, however, neither invariable nor irreversible, for, as discussed previously, the placenta can continue to increase its size considerably if faced with an unfavourable maternal environment whereas the potential for a recrudescence of growth is clearly seen in the proliferative response to ischaemic syncytial damage. Those arguing that a decreased placental growth rate during late pregnancy is evidence of senescence often appear to be comparing the placenta with an organ such as the gut, in which continuing viability is dependent upon a constantly replicating stem cell layer producing short-lived, post-mitotic cells. A more apt comparison would be with an organ such as the liver, which is formed largely of long-lived, post-mitotic cells and which, once the most favourable size has been reached to meet the metabolic demands placed upon it, shows little evidence of cell replication while retaining a latent potentiality for growth activity. Certainly there seems no reason why the placenta should continue to grow once it has reached a size sufficient to meet adequately its transfer function, and the term placenta, with its considerable physiologic reserve capacity, has more than fulfilled this aim.

## Placental infection

If the placenta is taken to include the membranes, then infection may reach the organ either from the maternal bloodstream or from the endometrium to produce a villitis, or by ascent of organisms from the birth canal with a resultant chorioamnionitis.

A predominantly villous inflammation can be due to placental involvement in maternal infections such as rubella, toxoplasmosis, listeriosis, syphilis, or cytomegalovirus disease (Blanc 1981), but such conditions account for only a very small proportion of cases of villitis, the vast majority of which are of unknown aetiology (Russell 1980). The incidence of villitis in unselected series of placentas in the UK, the USA and Australia is in the region of 5 to 8 per cent, though an incidence of 24 per cent has been reported from Argentina (Labarrere *et al.* 1982). There appears to be a clear correlation between the presence of a villitis and intrauterine growth retardation and there has been a tendency to attribute the deficient fetal growth to damage inflicted on the placenta by the inflammatory process. Most cases of villitis are, however, of a focal nature with only a small, widely scattered, proportion of the villous population showing any evidence of either an active or a healed inflammatory lesion, and this degree of villous damage is unlikely to impair, let alone dissipate, the functional reserve capacity of the placenta. Occasional instances of a widespread, diffuse, necrotizing villitis are encountered (Russell & Atkinson 1980) and these would certainly decrease placental efficiency; a villitis of this extent is, however, most exceptional. It seems unlikely, therefore, that the association between villitis and fetal growth retardation can be explained simply in terms of placental damage and the most probable basis for this relationship is that a villitis is commonly an indication of fetal infection. Although there is a widespread faith in the placenta as a barrier to fetal infection, it appears that virtually all organisms can in fact breach it. The placenta acts largely as a simple, non-specific barrier, which delays, rather than prevents, the passage of organisms to the fetus. The effects of fetal infection vary with the stage of gestation, but it is probable that infection during the later stages of pregnancy, which is known to inhibit fetal DNA synthesis, will lead to a failure of adequate growth.

The only obvious exception to this general rule is maternal malaria. In endemic areas malarial infection of the placenta is common and is frequently associated with fetal growth retardation, but transplacental passage of the parasite is rare. In this condition, however, there is a massive accumulation of monocytes in the intervillous space which almost certainly impedes maternal blood flow through the placenta (Galbraith *et al.* 1980).

It is generally agreed that a chorioamnionitis is due to an ascending bacterial, fungal, or viral infection of the membranes and it is further agreed that prolonged membrane rupture is associated with a high incidence of chorioamnionitis and that chorioamnionitis is frequently found in the placentas of prematurely delivered infants. It remains controversial, however, whether chorioamnionitis is a precipitating cause or a complication of premature labour and whether there is a significant incidence of chorioamnionitis in cases without prolonged membrane rupture. Other still-debated questions about chorioamnionitis are the incidence of amniotic fluid infection in the presence of intact membranes and the relationship between coitus in late pregnancy and inflammation of the membranes.

## Toxic damage to the placenta

Remarkably little is known about the possible injurious effects on the placenta of toxins, drugs, or environmental pollutants. The only example of toxic damage that has been adequately studied is that of the effects of maternal cigarette smoking, an interest stimulated by the established association between maternal smoking and low birth weight. The placentas of cigarette smokers show evidence of ischaemic damage, which is probably due to the vasoconstrictive effects of nicotine on the uterine vasculature (van der Veen & Fox 1982). Focal cytotrophoblastic and endothelial cell necrosis are also found and it has been suggested that these latter lesions could be because of the effects of cadmium in tobacco smoke, for cadmium is known to cause placental necrosis in experimental animals and is found in much higher concentration in the placentas of smokers than in those from non-smokers (Di Sant'Agnese *et al.* 1983). The functional consequences of placental damage caused by cigarette smoke are, however, almost certainly nullified by the compensatory hyperplasia that is a feature of the smoker's placenta (Christianson 1979) and the deficiency of fetal growth is probably because of the direct effects of nicotine on the uterine vasculature and of carbon monoxide on the fetus.

## Immunopathology of the placenta

The placenta contains paternal antigens and is thus an allograft. It is therefore possible that placental damage could be due to a form of graft rejection. Such a rejection would imply a breakdown of the mechanisms that allow the placenta to flourish as a graft, and although these are still not fully elucidated some understanding of this immunologic paradox has been gained in recent years (Faulk & Johnson 1980). First, it is now established that villous trophoblast does not express antigens of the major histocompatibility complex, a deficiency that may protect trophoblast from recognition by maternal immunocytes and from cytotoxic immune reactions. It must be admitted, however, that the significance of this particular finding has been diluted by the more recent description of HLA antigens on extravillous trophoblast (Sunderland *et al.* 1982). There is, however, evidence that the HLA antigen in extravillous trophoblast is of a novel nature and not functioning as a true transplantation antigen. Second, the villous trophoblast contains a surface antigen that blocks rejection reactions by maternal lymphocytes. Third, blocking antibodies are present in the serum of pregnant women, which inhibit the cytotoxic effect of maternal lymphocytes against cultured trophoblastic tissue. Other factors, such as the relative immunologic privilege conferred by decidua or the immunosuppressive effect of placental hormones, appear to be of lesser or only transitory importance.

Evidence that these protective mechanisms sometimes fail is scanty. There are certainly no grounds for believing that either normal or premature labour is caused by a graft rejection process but there is a widespread belief that some form of immunologically mediated attack on placental tissue is an important factor in the pathogenesis of pre-eclampsia. It is usually thought to be an oversimplification to regard such an attack as being directly comparable to an allograft rejection, for women who develop anti-HLA antibodies during pregnancy have a low incidence of pre-eclampsia and the placenta of the pre-eclamptic woman does not show any morphologic features suggestive of a graft reaction. On the other hand, prior blood transfusion, which appears to protect transplanted kidneys from rejection, also offers some protection against the development of pre-eclampsia, and the histologic changes seen in the uteroplacental vessels in pre-eclampsia resemble those noted in the vessels of rejected renal transplants. Claims that antitrophoblastic antibodies or circulating immune complexes play a role in the pathogenesis of pre-eclampsia are currently controversial. Electron microscopic evidence of immune complex deposition in the placenta is, however, not seen and while immunohistologic studies have shown an increased amount of the complement factors C3 and C4 on the trophoblastic basement membrane of placentas from pre-eclamptic women (Faulk & Johnson 1980), no deposition of immunoglobulins has been detected.

There is, however, a contrasting view that pre-eclampsia represents a failure, rather than an overactivity, of the maternal immune system, evidence for this including the low proportion of pre-eclamptic women with anti-HLA antibodies, a higher than expected incidence of HLA compatibilities between mother and father in pre-eclamptic pregnancies, and reduced lymphocyte reactivity in women with this disease. A failure of maternal immunologic recognition of paternal antigens expressed in trophoblast appears to be another important factor in some women who repetitively abort. In such cases there is an unusual degree of sharing of HLA antigens between husband and wife and there is a failure of development of maternal blocking antibodies. It is possible that, as trophoblastic antigens are allotypic, certain trophoblastic antigens are coded by specific HLA loci, and if there is an excessive parental sharing of such loci the mother is unable to recognize trophoblast as an alien tissue (Taylor & Faulk 1981). Maternal blocking factors are therefore not developed, there is no inhibition of cell-mediated immune reactions, and the woman aborts, though the exact mechanism for this is still unknown.

### Extravillous trophoblast and the pathology of the uteroplacental vessels

It is difficult to accept that most cases of placental insufficiency are caused by intrinsic placental damage and it is becoming increasingly clear that the common factor that runs as a thread through most cases of presumed placental inadequacy is a reduced maternal blood flow to the fetoplacental unit. It has been previously pointed out that the placenta establishes its own blood supply as a result of invasion of the spiral arteries in the placental bed by extravillous trophoblast, this process occurring in two stages. The factors controlling and limiting intravascular invasion by extravillous trophoblast are unknown but the crucial importance of this process is shown by the finding that in women destined to develop pre-eclampsia in the later stages of their pregnancy there is a partial failure of placentation which results in a markedly restricted blood flow to the placenta. This failure has two components: firstly, whilst in a normal pregnancy all the spiral arteries in the placental bed are invaded by trophoblast this process occurs in only a proportion of these vessels in patients who later develop pre-eclampsia, a significant fraction of the placental bed arteries showing a complete absence of physiological change (Khong *et al.* 1986). Secondly, in those arteries which are invaded by extravillous trophoblast the first stage in this process occurs quite normally with trophoblast evoking physiological changes in their intradecidual segments but there is subsequently a complete failure of the second stage with endovascular trophoblast failing to advance into the intramyometrial portion of these vessels (Robertson *et al.* 1967, 1975). Hence in these women there is an incomplete transformation of the spiral arteries to uteroplacental vessels and this abnormality, with its consequent restriction of maternal uteroplacental blood flow, is in itself an adequate cause for all the placental abnormalities and all the fetal complications seen in pre-eclampsia.

Pre-eclampsia is not the sole instance of the serious consequences of inadequate placentation for it is now becoming clear that a similar defective invasion of the spiral arteries by extravillous trophoblast is also a feature of many cases of normotensive intrauterine fetal growth retardation, the deficit in fetal growth being due to the reduced maternal supply of oxygen and nutrients (Robertson *et al.* 1981). Placentas from such cases show evidence of ischaemic damage on electron microscopy (van der Veen & Fox 1983). Experimentally induced limitation of maternal blood flow in animals results in an unduly small fetus (O'Shaughnessy 1981). Haemodynamic studies have demonstrated a significantly reduced maternal blood flow to the placenta in many cases of fetal growth retardation (Lunell *et al.* 1979). Although some have observed occlusive atheroma-like lesions in the spiral vessels in cases of intrauterine growth retardation (Sheppard & Bonnar 1976), others have failed to confirm this finding (Brosens *et al.* 1977) and there is more general agreement that in many, but not all cases of intrauterine growth retardation there is either a partial or complete failure of cytotrophoblastic invasion and normal physiologic changes in the intramyometrial segments of the spiral arteries (Robertson *et al.* 1981), a situation akin to that found in pre-eclampsia.

It is clear therefore that most cases of apparent placental insufficiency are in fact examples of maternal vascular insufficiency. It may appear pedantic to some to draw this distinction but the use of the term placental insufficiency gives the obstetrician a false sense of having identified, or at least localized, the abnormality, induces a mood of therapeutic nihilism, and directs research along unrewarding pathways.

### Conclusion

The placenta is a vigorous, energetic, versatile organ with a considerable physiologic reserve capacity. Most pathologic lesions of the placenta are functionally irrelevant and it is doubtful if the placenta often, or ever, becomes insufficient. Attention is being increasingly directed to the interaction of extravillous trophoblast and maternal tissues during placentation and it is becoming clear that many of the ills that may beset a pregnancy have their origin in an abnormal interrelationship between fetal and maternal tissues during the early stages of gestation.

## References

Adamson K. & Myers R.E. (1975) Circulation in the intervillous space: obstetrical considerations in fetal deprivation. In *The Placenta and its Maternal Supply Line*, (Ed. by P. Gruenwald), pp. 158–77. Medical and Technical Publishing, Lancaster.

Aherne W. (1975) Morphometry. In *The Placenta and its Maternal Supply Line*, (Ed. by P. Gruenwald), pp. 80–97. Medical and Technical Publishing, Lancaster.

Amstutz E. (1960) Beobachtungen über die Refung der Chorionzotten in der menslichen Plazenta mit beswonderer Berückichtigung der Epithelplatten. *Acta Anatomica*, **42**, 12–30.

Blanc W.A. (1981) Pathology of the placenta, membranes and umbilical cord in arterial, fungal and viral infections in man. In *Perinatal Diseases*, (Ed. by R.L. Naeye, J.H. Kissane & N. Kaufman), p. 67–132. Williams & Wilkins, Baltimore.

Bleker O.P., Kloosterman G.J., Mieras D.J., Oosting J. & Sallé H.J.A. (1975) Intervillous space during uterine contractions in human subjects: an ultrasonic study. *American Journal of Obstetrics and Gynecology*, **123**, 697–9.

Boyd J.D. & Hamilton W.J. (1970) *The Human Placenta*. Heffer, Cambridge.

Brosens I., Robertson W.B. & Dixon H.G. (1967) The physiological response of the vessels of the placental bed in normal pregnancy. *Journal of Pathology and Bacteriology*, **93**, 569–79.

Brosens I., Dixon H.G. & Robertson W.B. (1977) Fetal growth retardation and the arteries of the placental bed. *British Journal of Obstetrics and Gynaecology* **84**, 656–65.

Bulmer J.N. & Johnson P.M. (1985) Antigen expression by trophoblast populations in the human placenta and their possible immunobiological relevance. *Placenta*, **6**, 127–40.

Burgos M.H. & Rodriguez E.M. (1966) Specialized zones in the trophoblast of the human term placenta. *American Journal of Obstetrics and Gynecology*, **96**, 342–56.

Cantle S.J., Kaufmann P., Luckhardt M. & Schweikhart G. (1987) Interpretation of syncytial sprouts and bridges in the human placenta. *Placenta*, **8**, 221–34.

Castelucci M., Celona A., Bartels H., Steininger B., Benedetto V. & Kaufman P. (1987) Mitoses of the Hofbauer cell: possible implications for a fetal macrophage. *Placenta*, **8**, 65–76.

Castellucci M., Zaccheo D. & Pescetto G. (1980) A three-dimensional study of the normal human placental villous core. I. The Hofbauer cells. *Cell and Tissue Research*, **210**, 235–47.

Christianson R. E. (1979) Gross differences observed in the placentae of smokers and non-smokers. *American Journal of Epidemiology*, **110**, 178–87.

Dearden I. & Ockleford C.D. (1983) Structure of human trophoblast: correlation with function. In *Biology of Trophoblast*, (Ed. by Y.W. Loke & A. Whyte), pp. 69–110. Elsevier, Amsterdam.

Demir R. & Erbengi T. (1984) Some new findings about Hofbauer cells in the chorionic villi of the human placenta. *Acta Anatomica*, **119**, 18–26.

Di Sant'Agnese P.A., Jensen K.D., Levin A. & Miller R.K. (1983) Placental toxicity of cadmium in the rat: An ultrastructural study. *Placenta*, **4**, 149–64.

Enders A.C. (1965) A comparative study of the fine structure of the trophoblast in several hemochorial placentae. *American Journal of Anatomy*, **116**, 29–67.

Faulk W.P. & Johnson P.M. (1980) Immunological studies of human placentae: Basic and practical implications. In *Recent Advances in Clinical Immunology 2*, (Ed. by R.A. Thompson), p. 1. Churchill Livingstone, Edinburgh.

Fox H. (1967) The incidence and significance of Hofbauer cells in the mature placenta. *Journal of Pathology of Bacteriology*, **93**, 710–17.

Fox H. (1978) *Pathology of the Placenta*. Saunders, Philadelphia.

Fox H. (1979) The placenta as a model for organ ageing. In *Placenta—a Neglected Experimental Animal*, (Ed. by P. Beaconsfield & C. Villee), pp. 351–78. Pergamon Press, Oxford.

Fox H. (1985) Placental structure. In *Scientific Basis of Obstetrics and Gynaecology*, 3rd edn (Ed. by R.R. Macdonald), pp. 1–28. Churchill Livingstone, Edinburgh.

Fox H. (1986) Development of the placenta and membranes. In *Basic Sciences in Obstetrics and Gynaecology*, (Ed. by J. Dewhurst, M. De Swiet & G. Chamberlain), pp. 34–41. Churchill Livingstone, Edinburgh.

Fox H. & Agrofojo-Blanco A. (1974) Scanning electron microscopy of the human placenta in normal and abnormal pregnancies. *European Journal of Obstetrics, Gynecology and Reproductive Biology*, **4**, 45–50.

Fox H. & Kharkongor N.F. (1969) Enzyme histochemistry of the Hofbauer cells of the human placenta. *Journal of Obstetrics and Gynaecology of the British Commonwealth*, **76**, 918–21.

Fox H. & Sen D.K. (1972) Placenta extrachorialis: A clinicopathological study. *Journal of Obstetrics and Gynaecology of the British Commonwealth*, **79**, 32–5.

Freese U.E. (1966) The fetal–maternal circulation of the placenta. I. Histomorphologic, placental injection and X-ray cinematographic studies on human placenta. *American Journal of Obstetrics and Gynecology*, **94**, 354–60.

Galbraith R.M., Fox H., Hsi B., Galbraith G.M.P., Bray R.S. & Faulk W.P. (1980) The human materno-fetal relationship in malaria. II. Histological, ultrastructural and immunopathological studies of the placenta. *Transactions of the Royal Society of Tropical Medicine and Hygiene*, **74**, 61–72.

Galton M. (1962) DNA content of placental nuclei. *Journal of Cell Biology*, **13**, 183–203.

Gaunt M. & Ockleford C.D. (1986) Microinjection of human placenta: 2. Biological application. *Placenta*, **7**, 325–31.

Geier G., Schuhmann R. & Kraus H. (1975) Regional unterschiedliche Zellproliferation innerhalb der Plazentenone reifer menschlicher Plazenten: autoradiographische Untersuchungen. *Archiv für Gynäkologie*, **218**, 31–7.

Getzowa S. & Sodowsky A. (1950) On the structure of the human placenta with full-term and immature foetus, living or dead. *Journal of Obstetrics and Gynaecology of the British Empire*, **57**, 388–96.

Gosseye S. & Fox H. (1984) An immunohistological comparison of the secretory capacity of villous and extravillous trophoblast in the human placenta. *Placenta*, **5**, 329–48.

Gruenwald P. (1973) Lobular structure of hemochorial primate placentas, and its relation to maternal vessels. *American Journal of Anatomy*, **136**, 133–52.

Haigh M. & Fox H. (1984) The human placenta does not contain lipofuscin pigment. *Placenta*, **5**, 459–64.

Jones C.J.P. & Fox H. (1977) Syncytial knots and intervillous bridges in the human placenta: an ultrastructural study. *Journal of Anatomy*, **124**, 275–86.

Jones C.J.P. & Fox H. (1980) An ultrastructural and ultrahistochemical study of the human placenta in maternal pre-eclampsia. *Placenta*, **1**, 61–76.

Kaufmann P., Bruns U., Leiser R., Luckhardt M. & Winterhager E. (1985) The fetal vascularisation of term human placental villi. II. Intermediate and terminal villi. *Anatomy and Embryology*, **173**, 203–14.

Khong T.Y., de Wolf F., Robertson W.B. & Brosens I. (1986) Inadequate maternal vascular response to placentation in pregnancies complicated by pre-eclampsia and by small-for-gestational-age infants. *British Journal of Obstetrics and Gynaecology*, **93**, 1049–59.

Kurman R.J., Main C.S. & Chen H.-H. (1984) Intermediate trophoblast: a distinctive form of trophoblast with specific morphological, biochemical and functional features. *Placenta*, **5**, 349–70.

Küsterman W. (1981) Uber 'Proliferationaknoten' und 'syncytialknoten' der menschlichen plazenta. *Anatomischer Anzeiger*, **150**, 144–57.

Labarrere C., Althabe O. & Telenta M. (1982) Chronic villitis of unknown aetiology in placentae of idiopathic small for gestational age infants. *Placenta*, **3**, 309–18.

Ladermacher D.S., Vermeulen R.C.W., Harten J.J. & Arts N.F.T. (1981) Circumvallate placenta and congenital malformation. *Lancet*, **ii**, 737.

Lemtis H. (1970) Physiologie der Plazenta. *Fortschritte der Geburtshilfe und Gynäkologie*, **41**, 1–52.

Lorijn R.H.V. & Longo L.D. (1980) Clinical and physiologic implications of increased fetal oxygen consumption. *American Journal of Obstetrics and Gynecology*, **136**, 451–7.

Lunell N.O., Sarby B., Lewender R. & Nylund R.L. (1979) Comparison of uteroplacental blood flow in normal and in intrauterine growth retarded pregnancy. *Gynecologic and Obstetrical Investigation*, **10**, 106–18.

Moll W. (1981) Physiologie der maternen placentaren Durchblutung. In *Die Plazenta des Menshen*, (Ed. by V. Becker, Th.H. Schiebler & F. Kubli), pp. 172–94. Thieme, Stuttgart.

Moll W., Zunzell W. & Herburger J. (1975) Hemodynamic implications of hemochorial placentation. *European Journal of Obstetrics, Gynecology and Reproductive Biology*, **5**, 67–74.

Moskalewski S., Ptak W. & Czernik Z. (1975) Demonstration of cells with IgG receptor in human placenta. *Biology of the Neonate*, **26**, 269–73.

O'Shaughnessy E.W. (1981) Uterine blood flow and fetal growth. In *Fetal Growth Retardation*, (Ed. by F.A. van Assche & W.B. Robertson), pp. 101–16. Churchill Livingstone, Edinburgh.

Pijnenborg R., Bland J.M., Robertson W.B. & Brosens I. (1983) Uteroplacental arterial changes related to interstitial trophoblast migration in early human pregnancy. *Placenta*, **4**, 397–414.

Pijnenborg R., Bland J.M., Robertson W.B., Dixon G. & Brosens I. (1981) The pattern of interstitial trophoblastic invasion of the myometrium in early human pregnancy. *Placenta*, **2**, 303–15.

Ramsey E.M. (1959) Circulation in the placenta. In *Gestation: Transactions of the Fifth Conference*, (Ed. by C.A. Villee), pp. 77–107. Macy Foundation, New York.

Ramsey E.M. (1965) Circulation of the placenta. *Birth Defects, Original Articles Series*, **1**, 5–12.

Ramsey E.M. (1975) Discussion of Gruenwald P. *European Journal of Obstetrics, Gynecology and Reproductive Biology*, **5**, 31.

Ramsey E.M. & Donner M.W. (1980) *Placental Vasculature and Circulation*. Thieme, Stuttgart.

Redman C.W., McMichael A.J., Stirrat G.M., Sunderland C.A. & Ting A. (1984) Class I major histocompatibility complex antigens on human extra-villous trophoblast. *Immunology*, **52**, 457–68.

Reynolds S.R.M. (1966) Formation of fetal cotyledons in the hemochorial placenta: a theoretical consideration of the functional implications of such an arrangement. *American Journal of Obstetrics and Gynecology*, **94**, 425–39.

Richart R. (1961) Studies of placental morphogenesis I. Radiographic studies of human placenta utilizing tritiated thymidine. *Proceedings of the Society for Experimental Biology and Medicine*, **106**, 829–31.

Robertson W.B., Brosens I. & Dixon H.G. (1967) The pathological response of the vessels of the placental bed in hypertensive pregnancy. *Journal of Pathology and Bacteriology*, **93**, 581–92.

Robertson W.B., Brosens I. & Dixon H.G. (1975) Uteroplacental vascular pathology. *European Journal of Obstetrics, Gynecology and Reproductive Biology*, **5**, 47–65.

Robertson W.B., Brosens I.A. & Dixon H.G. (1981) Maternal blood supply in fetal growth retardation. In *Fetal Growth Retardation*, (Ed. by A. van Assche & W.B. Robertson), pp. 126–38. Churchill Livingstone, Edinburgh.

Robinson J.S., Kingstone E.J., Jones C.T. & Thorburn G.D. (1979) Studies of experimental growth retardation in sheep: the effect of removal of endometrial caruncles on fetal size and metabolism. *Journal of Developmental Physiology*, **1**, 379–98.

Russell P. (1980) Inflammatory lesions of the human placenta. III. The histopathology of villitis of unknown aetiology. *Placenta*, **1**, 227–44.

Russell P. & Atkinson K. (1980) Recurrent reproductive failure due to severe placental villitis of unknown etiology. *Journal of Reproductive Medicine*, **24**, 93–8.

Sands J. & Dobbing J. (1985) Continuing growth and development of the third trimester human placenta. *Placenta*, **6**, 13–22.

Schumann R. (1981) Plazenten: Begriff, Entstehung, funktionelle Anatomie. In *Die Plazenta des Menschen*, (Ed. by V. Becker, Th.H. Schiebler & F. Kubli), pp. 199–207. Thieme, Stuttgart.

Sheppard B.L. & Bonnar J. (1976) The ultrastructure of the arterial supply of the human placenta in pregnancy complicated by fetal growth retardation. *British Journal of Obstetrics and Gynaecology*, **83**, 948–59.

Sunderland C.A., Redman C.W.G. & Stirrat G.M. (1982) HLA-A, B, C antigens are expressed on non-villous trophoblast of the early human placenta. *Journal of Immunology*, **127**, 2614.

Taylor C. & Faulk W.P. (1981) Prevention of recurrent abortion with leucocyte transfusions. *Lancet*, **2**, 68–70.

Uyanwah-Akpom W.P. & Fox H. (1977) The clinical significance of marginal and velamentous insertion of the cord. *British Journal of Obstetrics and Gynaecology*, **84**, 941–3.

van der Veen F. & Fox H. (1982) The effects of cigarette smoking on the human placenta: A light and electron microscopic study. *Placenta*, **3**, 243–56.

van der Veen F. & Fox H. (1983) The human placenta in idiopathic intrauterine growth retardation: A light and electron microscopic study. *Placenta*, **4**, 65–78.

Voland J.R., Frisman D.M. & Baird S.M. (1986) Presence of an endothelial antigen on the syncytiotrophoblast of human chorionic villi: detection by a monoclonal antibody. *American Journal of Reproductive Immunology and Microbiology*, **11**, 24–30.

Wigglesworth J.S. (1967) Vascular organisation of the human placenta. *Nature*, **216**, 1120–1.

Wilkin P. (1965) *Pathologie du Placenta*. Masson, Paris.

de Wolf F., de Wolf-Peeters C. & Brosens I. (1973) Ultrastructure of the spiral arteries in the human placental bed at the end of normal pregnancy. *American Journal of Obstetrics and Gynecology*, **117**, 833–48.

Wood D.L. & Malan A.F. (1978) The site of umbilical cord insertion and birthweight. *British Journal of Obstetrics and Gynaecology*, **85**, 332–3.

# 4: Endocrinology and metabolism in early pregnancy

J. GEDIS GRUDZINSKAS



The synthesis and secretion of human chorionic gonadotrophin (hCG) by the conceptus at implantation is a milestone in a series of subsequent endocrine and metabolic changes which are involved in adaptation to the pregnant state. These changes can be exploited clinically by the measurement of hormones and proteins in peripheral blood, urine or amniotic fluid. Typically, the detection of hCG in maternal blood or urine is the basis of pregnancy diagnosis by biochemical methods. In addition to the increasing synthesis of gonadal steroids, a systematic examination of the fetus, amniotic fluid, placenta, decidua and maternal blood has revealed a new generation of proteins which may be used in the diagnosis of early pregnancy and its failure (Table 4.1). For example, measurements of Schwangerschafts protein 1 (SP1) can be used in the biochemical diagnosis of pregnancy (Grudzinskas *et al.* 1977), and recent reports have described consistently depressed levels of pregnancy-associated plasma protein A (PAPP-A) in early pregnancy failure (Westergaard *et al.* 1985).

Elevated maternal serum alpha-fetoprotein (AFP) levels may indicate fetal spina bifida, whereas a depressed level is associated with an increased risk of trisomy 21 (Wald *et al.* 1988). Furthermore, the recent identification of secretory proteins of endometrial and decidual origin holds the promise of the first non-invasive indices of function of these tissues. This chapter deals with recent developments in measurements of hormones and proteins of fetal, maternal and placental origin in normal and abnormal early pregnancy which may be clinically useful.

**Table 4.1** Major fetal, trophoblast and decidual proteins identified in early pregnancy

| |
|---|
| *Fetal* |
| Alpha-fetoprotein (AFP) |
| Fetal antigen 1 (FA-1) |
| Fetal antigen 2 (FA-2) |
| |
| *Trophoblast* |
| Human chorionic gonadotrophin (hCG) |
| Schwangerschaftsprotein 1 (SP1) |
| Human placental lactogen (hPL) |
| Pregnancy-associated plasma protein A (PAPP-A) |
| Placental protein 5 (PP5) |
| |
| *Decidual or endometrial* |
| Insulin-like growth factor binding protein (IGF-bp: $a_1$PEG, PP12, $a_1$PAMG) |
| Progestogen-dependent endometrial protein (PEP: $a_2$ PEG, PP14, $a_2$CMG, $a_2$PAMG, AUP) |

## Diagnosis of pregnancy

The early diagnosis of pregnancy depends on the detection of hCG in maternal urine, or 1–2 days earlier in blood. The current developments in assay technology have contributed to the resolution of problems of potential non-specific results. However, it must be recognized that highly sensitive assays have shown the ubiquitous nature of hCG at low concentrations (<5 IU/l), and in clinical practice a single estimation of hCG should only be considered indicative of pregnancy if it is greater than 25 IU/l or if a lower level of hCG is seen to increase twofold at an interval of 3 days (Jones *et al.* 1983). If hCG has been given therapeutically, estimations should be delayed until clearance of the exogenous hCG has occurred, possibly delaying the diagnosis by up to 14 days. In this circumstance, assays for other proteins of placental origin, namely SP1, may be appropriate. Other pregnancy-associated proteins, such as human placental lactogen (hPL), pregnancy-associated plasma protein A (PAPP-A) and placental protein 5 (PP5), are not contenders as diagnostic tests since they do not appear in the maternal blood until after 6 weeks of amenorrhoea. Finally, hCG results immediately after implantation should be interpreted with care; the sooner the diagnosis is made, the less likely is

**Table 4.2** Pregnancy outcome in relation to time of diagnosis

| Time of diagnosis | Likelihood of normal outcome (per cent) |
|---|---|
| Pre-implantation | 25–30 |
| Post-implantation | 43–60 |
| Six weeks' amenorrhoea | 85–90 |
| Second trimester | 95 |
| Third trimester | 98 |

the outcome to be normal (Table 4.2) given the very high rate of spontaneous pregnancy failure in the peri-implantation period (see later).

## Normal early pregnancy

The apparent trigger for synthesis of hCG by the conceptus is implantation. The stimulus for the production of other placental products, such as hPL, SP1 and PAPP-A, is unclear but is likely to include implantation and other as yet unrecognized events. SP1 secretion into the maternal circulation appears likely to be simultaneous with implantation and the trends in blood concentration seem to parallel the growth rate curve of functioning trophoblast (Grudzinskas *et al.* 1977; Lenton *et al.* 1981; Ahmed & Klopper 1985; Figure 4.1). In normal pregnancy this pattern contrasts with that of hCG, but is similar to hPL, PAPP-A and PP5. The synthesis of SP1, at least for the initial weeks of pregnancy, seems to be independent of the presence of an embryo or fetus as seen in women with hydatidiform mole, and also of the site of implantation, as seen in women with ectopic gestation. In normal pregnancy the doubling times for hCG and SP1 are quite similar; concentrations of hCG and SP1 double in 2–3 days in the first 6 weeks of pregnancy (Lenton *et al.* 1981).

The disappearance rates of these molecules after removal of the placenta are also equivalent (40–60 h). Curiously, there is not an extensive literature on hPL in early pregnancy, and this hormone is not considered to be useful as a pregnancy test (Letchworth 1976). Blood levels of hPL increase as pregnancy advances, and have a relationship to functioning trophoblast mass. Circulating PAPP-A can be detected in the maternal circulation consistently 28 days after conception in singleton pregnancies, but the relatively late appearance of this molecule in the peripheral blood also precludes it from use as a primary diagnostic test for pregnancy (Chemnitz *et al.* 1986; Figure 4.2). PAPP-A levels increase throughout gestation with a main doubling time of 4.9 days during the first trimester; the disappearance rate after removal of the placenta is several days (Sinosich 1985).

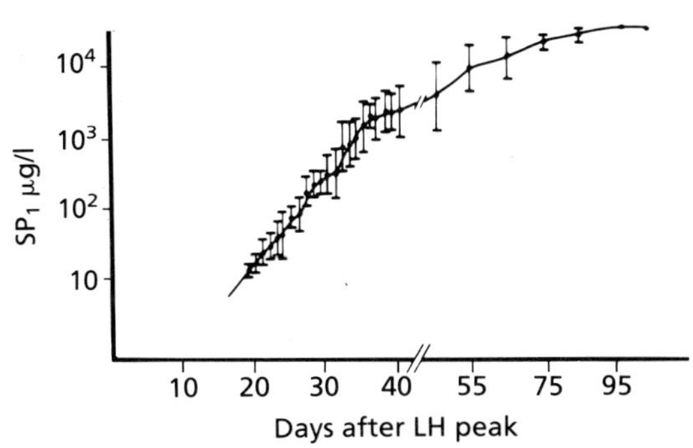


**Fig. 4.1** Mean serum SP1 levels in nine women in the first trimester of normal pregnancy (from Lenton *et al.* 1981, by permission from *Acta Obstetrica et Gynecologica Scandinavica*).

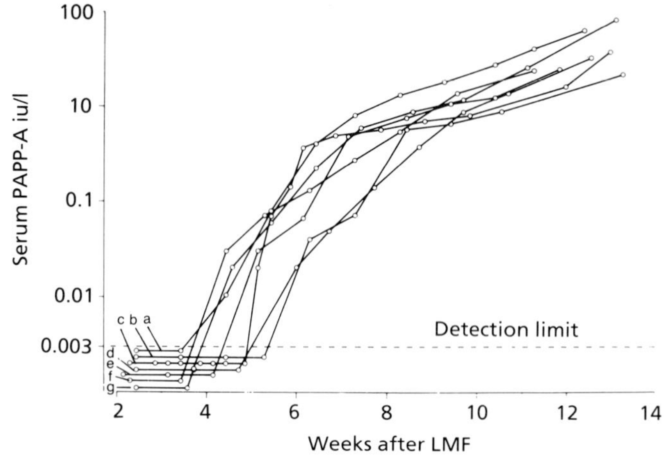


**Fig. 4.2** Serum PAPP-A levels in seven women in the first trimester of normal pregnancy (from Chemnitz *et al.* 1986, by permission from *British Journal of Obstetrics and Gynaecology*).

The production of oestradiol and progesterone is transferred from the corpus luteum of pregnancy to the fetoplacental unit in the middle of the first trimester (Klopper 1985). The synthesis of AFP by embryonal endodermal tissues is reflected by an increase in circulating levels during the first trimester; substantial amounts of AFP are detected consistently after 10 weeks' gestation (Kunz & Keller 1976). Synthesis of the secretory proteins of the endometrium may parallel the morphological changes which this tissue undergoes (Bell 1986). Progestogen-dependent endometrial protein (PEP; also known as PP14; see Table 4.1) which is derived from the glandular epithelium of the endometrium has trends in blood levels during pregnancy which bear a striking resemblance to hCG. By contrast, insulin-like growth factor binding protein (IGF-bp), which is derived from stromal cells of the gestational endometrium, is reported to have peak levels in mid-pregnancy (Bell, 1989).

## Control of synthesis and secretion

The mechanisms which control the synthesis of proteins of trophoblastic origin are poorly understood; uteroplacental perfusion probably plays a major role, influencing synthesis and secretion according to the law of mass action (Chard & Grudzinskas 1985). Nevertheless, it is possible to draw some conclusions on the possible effects of the ovary, the embryo and the endometrium. Firstly, following successful intrauterine pregnancy in women participating in embryo donation programmes, pregnancy seems to be dependent of ovarian support only in as much as is provided by the synthetic oestrogens and progestagens administered for the first 8–9 weeks of the pregnancies of women with ovarian failure, or after bilateral oophorectomy (Lutjen *et al.* 1984). Secondly, whereas depressed levels of some trophoblastic proteins and hormones are seen when complications of early pregnancy become evident clinically, the initiation of synthesis and secretion appears to be unrelated to the presence of the embryo, as evidenced in blighted ovum and hydatidiform mole. Thirdly, the site of implantation and presumably the interaction between the trophoblast and gestational endometrium seem to be less relevant for the majority of the substances considered here, at least in the earliest days of pregnancy. Circulating placental hormones and proteins have been consistently observed in ectopic gestation, but the abnormalities in synthesis have varied widely, the earliest and greatest difference being seen for progesterone, PAPP-A and PEP, and the least for hCG (Sinosich *et al.* 1985). Finally, with the possible exception of PAPP-A in association with Cornelia de Lange syndrome, fetal congenital abnormalities are not related to changes in circulating levels of trophoblastic proteins in either direction, since normal pregnancy outcome has been reported in association with the apparent absence of hPL and SP1 (Westergaard *et al.* 1983). Gross elevations of hCG and SP1 in amniotic fluid have been reported in pregnancies complicated by Meckel's syndrome, but these changes are not reflected in the maternal circulation (Heikinheimo *et al.* 1982). By contrast, the metabolism of progesterone and oestrogen in pregnancy is well described, and the dramatic changes in ovarian hormones observed in early pregnancy, given the work of Lutjen and his colleagues (1984), is presumably part of the maternal response to pregnancy rather than a primary phenomenon. The information on endometrial and decidual proteins is less extensive (for reviews see Bell 1988, 1989; Huhtala *et al.* 1988), but it is likely that PEP and IGF-bp synthesis is modulated by progesterone.

## Complications of early pregnancy

### Early pregnancy failure

The chances of a woman desirous of pregnancy producing a viable offspring in any one ovarian cycle is approximately 25 per cent. Detailed studies using sensitive biochemical tests confirm ovulation and pregnancy have occurred spontaneously, or whether they resulted from an *in vitro* fertilization–embryo transfer (IVF–ET) programme (Table 4.2).

The incidence of clinically obvious miscarriage is 10–15 per cent, whether fertilization occurred *in vivo* or *in vitro*. Estimates of the incidence of this phenomenon vary from 8 to 55 per cent (for review see Grudzinskas *et al.* 1986). The work of Hertig and his colleagues (1952), together with the calculations of Roberts & Lowe (1975), stimulated these studies. Differences in clinical study design, assay technology, and study groups account for the discordance in the literature. A major issue is the specificity of the substances measured as an index of trophoblastic activity. In this respect, hCG estimations must still be considered as superior to those of SP1 (unless hCG has been given therapeutically). By contrast, ultrasonic findings such as uterine distension or a gestational sac cannot be considered as specific signs of pregnancy (Stabile *et al.* 1988a).

### Threatened and spontaneous miscarriage

Circulating levels of hormones and proteins of fetal, trophoblastic and maternal origin have been used to predict the outcome in women with vaginal bleeding in early pregnancy (Niven *et al.* 1972; Nygren *et al.* 1973; Garoff & Seppala 1975; Kunz & Keller 1976; Braunstein *et al.* 1978; Damber *et al.* 1978; Javanovic *et al.* 1978; Schultz-Larsen & Hertz 1978; Jouppila *et al.* 1979; Masson *et al.* 1983a,b; Salem *et al.* 1984). As ultrasound examination has now revolutionized this practice, some of these tests are probably obsolete if fetal life can be demonstrated by ultrasound (Hertz *et al.* 1980; Jouppila *et al.* 1980a,b; Stabile *et al.* 1987). Nevertheless, a proportion of patients in whom fetal heart action has been demonstrated will spontaneously miscarry. We have previously described serum levels of hPL, SP1, PAPP-A, progesterone, oestradiol, AFP and pregnancy-zone protein (PZP) in this condition. In the 108 patients in whom the history and clinical findings were diagnostic of threatened miscarriage (Westergaard *et al.* 1985) ultrasound revealed a fetal heart action in 77 women, whereas examination during the first week of study gave no clearcut evidence of fetal life in the remaining 31 patients. Ultrasound scans were done at weekly intervals for 3 weeks and every 2 weeks thereafter, unless otherwise indicated by vaginal bleeding and maternal venous blood was obtained at each ultrasound scan. Spontaneous miscarriage occurred in 42 pregnancies, 31 of which showed no sign of fetal heart action on repeated scan examination. In the remaining 11 patients, the fetal heart action was observed repeatedly until miscarriage occurred. The sensitivity, predictive values and relative risk of normal and abnormal levels of the biochemical indices measured in the first sample, and in all samples in relation to the scan findings in the women who aborted revealed that the predictive value of an abnormal level in the sample obtained at presentation was greatest for PAPP-A, particularly if there was scan evidence of fetal life (54 per cent). When all abnormal results were considered, the predictive value was highest for AFP and PAPP-A.

The differences between the indices, both in single and serial samples, were less if the ultrasound findings were not included. However, when ultrasound demonstrated a live fetus, the predictive value of a normal test was highest (99 per cent) for PAPP-A estimations. The relative risk of miscarriage was highest for depressed levels of PAPP-A, being three times greater than the other biochemical indices if the fetus was alive, and five to ten times greater regardless of the ultrasound findings. All the 11 women who had evidence of a live fetus but subsequently miscarried had depressed PAPP-A levels, levels being abnormal at least 4 weeks before miscarriage in four patients and in every sample obtained in the other seven.

By contrast, the levels of the other substances measured generally remained within the normal range — the only exception was AFP. We have attempted to repeat this study and examine many of the unanswered questions concerning the value of biochemical tests relative to ultrasound in women presenting with threatened miscarriage (Grudzinskas *et al.* 1988).

It is now possible to conclude, first, if the fetal heart action was not evident ultrasonically, after 7 weeks gestation or if the gestational sac volume is greater than 3 ml, that depressed levels of hCG, hPL, SP1, PAPP-A, oestradiol, progesterone and AFP will be providing the clinician with no additional information; and second, spontaneous miscarriage after the observation of the embryonic or fetal heart action is an extremely uncommon event, and that in this small group the levels of these hormones and proteins will be in the normal range, the possible exception being PAPP-A.

Finally, recent studies in women with apparently normal pregnancies at 6–10 weeks gestation, with a live structurally normal fetus seen ultrasonically studied (whilst awaiting chorionic villus sampling because of concern of fetal chromosomal abnormalities) have revealed depressed levels of at least serum AFP, PAPP-A and to a lesser degree hCG within 2–3 weeks of spontaneous miscarriage (B. Brambati, J.G. Grudzinskas and T. Chard, pers. obs.). As most of these aborted fetuses had or were likely to have an abnormal karyotype, measurements of hormones and proteins in the first trimester may identify this particular risk group as do AFP and oestriol measurements in the second trimester.

## Anembryonic pregnancy

Early arrest of embryonic development permits an examination of the contribution of the growing conceptus to the control of hormone and protein synthesis by the trophoblast. Stabile and her colleagues (1989) have described the unambiguous diagnosis of this condition ultrasonically in relation to gestational age (7 weeks) and an estimation of gestational sac volume (3 ml). If the embryonic heart action cannot be seen in a sac greater than 3 ml in size, the diagnosis can be confidently made. Prior to this time, measurements of serum hCG and SP1 have a specificity in excess of 90 per cent in the exclusion of this condition. Curiously, serum AFP levels are within the normal range in a substantial number of women with this condition suggesting that an embryo has been in evidence at sometime and that the term anembryonic pregnancy is a misnomer (Stabile *et al.* 1989).

Mean levels of circulating hCG have also been shown to be depressed at 4 weeks' gestation in a group of women studied prospectively at a subfertility clinic; mean levels of maternal PAPP-A, oestradiol and progesterone fell some 3 weeks later (Yovich *et al.* 1986). Regardless of the pathogenesis of this condition these findings confirm that a deviation from the normal rise in blood levels of hCG is highly suggestive of failed pregnancy at a time before ultrasound can provide useful information (i.e. in the absence of fetal heart action).

## Ectopic pregnancy

The use of biochemical tests in this condition has been reviewed (Kadar 1983) confirming the value of assays capable of detecting the very low levels of hCG present in this condition. hCG tests alert the clinician to the possibility of a pregnancy-related disorder if it is detected, and virtually exclude the diagnosis if a negative result (i.e. <25 IU/l) is obtained.

Furthermore, Stabile and her colleagues (1988b) have reported a sensitivity of 100 per cent if estimations of hCG are used in conjunction with ultrasound to make the diagnosis. Quantitative estimations of hCG may also be of some value, since depressed levels are commonly seen in ectopic gestation and in conjunction with ultrasonic examination can often distinguish between normal or failed intrauterine pregnancy and ectopic gestation (Pittaway *et al.* 1985). The use of a discriminatory zone for hCG in conjunction with ultrasound can also be most helpful. If levels of hCG are greater than 6500 IU/l, ultrasound examination should reveal the presence of a live embryo *in utero*; if this is not the case, failed pregnancy, in particular ectopic gestation, should be suspected (Kadar 1983; Rottem & Timor-Tritsch 1988).

The data on SP1 are similar to that on hCG, while the findings with PAPP-A levels suggest that secretion is more severely compromised in this condition (Chemnitz *et al.* 1984; Sinosich *et al.* 1985). A preliminary report has shown that PAPP-A levels were depressed in all 17 women with ectopic gestation, with PAPP-A being detectable in only two women (Sinosich *et al.* 1985). Our study examined 60 women with surgically

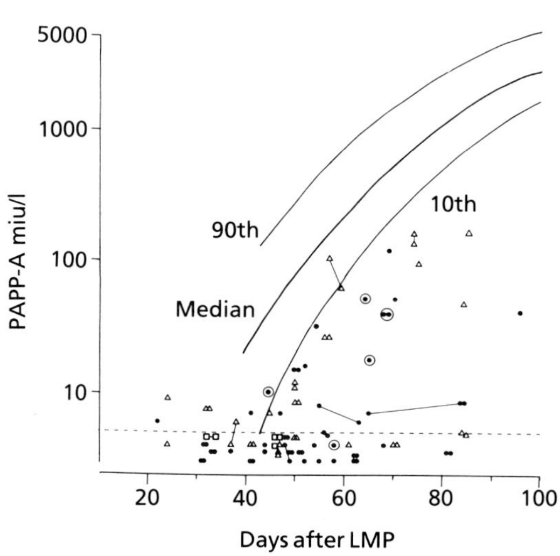


**Fig. 4.3** Circulating PAPP-A levels in 60 women with ectopic gestation in relation to the normal range. The encircled symbols indicate that fetal tissue was identified (from Stabile *et al.* 1988b, by permission from Springer-Verlag).

proven ectopic pregnancy, in whom circulating PAPP-A was detected in only 30 and levels being depressed in 24 women (Figure 4.3) (Stabile *et al.* 1988b). Thus the synthesis of PAPP-A is severely compromised in ectopic gestation.

In addition, Westergaard and his colleagues (1988) have examined serum levels of oestradiol 17β, progesterone, and the major secretory protein of the gestational endometrium (PP14; see Table 4.1) in these women, observing depressed levels, in particular, of progesterone and PP14. They concluded that it was not possible to distinguish between failed intrauterine pregnancy and ectopic gestation by the measurement of serum hormones and proteins, but that it could be possible to exclude the possibility of ectopic pregnancy by these measurements. At the time of clinical presentation, firstly, the presence of hCG would alert the clinician to the possibility of a pregnancy-related disorder; secondly, normal levels of either progesterone, or PAPP-A, or PP14 would indicate a normal intrauterine pregnancy, thereby making the possibility of ectopic pregnancy extremely remote (Stabile *et al.* 1988b).

## Trophoblastic disease

Trophoblastic tissue in hydatidiform mole maintains its ability to synthesize hormones and proteins, and although this capacity is reduced for hPL and steroids, it is usually greater for hCG.

Since the risk of choriocarcinoma is higher in women in the presence of excessive hCG secretion in gestational trophoblast tumours (Newlands 1983), we have evaluated measurements of proteins specifically synthesized by trophoblastic tissue (e.g. SP1, PP5 and PAPP-A) in this con-

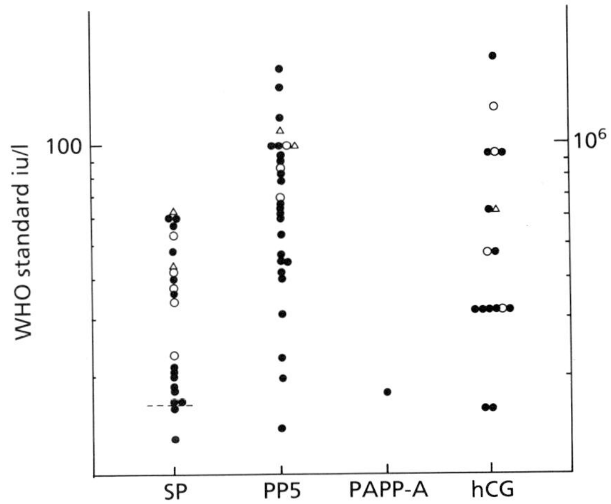


**Fig. 4.4** Serum SP1, PP5, PAPP-A and hCG levels in 31 women with gestational trophoblastic disease before treatment: hydatidiform mole; choriocarcinoma, ○ = lung metastases, △ = --- 16.5 IU/l WHO standard 78/610. Levels of SP1, PP5, PAPP-A <IU/l or hCG <100 000 IU/l not shown (from Tsakok *et al.* 1983, by permission from *British Journal of Obstetrics and Gynaecology*).

text. In untreated hydatidiform mole whereas reduced levels of PAPP-A have been observed in women prior to treatment, elevated levels of circulating SP1 and PP5 are seen (Figure 4.4; Tsakok *et al.* 1983). High SP1 levels were seen in a larger proportion of women who developed subsequent malignant disease. Than and his colleagues (1988) observed high serum concentration of PP14 in women prior to treatment for hydatidiform mole which fell quickly after evacuation. Circulating PP14 was not seen in women with choriocarcinoma. In patients with extensive choriocarcinoma, serum SP1 levels are usually lower than in benign disease and circulating PP5 cannot be detected (Seppala *et al.* 1979; Lee *et al.* 1981, 1982; Soma *et al.* 1981). Although the place of hCG estimation in the monitoring of women with this disease is firmly established, estimations of endometrial or trophoblastic-specific proteins may give further insight into the pathogenesis of this condition.

## Prenatal diagnosis: chorionic villus sampling

Miscarriage occurring in women before chorionic villus sampling (CVS), immediately and several weeks after the procedure, has been examined to determine whether the pregnancies which failed were destined to miscarry or whether the miscarriage was a direct result of the surgical procedure.

In some women with an apparently normal live fetus as evidenced ultrasonically, prior to CVS (6–9 weeks gestation) who will miscarry spontaneously before CVS, depressed serum levels of AFP, PAPP-A and hCG have been observed in the majority (B. Brambati, T. Chard and J.G. Grudzinskas, pers. obs.). An abnormal karyotype was evident in the abortus tissue examined from the majority of cases. Wald and his colleagues (1988) have also reported substantial differences in serum AFP and oestriol measurements between those women who are more likely to have a fetus affected by Down's syndrome and those who are not. Whereas the overlap in hormone levels between the two groups is substantial, nevertheless the differences are sufficiently large to be able to increase the identification of women who will have a Down's syndrome to 60 per cent of cases. These women will be offered fetal karyotyping on the basis of their increased risk.

Ward and his colleagues (1985) examined serum levels of AFP, hCG, SP1 and PAPP-A before and 6 h after villus sampling in 20 women. In the majority, AFP levels rose after sampling. Depressed or elevated preoperative levels of AFP, hCG and PAPP-A were associated with fetal anomalies and pregnancy loss in seven of the eleven pregnancies which did not progress. All pregnancies but one (missed abortion) were apparently normal when assessed by ultrasound, and the two highest levels of hCG were seen in the pregnancies in which the fetus was homozygous for alpha- and beta-thalassaemia. Similar observations have been made for hPL and SP1 in pregnancies complicated by hydrops fetalis in late pregnancy (Bellman *et al.* 1980).

We have subsequently confirmed that serum AFP levels usually rise within 30 min of CVS (Knott *et al.* 1988) and that the fluctuations in proteins and hormones of trophoblastic origin following CVS are insufficient to invalidate their use in the assessment of this particular function of the placenta (Stabile *et al.* 1988c).

## Conclusion

Ultrasonic examination has contributed substantially to precise assessment of early pregnancy. Nevertheless, hCG estimations are still the mainstay of the diagnosis of early pregnancy and, when used in conjunction with ultrasound, provide valuable clinical information prior to 6 weeks gestation.

After the detection of the embryonic heart action at 6–7 weeks gestation, spontaneous miscarriage is very uncommon. In some women with apparently unremarkable pregnancies but who will miscarry within a few weeks, depressed levels of AFP, hCG and PAPP-A have been observed, but it is still unclear whether this information can be exploited by the clinician. In women presenting with vaginal bleeding after 7 weeks gestation, if the fetal heart action is seen, apparently only PAPP-A measurement may predict the small group who will subsequently miscarry.

In women suspected of having ectopic gestation, whereas the detection of hCG will indicate pregnancy, high levels of progesterone or PEP, may exclude this life threatening condition and depressed levels of PAPP-A may increase the possibility. However, these measurements should be performed in conjunction with hCG, if ultrasonic examination has not been helpful.

The identification of secretory proteins of endometrium and decidua which can be measured in the uterine lumen and maternal blood encourages the inclusion IGF-bp and PEP as active rather than passive participants in the reproductive axis. Since these tissues produce hormones, lipids and proteins which act locally and distally, it is possible to consider the endometrium or decidua as an endocrine organ (Healey & Hodgen 1983; Grudzinskas 1987; Bell 1988). The ability to measure these substances, in particular IGF-bp and progestogen-dependent endometrial protein, may provide not only a non-invasive test of endometrial function in the assessment of fertility, but also an index of endometrial and decidual function in the earliest days and weeks of pregnancy.

## References

Ahmed A.G. & Klopper A. (1985) Concomitant secretion of Schwangerschaftsprotein and human chorionic gonadotrophin following conception. *Clinical Endocrinology*, **23**, 677–81.

Bell S.C. (1986) Secretory endometrial and decidual proteins: studies on clinical significance of a maternally derived group of pregnancy associated serum proteins. *Human Reproduction*, **1**, 129–43.

Bell S.C. (1988) Synthesis and secretion of proteins by the endometrium and decidua.

In *Implantation*, (Ed. by M.G. Chapman, J.G. Grudzinskas & T. Chard), pp. 95–118. Springer Verlag, London.

Bell S.C. (1989) Decidualisation and insulin-like growth factor (IGF) binding protein: implications for its role in stromal cell differentiation and the decidual cell in haemochorial placentation. *Human Reproduction*, **4**, 125–30.

Bellman O., Tebbe J., Lang N. & Baur M.P. (1980) Determination of SP1 and hPL for predicting perinatal asphyxia. In *The Human Placenta: Proteins and Hormones*, (Ed. by A. Klopper, A. Genazzani & P.G. Crosignani), pp. 99–108. Academic Press, London.

Braunstein G.D., Karow W.G., Gentry W.C., Rasor I. & Wade M.M. (1978) First trimester chorionic gonadotrophin measurements as an aid in the diagnosis of early pregnancy disorders. *American Journal of Obstetrics and Gynecology*, **143**, 25–32.

Chard T. & Grudzinskas J.G. (1985) Placental and pregnancy-associated proteins: control mechanisms and clinical application. In *Proteins of the Placenta*, (Ed. by P. Bischof & A. Klopper), pp. 104–113. Karger, Basel.

Chemnitz J., Folkersen J., Teisner B. *et al.* (1986) Comparison of different antibody preparations against pregnancy-associated plasma protein A (PAPP-A) for use in localisation and immunoassay studies. *British Journal of Obstetrics and Gynaecology*, **93**, 111–18.

Chemnitz J., Tornehave D., Teisner B., Poulsen H.K. & Westergaard J.G. (1984) The localisation of pregnancy proteins (hPL, SP1 and PAPP-A) in intra- and extrauterine pregnancies. *Placenta*, **5**, 489–94.

Damber M.G., von Schoultz B., Solheim F., Strigbrand T. & Carlstrom K. (1978) Prognostic value of the pregnancy zone protein during early pregnancy in spontaneous abortion. *Obstetrics and Gynecology*, **51**, 677–81.

Garoff L. & Seppala M. (1975) Prediction of fetal outcome in threatened abortion by maternal serum placental lactogen and alphafetoprotein. *American Journal of Obstetrics and Gynecology*, **121**, 257–61.

Grudzinskas J.G. (1987) Secretory proteins of the endometrium. *Tokyo Medical College Journal*, **45**, 170–5.

Grudzinskas J.G., Gordon Y.B., Jeffrey D. & Chard T. (1977) Specific and sensitive determination of pregnancy specific beta-1 glycoprotein by radioimmunoassay. *Lancet*, **i**, 333–5.

Grudzinskas J.G., Stabile I. & Campbell S. (1988) Early pregnancy failure: biochemical and biophysical assessment. In *Early Pregnancy Loss Mechanisms and Treatment*, (Ed. by R.W. Beard & F. Sharp), pp. 183–90. RCOG, London.

Grudzinskas J.G., Westergaard J.G. & Teisner B. (1985) Pregnancy-associated plasma protein A in normal and abnormal pregnancies. In *Proteins of the Placenta*, (Ed. by P. Bischof & A. Klopper), pp. 184–97. Karger, Basel.

Grudzinskas J.G., Westergaard J.G. & Teisner B. (1986) Biochemical assessment of placental function: early pregnancy. *Clinics in Obstetrics and Gynaecology*, **13**, 553–69.

Healey D.L. & Hodgen G. (1983) Endocrinology of the endometrium. *Obstetric and Gynaecological Survey*, **38**, 509–30.

Heikinheimo M., Wahlstrom T., Aula P. & Seppala M. (1982) Pregnancy specific beta-1 glycoprotein in amniotic fluid. In *Pregnancy Proteins: Biology, Chemistry and Clinical Application*, (Ed. by J.G. Grudzinskas, B. Teisner & M. Seppala), pp. 215–21. Academic Press, Sydney.

Hertig A.T., Rock J., Adams E.C. & Menkin E.C. (1952) Thirty-four fertilized human ova, good, bad and indifferent recovered from 210 women of known fertility. *Paediatrics*, **23**, 202–11.

Hertz J.B., Mantoni M. & Svenstrup B. (1980) Threatened abortion studies by estradiol-17-beta in serum and ultrasound. *Obstetrics and Gynecology*, **55**, 324–8.

Huhtala M.L., Seppala M., Julkunen M. & Koistinen R. (1988) Characterisation, biological action and clinical studies of endometrial proteins. In *Implantation*, (Ed. by M.G. Chapman, J.G. Grudzinskas & T. Chard), pp. 119–34. Springer-Verlag, London.

Huisjes J.J. (1984) Spontaneous abortion. In *Current Review in Obstetrics and Gynaecology*, (Ed. by T. Lind), pp. 132–6. Churchill Livingstone, London.

Jones H.W., Acosta A.A., Andrews M.C. *et al.* (1983) What is pregnancy? A question for *in vitro* fertilisation. *Fertility and Sterility*, **40**, 728–33.

Jouppila P., Huhtaniemi I. & Tapanainen J. (1980b) Early pregnancy failure: study by ultrasonic and hormonal methods. *Obstetrics and Gynecology*, **55**, 42–7.

Jouppila P., Seppala M. & Chard T. (1980a) Pregnancy-specific beta-1 glycoprotein in complications of early pregnancy. *Lancet*, **i**, 667–8.

Jouppila P., Tapanainen J. & Huhtaniemi I. (1979) Plasma hCG levels in patients with bleeding in the first and second trimesters of pregnancy. *British Journal of Obstetrics and Gynaecology*, **86**, 343–9.

Jovanovic L., Dawood M.Y., Landesmann R. & Saxena B.B. (1978) Hormonal profile as a prognostic index of early threatened abortion. *American Journal of Obstetrics and Gynecology*, **130**, 274–8.

Kadar N. (1983) Ectopic pregnancy. In *Progress in Obstetrics and Gynaecology*, Vol 3 (Ed. by J. Studd), pp. 305–23. Churchill Livingstone, Edinburgh.

Klopper A. (1985) Steroids in pregnancy. In *Clinical Reproductive Endocrinology*, (Ed. by R.P. Shearman), pp. 209–23. Churchill Livingstone, Edinburgh.

Kunz J. & Keller P.J. (1976) hPL, oestradiol, progesterone and AFP in patients with threatened abortion. *British Journal of Obstetrics and Gynaecology*, **83**, 640–4.

Lee J.N., Salem H.T., Al-Ani A.T.M. *et al.* (1981) Circulating concentrations of specific placental proteins (human chorionic gonadotrophin, pregnancy-specific beta-1 glycoprotein and placental protein 5) in untreated gestational trophoblastic tumours. *American Journal of Obstetrics and Gynecology*, **39**, 702–4.

Lee J.N., Salem H.T., Chard T., Huang S.C. & Ouyang P.C. (1982) Circulating placental proteins (hCG, SP1 and PP5) in trophoblastic disease. *British Journal of Obstetrics and Gynaecology*, **89**, 69–72.

Lenton A.E., Grudzinskas J.G., Gordon Y.B., Chard T. & Cooke I.D. (1981) Pregnancy specific beta-1 glycoprotein and chorionic gonadotrophin in early pregnancy. *Acta Obstetricia et Gynecologica Scandinavica*, **60**, 489–92.

Letchworth A.T. (1976) Human placental lactogen assay as a guide to fetal wellbeing. In *Plasma Hormone Assays in Evaluation of Fetal Wellbeing*, (Ed. by A. Klopper), pp. 147–73. Churchill Livingstone, Edinburgh.

Lutjen C., Trouson A., Leeton J., Findlay J., Wood C. & Renou P. (1984) The establishment and maintenance of pregnancy using *in-vitro* fertilisation and embryo donation in a patient with primary ovarian failure. *Nature*, **307**, 174–5.

Masson G.M., Anthony F. & Wilson M.S. (1983b) Value of Schwangerschaftsprotein 1 (SP1) and pregnancy associated plasma protein (PAPP-A) in the clinical management of threatened abortion. *British Journal of Obstetrics and Gynaecology*, **90**, 146–9.

Masson G.M., Anthony F., Wilson M.S. & Lindsay K. (1983a) Comparison of serum and urine hCG levels with SP1 and PAPP-A levels in patients with first-trimester vaginal bleeding. *Obstetrics and Gynecology*, **61**, 223–6.

Newlands E.S. (1983) Treatment of trophoblastic disease. In *Progress in Obstetrics and Gynaecology*, Vol 3 (Ed. by J. Studd), pp. 158–74. Churchill Livingstone, Edinburgh.

Niven P.A.R., Landon J. & Chard T. (1972) Placental lactogen levels as a guide to outcome of threatened abortion. *British Medical Journal*, **iii**, 799–801.

Nygren K.G., Johansson E.D.G. & Wide L. (1973) Evaluation of the prognosis of threatened abortion from the peripheral levels of plasma progesterone, oestradiol and human chorionic gonadotrophin. *American Journal of Obstetrics and Gynecology*, **116**, 916–22.

Pittaway D.E., Wentz A.C., Maxon W.S., Herbert C., Daniell J. & Fleischer A.C. (1985) The efficacy of early pregnancy monitoring with serial chorionic gonadotrophin determinations and realtime ultrasonography in an infertile population. *Fertility and Sterility*, **44**, 190–4.

Roberts C.J. & Lowe C.R. (1975) Where have all the conceptions gone? *Lancet*, **i**, 498–9.

Rottem S. & Timor-Tritsch I.E. (1988) In *Transvaginal Ultrasonography*, (Ed. by I.E. Timor-Tritsch & S. Rottem), pp. 125–42. Heinemann Medical Books, London.

Salem H.T., Ghaneimah S.A., Shabaan M.M. & Chard T. (1984) Prognostic value of biochemical tests in the assessment of fetal outcome in threatened abortion. *British Journal of Obstetrics and Gynaecology*, **91**, 382–5.

Schultz-Larsen P. & Hertz J.B. (1978) The predictive value of pregnancy specific beta-1 glycoprotein in threatened abortion. *European Journal of Obstetrics, Gynecology and Reproductive Biology*, **8**, 253–7.

Seppala M., Wahlstrom T. & Bohn H. (1979) Circulating levels and tissue localisation of placental protein 5 (PP5) in pregnancy and trophoblastic disease: absence of PP5 expression in the malignant trophoblast. *International Journal of Cancer*, **24**, 6–10.

Sinosich M.J. (1985) Biological role of pregnancy-associated plasma protein A in human reproduction. In *Proteins of the Placenta*, (Ed. by P. Bischof & A. Klopper), pp. 158–84. Karger, Basel.

Sinosich M.J., Ferrier A., Teisner B. *et al.* (1985) Circulating pregnancy-associated plasma A and its tissue concentration in tubal ectopic gestation. *Journal of Clinical Reproduction and Fertility*, **3**, 311–17.

Soma H., Kikuchi M., Takayama M. *et al.* (1981) Concentrations of SP1 and beta-hCG in serum and cerebrospinal fluid and concentrations of hCG in urine in patients with trophoblastic tumour. *Archives of Gynecology*, **230**, 321–7.

Stabile I., Campbell S. & Grudzinskas J.G. (1988a) Can ultrasound reliably diagnose ectopic pregnancy? *British Journal of Obstetrics and Gynaecology*, **95**, 1247–52.

Stabile I., Grudzinskas J.G. & Campbell S. (1987) Ultrasonic assessment of complications during first trimester of pregnancy. *Lancet*, **ii**, 1237–40.

Stabile I., Olajide F., Chard T. & Grudzinskas J.G. (1989) Maternal serum alphafetoprotein levels in anembryonic pregnancy. *Human Reproduction*, **4**, 204–5.

Stabile I., Warren R., Rodeck C. & Grudzinskas J.G. (1988c) Measurements of placental, decidual and fetal proteins before and after chorionic villus sampling. *Prenatal Diagnosis*, **8**, 387–96.

Stabile I., Westergaard J.G. & Grudzinskas J.G. (1988b) Ectopic pregnancy: diagnostic aspects. In *Implantation: Biological and Clinical Aspects*, (Ed. by M.G. Chapman, J.G. Grudzinskas & T. Chard), pp. 229–38. Springer Verlag, London.

Than G.N., Tatra G., Szabo D.G., Csaba K. & Bohutt (1988) Beta lactoglobulin homologue placental protein 14 (PP14) in serum of patients with trophoblastic disease and non-trophoblastic gynaecological malignancy. *Archives of Gynaecology*, **243**, 131–7.

Tsakok F.T.M., Koh M., Ratnam S.S. *et al.* (1983) Pregnancy associated proteins in trophoblastic disease. *British Journal of Obstetrics and Gynaecology*, **90**, 483–6.

Wald N.J., Cuckle H.S., Densem W. *et al.* (1988) Maternal serum screening for Down's syndrome in early pregnancy *British Medical Journal*, **ii**, 883–7.

Ward R.H.T., Grudzinskas J.G., Bolton A.E. *et al.* (1985) Fetoplacental products as a prognostic guide following chorionic villus sampling. In *First Trimester Diagnosis*, (Ed. by M. Fraccaro, G. Simoni & B. Brambati), pp. 73–6. Springer-Verlag, Berlin.

Westergaard J.G., Chemnitz J., Teisner B. *et al.* (1983) Pregnancy-associated plasma protein A — a possible marker in the classification and diagnosis of Cornelia de Lange syndrome. *Prenatal Diagnosis*, **3**, 225–32.

Westergaard J.G., Teisner B., Sinosich M.J., Madsen L.T. & Grudzinskas J.G. (1985) Does ultrasound examination render biochemical tests obsolete in the prediction of early pregnancy failure? *British Journal of Obstetrics and Gynaecology*, **92**, 77–83.

Westergaard J.G., Teisner B., Stabile I. & Grudzinskas J.G. (1988) Ectopic pregnancy: diagnostic aspects. Protein and hormone measurements in ectopic gestation. In *Endometrial and Placental Proteins: Basic Concepts and Clinical Applications*, (Ed. by S. Tomoda, S. Mizutani, O. Narita & A. Klopper), pp. 615–22. VSP International Science Publishers, Netherlands.

Yovich J.L., McColin J.C., Willcox D.L., Grudzinskas J.G. & Bolton A.E. (1986) The prognostic value of beta hCG, PAPP-A, oestradiol and progesterone in early human pregnancies and the effect of medroxy progesterone acetate. *Australia and New Zealand Journal of Obstetrics and Gynaecology*, **26**, 59–64.

# 5: The measurement of fetal growth

JAMES P. NEILSON



Clinical assessment of fetal size by abdominal palpation is not to be dismissed. In developed countries it is the primary method of assessment while in many parts of the developing world it is the only method available. Direct comparisons of clinical assessment with ultrasonography are rare. However, we have found that when the observer, whether midwife or obstetrician, is required to write down a numerical estimate of fetal weight based on clinical examination, the results are not significantly less good than those obtained by ultrasound measurement of the abdominal circumference, and indeed may actually be better in large babies (Hanretty *et al.* 1990). Likewise, when the examiner is obliged to make a numerical record after simple tape measurement of symphysis–fundal height, the correct identification of small-for-gestational age fetuses may approach 80 per cent (Pearce & Campbell 1987). However, because of its ability to image soft tissues, ultrasound is the method which gives us most information about fetal size and shape and, through repeated examinations, the greatest insight into the physiology and pathophysiology of fetal growth. In addition, ultrasound is versatile and gives information about many more facets of fetal status than merely an estimate of overall size; it is, therefore, the subject of this chapter.

## Fetal measurements

Descriptions of new fetal measurements by ultrasound have rapidly outstripped a critical assessment of their value in practice. It is, therefore, appropriate to start by considering the range of different measurements now possible, and then to discuss the purposes to which they may be put. Technique of measurement has been described in great detail recently by Kurtz & Goldberg (1988) whose book is recommended to the interested reader.

## The head

The biparietal diameter was the first fetal dimension to be measured by ultrasound. A simple A-mode technique was used to demonstrate, on an oscilloscope, reflections of the ultrasound beam by anterior and posterior walls of the skull and, in the midline, by the falx cerebri (Willocks *et al.* 1964). With the evolution of the static B-scanner, the combined A and B-mode technique (Campbell 1968) was developed to give greater sophistication to measurement of the biparietal diameter. These complex and cumbersome machines gave way in turn to real-time systems with which manufacturers have, in recent years, achieved enormous improvements in resolution and quality of imaging. Nowadays, the biparietal diameter is measured on a transverse section of the fetal head identified by appropriate anatomical landmarks in the brain (Figure 5.1).

Although the biparietal diameter can be quite correctly measured in several different planes, it is best measured in the occipito-frontal plane in which the head circumference or area may also be measured. Most modern electronic measuring systems give figures simultaneously for both

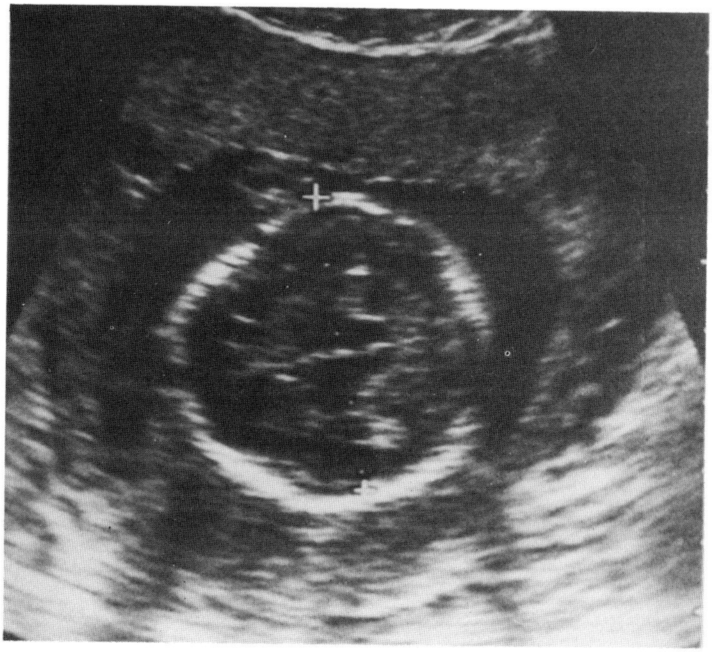

**Fig. 5.1** Biparietal diameter, measured at the level of the thalamus on a section of the fetal head that includes the cavum septum pellucidum.

area and circumference, and although, using some systems, area measurement is theoretically more accurate, this seems to make little difference in practice. Head circumference or area measurements are of particular value when fetal head shape is unusual as in dolichocephaly (very narrow) or brachycephaly (very round). In these cases the biparietal diameter does not represent accurately overall head size. The cephalic index (ratio of biparietal diameter to occipito-frontal diameter expressed as a percentage) allows a quantitative assessment of head shape. Dolichocephaly may be associated with breech presentation and with oligohydramnios and is not, in itself, a sinister finding.

As imaging has improved to allow more anatomical detail to be seen, the number of descriptions of different fetal head measurements has increased. Parts of the ventricular system in the brain can be seen, for example, and distances measured from the bodies and from the anterior and posterior horns to the midline. The cerebellum is readily identified except in late pregnancy and its transverse dimensions may be measured (Figure 5.2). Immediately posterior to the cerebellum lies the cisterna magna; this also may be measured. The binocular distance stretches from the outer margin of one orbit to that of the other (Figure 5.3).

## The trunk

Measurement of the trunk started with measurement of the thorax but the main thrust to development came with Campbell's description of the abdominal section, at the level of the fetal liver, which is identified by the presence of the umbilical vein (Figure 5.4) (Campbell & Wilkin 1975).

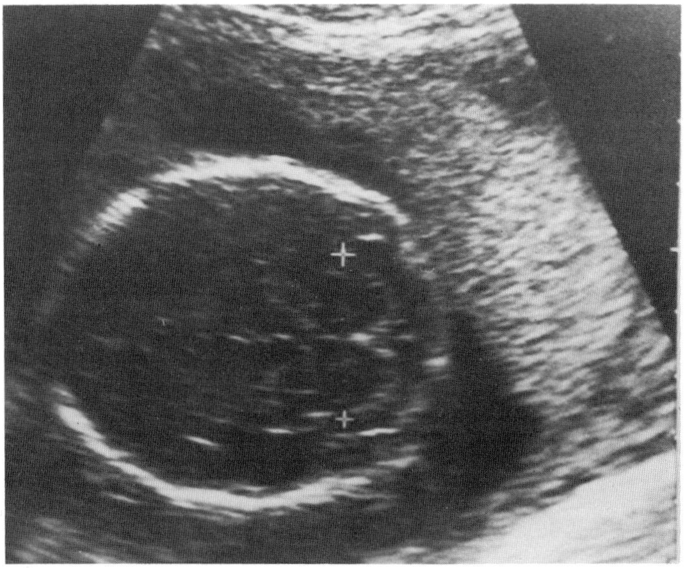

**Fig. 5.2** Transcerebellar diameter. The normal cerebellum has a characteristic dumb-bell shape.

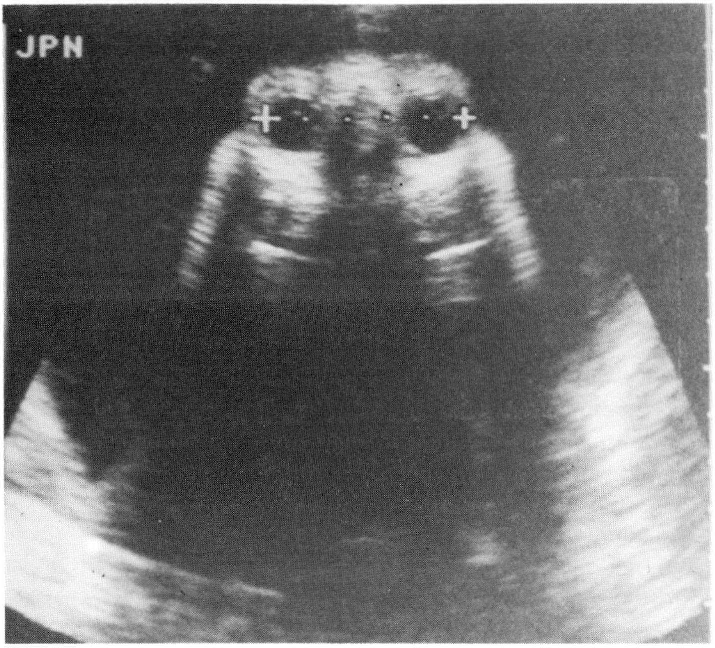


**Fig. 5.3** Binocular diameter, measured between the outer margins of each orbit.

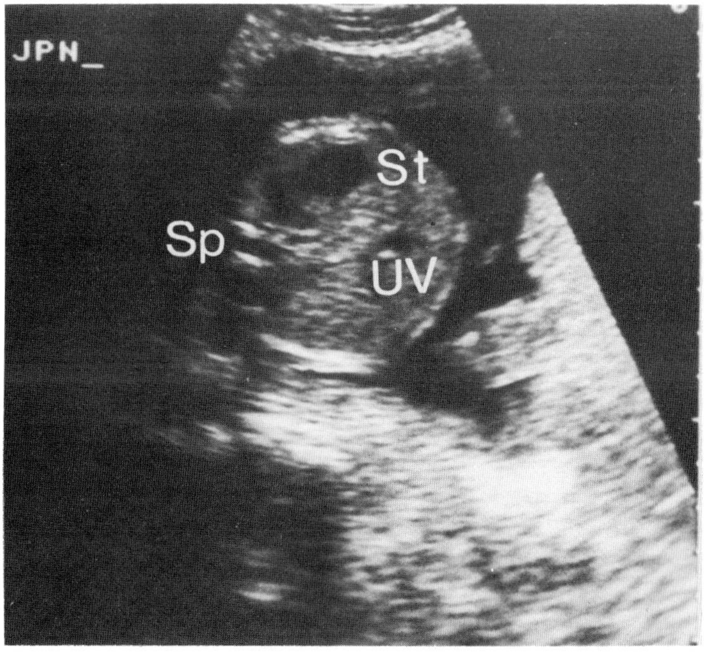


**Fig. 5.4** Abdominal section (Sp, spine; St, stomach; UV, umbilical vein).

Area or circumference abdominal measurements have proved preferable to simple linear measurements (Neilson *et al.* 1980). Abdominal measurements, which are more reproducible than thoracic measurements, are generally preferred although, as will be discussed, there are specific circumstances in which thoracic measurement may be valuable (Nimrod *et al.* 1986).

Normal values have been published for the dimensions of a number of organs found in the trunk. These include the heart (best studied by real-time B-mode and M-mode ultrasound), the liver (Vintzileos *et al.* 1985a), the spleen (Schmidt *et al.* 1985), the kidneys (Grannum *et al.* 1980), and even the adrenal gland (Lewis *et al.* 1982). The volume of urine in the fetal bladder may be estimated and the rate of urine production thus calculated from repeated observations (Wladimiroff & Campbell 1974). The lumen of the large bowel may be measured (Goldstein *et al.* 1987a).

## The limbs

The length of the long bones of the fetus are readily measured, although patience is required when the fetus is moving, and it is important that the angle of ultrasound beam to long axis of bone should be approximately 90°. Normal values have been described for femur (Figure 5.5), tibia, fibula, humerus, ulna, and radius (Jeanty *et al.* 1984; Merz *et al.* 1987), and also (on the subject of bone) for the clavicle (Yarkoni *et al.* 1985). The volume of the fetal limbs may be estimated (Jeanty *et al.* 1985) and the length of the feet measured (Mercer *et al.* 1987). Limb measurements have been performed not only for direct purposes but also as indices of overall fetal length (e.g. femoral length; Vintzileos *et al.* 1984) or soft tissue mass (e.g. thigh circumference; Deter *et al.* 1986a).

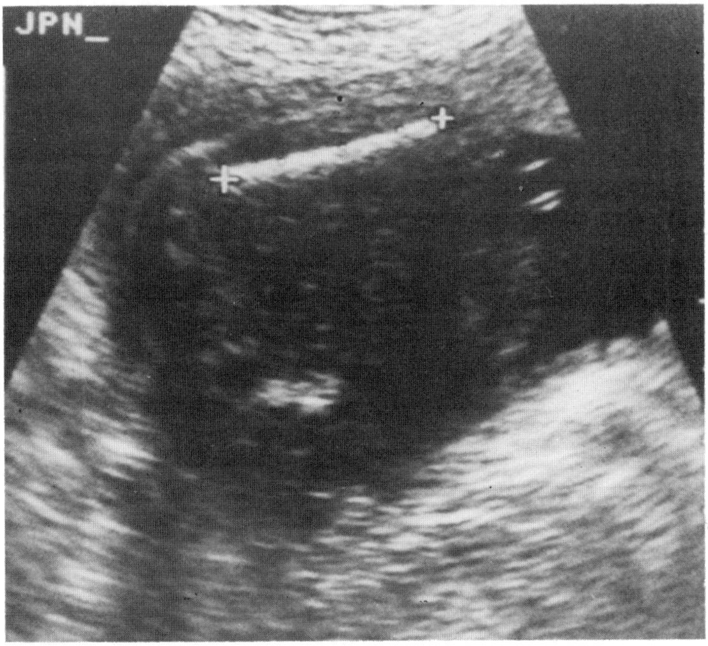


**Fig. 5.5** Femur length.

## Other measurements

It is, of course, important to consider the fetus in the context of its environment. Thus, the other contents of the gravid uterus have also been studied using ultrasound; this has sometimes proved fruitful.

### Amniotic fluid

The amount of amniotic fluid may be assessed subjectively or objectively. Subjective assessment, which is based on an overall impression with special attention paid to fluid between the limbs, is, because of the irregular (and changing) distribution of fluid around the fetus, not unreasonable; it certainly seems to be a replicable examination by both the same and also by different observers (Halperin *et al.* 1985). Attempts have inevitably been made to quantitate the amount of amniotic fluid. Various approaches have been used, mainly concentrating on the largest visible pool of amniotic fluid. Calculation of an average diameter of the pool (from one vertical and two horizontal measurements) gives a more replicable result than does simply measuring the vertical diameter alone (Patterson *et al.* 1987). Despite this, the maximum vertical diameter of the largest pool is now a commonly used parameter. It has been suggested that a distance of less than 2 cm (Figure 5.6) indicates oligohydramnios (Chamberlain *et al.* 1984a), while one of 8 cm or greater (Figure 5.7) indicates polyhydramnios (Chamberlain *et al.* 1984b).

### The placenta

There are a number of factors which can influence ultrasound measurement of the thickness of the placenta (Hoddick *et al.* 1985). These in-

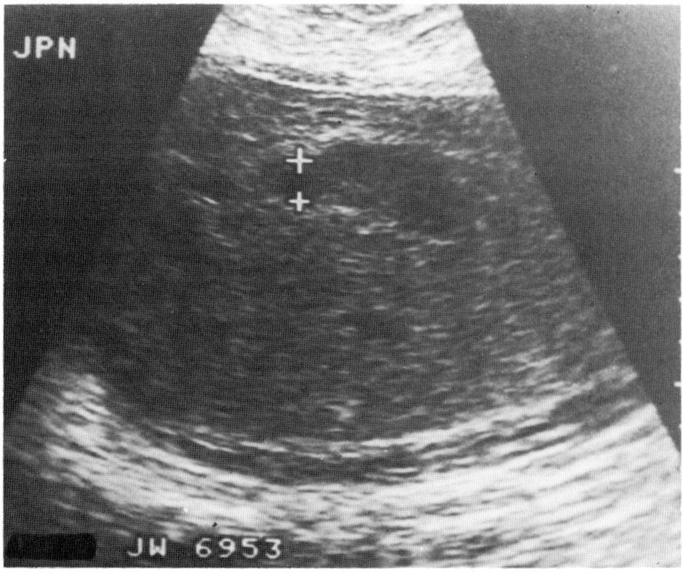


**Fig. 5.6** Vertical depth of largest pool of amniotic fluid in a case of oligohydramnios associated with severe fetal growth retardation (depth 9 mm).

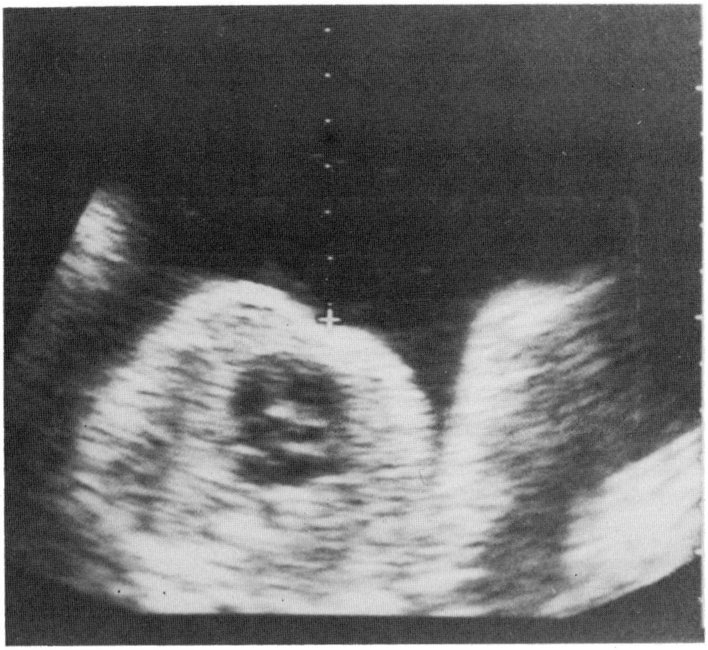

**Fig. 5.7** Vertical depth of largest pool of amniotic fluid in a case of polyhydramnios due to oesophageal atresia (depth 93 mm).

clude gestational age, polyhydramnios and uterine contractions, and this measurement has never found a proper niche in the armamentarium of the ultrasonographer. Likewise, estimation of placental volume, which was an early focus of investigation by ultrasound (Hellmann *et al.* 1970) and which has also been studied more recently (Geirsson, 1986; Wolf *et al.* 1987), has not become popular. Of more interest than the physical dimensions of the placenta has been its acoustic texture — its appearance on ultrasound examination. This has been known for some time to change with increasing gestation and these features have been attributed to placental ageing. The changes seen were classified by Grannum and colleagues (1979) who suggested that advanced textural grades correlated well with fetal lung maturation. This was not fully confirmed by subsequent study but placental grading has remained as a method of assessment in potentially compromised pregnancies and it may have an additional role as a screening technique.

## The uterus

Measurement of total intrauterine volume, which was popular at one time in the USA, was prompted by the fact that small-for-gestational age fetuses tend to have small placentas and diminished amniotic fluid volume (Gohari *et al.* 1977). However, even when measured using a complex and time-consuming planimetric technique, it did not prove more sensitive than simple fetal measurements (Geirsson 1986) and it fell into disfavour.

## The purpose of measurement

Fetal measurement can fulfil a number of purposes and not merely assist identification of fetuses that are insufficiently grown.

### Gestational age assessment

An accurate knowledge of gestational age is vital for the optimal interpretation of the results of most forms of fetal assessment (including clinical assessment) in later pregnancy. This is especially true for fetal measurement. The use of ultrasound to assess gestational age is based on the thesis that, in early pregnancy, fetal growth is rapid, there is little biological variation in size, and pathological growth retardation is uncommon. The age of the pregnancy can therefore be estimated by measurement of the fetus. During the first trimester, crown–rump length is measured and this has been reported as accurate in determining gestational age to within 5 days in 95 per cent of cases (Robinson & Fleming 1975). After 13 weeks varying flexion of the fetal trunk makes this measurement less reliable and, instead, the biparietal diameter is measured. This, when carried out before 18 weeks, predicts the date of delivery to within 2 weeks in 89 per cent of cases (Campbell 1976). Measurement of femoral length (or more accurately, femoral diaphysis length, because the greater trochanter and condyles do not calcify *in utero* and are not measured) appears to be of similar accuracy as the biparietal diameter (O'Brien *et al.* 1981). This is a particularly useful alternative when the fetal head is in an unsuitable position for measurement. Measurement of the transverse cerebellar diameter may be useful when fetal head shape is unusual (Goldstein *et al.* 1987b) and fetal foot length may also have an occasional role in estimating gestational age (Mercer *et al.* 1987). Measurement of any part of the fetus is of no value after 30 weeks in assessing gestational age.

Gestational age assessment is one area of obstetric ultrasound in which it has proven difficult to identify a suitable gold standard against which to test the validity of the technique. There has been a circular tendency by some authors to compile normal standards from the study of pregnancies in women who present with certain menstrual dates and then advocate the use of these measurements in all pregnancies because of the uncertainty of the date of the last menstrual period as an accurate index of gestational age in many women. There was a need for the definitive study of pregnancies with known dates of conception based on prior ultrasound monitoring of the Graafian follicle, or basal body temperature charts, or both. Such a study has recently been reported by MacGregor and colleagues (1987) who found that 95 per cent of estimates of gestational age by crown–rump length measurement were within 9 per cent of the actual gestational age. This represents reasonable accuracy. These authors have suggested that previous standards (Robinson & Fleming 1975) might underestimate gestational age by, on average, only 3 days.

There is a case for the routine ultrasound examination of all pregnancies at an early stage because of the importance of gestational age assessment and because it is not possible to predict with confidence all those in which this information will be vital later (at a time when gestational age can no longer be assessed accurately by ultrasound or any other technique). Such pregnancies will include those to be complicated by fetal growth retardation. Routine ultrasonography during early pregnancy has the main purpose to check gestational age although the detection of multiple pregnancies and of some fetal malformations may also result. Such screening has been evaluated on a limited basis by randomized controlled trials and these have been reviewed elsewhere (Neilson & Grant 1989). The use of routine ultrasonography in early pregnancy certainly results in a decreased rate of induction of labour for perceived post-term pregnancy (Eik-Nes *et al.* 1984; Waldenstrom *et al.* 1988) presumably because of more accurate dating. Other advantages which were predicted to result from this policy have not as yet been confirmed by scientific study and there remains a need for larger randomized trials than have been performed hitherto.

## Detection of the small-for-gestational age fetus

The terms *small-for-gestational age* and *growth retarded* are frequently, but wrongly, used as synonyms. Small-for-gestational age is a statistical concept useful both because it is easily determined as long as gestational age and birth weight are known and appropriate criteria agreed to separate normal from abnormal, and also because it undoubtedly identifies a group of babies at increased perinatal risk. The major risks are of death (especially intrauterine), intrapartum asphyxia, neonatal hypoglycaemia and possibly long-term neurological and intellectual impairment. Large epidemiological studies have emphasized both the important contribution that this group of babies makes to the perinatal mortality rate (McIlwaine *et al.* 1979; Northern Regional Group 1984) and also the frequent failure to identify such fetuses during routine antenatal care (Rosenberg *et al.* 1982). Disadvantages of the small-for-gestational age concept include the probability that birth weight for gestational age charts (upon which the classification is based) do not accurately reflect intrauterine standards of size, and that the separation of normality from abnormality by arbitrary (and varying) criteria ensures a small-for-gestational age group of great heterogeneity. Thus are included babies that have major malformations, those malnourished through uteroplacental insufficiency, and others that are small merely because of their genetic endowment. A large number of factors may operate to produce a small-for-gestational age baby, and the perinatal risks applicable to the group as a whole are not equally applicable to individual fetuses. Despite the shortcomings of the small-for-gestational age concept it remains the gold standard against which most new ultrasound measurements have been evaluated.

Campbell & Dewhurst (1971) showed that up to 73 per cent of small-for-gestational age babies could be identified by repeated measurement of the biparietal diameter and for many years this was the standard ultrasound technique used in high risk pregnancies. However, it is relatively insensitive because of the brain sparing effect. If the organ weights of small-for-gestational age babies are compared with those of controls, of either similar body weight or gestational age, it is found that the organs most diminished in weight are the thymus, spleen and liver (Gruenwald 1974). In contrast, brain weight is very much less reduced. Thus, in performing biparietal cephalometry, the ultrasonographer measures an index of the size of the fetal organ least affected (in terms of size, not necessarily of function) by the process of growth retardation. This appeared illogical and it was predicted that the measurement of other fetal organs and dimensions would prove more sensitive. This was confirmed on prospective study. Thus, Neilson and colleagues (1980) studied 474 pregnancies at between 34 and 36 weeks and compared the effectiveness of several fetal measurements — of head, trunk and length, singly and in combination — in predicting babies that were small-for-gestational age at birth. Trunk measurements were found, as had been predicted, to be more sensitive than head measurements; the best single measurement was the abdominal circumference with a sensitivity of 81 per cent and a specificity of 89 per cent. The abdominal circumference (or area) remains the best single measurement for identifying small-for-gestational age fetuses. We await the results of the newer measurements in large, broadly based populations to see if any will prove superior.

## Identification of fetal growth retardation

Fetal growth retardation is more difficult to define than is the state of being small-for-gestational age. A reasonable working definition is the failure of a fetus to achieve its intrinsic growth potential through lack of nutritional support. Although it has proven difficult to apply a numerical definition to this concept, all obstetricians and neonatal paediatricians recognize the characteristic features of these babies, described by Clifford (1954) in his study of post-term pregnancies, as wasted, often associated with meconium staining of the amniotic fluid, and prone to become asphyxiated during labour. The important point to stress here is that just as small-for-gestational age babies may not necessarily be growth retarded, so the genuinely growth retarded fetus, who has stopped growing because of uteroplacental insufficiency, may not have been deflected into the small-for-gestational age zone. It is possible that many babies who experience growth retardation in late pregnancy, but who are not small-for-gestational age, have sufficient reserve so that they are not placed at substantial perinatal risk; on the other hand, this phenomenon may be responsible for some intrauterine deaths which presently go unexplained because the growth problem is unrecognized since the baby is not small-for-gestational age. Clarification is urgently required both for clinical purposes and also to permit more appropriate evaluation of fetal measurement as well as of new techniques such as Doppler ultrasound (Neilson 1987). This should be an important focus for perinatal research.

Because diagnostic ultrasound provides the ideal tool for monitoring the rate of growth in individual fetuses, it is the definitive method for detecting growth retardation. It has to be admitted, however, that the use of ultrasound to assess individual growth patterns has received surprisingly little attention — certainly less than the subject deserves. Less concentration on the identification of small-for-gestational age fetuses by cross-sectional study and a reversal of the current obsession with attempts to predict fetal weight would release research time and energy to study longitudinal growth.

Deter and colleagues (1986) have proposed that the growth potential of individual fetuses could be assessed by two measurements during the second trimester separated by several weeks, e.g. at 20 and 28 weeks. The rate of growth derived from these could then be projected into the third trimester and significant slowing from this rate could then be detected by subsequent measurement. This approach concentrating on growth rather than size, and using each fetus as its own control, is attractive; however, the fact that growth retardation may start in the second trimester poses obvious difficulties.

Using serial measurement of the biparietal diameter, attempts were made to establish pathogenesis by demonstrating different patterns of growth among small-for-gestational age fetuses (Campbell 1974). Those showing abrupt cessation of previously normal growth were thought to be genuinely growth retarded (as a result of uteroplacental insufficiency) while those showing early departure from normal limits of growth but continuing until delivery were deemed to have low growth potential, sometimes in association with abnormality. The calculation of head–abdomen circumference ratios was proposed as a useful method of further differentiating these two groups (Campbell & Thoms 1977) based on the hypothesis that those babies which are genuinely growth retarded will show evidence of brain sparing and thus have disproportionately high head–abdomen ratios. While there was a higher incidence of intrapartum fetal distress and operative delivery in the asymmetrical group, the perinatal mortality rate and incidence of low Apgar scores were similar (and high) in both groups (Campbell & Thoms 1977). It thus appears that calculation of the head–abdomen ratio has a limited role in fetal assessment: the demonstration of asymmetry suggests, but does not prove, uteroplacental insufficiency; the demonstration of a symmetrically small-for-gestational age fetus indicates the need to exclude abnormality, but this pattern is also seen in some perfectly normal babies and some with genuine growth retardation (Davies *et al.* 1979).

An alternative approach is to concentrate on wasting. The ponderal index is calculated from the formula:

$$\text{birth weight} \times 100/(\text{crown–heel length})^3$$

It has been used for some time by paediatricians to estimate the degree of intrauterine malnutrition experienced by the growth retarded neonate. Attempts have recently been made to calculate the fetal ponderal index from ultrasound measurement. The most popular technique has been to calculate a ratio of femur length to abdominal circumference (Vintzileos *et al.* 1985b; Divon *et al.* 1986); the wasted fetus will be expected to have a high ratio. These ratios appear to be constant over different gestational ages in normally grown fetuses, so they may have a very useful role when growth retardation is suspected but gestational age is not certain. Yagel and colleagues (1987) investigated a slightly different form of fetal ponderal index by dividing the estimated weight by the femoral length cubed. This appeared to provide useful prognostic information after fetuses were identified as small-for-gestational age. Estimation of amniotic fluid volume by ultrasonography also helps separate the healthy from the unhealthy among the small-for-gestational age group (Chamberlain *et al.* 1984a).

## Estimation of fetal weight

This is a subject which, in the opinion of the author, has received an inordinate amount of attention by ultrasonographers. Formulas exist to estimate fetal weight from abdominal measurements (Campbell & Wilkin 1975), abdominal and head measurements (Shepard *et al.* 1982), and abdominal, head and femur measurements (Hadlock *et al.* 1985). Many other authors have reported on minor variations of these approaches. As a generalization, the estimates tend to be accurate to within 10 to 15 per cent of the actual weight and therefore may, at times, give clearly inaccurate predictions. An estimate of fetal weight may be useful in managing women who have had a Caesarean section previously, those with a fetus presenting by the breech, and in managing preterm labour, although gestational age gives better prognostic information (Verloove-Vanhorick *et al.* 1986). In the investigation of the small-for-gestational age fetus, measurements are best compared to normal intrauterine standards rather than converted to an estimate of fetal weight and then plotted on a birth weight for gestational age chart.

## Detection of anomalies

Fetal measurement can contribute to the identification of a number of malformations. Thus, calculation of the ventricular–hemispheric ratios will assist the diagnosis of hydrocephalus (Nicolaides & Campbell 1987) while measurements of the fetal head may identify microcephaly (Chervenak *et al.* 1987) although the latter diagnosis may not be possible until late in the second trimester. Measurements of the thoracic dimensions may help identify spondylothoracic dysplasia (Chitkara *et al.* 1987) while long bone measurements can identify skeletal dysplasias. It has been reported that fetal trisomy 21 can be identified non-invasively by measurement of the soft tissue thickness at the neck (Benacceraf & Frigoletto 1987). This has not, however, been confirmed by others (Toi *et al.* 1987) and, whilst awaiting validation, this technique should not be used for screening for Down's syndrome.

### Detection of pulmonary hypoplasia

Fetal pulmonary hypoplasia is associated with prolonged oligohydramnios during the second trimester of pregnancy, and with early neonatal death. Accurate prediction of this complication could assist the management of pregnancies in which early spontaneous rupture of the membranes has occurred during mid-pregnancy. It has been suggested that a sustained absence of fetal breathing (as demonstrated by real-time ultrasonography) is highly predictive of lung hypoplasia (Blott *et al.* 1987) although this is disputed by others (Moessinger *et al.* 1987) and this interesting observation awaits confirmation. Measurement of the thoracic circumference (at the level of the lungs) by ultrasound may be of value (Nimrod *et al.* 1986) although, because there is overlap in results between fetuses with pulmonary hypoplasia and those that are small-for-gestational age, the ratio of thoracic to abdominal circumferences may give better discrimination (Johnson *et al.* 1987). While there remains diagnostic doubt, it is prudent to be cautious in advising termination of pregnancy after very early rupture of the membranes.

## Screening

The use of ultrasound as a screening technique applied to all pregnancies in the early stages has been discussed already. Routine late pregnancy ultrasonography, with its main purpose to detect the clinically unsuspected small-for-gestational age fetus, has also been studied. The ideal method to evaluate ultrasound screening (as other forms of fetal assessment) is by randomized controlled trial to avoid selection biases, and to control for unknown as well as known influencing variables. Four randomized controlled trials of routine late pregnancy ultrasonography have been published (Bakkateig *et al.* 1984; Eik-Nes *et al.* 1984; Neilson *et al.* 1984; Secher *et al.* 1987). These studies took different forms, used different ultrasound techniques, and were associated with great variation in sensitivity in identifying small-for-gestational age fetuses — from 25 per cent (Bakkateig *et al.* 1984) to 94 per cent (Neilson *et al.* 1984). Combining the results of these trials to give a consensus view, by meta-analysis, does not encourage the use of routine measurement of all fetuses by ultrasound in late pregnancy as no clear benefit has been demonstrated in improving fetal outcome or obstetric management (Neilson & Grant 1989). Fetal measurement should continue to be confined to those situations in which it is indicated for specific clinical reasons.

In contrast, another randomized controlled trial (of routine placental texture grading by ultrasound in late pregnancy) has suggested that this examination may improve fetal outcome. Proud and Grant (1987) studied 2000 pregnancies and found that among those in which the placental grade was reported to the clinical staff, there were fewer perinatal deaths, neonatal convulsions and low Apgar scores at 5 min. Whether further studies will confirm the desirability of this technique for screening remains to be seen; in the mean time, it is useful for the ultrasonographer to report placental texture grade at any examination performed for specific reasons during the third trimester.

## Multiple pregnancies

There has been much debate about whether ordinary singleton or separate twin standards of growth, size and birth weight should be applied to twins. The differing views on this depend on whether the generally smaller size of twin fetuses is seen as a physiological or a pathological phenomenon. There is no obvious physiological reason why dizygotic twins should have diminished growth potential compared with singletons, so there is certainly an argument for applying normal singleton standards to at least these twins. Our studies of abdominal circumference measurements by ultrasound in twin pregnancies showed no difference between monozygotic and dizygotic pregnancies from 16 weeks (Neilson & Hastie 1988) and this would suggest that the same standards may be relevant to monozygotic pregnancies as well. Others, however, have described differences between monozygotic and dizygotic pairs from mid-pregnancy onwards (Grennert *et al.* 1980) and this requires further study. In the mean time, the high perinatal loss rate associated with multiple pregnancy should prevent clinical complacency when a twin fetus is found to be small-for-gestational age.

Although (accepting singleton standards as appropriate) many twins are small-for-gestational age (Manlan & Scott 1978), it is especially difficult to identify them antenatally by clinical examination (Neilson *et al.* 1988). Ultrasound therefore should play an important role. However, serial biparietal cephalometry has proved even less sensitive in identifying the small-for-gestational age fetus in twin pregnancies than in singleton (Neilson 1981), probably because of the added technical difficulties of accurate head measurement in late twin pregnancy. This technique is not therefore recommended. Abdominal measurements are satisfactory in predicting twins that are small-for-gestational age at birth (Neilson 1981; Secher *et al.* 1985) although the results are probably less good than in singleton pregnancies. This may result from artificially increased measured dimensions due to mechanical trunk flexion in late pregnancy from overcrowding (Neilson 1988).

Many reports on fetal measurement have concentrated solely on the difference in size between twins. Whilst discordancy of size is important to note, this general approach is illogical because growth retardation may affect one or both of twins, and use of the other twin as the only standard to assess growth or size may be very misleading. Divergent growth is one feature of the twin–twin transfusion syndrome although it is, by no means, confined to it. The syndrome is though to result from unbalanced blood flow through vascular anastomoses in monochorionic placentas and, in its most florid form, it is readily identifiable by ultrasound examination (Wittmann *et al.* 1981). Whether less extreme forms of the condition may be detected by fetal measurement alone requires further study, with careful attention to stringent diagnostic criteria (Danskin & Neilson 1989). We have been unable to demonstrate any difference in abdominal circumference measurement between monozygotic/monochorionic and monozygotic/dichorionic pregnancies (Neilson *et al.* 1989). Since vascular anastomoses are almost universal in monochorionic placentas and virtually never present in dichorionic placentas, vascular anastomoses may not have an important effect on fetal growth in the absence of the florid form of the syndrome.

## References

Bakkateig L.S., Eik-Nes S.H., Jacobsen G., Ulstein M.K., Brodtkors C.J., Balstad P., Eriksen B.C. & Jorgensen N.P. (1984) Randomized controlled trial of ultrasonographic screening in pregnancy. *Lancet*, **ii**, 207–11.

Benacerraf B.R. & Frigoletto F.D. (1987) Soft tissue fold in the second-trimester fetus: standards for normal measurements compared with those in Down syndrome. *American Journal of Obstetrics and Gynecology*, **157**, 1146–9.

Blott M., Greenough A., Nicolaides K.H., Moscoso G., Gibb D. & Campbell S. (1987) Fetal breathing movements as predictor of favourable outcome after oligohydramnios due to membrane rupture in the second trimester. *Lancet*, **ii**, 129–31.

Campbell S. (1968) An improved method of fetal cephalometry by ultrasound. *Journal of Obstetrics and Gynecology of the British Commonwealth*, **75**, 568–76.

Campbell S. (1974) Fetal growth. *Clinics in Obstetrics and Gynecology*, **1**, 41–65.

Campbell S. (1976) Fetal growth. In *Fetal Physiology and Medicine*, (Ed. by R.W. Beard & P.W. Nathanielszw), pp. 271–301. Saunders, London.

Campbell S. & Dewhurst C.J. (1971) Diagnosis of the small-for-dates fetus by serial ultrasonic cephalometry. *Lancet*, **ii**, 1002–6.

Campbell S. & Thoms A. (1977) Ultrasonic measurement of the fetal head to abdomen circumference ratio in the assessment of growth retardation. *British Journal of Obstetrics and Gynaecology*, **84**, 165–74.

Campbell S. & Wilkin D. (1975) Ultrasonic measurement of fetal circumference in the estimation of fetal weight. *British Journal of Obstetrics and Gynaecology*, **82**, 689–97.

Chamberlain P.F., Manning F.A., Morrison I., Harman C.R. & Lange I. (1984a) Ultrasound evaluation of amniotic fluid volume 1. The relationship of marginal and decreased amniotic fluid volumes to perinatal outcome. *American Journal of Obstetrics and Gynecology*, **150**, 245–9.

Chamberlain P.F., Manning F.A., Morrison I., Harman C.R. & Lange I. (1984b) Ultrasound evaluation of amniotic fluid volume 2. The relationship of increased amniotic fluid volume to perinatal outcome. *American Journal of Obstetrics and Gynecology*, **150**, 250–4.

Chervenak F.A., Rosenberg J., Brightman R.C., Chitkara U. & Jeanty P. (1987) A prospective study of the accuracy of ultrasound in predicting microcephaly. *Obstetrics and Gynecology*, **69**, 908–10.

Chitkara U., Rosenberg J., Chervenak F.A., Berkowitz G.S., Levine R., Fagerstrom R.M., Walker B. & Berkowitz R.L. (1987) Prenatal sonographic assessment of the fetal thorax: normal values. *American Journal of Obstetrics and Gynecology*, **156**, 1069–74.

Clifford S.H. (1954) Postmaturity with placental dysfunction. *Journal of Pediatrics*, **44**, 1–13.

Danskin F.H. & Neilson J.P. (1989) The twin to twin transfusion syndrome: what are diagnostic criteria? *American Journal of Obstetrics and Gynecology*, suitable **161**, 365–9.

Davies D.P., Platts P., Pritchard J.M. & Wilkinson P.W. (1979) Nutritional status of light-for-dates infants at birth and its influence on early postnatal growth. *Archives of Disease in Childhood*, **54**, 703–6.

Deter R.L., Rossavik I.K., Harrist R.B. & Hadlock F.P. (1986b) Mathematic modeling of fetal growth: development of individual growth curve standards. *Obstetrics and Gynecology*, **68**, 156–61.

Divon M.Y., Chamberlain P.F., Sipos L., Manning F.A. & Platt L.D. (1986) Identification of the small for gestational age fetus with the use of gestational age-independent indices of fetal growth. *American Journal of Obstetrics and Gynecology*, **155**, 1197–1201.

Eik-Nes S.H., Okland O., Aure J.C. & Ulstein M. (1984) Ultrasound screening in pregnancy: a randomised controlled trial. *Lancet*, **i**, 1347.

Geirsson R.T. (1986) Intrauterine volume in pregnancy. *Acta Obstetricia et Gynecologica Scandinavica*, Suppl. 136.

Gohari P., Berkowitz R.L. & Hobbins J.C. (1977) Prediction of intrauterine growth retardation by determination of total intrauterine volume. *American Journal of Obstetrics and Gynecology*, **127**, 255–60.

Goldstein I., Lockwood C. & Hobbins J.C. (1987a) Ultrasound assessment of fetal intestinal development in the evaluation of gestational age. *Obstetrics and Gynecology*, **70**, 682–6.

Goldstein I., Reece A., Pilu G., Bovicelli L. & Hobbins J.C. (1987b) Cerebellar measurements with ultrasonography in the evaluation of fetal growth and development. *American Journal of Obstetrics and Gynecology*, **156**, 1065–9.

Grannum P.A.T., Berkowitz R.L. & Hobbins J.C. (1979) The ultrasonic changes in the maturing placenta and their relation to fetal pulmonic maturity. *American Journal of Obstetrics and Gynecology*, **133**, 915–22.

Grannum P., Bracken M., Silverman R. & Hobbins J.C. (1980) Assessment of fetal kidney size in normal gestation by comparison of ratio of kidney circumference to abdominal circumference. *American Journal of Obstetrics and Gynecology*, **136**, 249–54.

Grennert L., Persson P-H., Gennser G. & Gullberg B. (1980) Zygosity and the intrauterine growth of twins. *Obstetrics and Gynecology*, **55**, 684–7.

Gruenwald P. (1974) Pathology of the fetus and its supply line. In *Size at Birth*, pp. 3–19. Associated Scientific Publishers, Amsterdam.

Hadlock F.P., Harrist R.B., Sharman R.S., Deter R.L. & Park S.K. (1985) Estimation of fetal weight with the use of head, body and femur measurements — a prospective study. *American Journal of Obstetrics and Gynecology*, **151**, 333–7.

Halperin M.E., Fong K.W., Zalev A.H. & Goldsmith C.H. (1985) Reliability of amniotic fluid volume estimation from ultrasonograms. Intraobserver and interobserver variation before and after the establishment of criteria. *American Journal of Obstetrics and Gynecology*, **153**, 264–7.

Hanretty K.P., Neilson J.P. & Fleming J.E.E. (1990) Re-evaluation of clinical estimation of fetal weight: a comparison with ultrasound. *Journal of Obstetrics and Gynaecology* (in press).

Hellman L.M., Kobayashi M., Tolles W.E. & Cromb E. (1970) Ultrasonic studies on the volumetric growth of the human placenta. *American Journal of Obstetrics and Gynecology*, **108**, 740–8.

Hoddick W.K., Mahony B.S., Callen P.W. & Filly R.A. (1985) Placental thickness. *Journal of Ultrasound in Medicine*, **4**, 479–82.

Jeanty P., Rodesch F., Delbeke D. & Dumont J.E. (1984) Estimation of gestational age by measurement of fetal long bones. *Journal of Ultrasound in Medicine*, **3**, 75–9.

Jeanty P., Romero R. & Hobbins J.C. (1985) Fetal limb volume: a new parameter to assess fetal growth and nutrition. *Journal of Ultrasound in Medicine*, **4**, 273–82.

Johnson A., Callan N.A., Bhutani V.K., Colmorgen G.H.C., Weiner S. & Bolognese R.J. (1987) Ultrasonic ratio of fetal thoracic to abdominal circumference: an association with fetal pulmonary hypoplasia. *American Journal of Obstetrics and Gynecology*, **157**, 764–9.

Kurtz A.B. & Goldberg B.B. (1988) *Obstetrical Measurements in Ultrasound. A Reference Manual*. Year Book Publishers Inc., Chicago.

Lewis E., Kurtz A.B., Dubbins P.A., Wapner R.J. & Goldberg B.B. (1982) Real-time ultrasonographic evaluation of normal fetal adrenal glands. *Journal of Ultrasound in*

*Medicine*, **1**, 265–70.

MacGregor S.N., Tamura R.K., Sabbagha R.E., Minogue J.P., Gibson M.E. & Hoffman D.I. (1987) Underestimation of gestational age by conventional crown–rump length dating curves. *Obstetrics and Gynecology*, **70**, 344–8.

McIlwaine G.M., Howat R.C.L., Dunn F. & Macnaughton M.C. (1979) The Scottish perinatal mortality survey. *British Medical Journal*, **2**, 1103–6.

Manlan G. & Scott K.E. (1978) Contribution of twin pregnancy to perinatal mortality and fetal growth retardation: reversal of growth retardation after birth. *Canadian Medical Association Journal*, **118**, 365–8.

Mercer B.M., Siklar S., Shariatmadar A., Gillieson M.S. & D'Alton M.E. (1987) Fetal foot length as a predictor of gestational age. *American Journal of Obstetrics and Gynecology*, **156**, 350–5.

Merz E., Kim-Kern M-S. & Pehl S. (1987) Ultrasonic mensuration of fetal limbs in the second and third trimesters. *Journal of Clinical Ultrasound*, **15**, 175–83.

Moessinger A.C., Fox H.E., Higgins A., Rey H.R. & Haideri M.A. (1987) Fetal breathing movements are not a reliable predictor of continued lung development in pregnancies complicated by oligohydramnios. *Lancet*, **ii**, 1297–1300.

Neilson J.P. (1981) Detection of the small-for-dates twin fetus by ultrasound. *British Journal of Obstetrics and Gynaecology*, **88**, 27–32.

Neilson J.P. (1987) Doppler ultrasound. *British Journal of Obstetrics and Gynaecology*, **94**, 929–34.

Neilson J.P. (1988) Fetal growth in twin pregnancies. *Acta Geneticae Medicae et Gemellologiae*, **37**, 35–9.

Neilson J.P., Danskin F. & Hastie S.J. (1989) Monozygotic twin pregnancy: diagnostic and Doppler ultrasound studies. *British Journal of Obstetrics and Gynaecology*, (in press).

Neilson J.P. & Grant A. (1989) Ultrasound examinations in pregnancy. In *Effective Care in Pregnancy and Childbirth*, (Ed. by M. Enkin, M. Keirse & I. Chalmers), pp. 419–39. Oxford University Press, Oxford.

Neilson J.P. & Hastie S.J. (1988) Ultrasound studies of monozygotic and dizygotic twin pregnancies. In *Fetal and Neonatal Development*, (Ed. by C.T. Jones), pp. 541–3. Perinatology Press, New York.

Neilson J.P., Munjanja S.P. & Whitfield C.R. (1984) Screening for the small-for-dates fetus: a controlled trial. *British Medical Journal*, **289**, 1179–82.

Neilson J.P., Verkuyl D.A.A. & Bannerman C. (1988) Tape measurement of symphysis–fundal height in twin pregnancies. *British Journal of Obstetrics and Gynaecology*, **95**, 1054–9.

Neilson J.P., Whitfield C.R. & Aitchison T.C. (1980) Screening for the small-for-dates fetus: a two-stage ultrasound examination schedule. *British Medical Journal*, **280**, 1203–6.

Nicolaides K.H. & Campbell S. (1987) Diagnosis and management of fetal malformations. *Baillière's Clinical Obstetrics and Gynaecology*, **1**, 591–622.

Nimrod C., Davies D., Iwanicki S., Harder J., Persaud D. & Nicholson S. (1986) Ultrasound prediction of pulmonary hypoplasia. *Obstetrics and Gynecology*, **68**, 495–7.

Northern Regional Health Authority Coordinating Group (1984) Perinatal mortality; a continuing collaborative regional survey. *British Medical Journal*, **288**, 1717–20.

O'Brien G.D., Queenan J.T. & Campbell S. (1981) Assessment of gestational age in the second trimester by real-time ultrasound measurement of the femur length. *American Journal of Obstetrics and Gynecology*, **139**, 540–5.

Patterson R.M., Prihoda T.J. & Pouliot M.R. (1987) Sonographic amniotic fluid measurement and fetal growth retardation: a reappraisal. *American Journal of Obstetrics and Gynecology*, **157**, 1406–10.

Pearce J.M. & Campbell S. (1987) A comparison of symphysis–fundal height and ultrasound as screening tests for light-for-gestational age infants. *British Journal of Obstetrics and Gynaecology*, **94**, 100–4.

Proud J. & Grant A. (1987) Third trimester placental grading by ultrasonography as a test of fetal wellbeing. *British Medical Journal*, **294**, 1641–4.

Robinson H.P. & Fleming J.E.E. (1975) A critical evaluation of sonar 'crown–rump length' measurements. *British Journal of Obstetrics and Gynaecology*, **82**, 702–10.

Rosenberg K., Grant J.M. & Hepburn M. (1982) Antenatal detection of growth retardation: actual practice in a large maternity hospital. *British Journal of Obstetrics and Gynaecology*, **89**, 12–15.

Schmidt W., Yarkoni S., Jeanty P., Grannum P. & Hobbins J.C. (1985) Sonographic measurements of the fetal spleen: clinical implications. *Journal of Ultrasound in Medicine*, **4**, 667–72.

Secher N.J., Hansen P.K., Lenstrup C., Eriksen P.S. & Morsing G. (1987) A randomised study of fetal abdominal diameter and fetal weight estimation for detection of light-for-gestation infants in low-risk pregnancies. *British Journal of Obstetrics and Gynaecology*, **94**, 105–9.

Secher N.J., Kaern J. & Hansen P.K. (1985) Intrauterine growth in twin pregnancies: prediction of fetal growth retardation. *Obstetrics and Gynecology*, **66**, 63–8.

Shepard M.J., Richards V.A., Berkowitz R.L., Warsof S.L. & Hobbins J.C. (1982) An evaluation of two equations for predicting fetal weight by ultrasound. *American Journal of Obstetrics and Gynecology*, **142**, 47–54.

Toi A., Simpson G.F. & Filly R.A. (1987) Ultrasonically evident fetal nuchal thickening: is it specific for Down syndrome? *American Journal of Obstetrics and Gynecology*, **156**, 150–3.

Verloove-Vanhorick S.P., Verwey R.A., Braud R., Bennebroek Gravenhorst J., Keirse M.J.N.C. & Ruys J.H. (1986) Neonatal mortality risk in relation to gestational age and birthweight. *Lancet*, **i**, 55–7.

Vintzileos A.M., Neckles S., Campbell W.A., Andreoli J.W., Kaplan B.M. & Nochimson D.J. (1985a) Fetal liver measurements during normal pregnancy *Obstetrics and Gynecology*, **66**, 477–80.

Vintzileos A.M., Neckles S., Campbell W.A., Andreoli J.W., Kaplan B.M. & Nochimson D.J. (1985b) Three fetal ponderal indexes in normal pregnancy. *Obstetrics and Gynecology*, **65**, 807–11.

Waldenstrom U., Axelsson O., Nilsson S., Eklund G., Fall O., Lindberg S. & Sjodin Y. (1988) Effects of routine one-stage ultrasound screening in pregnancy: a randomised controlled trial. *Lancet*, **ii**, 585–8.

Willocks J., Donald I., Duggan T.C. & Day N. (1964) Foetal cephalometry by ultrasound. *Journal of Obstetrics and Gynaecology of the British Commonwealth*, **71**, 11–20.

Wittmann B.K., Baldwin V.J. & Nichol B. (1981) Antenatal diagnosis of twin transfusion syndrome. *Obstetrics and Gynecology*, **58**, 123–7.

Wladimiroff J.W. & Campbell S. (1974) Fetal urine production rates in normal and complicated pregnancy. *Lancet*, **i**, 151–4.

Wolf H., Oosting H. & Treffers P.E. (1987) Placental volume measurement by ultrasonography: evaluation of the method. *American Journal of Obstetrics and Gynecology*, **156**, 1191–4.

Yagel S., Zacut D., Igelstein S., Palti Z., Hurwitz A. & Rosenn B. (1987) *In utero* ponderal index as a prognostic factor in the evaluation of intrauterine growth retardation. *American Journal of Obstetrics and Gynecology*, **157**, 415–19.

Yarkoni S., Schmidt W., Jeanty P., Reece E.A. & Hobbins J.C. (1985) Clavicular measurement: a new biometric parameter for fetal evaluation. *Journal of Ultrasound in Medicine*, **4**, 467–70.

# 6: Uteroplacental and fetal blood flow

PETER J. McPARLAND AND J. MALCOLM PEARCE



One of the most important landmarks in perinatal medicine was the introduction of ultrasound by Ian Donald in 1958. Prior to this the human fetus was inaccessible to study apart from the fetal movements perceived by the mother and by auscultation with a simple stethoscope. Since the advent of ultrasound, perinatal medicine has dramatically changed from an art to a science. Doppler ultrasound represents the third major application of ultrasound to obstetrics. Unlike the other two — real-time ultrasound scanning and external cardiotocography — Doppler ultrasound appears to be undergoing careful evaluation in order to clearly define its role in clinical practice.

The use of Doppler ultrasound was first described in 1959 by Satomura when he reported the transcutaneous detection of blood flow velocity patterns in superficial arteries in adults. Nearly two decades passed before Doppler ultrasound of fetal blood flow was described

(Fitzgerald & Drumm 1977). The past decade has seen an escalating interest in Doppler ultrasound as it provides non-invasive access to the uteroplacental and fetal circulation. This chapter attempts to summarize the current state of knowledge, and will briefly describe the anatomical and historical aspects of uteroplacental and fetal blood flow measurement, before discussing the clinical application of Doppler ultrasound.

## Anatomical aspects

### Uteroplacental circulation

The uterine artery arises from the internal iliac artery and having crossed in front of the ureter penetrates the uterine musculature between the layers of the broad ligament. It then continues through the outer one-third of the myometrium before dividing into arcuate arteries which run circumferentially around and parallel to the surface of the uterus. The radial arteries arise from the arcuate arteries at approximately right angles and divide into 100–150 spiral arteries and also into basal arteries (Brosens & Dixon 1966) (Figure 6.1). The basal arteries supply the myometrium and basal endometrium and undergo only minor changes during pregnancy.

In normal pregnancy the decidual and the myometrial portion of each spiral artery is invaded by trophoblast in two stages. In the first trimester the decidual portion is invaded, with the myometrial portion being invaded in the second trimester. Trophoblastic invasion replaces much of the internal lining of the endothelium resulting in the loss of musculo-elastic tissue converting these arteries into large funnel-shaped vessels (Figure 6.2) which can accommodate the massive increase in blood flow from 2–10 ml/min in the non-pregnant endometrium, to 600–800 ml/min which empties into the intervillous space in pregnancy.

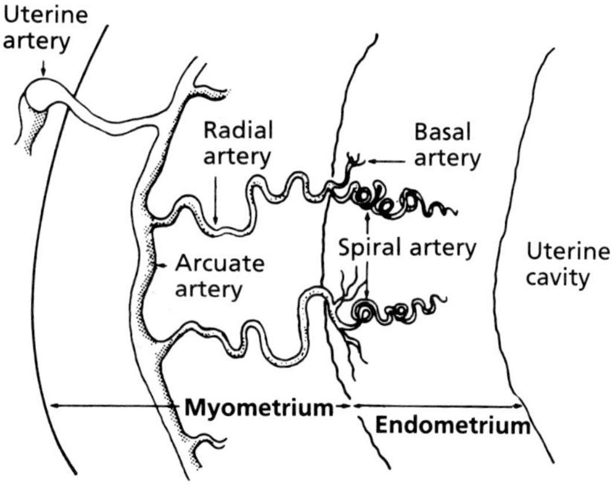


**Fig. 6.1** Anatomy of the arterial supply to the non-pregnant endometrium

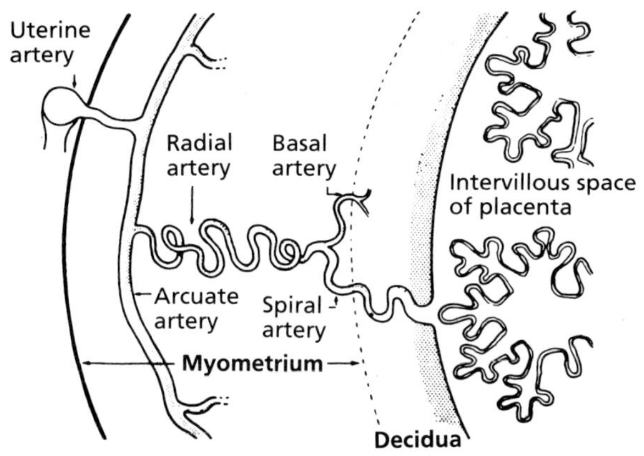


**Fig. 6.2** Anatomy of the arterial supply to the placenta in normal pregnancy

## Umbilical circulation

The definitive architecture of the placenta is established by the end of the first trimester but the placenta continues to grow and becomes subdivided into 15–30 cotyledons by septa formed by a combination of the trophoblast and decidual elements. The umbilical arteries wind around the fetal bladder to reach the umbilicus and from there progress to the placenta. They then anastomose at the chorionic plate and thence they split up into cotyledonary branches. These cotyledonary arteries are end vessels with three orders of arterial divisions. There are no anastomoses between arteries in the same or contiguous cotyledons. The basic configuration of the arterial tree is completely developed in the first trimester with the number of cotyledons remaining constant from approximately 16 weeks. After this time placental growth is characterized by a continuous proliferation of the terminal capillary bed. This peripheral growing-end comprises an extensive capillary network with small sprouting capillary units covered by a thin layer of syncytium. These sprouts are the chorionic villi where oxygen and metabolites are exchanged. New syncytial buds, vascularized with capillary sprouts from older villi, are continuously formed until term (Gruenwald 1972) although the rate of proliferation slows down in the last trimester.

## The intervillous space

Maternal blood enters the intervillous space (IVS) under high pressure. The pressures responsible for perfusion are approximately 90 mmHg at the level of the uteroplacental artery, 25 mmHg in the spiral artery and 15–20 mmHg in the IVS. The blood is directed towards the chorionic plate which forms the roof of the IVS. Dampening pressure results and the blood slowly flows round and over the surface of the villi allowing metabolic and gaseous exchange. The maternal blood is then returned to the floor of the IVS where it drains into the endometrial veins. Once fetomaternal gas exchange has occurred, the fetal blood returns to the fetal heart via the umbilical vein.

## Historical methods of measuring blood flow in pregnancy

### Uteroplacental blood flow measurement

#### DIRECT METHODS

Two types of direct method have been used for measuring uterine flow, by venous outflow or arterial inflow. The first recorded measurement was performed by Barcroft *et al.* (1933). They cannulated the common iliac vein in pregnant rabbits after removing the bladder, vagina and rectum and after tying all other pelvic veins so that all uterine venous blood flow drained through a cannula in the external iliac vein and could thus be measured.

The next development was of flowmeters where, at laparotomy, one or both uterine arteries were cannulated at the uterocervical junction, with the other end of the cannula connected to the left carotid artery. Incorporated in the loop system was a flowmeter which contained a float that was displaced vertically in proportion to the rate of flow (Ahlquist 1950).

This led to development of electromagnetic flowmeters which are of either the cannulated or the more popular cuffed variety. The placement of the cuff may in itself produce an artefact by compressing the vessel and this technique does not measure the entire uterine flow because the placenta may have several arterial inputs. There is also no differentiation between flow to the supporting arteries and of that to the placenta. Attempts to determine the rate of blood flow by following volume change of the uterus enclosed in a plethysmograph have not met with significant success. The main difficulty was the anatomical problem of achieving a tight fit between the uterus and the oncometer without impeding the uterine blood flow.

#### INDIRECT METHODS

Indirect measurements of uterine blood flow include the application of the Fick principle, isotope clearance and changes in heat conductivity. The Fick principle has been applied to the uteroplacental circulation using a diffusible inert gas, nitrous oxide (Assali *et al.* 1953). Huckabee *et al.* (1961) used 4-amino-antipyrine instead of nitrous oxide to measure uterine blood flow in goats as it attains equilibrium much more rapidly in maternal blood, the fetus and the placenta (Metcalfe *et al.* 1959) and a period of 15–20 min is all that is required compared with several hours for nitrous oxide.

One of the better methods described initially by Rudolph & Heymann (1967) and modified by Makowski *et al.* (1968) uses radioactive microspheres which are injected into the arterial circulation. If the spheres are well mixed with the blood and are too large to pass through the precapillary arterioles, they will then be distributed in accordance with the arterial blood flow. If a representative arterial sample can be drawn, then the blood flow to any organ can be obtained by multiplying the number of spheres found in that organ by a flow factor, which consists of the withdrawal rate divided by the number of spheres observed in the representative arterial sample.

By far the widest experience on measuring uteroplacental blood flow in humans is by the use of isotopes injected intravenously, into the myometrium or directly into the IVS through the abdominal wall. The rate of disappearance of the isotope is usually measured by a scintillation counter located over the site of interest. The results are difficult to interpret quantitatively but are useful when flow is very much reduced in particular circumstances or to study the effects of certain manoeuvres upon a steady state. The two most widely reported isotopes are sodium-24 and xenon-133.

Using this technique McClure-Brown & Veall (1953) found prolonged clearance times of sodium-24 from the IVS in hypertensive women. The same finding was reported by Dixon *et al.* (1963) who went on to show that the delay in clearance was proportional to the degree of hypertension. Using isotope washout techniques Clavero-Nunez (1980), Wolfson & Blake (1975) and Lunnell *et al.* (1979) have found evidence of reduced placental blood flow in association with fetal growth retardation.

## Fetal umbilical blood flow measurement

The fetal circulation is even less accessible to blood flow measurement than the uteroplacental circulation. The first attempt to measure umbilical blood flow was by Cooper & Greenfield (1949). An exteriorized fetal lamb with its cord intact was wholly immersed in a bath of warm saline arranged as a plethysmograph. Umbilical blood flow was then calculated from the reduction in fetal volume consequent upon arterial bleeding into the placenta with the umbilical vein occluded. They repeated their experiments in a 15 week human fetus (Greenfield *et al.* 1951) and obtained a value of 45 ml/min/kg.

The next method which was used for measuring total umbilical blood flow was to insert a flowmeter to the intra-abdominal umbilical vein. The disadvantage is that a laparotomy must be performed. Several types of flowmeter have been used with the electromagnetic flowmeter proving most reliable. Umbilical flow measurement measured by this method ranges from 132 to 260 ml/min/kg in mature fetal lambs. Values of 110 ml/min/kg were reported using a cuff electronic flowmeter in the human fetus, in mothers anaesthetized just prior to the termination of pregnancy via hysterotomy (Assali *et al.* 1960). The introduction of electromagnetic flowmeters gave mean umbilical flow rates of 138 ml/min/kg (Kirschbaum *et al.* 1967) to 170 ml/min/kg (Dawes & Mott 1964).

Further attempts were made using thermodilutional techniques to determine umbilical venous flow in newborn babies while the placenta was still attached and the cord still pulsating. Stembera *et al.* (1965) obtained estimates of a mean flow rate of 75 ml/min/kg whilst McCallum (1977) obtained a mean estimate of 171 ml/min/kg. Clavero *et al.* (1973) injected xenon into the intervillous space of intact human pregnancies and estimated fetoplacental blood flow by means of a scintillation counter to be between 900–1900 ml/min/kg. This is grossly different from all other studies and presumably reflects the difficulty in estimating clearance rates.

The only other indirect method of measuring umbilical blood flow makes use of the Fick principle. The preliminary work involved infusing urea into pregnant sheep and measuring the umbilical arteriovenous difference and by calculating the quantity of urea transferred to the fetus, mean umbilical flow could be calculated. These experiments were repeated by Meschia *et al.* (1965) and Crenshaw *et al.* (1968). Values of 164–302 ml/min/kg were obtained.

Makowski *et al.* (1968) showed agreement between the steady-state diffusion method using urea or antipyrine and the isotope-labelled microsphere method both applied in acute experiments *in utero*, but their figures were lower (135 ml/min/kg). Despite the mentioned difficulties of the techniques and the various experimental conditions there is reasonable agreement amongst results obtained for umbilical blood flow.

However, all of these techniques are relatively invasive and therefore not applicable or practical in the clinical setting. Numerous problems also exist when relating animal data to the human including the difference in placentation that exists between species and the effects of anaesthesia and surgical procedures.

The introduction of Doppler ultrasound technology promised non-invasive, probably safe, repeatable assessment of human and fetal blood flow and therefore might yield more direct information on the pathophysiology of vascular insufficiency.

## The Doppler principle

Christian Johann Doppler (1803–1853) studied the light emitted by stars. He observed that the light from a star moving away from the earth turned to red whereas the light of an approaching star turned to blue. In 1842, he postulated that there was a change in the observed colour (frequency) when there was a change in the relative position between the light source and the observer. This shift in the observed frequencies of waves from moving sources is called the Doppler effect or shift.

Buys Ballot (1817–1890) was the first to demonstrate the validity of the Doppler principle for acoustic waves. He demonstrated that the sound

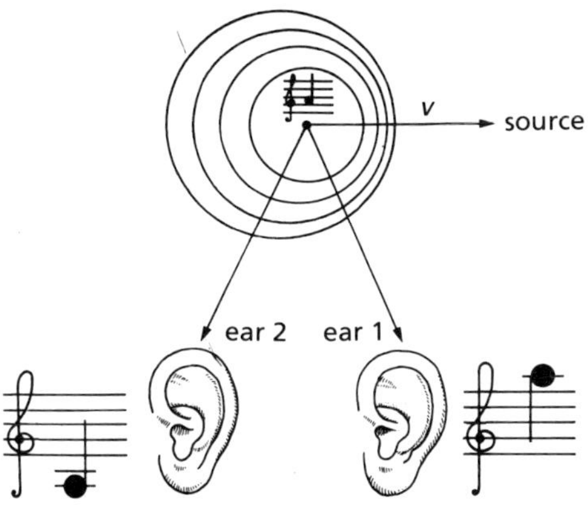


**Fig. 6.3** The Doppler effect. If a source of sound is moving with a velocity *v* the number of wavefronts reaching observer (ear 1) per second increases as the source of the sound approaches the observer and the pitch (tone) of the sound appears to increase. Conversely, a second observer (ear 2) situated away from the direction of sound receives fewer wavefronts per second as the source of sound moves away and the pitch of the sound therefore falls.

of a trumpet player sitting on a moving train and playing a constant pitch was observed to be higher as the train approached and lower after it had passed. The Doppler effect is illustrated in Figure 6.3.

If a Doppler transducer emits a beam of ultrasonic waves into the body, wave reflection occurs at tissue boundaries which have a difference in acoustic impedance. Echoes from stationary boundaries are returned with the same frequency as the emitted beam, whereas echoes from moving particles such as groups of red blood cells undergo a frequency change (Doppler shift) which is proportional to the velocity of the moving particles. The Doppler shift is given by the formula

$$fd = \frac{2fv \cos \theta}{c}$$

where $fd$ is the Doppler shift, $v$ is the velocity of the moving target, $\theta$ is the angle between the ultrasound beam and the direction of movement, $f$ is the transmitted frequency, and c is the velocity of sound in tissue, generally assumed to be 1540 m/s.

It follows that if the ultrasound beam is at right angles to the blood vessel there will be no Doppler shift ($\cos 90° = 0$) and that the maximum Doppler shift occurs at 0°. Doppler shifts from human blood flow are in the order of 0–10 kHz which coincidentally falls within the audible range and can therefore be monitored by a loudspeaker. These audible signals can also be fed into on-line signal processing systems such as the real-time spectrum analyser (Coghlan & Taylor 1976). The visual signal that is produced is known as the flow velocity waveform, each part of which is the result of a spectrum of Doppler shifted signals.

## Doppler equipment

Doppler signals may be obtained by two types of devices:

1 Continuous wave Doppler ultrasound.
2 Pulsed wave Doppler ultrasound.

### Continuous wave Doppler ultrasound

Continuous wave (CW) machines employ two crystals, one for transmitting the signal and one for receiving returning ultrasound waves (Figure 6.4). They usually operate at frequencies ranging between 2–10 MHz. Because it transmits and receives continuously, CW Doppler equipment is unable to discriminate between signals coming from different depths. These machines are simple to operate, easily portable, have low output sound intensities (see later) and are relatively inexpensive.

When using this equipment the operator relies on pattern recognition, which is both audible and visual. Umbilical and uteroplacental vessels have characteristic waveforms both in normal and pathological pregnancies. Continuous wave Doppler is not reliable for studying the fetal aorta or carotid artery.

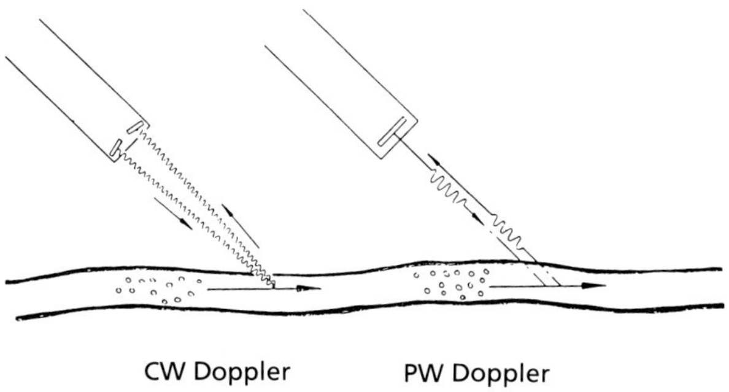


**Fig. 6.4** Continuous wave (CW) Doppler ultrasound employs two crystals in the probe, one for transmitting the signal and one for receiving the returning echo. Pulsed wave (PW) Doppler ultrasound uses only one crystal which is used alternately for transmission and reception.

### Pulsed wave Doppler ultrasound

Pulsed Doppler only uses one crystal which is used alternatively for transmission and reception (Figure 6.4). A short burst of waves are transmitted and then the crystal is switched over to the receiver mode which picks up the returning echoes. The major advantage over continuous wave Doppler ultrasound is that it is capable of separating signals coming from different depths by the positioning of a sample volume. The sample volume may be thought of as a region, some distance in front of the transducer, from which all returning echoes must have originated. In order to place the sample volume within the vessel to be studied, pulsed wave Doppler machines are usually combined to a real-time ultrasound apparatus — a duplex, pulsed Doppler system. Thus the major disadvantages of continuous wave of poor orientation in space and of lack of depth selectivity are overcome by this system. They are however considerably more expensive, less mobile and often have a higher output sound intensity.

Colour flow equipment is the most recently developed method utilizing pulsed Doppler ultrasound. The basic principle was first developed for military use in moving target identification radar. The comparison of consecutive images, based on the subtraction of images obtained from the same area at different intervals is the simplest method for identifying moving objects or reflections. When two subsequent two dimensional images are subtracted, the non-moving reflections vanish and only the subsequent positions of moving reflections appear in the image.

By applying the moving target identification principle using sound waves instead of radio waves blood flow in the heart or large vessels can be displayed. Colour flow mapping displays direction of blood flow in three different formats: Doppler signals away from the transducer are seen in increasing shades of blue; and those towards the transducer are seen in shades of red with a mosaic pattern of red–orange or blue–green representing flow in several directions, suggesting turbulence. The sample volume of the pulsed Doppler equipment can then be accurately placed over the study vessel and the flow velocity waveform displayed.

The value of colour flow mapping has already been recognized in the diagnoses of congenital and acquired heart disease in adults and children and preliminary reports suggest it may be useful in antenatal diagnosis of congenital heart abnormalities (De Vore *et al.* 1987; Kurjak *et al.* 1987).

## Safety of Doppler ultrasound

The question of safety of Doppler ultrasound has been investigated and widely discussed. Biological effects such as cavitation have been described experimentally, but no such effects have ever been described in mammalian tissues exposed to ultrasound intensities below 100 $mW/cm^2$ (spatial peak, temporal average values). The American Institute for Ultrasound in Medicine and the WHO have set a safety standard for maximum power intensity of 100 $mW/cm^2$. There has been no clinical observation of harmful effects of Doppler ultrasound upon the fetus or mother to date. Typical power levels of continuous wave Doppler machines range from 10 to 25 $mW/cm^2$. Pulsed Doppler systems however often produce considerably higher output intensities and the application of pulsed Doppler systems designed for use in other areas of clinical investigation, e.g. adult cardiology should only be used in pregnancy having ensured that the recommended guidelines are satisfied.

## Quantitative flow

Estimation of volume flow in the fetal circulation requires duplex pulsed Doppler equipment. Real-time ultrasound is necessary for visualization of the study vessel and also to allow for measurement of the angle between the study vessel and the insonation beam. As the transmitted frequency ($f$) and speed of sound in tissue are known, once this angle ($\theta$) is estimated blood velocity can be calculated. This is done by positioning an angle bar on the screen parallel to the axis of the vessel.

There are however several inherent problems in flow velocity measurement. The Doppler shift is directly proportional to the cosine of the angle of insonation of the vessel. Experience indicates that accuracy of the order of 3° can be achieved when a reasonable length of straight vessel can be visualized. The effect of this error when the angle is small (e.g. 3 per cent at 30°) is small but it becomes significantly larger at angles greater than 60° (e.g. 16 per cent at 70°).

In order to calculate volume flow the diameter of the vessel must be known. Any errors in vessel diameter measurement will be squared in the volume flow calculation

$$Q = v\pi r^2$$

where $Q$ is the volume flow in ml/min, $v$ is the mean velocity, and $r$ is the radius of the vessel. In addition, pulsatile changes in diameter of approximately 15 per cent occur over the cardiac cycle, all vessels are not entirely circular in cross-section and difficulty exists in measuring the exact diameter of the vessel. To express volume flow in terms of weight (ml/min/kg) estimates of fetal weight are required. These estimates carry an additional 10–15 per cent error.

The potential inaccuracies with Doppler volume flow measurement are discussed in detail elsewhere (Griffin *et al.* 1983b; Eik-Nes *et al.* 1984; Gill 1985).

## Clinical studies

### THE UMBILICAL VEIN

The errors and variations described may result in a cumulative error of up to 50 per cent and clinical use of these measurements are unlikely to be helpful as a result.

Several studies of normal pregnant women have evaluated umbilical venous flow per kilogram. These measurements were made in the third trimester and most agree that third trimester flow per kilogram decreases towards term. The results are summarized in Table 6.1. The average flow per kilogram was 110–120 ml/min/kg which agrees with the classic work by Assali *et al.* (1960).

Jouppila & Kirkinen (1984a,b) and Gill *et al.* (1984) have demonstrated a reduction in flow in growth retarded fetuses. The latter group showed that reduced umbilical venous blood flow was more sensitive than either biparietal diameter and biochemical methods (serum oestriols or human placental lactogen) in the prediction of small-for-gestational

**Table 6.1** Blood flow in the fetal thoracic aorta and umbilical vein (ml/min/kg, mean ±SD)

| Reference | Number of cases | Gestational age (weeks) | Descending aorta | Umbilical vein |
|---|---|---|---|---|
| Eik-Nes *et al.* (1980) | 26 | 32–41 | 191±12* | 110±6* |
| Gill *et al.* (1981) | 47 | 22–35<br>35–40 | | 120±20<br>100±30 |
| Wladimiroff & McGhie (1981) | 4 | 34–40 | 168–179 | |
| Kurjak & Rajhvajn (1982) | 63 | 30–41 | | 107 |
| Joupilla & Kirkinen (1984a) | | 30–40 | | 90–110 |
| Griffin *et al.* (1983a) | 65<br>45 | 28–40 | 277±85 | 122±42 |
| Van Lierde *et al.* (1984a) | 20 | 37–40 | 216±24 | 117±16 |
| Marsal *et al.* (1984a) | 64 | 27–40 | 238±40 | |
| Gill *et al.* (1984) | 95 | 32–40 | | 110–120 |
| Tonge *et al.* (1984) | 33 | 28–40 | 232±78 | |
| Erskine & Ritchie (1985b) | 71 | 28–40 | 206±72 | |
| Eldridge *et al.* (1985) | 18 | 16–40 | 184±35 | |
| Lingman & Marsal (1986a) | 21 | 28–40 | 213–238 | |
| Gerson *et al.* (1987) | 209 | 20<br>30<br>40 | | 153<br>131<br>108 |

* ± SEM

age (SGA) infants. However, neither of these latter methods are particularly sensitive in the prediction of SGA infants.

### THE AORTA

Eik-Nes *et al.* (1980) first reported on Doppler measurements from the fetal descending aorta. Measurements of flow are best obtained from the descending aorta as flow is not turbulent due to absence of branches.

The fetal aortic blood flow, both in the thoracic descending aorta and in the abdominal aorta increases with gestational age up to 36–37 weeks gestation after which a plateau is reached or a slight decrease in flow may occur (Lingman & Marsal 1986a). When related to fetal weight a slight decrease occurs in the last trimester. Table 6.1 summarizes the published data on flow measurements in the aorta.

A study of 159 singleton pregnancies at risk for intrauterine growth retardation (IUGR) showed mean volume blood flow to be lower in growth retarded infants (Laurin *et al.* 1987b). However, the predictive value of quantitative blood flow is poor (Laurin *et al.* 1987a). Similar conclusions were reached by Griffin *et al.* (1983a) and Erskine & Ritchie (1985b). However, peak velocity measurements which are unaffected by vessel diameter and fetal weight estimates may be of clinical value in selected situations, such as rhesus isoimmunization, cardiac arrhythmias (see later) and in monitoring high risk pregnancies. Using cordocentesis in SGA fetuses Soothill *et al.* (1986) demonstrated that a decrease in aortic blood velocity is associated with fetal hypoxia, acidosis, hypercapnoea and hyperlacticaemia. In an attempt to treat the hypoxic growth retarded fetus considered too premature to deliver, the administration of maternal oxygen was associated with a substantial rise in the mean blood velocity in the fetal aorta. These studies nicely complement the work by Peeters *et al.* (1979). They showed that when the inspired oxygen of pregnant sheep is reduced, fetuses are made hypoxic and blood is diverted to the most vital organs such as the brain and heart, and the supply to the rest of the body falls.

Umbilical and aortic volume flow measurements have not achieved widespread popularity because of the necessity of using duplex equipment in addition to the large inherent error in measurements of volume flow. Attention has therefore turned to study of the flow velocity waveform in an attempt to overcome the appreciable methodological errors inherent in quantitative flow measurement.

## Qualitative flow

It quickly became apparent that the maximum frequency outline of the flow velocity waveform (FVW) yielded valuable clinical information.

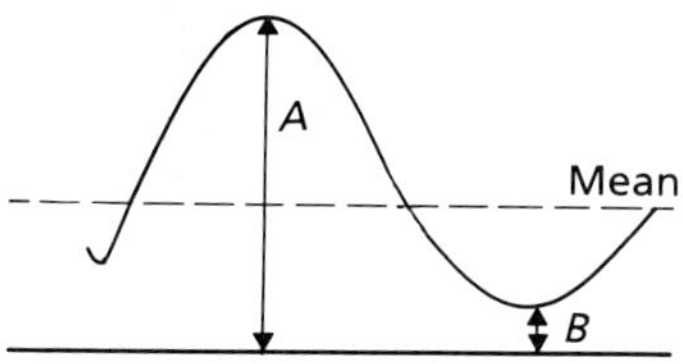


**Fig. 6.5** The indices used to describe the maximum frequency outline.

$\frac{A}{B}$ = A/B ratio (Stuart *et al.* 1980)

$\frac{A - B}{A}$ = Resistance index (Pourcelot 1974)

$\frac{A - B}{\text{Mean}}$ = Pulsatility index (Gosling & King 1975)

The indices used to describe the FVW have been derived from the use of such waveforms in the investigation of peripheral vascular disease and of carotid flow in the adult. The indices used to describe the FVW are illustrated in Figure 6.5. The advantage of utilizing the FVW is that the major sources of error in measurement are removed. All the indices are angle independent as they compare one part of the maximum frequency outline with another and therefore allow comparison between waveforms. Measurement of fetal vessel diameter and weight are unnecessary. All of these indices are readily calculated by computer. It is likely that different methods of analysing waveforms will emerge such as the frequency index profile (Campbell *et al.* 1983) and relative flow index (Thompson *et al.* 1986) which merit further evaluation.

## The flow velocity waveform

The shape of the waveform reflects the pulsatile nature of blood flow in an artery. Fetal cardiac contraction causes a force in the form of pressure to be applied to the blood cells in the aorta and umbilical arteries. A high forward pressure gradient is generated and the blood cells accelerate rapidly producing the rising slope of the waveform. The rate of acceleration depends on the density of the blood, the elasticity of the vessel wall and on the pressure of gradient generated (McDonald 1974). As the pressure gradient moves distally the gradient is reversed, acceleration ceases, the blood reaches its highest systolic velocity (A) and then decelerates resulting in the descending slope of the waveform (Figure 6.5). The velocity at the end of diastole (B) and the rate of deceleration reflect peripheral resistance. Where peripheral resistance is low, as in normal pregnancy in both the uteroplacental and umbilical circulations, forward flow continues throughout diastole whereas in the femoral artery where peripheral resistance is high, forward flow ceases, the waveform descends to the baseline and reverse flow may occur during part of diastole.

## Other factors affecting the flow velocity waveform

### HEART RATE

If the heart rate slows then the value of the end-diastolic frequency is likely to fall, giving a corresponding increase in A/B ratio, resistance index (RI) and pulsatility index (PI). Conversely, if the fetal heart rate accelerates the end-diastolic frequencies may increase thus lowering the A/B, RI and PI. Several studies addressing the relation between fetal heart rate (FHR) and FVW have recently been published.

In the fetal circulation Mires *et al.* (1987) reported a significant negative correlation ($r = -0.49$) between umbilical artery A/B ratio and instantaneous fetal heart rate and suggested that A/B ratios should be corrected for FHR even within the normal range (120–160 b.p.m.). Other studies however have suggested that umbilical artery A/B ratios were independent of fetal heart rate within the normal range (Thompson *et al.* 1986, 1988a; Gagnon *et al.* 1988; Gudmundsson & Marsal 1988a). However the A/B ratio is likely to be lowered in the presence of fetal tachycardia (>160 b.p.m.) and elevated in the presence of fetal bradycardia (<120 b.p.m.).

On the maternal side, heart rate does not appear to significantly alter the uteroplacental waveforms over the clinically normal range (Pearce 1987).

### FETAL BREATHING

Fetal respiratory movements profoundly affect the peak systolic and diastolic frequencies in addition to altering the length of the cardiac cycle. The flow velocity in the fetal aorta significantly increased during fetal breathing movements (Marsal *et al.* 1984a). Therefore, flow velocity waveforms should only be recorded during fetal apnoea.

### BLOOD VISCOSITY

There appears to be an increase in the A/B ratio with an increase in whole blood viscosity at high shear but not at low shear rates (Giles & Trudinger 1986). In the maternal circulation however small changes in viscosity do not appear to influence the flow velocity waveform (Steel *et al.* 1988a) suggesting that changes in vascular architecture are more important. Similar conclusions were reached by the same group when studying the fetal circulation (Steel *et al.* 1988b).

### BEHAVIOURAL STATES

There is now clear evidence for the existence of behavioural states in the human fetus in late pregnancy (Nijhuis *et al.* 1982). The relationship between aortic, umbilical and carotid artery FVW in different behavioural states in both normal and abnormal pregnancies has been investigated (Van Eyck *et al.* 1985, 1986, 1987, 1988). Based on the marked changes in fetal heart rate patterns and incidence of fetal body movements between different behavioural states, it is likely that these changes are associated with alterations in fetal cardiovascular performance and peripheral resistance which may affect the FVW; therefore Doppler studies should probably be performed in the absence of body movements to allow for direct comparison between studies.

### TYPE OF EQUIPMENT

Several studies have compared pulsed and continuous wave Doppler ultrasound and have demonstrated no differences in indices obtained from FVW of the umbilical artery (Brar *et al.* 1988a; Mehalek *et al.* 1988; Van Vugt *et al.* 1988) between the two methods.

## Which index?

There is no real consensus as to which index yields the most information. The A/B ratio, PI and RI are very highly correlated (Thompson *et al.* 1986, 1988b; Mulders *et al.* 1987; Pearce *et al.* 1988). For RI and A/B ratio this is not suprising as they are related by the equation A/B = (1/1 − RI). In the clinical setting it is unlikely that one index offers any clear advantage over the others.

In the study of the aortic blood FVW the diastolic part has the best predictive capacity and some groups have described the FVW based on whether frequencies are present or absent in end-diastole (Laurin *et al.* 1987a; Marsal & Persson 1988). In the absence of end-diastolic frequencies (EDF) the A/B ratio becomes infinity whilst the RI becomes unity. It is therefore both logical and effective to simply report that there is loss of end-diastolic frequencies.

## The umbilical artery in normal pregnancy

The umbilical artery is the most studied vessel in the fetal circulation because of the ease in obtaining waveforms with inexpensive, continuous wave equipment. Reference ranges for changes in indices with gestational age have been published by many groups (Stuart *et al.* 1980; Fitzgerald *et al.* 1984; Reuwer *et al.* 1984; Schulman *et al.* 1984; Erskine & Ritchie 1985a; Trudinger *et al.* 1985a; Pearce 1987; Van Vugt *et al.* 1987; Wladimiroff *et al.* 1987; Al-Ghazali *et al.* 1988; Gudmundsson & Marsal 1988a; Thompson *et al.* 1988a).

Although there are minor differences, all indices show remarkable stability in all studies, with all three indices (A/B, PI and RI) showing a decrease with advancing gestational age in normal pregnancy. This decrease in indices indicates a reduction in placental peripheral resistance

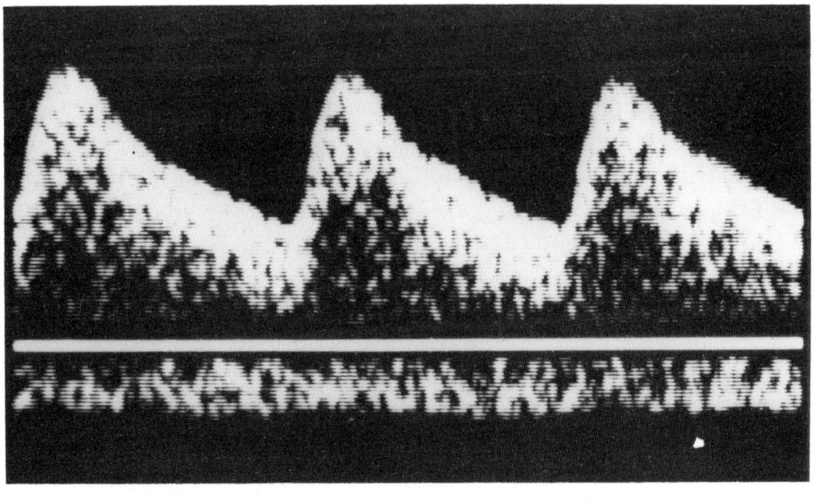

**Fig. 6.6** A normal flow velocity waveform from the umbilical artery.

probably at the level of the arterioles of the tertiary stem villi (Dawes 1968). Development of such vessels is known to continue well into the third trimester (Gruenwald 1972; Kaufman *et al.* 1979) and probably accounts for the reduction in peripheral resistance.

The normal umbilical artery flow velocity waveform is characterized by high end-diastolic frequencies in relation to peak systolic frequencies and is illustrated in Figure 6.6.

## The umbilical artery in complicated pregnancies

It quickly became apparent that waveforms obtained from compromised fetuses were characterized by low end-diastolic frequencies (McCallum *et al.* 1978; Stuart *et al.* 1980; Fitzgerald *et al.* 1984; Schulman *et al.* 1984). Most of the published work has assessed the ability of abnormal umbilical artery FVW to predict small-for-gestational age fetuses. This is not an ideal endpoint to evaluate a new technique, but undoubtedly identifies a group with a significantly higher perinatal mortality rate than appropriately grown fetuses (Dobson *et al.* 1981).

When applied to a mixed risk or high risk group an abnormal umbilical artery FVW identifies SGA fetuses with a sensitivity of 45–87 per cent depending on the prevalance of the condition (Table 6.2). The wide range in sensitivity and specificity values may be partly explained by different study populations, use of different birth weight nomograms, varying study to delivery intervals and different cut-off points to define abnormality.

Sensitivity and specificities are directly related to prevalence and when umbilical artery FVW were used to predict SGA/IUGR fetuses, in a large unselected group of 2097 pregnancies where the prevalence of these complications is considerably less than the studies outlined in Table 6.1, disappointing results were obtained (Beattie *et al.* 1988). The sensitivity was 20–31 per cent, specificity 85–94 per cent and positive predictive value 10–15 per cent.

It seems likely that umbilical artery velocimetry offers no major advantages over ultrasound in the prediction of SGA/IUGR fetuses. Indeed, the use of the ratio of two morphological measurements using ultrasound gives a more impressive prediction of the SGA fetus (Neilson *et al.* 1980). Several studies directly comparing ultrasound with Doppler studies have been recently published. Although Gaziano *et al.* (1988) demonstrated that Doppler studies were as good as ultrasound in the prediction of SGA two further studies showed real-time ultrasound to be a better predictor of the SGA fetus (Berkowitz *et al.* 1988a; Divon *et al.* 1988).

It is likely that Doppler studies of the umbilical artery will be more useful applied as a secondary screening test in those pregnancies identified by real-time ultrasound as being SGA or growth retarded (Berkowitz *et al.* 1988b). Better predictive values were obtained by several groups when Doppler studies were used to recognize various different measures of morbidity. These studies are listed in Table 6.3.

Abnormal umbilical artery FVW have been demonstrated to predate

**Table 6.2** Summary of published data on abnormal umbilical artery A/B ratios in the prediction of SGA

| Reference | Number and type | Outcome variable | Prevalence (per cent) | Sensitivity (per cent) | Specificity (per cent) | Predictive value positive test (per cent) | Kappa |
|---|---|---|---|---|---|---|---|
| Fitzgerald *et al.* (1984) | 221 mixed | Birth weight <10th centile | 10 | 77 | | | |
| Trudinger *et al.* (1985a) | 136 high risk | Birth weight <10th centile | 32 | 74 | 74 | 57 | 0.45 |
| Fleischer *et al.* (1985) | 189 mixed | Birth weight <10th centile | 17<br>31 | 78<br>87 | 83<br>81 | 49<br>67 | 0.50<br>0.63 |
| Trudinger *et al.* (1986) | 170 high risk | Birth weight <10th centile | 28 | 66 | 85 | 62 | 0.50 |
| | | Birth weight <5th centile | 14 | 71 | 77 | 34 | 0.33 |
| Arduini *et al.* (1987a) | 75 high risk | Birth weight <10th centile | 31 | 61 | 73 | 50 | 0.32 |
| Van Vugt *et al.* (1987) | 36 mixed | IUGR | 25 | 78 | 82 | 58 | 0.53 |
| Berkowitz *et al.* (1988a) | 168 high risk | Birth weight <10th centile | 25 | 45 | 89 | 58 | 0.35 |
| Divon *et al.* (1988) | 127 high risk | Birth weight <10th centile | 35 | 49 | 94 | 81 | 0.41 |

The Kappa index is a ratio denoting observed accuracy beyond chance. The index has a maximum value of 1.0; values above 0.8 suggest almost perfect agreement between test results and actual clinical state, values between 0.2 and 0.8 reflect fairly good agreement, and values below 0.2 suggest agreement by chance only.

**Table 6.3** Summary of published data on abnormal umbilical artery A/B ratios on adverse outcome

| Reference | Number and type | Outcome variable | Prevalence (per cent) | Sensitivity (per cent) | Specificity (per cent) | Predictive value positive test (per cent) | Kappa |
|---|---|---|---|---|---|---|---|
| Reuwer *et al.* (1987) | 46 high risk | IUGR | 61 | 100 | 89 | 93 | 0.91 |
| | | Fetal distress | 61 | 100 | 89 | 93 | 0.91 |
| | | IUD | | | | | |
| Rochelson *et al.* (1987a) | 54 | Abnormal CTG | 50 | 96 | 42 | 62 | 0.38 |
| | All <10th centile | PIH | 44 | 93 | 29 | 50 | 0.19 |
| | | CS (fetal distress) | 43 | 96 | 35 | 52 | 0.28 |
| | | NICU | 69 | 95 | 59 | 83 | 0.58 |
| | | IPPV | 24 | 100 | 29 | 31 | 0.17 |
| | | PMN | 1 | 100 | 25 | 14 | 0.07 |
| Marsal & Persson (1988) | 58 high risk | ODFD | 31 | 83 | 80 | 65 | 0.59 |

IUGR = birth weight <5th centile and/or ponderal index of <2.32 (ponderal index = weight/length$^2$).
IUD = intrauterine death.
PIH = pregnancy-induced hypertension.
CS = Caesarean section.
NICU = neonatal intensive care unit admission.
IPPV = intermittent positive pressure ventilation.
PNM = perinatal mortality.
ODFD = operative del. for fetal distress.

the onset of abnormal cardiotocography (CTG) in several studies, by up to 3–4 weeks (Schulman *et al.* 1984; Trudinger *et al.* 1985c, 1986; Reuwer *et al.* 1987; Rochelson *et al.* 1987a; Cameron *et al.* 1988; Haddad *et al.* 1988) and although Gilcs *et al.* (1986) showed that adverse fetal outcome was more efficiently predicted by the study of umbilical artery FVW when compared with CTG, further longitudinal studies are needed to establish the relationship between CTG and umbilical artery FVW. It is likely that Doppler studies will be of benefit in identifying truly compromised fetuses by reducing the number of false positive CTG as suggested by Farmakides *et al.* (1988a).

Having established a strong association between abnormal umbilical artery FVW and adverse perinatal outcome, before recommending its widespread introduction, prospective, randomized controlled trials need to be performed. To date only one such study on umbilical artery FVW alone has been reported. This study did not demonstrate that knowledge of Doppler waveforms improved morbidity or mortality but the authors suggested that they led to better obstetric decision making (Trudinger *et al.* 1987b).

## Loss of end-diastolic frequencies

This condition exists when the peripheral resistance in the placenta is increased to such an extent that forward flow through the umbilical artery is not achieved throughout the entire cardiac cycle (Figure 6.7) allowing less time for gaseous exchange. A more extreme abnormality exists when placental resistance is so high that flow in diastole is reversed; that is, blood flows back to the fetus. The loss of end-diastolic frequencies (EDF) is nearly always associated with abnormal pregnancy; however, it does not always indicate that the fetus is at immediate risk. Several cases

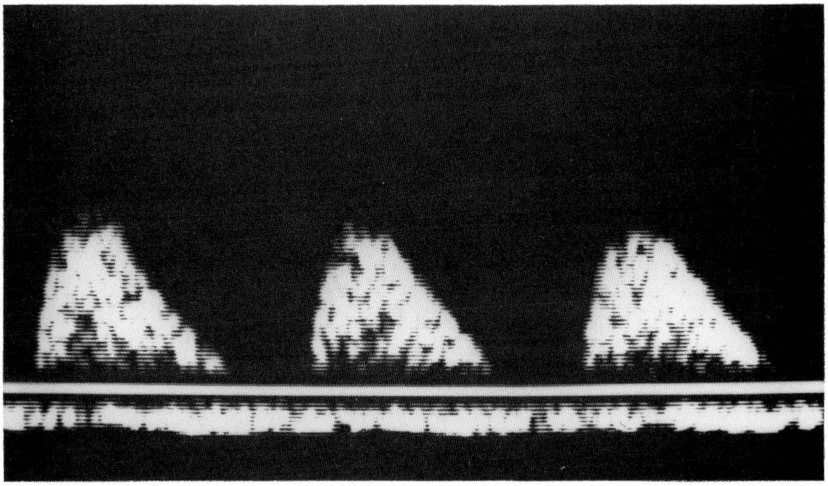

**Fig. 6.7** A flow velocity waveform from the umbilical artery demonstrating loss of end-diastolic frequencies.

of absent EDF for up to 6 weeks prior to delivery with good outcomes have been described (Johnstone *et al.* 1988). Thus delivery on the basis of absent EDF in the umbilical artery may not always be indicated as suggested by Woo *et al.* (1987a). Such a policy will result in unnecessary morbidity and mortality as a result of prematurity in some cases.

Further direct evidence that this represents a high risk situation has recently been published. Nicolaides *et al.* (1988) reported that only 7 (12 per cent) of 59 fetuses who were SGA with loss of EDF in the umbilical artery had normal oxygen tension and pH when umbilical venous blood was sampled using cordocentesis. The remainder (88 per cent) were either hypoxic or acidotic or both.

Table 6.4 summarizes the published data on pregnancies complicated by absence or reversal of EDF and undoubtedly identifies a very high risk fetus requiring intense fetal surveillance and in many cases, early delivery.

### Pathological correlation with umbilical waveforms

Giles *et al.* (1985a) have demonstrated a pathological basis to relate umbilical artery FVW and peripheral resistance. They reported a correlation between A/B ratios and placental microvascular anatomy. The modal counts of small muscular arteries in tertiary stem villi were significantly lower in patients with risk factors and an abnormally high A/B ratio when compared with patients who had similar risk factors and normal A/B ratios and with patients without risk factors who had normal A/B ratios. The tertiary stem villus counts did not vary between the groups. Similar findings have also been reported by McCowan *et al.* (1987b). Thus umbilical artery FVW appear to identify a specific placental lesion of vascular spasm and possible obliteration of the small muscular arteries of the tertiary stem villi.

## The uteroplacental circulation

In normal pregnancy, Doppler studies of the uteroplacental circulation show an increase in diastolic frequencies with advancing gestation up to about 22–24 weeks (Schulman *et al.* 1986; Pearce *et al.* 1988). This suggests a reduction in peripheral resistance and probably represents physiological trophoblastic invasion in the spiral arteries. A normal uteroplacental waveform is illustrated in Figure 6.8.

There is broad agreement amongst reported reference ranges although differences in methodology makes direct comparison difficult (Trudinger *et al.* 1985b; Schulman *et al.* 1986, 1987; Gudmundsson & Marsal 1988b; McCowan *et al.* 1988; Pearce *et al.* 1988; Rudelstorfer *et al.* 1988). There is however a difference between values obtained from vessels directly beneath the placenta and those on the opposite side of the placental site (Pearce *et al.* 1988). This may explain why average values obtained by Trudinger *et al.* (1985b) were lower as they obtained waveforms from

**Table 6.4** Summary of published data on fetuses with absent or reverse EDF in the umbilical artery

| Reference | Number | IUGR | Hypertension | Perinatal deaths | Comment |
|---|---|---|---|---|---|
| Fitzgerald *et al.* (1984) | 13 | 13 (100%) | — | 1 (10%) | |
| Erskine & Ritchie (1985a) | 2 | 2 (100%) | — | 1 (50%) | 1 IUD at 29/40 |
| Trudinger *et al.* (1985c) | 10 | — | — | 1 (10%) | All fetuses delivered before 32 weeks because of abnormal tests of fetal well-being |
| Rochelson *et al.* (1987b) | 15 | 8 (53%) | 11 (73%) | 8 (53%) | All 15 had evidence of hypoxia |
| Reuwer *et al.* (1987) | 17 | 17 (100%) | | 4 (24%) | 3 IUDs remaining 14 Caesarean section for fetal distress in labour |
| Woo *et al.* (1987a) | 9 | 6 (67%) | 5 (56%) | 8 (89%) | |
| McCowan *et al.* (1987a) | 8 | 8 (100%) | 5 (63%) | 3 (38%) | |
| Reed *et al.* (1987) | 14 | 11 (78%) | | 6 (42%) | 100% perinatal morbidity 57% Caesarean section for fetal distress |
| Arabin *et al.* (1988) | 30 | 30 (100%) | | 6 (20%) | 87% Caesarean section rate |
| Brar & Platt (1988) | 12 | 12 (100%) | 4 (25%) | 6 (50%) | All 12 reverse flow |
| Johnstone *et al.* (1988) | 24 | 22 (92%) | 17 (71%) | 4 (17%) | 83% Caesarean section rate |
| *Total* | 154 | 129/144 (90%) | 42/68 (62%) | 48/154 (31%) | |

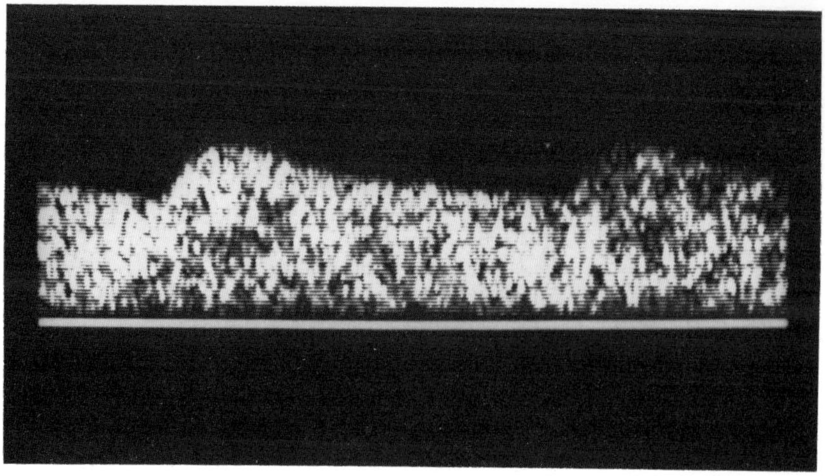

**Fig. 6.8** A normal flow velocity waveform from the uteroplacental circulation.

retroplacental vessels only. Others have averaged values obtained from either side of the uterus leaving the mean slightly above the mean on the placental side as defined by Pearce *et al.* (1988).

Flow velocity waveforms from the uteroplacental circulation appear to yield useful information in pregnancies complicated by hypertension and possibly IUGR. Several studies have shown an association between abnormal uteroplacental FVW (Figure 6.9) and adverse pregnancy outcome (Campbell *et al.* 1983; Fleischer *et al.* 1986). Campbell's group showed that pregnancy outcome was significantly worse in those patients with IUGR and hypertension with abnormal uteroplacental waveforms when compared to a similar group with normal waveforms. In a similar study of 71 hypertensive patients uteroplacental waveforms clearly divided the patients into normal and abnormal groups (Fleischer *et al.* 1986). Patients with abnormal FVW were more likely to develop an abnormal CTG, be delivered prematurely or to have a SGA infant at highly significant levels ($P < 0.001$). They suggested that uteroplacental waveforms accurately describe the pathophysiology of the uteroplacental circulation in that the positive and negative predictive values for pregnancy outcome were both more than 90 per cent.

Recently, a controversial case controlled study showed no significant differences in pulsatility index between hypertensive and normal pregnancies (Hanretty *et al.* 1988). This finding is probably explained mainly by the choice of the FVW with the lowest resistance to describe the uteroplacental circulation as opposed to the studies described which chose the waveform demonstrating the highest resistance or an average of the highest values obtained from both sides of the uterus. The most predictive FVW to use is probably the one with the highest resistance (Campbell *et al.* 1988).

Pearce (1987) has demonstrated that uteroplacental waveforms probably reflect the depth of trophoblastic invasion. He obtained placental bed

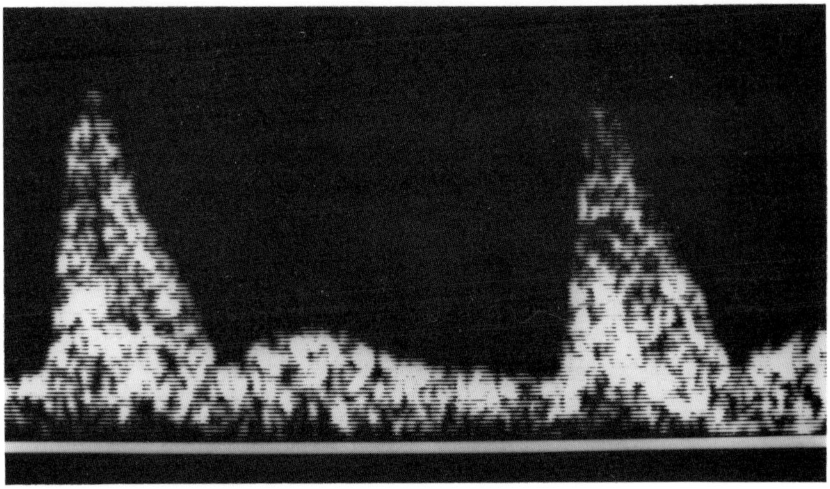

**Fig. 6.9** An abnormal flow velocity waveform from the uteroplacental circulation.

biopsies at Caesarean section in patients who had Doppler studies of the uteroplacental circulation performed in the preceding 24 hours. There was a highly significant difference in the resistance indices between those patients with pathological and physiological invasion in cases of pregnancy-induced hypertension.

As trophoblastic invasion is usually completed by 22 weeks (Brosens *et al.* 1967), it is theoretically possible that abnormal uteroplacental FVW that persist after this time may predict pregnancies at risk of developing complications resulting from inadequate uteroplacental perfusion. Several groups have performed studies to assess the potential role of uteroplacental waveforms as a screening test for IUGR and pregnancy-induced hypertension (PIH). The results are summarized in Table 6.5. These results suggest that uteroplacental waveforms obtained before 24 weeks identifies the majority of pregnancies that will subsequently become abnormal. In the largest study the prediction of pregnancy-induced hypertension alone was poor but nearly all cases of complicated PIH were identified (Steel *et al.* 1988b). These findings now offer the possibility of therapeutic intervention aimed at prevention.

## Aortic flow velocity waveforms in abnormal pregnancy

Qualitative analysis of FVW has been shown to be a better predictor of fetal outcome than quantitative analysis (Laurin *et al.* 1987a). In cases complicated by IUGR there is an increase in the pulsatility index obtained from the descending aorta (Griffin *et al.* 1984; Joupilla & Kirkinen 1984b, 1986; Tonge *et al.* 1986; Laurin *et al.* 1987a). The latter group defined four blood flow classes based on a combination of the pulsatility index and whether EDF were present or not. The absence of EDF was the best predictor of adverse fetal outcome. This confirmed previous suggestions that absent EDF in the aorta reflects fetal compromise. Jouppila & Kirkinen

**Table 6.5** Summary of published data on the ability of uteroplacental flow velocity waveforms to predict pregnancy-induced hypertension/IUGR

| Reference | Gestation weeks | Number of cases | Outcome measure | Sensitivity (per cent) | Specificity (per cent) | Predictive value | | Kappa |
|---|---|---|---|---|---|---|---|---|
| | | | | | | Positive (per cent) | Negative (per cent) | |
| Campbell *et al.* (1986) | 16–18 | 126 unselected | PIH and/or IUGR and/or fetal asphyxia | 68 | 69 | 42 | 87 | 0.31 |
| Arduini *et al.* (1987b) | 18–20 | 68 high risk | PIH | 64 | 84 | 70 | 80 | 0.48 |
| Mulders *et al.* (1988) | <32 | 73 unselected | SGA and/or fetal distress | 30 | 90 | 58 | 74 | 0.24 |
| Steel *et al.* (1988b) | 22–24 | 200 unselected | PIH with proteinuria and IUGR | 100 | 90 | 19 | 100 | 0.3 |

(1984b) described the absence of EDF in the aorta in nine pregnancies with evidence of chronic fetal hypoxia. In a group of growth retarded fetuses the absence of EDF in the aorta was associated with a higher incidence of Caesarean section for fetal distress, lower birth weight infants and a higher perinatal mortality and morbidity when compared with a well matched group but where EDF in the aorta was still present (Hackett *et al.* 1987a). The presence of reverse flow appears to represent very severe fetal compromise. Illyes & Gati (1988) described five fetuses with reverse diastolic frequencies in the aorta; all five died *in utero* within 24 hours.

Like the umbilical artery, abnormal aortic FVW may predate cardiotocographic abnormalities by up to several weeks (Griffin *et al.* 1984; Jouppila & Kirkinen 1984b; Laurin *et al.* 1987a, b; Cameron *et al.* 1988).

In summary, characteristic changes of the aortic FVW occur in compromised fetuses. The absence of EDF is the best indicator of fetal status. Although requiring pulsed Doppler ultrasound aortic FVW may prove to be a useful method of monitoring fetuses at risk of developing fetal distress and may also provide a method of monitoring circulatory responses to potential therapies.

### The fetal cerebral circulation

Pulsed Doppler ultrasound in combination with real-time ultrasound is required to study the carotid circulation. The common carotid (Marsal *et al.* 1984b), internal carotid (Wladimiroff *et al.* 1986) and middle cerebral artery (Kirkinen *et al.* 1987; Woo *et al.* 1987b) have been studied in the human. In normal pregnancy, waveforms from the internal carotid artery (ICA) are highly pulsatile but with continuous forward flow throughout the cardiac cycle. The pulsatility index in the fetal ICA in normal pregnancy remains fairly constant during the last trimester.

Blood flow to the brain has been shown, in fetal lambs, to increase with decreasing oxygen tension (Cohn *et al.* 1974; Kjellmer *et al.* 1974; Peeters *et al.* 1979). Similar changes appear to occur in the human in that, in cases complicated by IUGR, there is an increase in the diastolic flow component in the ICA thus lowering the PI (Wladimiroff *et al.* 1986). This lowering of the PI also occurs in the middle cerebral arteries (Kirkinen *et al.* 1987; Woo *et al.* 1987b). This suggests an increased peripheral vascular resistance with a compensatory increase in cerebral blood flow secondary to a lowering of the cerebral vascular resistance. These findings would also explain the well-known head sparing effect that occurs in growth retardation.

### Combined studies

Few studies have taken the logical approach of studying both the fetal and maternal circulations. As the fetal placenta is nourished by the maternal uteroplacental circulation it might be expected that knowledge of waveforms from both circulations would provide more information in complicated pregnancies.

Campbell *et al.* (1984) divided high risk patients into four groups based on whether the umbilical circulation was normal or abnormal and in each case whether the uteroplacental circulation was normal or abnormal. The worst perinatal outcome was observed when both circulations were abnormal. These findings were confirmed in further studies using a similar approach (Trudinger *et al.* 1985a; Ducey *et al.* 1987). The latter group suggested that hypertensive pregnancies should be classified on the basis of Doppler studies of both circulations because they so clearly identified those pregnancies at high risk of a poor outcome.

Recently, preliminary results of a randomized controlled trial of 509 pregnancies complicated by either hypertension or IUGR or both have been reported (McParland & Pearce 1988). On admission to hospital, patients were randomized into concealed or revealed (Doppler data made available to the clinician) groups. There was a significant reduction in perinatal deaths in the revealed group. As both groups were well matched this suggests that knowledge of abnormal waveforms from both circulations improved decision making with a resulting improved outcome. Conversely, in patients with normal waveforms from both circulations, knowledge of the Doppler data allowed clinicians to adopt a more conservative approach resulting in delivery being advantageously delayed by one week largely as a result of a lower induction rate. In addition antenatal hospitalization was significantly reduced (25.0 vs. 10.5 days) in the revealed group.

Doppler studies of both circulations have also been suggested to be beneficial in patients with severe second trimester oligohydramnios. The uteroplacental waveform is usually abnormal where oligohydramnios is associated with severe IUGR suggesting abnormal uteroplacental perfusion whereas when the uteroplacental waveforms were normal, oligohydramnios was associated with premature rupture of the membranes or was secondary to a renal abnormality (Hackett *et al.* 1987b).

## Other potential clinical applications

### Twin pregnancy

Doppler studies of the umbilical artery may be of use in monitoring twin pregnancies. When umbilical artery FVW have been studied a combination of real-time ultrasound and Doppler ultrasound are necessary in order to match the umbilical artery FVW with the appropriate fetus.

Although twins may have different growth rates the reference range for the A/B ratio for both twins is the same as for singleton pregnancies (Gerson *et al.* 1988). If both fetuses have normal umbilical artery FVW they are likely to achieve their full growth potential (Giles *et al.* 1985b). Table 6.6 outlines the published data on the ability of Doppler studies to predict adverse outcome. The studies are not directly comparable because

**Table 6.6** Summary of the published data on umbilical artery flow velocity waveforms and outcome in twin pregnancies

| Reference | Number of cases | Abnormal test | Outcome measure | Sensitivity (per cent) | Specificity (per cent) | Predictive value: Positive (per cent) | Predictive value: Negative (per cent) | Kappa |
|---|---|---|---|---|---|---|---|---|
| Giles *et al.* (1985b) | 71 | A/B >95th centile | SGA <10th centile | 70 | 72 | 72 | 70 | 0.42 |
| Farmakides *et al.* (1985) | 43 | A/B difference >0.4 | Birth weight difference >349 g | 73 | 82 | 69 | 85 | 0.55 |
| Saldana *et al.* (1985) | 68 | A/B difference >0.4 | Birth weight difference >349 g | 78 | 80 | 58 | 91 | 0.52 |
| Nimrod *et al.* (1987) | 30 | A/B difference >50% | Preterm delivery or birth weight difference >500 g, or SGA <10th centile, or admission to NICU | 50 | 82 | | | |

of differing criteria used to define abnormality and differing outcome measures but overall suggest that Doppler studies in twin pregnancy demonstrate acceptable values in predicting twin pregnancies with discordant growth or resulting in a SGA fetus.

Giles *et al.* (1985b) suggested that twin to twin transfusion syndrome (TTS) should be strongly suspected if a discrepancy in ultrasound size is found in the presence of two A/B ratios with similar values. However, a discrepancy in A/B values in a case of TTS has been reported (Erskine *et al.* 1986). Many factors are involved in TTS including the major vessel anatomy, the type and size of anastomotic beds and the relative cardiac outputs which probably explain the wide range of Doppler findings in eight cases of TTS described by Pretorius *et al.* (1988). Doppler studies are unlikely to be of clinical usefulness in diagnosing twin pregnancies with TTS but may well suggest that pathology exists and close evaluation is warranted.

## Labour

Qualitative assessment of uteroplacental and umbilical artery FVW in labouring patients has seen reported (Stuart *et al.* 1981; Janbu *et al.* 1985; Fleischer *et al.* 1987; Brar *et al.* 1988b). These studies suggest that placental resistance to umbilical flow is not affected by uterine contractions. In the uteroplacental circulation, as might be expected a reduction in flow was observed during uterine contraction. At present Doppler studies in labour have not been demonstrated to have a clinical role.

## Diabetes

Two studies have reported on the application of umbilical artery FVW in pregnancies complicated by diabetes. An elevated A/B ratio was associated with an increased incidence of stillbirths and neonatal morbidity (Bracero *et al.* 1986). In this study a positive correlation between the A/B ratio and serum glucose levels was demonstrated. Olofsson *et al.* (1987) reported Doppler data on 40 diabetic pregnancies. There was no difference in blood flow indices between poorly controlled and well controlled diabetic women. However, fetuses were more likely to become distressed in labour when there was an abnormal umbilical artery FVW. Although these authors recommend that Doppler studies should be performed in diabetic pregnancies as a method of fetal surveillance, the evidence that this will be beneficial is as yet unconvincing.

## Post-date pregnancies

Two small studies evaluating the role of umbilical artery FVW in pregnancies exceeding 41 weeks concluded that there was no difference in A/B ratios between those with or without complications and was therefore unlikely to be of benefit (Guidetti *et al.* 1987; Farmakides *et al.*

1988b). However, Rightmire & Campbell (1987) found umbilical artery resistance to be raised in post-date pregnancies (>42 weeks gestation) in which the ensuing labour was stressful to the fetus. A large study of 534 pregnancies exceeding 42 weeks concluded that abnormal umbilical artery FVW with end-diastolic frequencies were not predictive of fetal compromise; however, where there was absence of EDF this was highly predictive of fetal distress occurring in early labour requiring Caesarean section (Pearce & McParland 1988b).

## Rhesus disease

In Rhesus-isoimmunized pregnancies the fetus suffers from a progressive anaemia due to red cell destruction. Compensatory mechanisms probably include an increased cardiac output. It has been suggested that Doppler ultrasound studies might reflect the hyperdynamic cardiovascular changes that occur. High fetal umbilical venous blood flow rates have been reported in pregnancies complicated by Rhesus immunization (Kirkinen *et al.* 1983; Gill *et al.* 1984; Jouppila & Kirkinen 1984a). Furthermore, a significant negative correlation between umbilical vein blood flow and the cord haemoglobin level of the newborn infant indicated that flow may reflect the degree of anaemia (Kirkinen *et al.* 1983). Increased umbilical venous blood flow rates have been shown to be associated with increased perinatal mortality and morbidity (Gill *et al.* 1984). Rightmire *et al.* (1986) described the mean velocities from the thoracic aorta and found a significant negative correlation with haematocrit levels in affected fetuses.

It would appear that the anaemic fetus can maintain tissue oxygenation by means of a hyperdynamic circulation until the haemoglobin falls to less than 4 g/dl (Bilardo *et al.* 1986), when decompensation may occur with the onset of hydrops fetalis. Knowledge of fetal blood flow values should prove to be useful in monitoring the progress and evaluation of intrauterine transfusion in cases of moderate to severe Rhesus isoimmunization.

## Cardiac arrhythmias

Doppler ultrasound provides invaluable help in the diagnosis of fetal cardiac arrhythmias (Marsal *et al.* 1984a; Tonge *et al.* 1984, 1986; Lingman & Marsal 1986b). These fetuses have a high perinatal morbidity and mortality. Prior to the availability of Doppler ultrasound, diagnoses were made with M-mode electrocardiography or transabdominal fetal ECG study, both methods having limitations. The type of arrhythmia can often be diagnosed on the basis of simultaneous aortic and inferior vena caval Doppler recordings as they reflect ventricular and atrial events respectively.

It appears that large changes in fetal heart rate can be tolerated with the fetus maintaining a normal blood flow (Frank Starling effect) without developing cardiac failure. The functional limits of the fetal myocardium appear to be between 50 and 250 b.p.m. Outside of this range there is a fall off in aortic stroke volume and blood flow (Tonge *et al.* 1984). Aortic volume flow or velocity estimations can probably detect imminent fetal cardiac failure. With the increase in the diagnosis of fetal cardiac arrhythmias attempts at *in utero* therapy have become commonplace. The effects of drug therapy can be monitored and the optimal timing of delivery decided, with the help of Doppler findings.

### The effect of drugs

The potential of Doppler ultrasound to study the possible pharmacological effects on the fetal and uteroplacental circulation has begun to result in many early reports. The potential for studying these responses is enormous and may result in improved and more rational therapy.

The effects of various agents on uteroplacental and fetal blood flow have already been assessed in different clinical areas. Such agents include antihypertensive drugs, maternal oxygen, epidural and spinal anaesthesia, tocolytic agents, smoking (nicotine) and prostaglandins. The effect of posture and exercise has also recently been reported. Many of these studies are preliminary and we look forward to a wealth of literature over the next few years to provide us with useful information on the effect, on both uteroplacental and fetal circulations of drugs commonly used in pregnancy and labour that hitherto have been poorly understood.

## Conclusion

Doppler ultrasound provides a safe non-invasive method of studying blood flow in pregnancy. The inherent errors associated with quantitative flow, together with the need for pulsed Doppler apparatus has turned attention to qualitative analysis of the flow velocity waveform. Detailed studies of the evolution of changes of waveforms from the uteroplacental and fetal circulations should help to elucidate the pathophysiology of many complicated pregnancies and therefore improve the management of such high risk pregnancies. Abnormal umbilical artery FVW are more useful in predicting adverse fetal outcome than predicting the SGA or IUGR fetus. The loss of end-diastolic frequencies represents a very high risk situation and although the detection of this abnormality does not as yet clearly indicate the optimal time for intervention, many will require early delivery. Abnormal uteroplacental FVW appears to identify the compromised pregnancy at an earlier gestation than current methods offering the possibility of early therapeutic intervention.

Doppler ultrasound should prove invaluable in studying the effects of drugs and other therapeutic measures on both the fetal and maternal circulation and should therefore lead to more logical and rational therapy in complicated pregnancies.

There is an urgent need to standardize Doppler terminology to allow direct comparison of studies that are being carried out in an increasing number of centres. More sensitive methods of describing the information contained in the flow velocity waveform are necessary. Large longitudinal studies are needed to detect a predictable sequence of events and randomized controlled trials probably on a multi-centre basis are required to determine whether intervention based on Doppler findings actually improves outcome or, at least, improves obstetric decision making.

## References

Ahlquist R.P. (1950) The action of various drugs on the arterial blood flow of the pregnant canine uterus. *Journal of the American Pharmacology Association*, **39**, 370–3.

Al-Ghazali W., Chapman M.G. & Allan L.D. (1988) Doppler assessment of the cardiac and uteroplacental circulations in normal and complicated pregnancies *British Journal of Obstetrics and Gynaecology*, **95**, 575–80.

Arabin B., Siebert M., Jimenez E. & Saling E. (1988) Obstetrical characteristics of a loss of end-diastolic velocities in the fetal aorta and/or umbilical artery using Doppler ultrasound. *Gynecologic and Obstetric Investigation*, **25**, 173–80.

Arduini D., Rizzo G., Romanini C. & Mancuso S. (1987a) Fetal blood flow velocity waveforms as predictors of growth retardation. *Obstetrics and Gynecology*, **70**, 7–10.

Arduini D., Rizzo G., Romanini C. & Mancuso S. (1987b) Utero-placental blood flow velocity waveforms as predictors of pregnancy-induced hypertension. *European Journal of Obstetrics, Gynecology and Reproductive Biology*, **26**, 335–41.

Assali N.S., Douglass R.A., Baird W.W., Nicholson D.B. & Suyemoto R. (1953) Measurement of uterine blood flow and uterine metabolism. IV Results in normal pregnancy. *American Journal of Obstetrics and Gynecology*, **66**, 248–53.

Assali N.S., Rauramo L. & Peltonan T. (1960) Measurement of uterine and fetal blood flow and oxygen consumption in early human pregnancy. *American Journal of Obstetrics and Gynecology*, **79**, 86–98.

Barcroft J., Herkel W. & Hills S. (1933) The rate of blood flow and gaseous metabolism of the uterus during pregnancy. *Journal of Physiology*, **156**, 49–66.

Beattie B., Dornan J.C., Clements C.W.A. & McGrath B. (1988) Umbilical artery velocity waveform assessed as an antenatal screening tool for intrauterine growth and poor fetal outcome. *British Journal of Obstetrics and Gynaecology*, **95**, 534–5.

Berkowitz G.S., Chitkara U., Rosenberg J. *et al.* (1988a) Sonographic estimation of fetal weight and Doppler analysis of umbilical artery velocimetry in the prediction of intrauterine growth retardation: A prospective study. *American Journal of Obstetrics and Gynecology*, **158**, 1149–53.

Berkowitz G.S., Mehalek K.E., Chitkara U., Rosenberg J., Cogswell C. & Berkowitz R.L. (1988b) Doppler umbilical velocimetry in the prediction of adverse outcome in pregnancies at risk for intrauterine growth retardation. *Obstetrics and Gynecology*, **71**, 742–6.

Bilardo C.M., Soothill P.W., Nicolaides K.H., Rodeck C.M., & Campbell S. (1986) Fetal blood flow velocities in Rhesus isoimmunization (abstract). Obstetric and Neonatal Blood Flow, Biological Engineering Society, London, pp. 52–5.

Bracero L., Schulman H., Fleischer A., Farmakides G. & Rochelson B. (1986) Umbilical artery velocimetry in diabetes and pregnancy. *Obstetrics and Gynecology*, **68**, 654–8.

Brar H.S., Medearis A.L., DeVore G.R. & Platt L.D. (1988a) Fetal umbilical velocimetry using continuous wave and pulsed-wave Doppler ultrasound in high-risk pregnancies: a comparison of systolic to diastolic ratios. *Obstetrics and Gynecology*, **72**, 607–10.

Brar H.S. & Platt L.D. (1988) Reverse end-diastolic flow velocity on umbilical artery velocimetry in high-risk pregnancies: An ominous finding with adverse pregnancy outcome. *American Journal of Obstetrics and Gynecology*, **159**, 559–61.

Brar H.S., Platt L.D., DeVore G.R., Horenstein J. & Medearis A.L. (1988b) Qualitative assessment of maternal uterine and fetal umbilical artery blood flow and resistance in laboring patients by Doppler velocimetry. *American Journal of Obstetrics and Gynecology*, **158**, 952–6.

Brosens I. & Dixon H.G. (1966) Anatomy of the maternal side of the placenta. *Journal of Obstetrics and Gynaecology of the British Commonwealth*, **73**, 357–63.

Brosens I., Robertson W.B. & Dixon H.G. (1967) The physiological response of the vessel of the placental bed to normal pregnancy. *Journal of Pathology and Bacteriology*, **93**, 569–74.

Cameron A.D., Nicholson S.F., Nimrod C.A., Harder J.R. & Davies D.M. (1988) Doppler waveforms in the fetal aorta and umbilical artery in patients with hypertension in pregnancy. *American Journal of Obstetrics and Gynecology*, **158**, 339–45.

Campbell S., Griffin D. & Pearce J.M. (1983) New Doppler technique for assessing uteroplacental blood flow *Lancet*, **i**, 675–7

Campbell S., Hernandez C.J., Cohen-Overbeek T.A. & Pearce J.M.F. (1984) Assessment of fetoplacental and uteroplacental blood flow using duplex pulsed Doppler ultrasound in complicated pregnancies. *Journal of Perinatal Medicine*, **12**, 262–5.

Campbell S., Pearce J.M.F., Hackett G., Cohen-Overbeek T. & Hernandez C. (1986) Qualitative assessment of uteroplacental blood flow: early screening test for high-risk pregnancies. *Obstetrics and Gynecology*, **68**, 649–53.

Campbell S., Vyas S. & Bewley S. (1988) Doppler uteroplacental waveforms. *Lancet*, **ii**, 1287–8

Clavero J.A., Neguerude J. & Ortiz L. (1973) Bloodflow in the intervillous space and fetal blood flow. *American Journal of Obstetrics and Gynecology*, **116**, 340–6.

Clavero-Nunez J.A. (1980) Uteroplacental blood flow in pregnancy at term. In *Clinical Perinatology*, (Ed. by S. Aladjen, A.K. Brown & C. Sureau), pp. 123–39. Mosby, St Louis.

Coghlan B.A. & Taylor (1976) Directional Doppler techniques for detection of blood velocities. *Ultrasound in Medicine and Biology*, **2**, 171–81.

Cohn H.E., Sacks E.J., Heymann M.A. & Rudolph A.M. (1974) Cardiovascular responses to hypoxemia and acidemia in fetal lambs. *American Journal of Obstetrics and Gynecology*, **120**, 817–24.

Copper K.E. & Greenfield A.D. (1949) A method for measuring the blood flow in the umbilical vessels. *Journal of Physiology*, **108**, 167–76.

Grenshaw C., Huckabee W.E., Curet L.B., Mann L. & Barron D.H. (1968) A method for the estimation of the umbilical blood flow in unstressed sheep and goats with some results of its application. *Quarterly Journal of Experimental Physiology*, **53**, 65–75.

Dawes G.S. (1968) *Foetal and Neonatal Physiology*, pp. 66–78. Year Book, Chicago.

Dawes G.S. & Mott J.C. (1964) Changes in oxygen distribution and consumption in foetal lambs in the umbilical vessels. *Journal of Physiology*, **108**, 167–76.

De Vore G.R., Horenstein J., Siassi B. & Platt L.D. (1987) Fetal echocardiography VII Doppler color flow mapping: a new technique for the diagnosis of congenital heart disease. *American Journal of Obstetrics and Gynecology*, **156**, 1054–64.

Divon M.Y., Guidetti D.A., Braverman J.J., Oberlander E., Langer O. & Merkatz I.R. (1988) Intrauterine growth retardation — a prospective study of the diagnostic value of real-time sonography combined with umbilical artery flow velocimetry. *Obstetrics and Gynecology*, **72**, 611–14.

Dixon H.G., Browne J.C. & Davey D.A. (1963) Choriodecidual and myometrial blood flow. *Lancet*, **ii**, 369–73.

Dobson P.C., Abell D.A. & Beischer N.A. (1981) Mortality and morbidity of fetal growth retardation. *Australian Journal of Obstetrics and Gynaecology*, **21**, 69–72.

Ducey J., Schulman H., Farmakides G., Rochelson B., Bracero L., Fleischer A., Guzman E., Winter D. & Penny B. (1987) A classification of hypertension in pregnancy based on Doppler velocimetry. *American Journal of Obstetrics and Gyncology*, **157**, 680–5.

Eik-Nes S., Brubakk A.O. & Ulstein M. (1980) Measurement of human fetal blood flow. *British Medical Journal*, **1**, 283–4.

Eik-Nes S.M., Marsal K. & Kristofferson K. (1984) Methodology and basic problems related to blood flow studies in the human fetus. *Ultrasound in Medicine and Biology*, **10**, 329–38.

Eldridge M.W., Berman W. & Greene F.R. (1985) Serial echo Doppler measurements of human fetal abdominal aortic blood flow. *Journal of Ultrasound in Medicine*, **4**, 453–8.

Erskine R.L.A. & Ritchie J.W.K. (1985a) Umbilical artery blood flow characteristics in normal and growth-retarded fetuses. *British Journal of Obstetrics and Gynaecology*, **92**, 605–10.

Erskine R.L.A. & Ritchie J.W.K. (1985b) Quantitative measurement of fetal blood flow using Doppler ultrasound. *British Journal of Obstetrics and Gynaecology*, **92**, 600–4.

Erskine R.L.A., Ritchie J.W.K. & Murnaghan G.A. (1986) Antenatal diagnosis of placental anastomosis in a twin pregnancy using Doppler ultrasound. *British Journal of Obstetrics and Gynaecology*, **93**, 955–9.

Farmakides G., Schulman H., Saldana L.R., Bracero L.A., Fleischer A. & Rochelson B. (1985) Surveillance of twin pregnancy with umbilical arterial velocimetry. *American Journal of Obstetrics and Gynecology*, **153**, 789–92.

Farmakides G., Schulman H., Winter D., Ducey J., Guzman E. & Penny B. (1988a) Prenatal surveillance using nonstress testing and Doppler velocimetry. *Obstetrics and Gynecology*, **71**, 184–7.

Farmakides G., Schulman H., Ducey J. *et al.* (1988b) Uterine and umbilical artery Doppler velocimetry in postterm pregnancy. *Journal of Reproductive Medicine*, **33**, 259–61.

Fitzgerald D.E. & Drumm J.E. (1977) Non-invasive measurement of human fetal circulation using ultrasound: a new method. *British Medical Journal*, **2**, 1450–1.

Fitzgerald D.E., Stuart B., Drumm J.E. & Duignan N.M. (1984) The assessment of the feto-placental circulation with continuous wave Doppler ultrasound. *Ultrasound in Medicine and Biology*, **10**, 371–6.

Fleischer A., Anyaegbunam A.A., Schulman H., Farmakides G. & Randolph G. (1987) Uterine and umbilical artery velocimetry during normal labor. *American Journal of Obstetrics and Gynecology*, **157**, 40–3.

Fleischer A., Schulman H., Farmakides G., Bracero L., Blattner P. & Randolph G. (1985) Umbilical artery velocity waveforms and intrauterine growth retardation. *American Journal of Obstetrics and Gynecology*, **151**, 502–5.

Fleischer A., Schulman H., Farmakides G. *et al.* (1986) Uterine artery Doppler velocimetry in pregnant women with hypertension. *American Journal of Obstetrics and Gynecology*, **154**, 806–13.

Gagnon R., Morrow R., Ritchie K., Hunse C. & Patrick J. (1988) Umbilical and uterine artery blood flow velocities after vibratory acoustic stimulation. *American Journal of Obstetrics and Gynecology*, **159**, 574–8.

Gaziano E., Knox E., Wager G.P., Bendel R.P., Boyce D.J. & Olson J. (1988) The predictability of the small-for-gestational-age infant by real-time ultrasound-derived measurements combined with pulsed Doppler umbilical artery velocimetry. *American Journal of Obstetrics and Gynecology*, **158**, 1431–9.

Gerson A., Johnson A., Wallace D., Bottalico J., Weiner S. & Bolognese R. (1988) Umbilical arterial systolic/diastolic values in normal twin gestation. *Obstetrics and Gynecology*, **72**, 205–7.

Gerson A., Wallace D.M., Stiller R.J., Paul D., Weiner S. & Bolognese R.J. (1987) Doppler evaluation of umbilical venous and arterial blood flow in the second and third trimesters of normal pregnancy. *Obstetrics and Gynecology*, **70**, 622–6.

Giles W.B., Lingman G., Marsal K. & Trudinger B.J. (1986) Fetal volume blood flow and umbilical artery flow velocity waveform analysis: a comparison. *British Journal of Obstetrics and Gynaecology*, **93**, 461–5.

Giles W.B. & Trudinger B.J. (1986) Umbilical cord whole blood viscosity and the umbilical artery velocity time waveforms: a correlation. *British Journal of Obstetrics and Gynaecology*, **93**, 466–70.

Giles W.B., Trudinger B.J. & Baird P.J. (1985a) Fetal umbilical artery flow velocity waveforms and placental resistance: pathological correlation. *British Journal of Obstetrics and Gynaecology*, **92**, 31–8.

Giles W.B., Trudinger B.J. & Cook C.M. (1985b) Fetal umbilical artery flow velocity waveforms in twin pregnancies. *British Journal of Obstetrics and Gynaecology*, **92**, 490–7.

Gill R.J., Trudinger B.J., Garrett W.J., Kossoff G. & Warren P.S. (1981) Fetal umbilical venous flow measured *in utero* by pulsed Doppler and B-mode ultrasound. *American Journal of Obstetrics and Gynecology*, **139**, 720–5.

Gill R.W. (1985) Measurement of blood flow by ultrasound: Accuracy and sources of error. *Ultrasound in Medicine and Biology*, **11**, 625–41.

Gill R.W., Kossoff G., Warren P.S. & Garrett W.J. (1984) Umbilical venous flow in normal and complicated pregnancy. *Ultrasound in Medicine and Biology*, **10**, 349–55.

Gosling R.G. & King D.H. (1975) Ultrasonic angiology. In *Ultrasonic Angiology in Arteries and Veins*, (Ed. by A. Marcus & L. Adamson), pp. 61–98. Churchill Livingstone,

Edinburgh.

Greenfield A.D., Shepherd J.T. & Whelan R.F. (1951) The rate of blood flow in the umbilical cord. *Lancet*, **ii**, 422–4.

Griffin D., Bilardo K., Diaz J., Teague M. & Campbell S. (1983a) The measurement of human fetal blood flow with linear array pulsed Doppler duplex. *European Journal of Obstetrics, Gynecology and Reproductive Biology*, **15**, 426–30.

Griffin D., Bilardo K., Masini L., Diag-Recasers J., Pearce J.M., Wilson K. & Campbell S. (1984) Doppler blood flow waveforms in the descending thoracic aorta of the human fetus. *British Journal of Obstetrics and Gynaecology*, **91**, 997–1006.

Griffin D., Cohen-Overbeek T. & Campbell S. (1983b) Fetal and uteroplacental blood flow. *Clinics in Obstetrics and Gynaecology*, **10**, 565–601.

Gruenwald P. (1972) Expansion of placental site and maternal blood supply of primate placentae. *Anatomical Record*, **173**, 189–204.

Gudmundsson S. & Marsal K. (1988a) Umbilical artery and uteroplacental blood flow velocity waveforms in normal pregnancy — a cross-sectional study. *Acta Obstetricia et Gynecologica Scandinavica*, **67**, 347–54.

Gudmundsson S. & Marsal K. (1988b) Umbilical and uteroplacental blood flow velocity waveforms in pregnancies with fetal growth retardation. *European Journal of Obstetrics, Gynecology and Reproductive Biology*, **27**, 187–96.

Guidetti D.A., Divon M.Y., Cavalieri R.L., Langer O. & Merkatz I.R. (1987) Fetal umbilical artery flow velocimetry in postdate pregnancies. *American Journal of Obstetrics and Gynecology*, **157**, 1521–3.

Hackett, G.A., Campbell S., Gamsu H., Cohen-Overbeek T. & Pearce J.M.F. (1987a) Doppler studies in the growth retarded fetus and prediction of neonatal necrotising enterocolitis, haemorrhage, and neonatal morbidity. *British Medical Journal*, **294**, 13–16.

Hackett G.A., Nicolaides K.H. & Campbell S. (1987b) Doppler ultrasound assessment of fetal and uteroplacental circulations in severe second trimetster oligohydramnios. *British Journal of Obstetrics and Gynaecology*, **94**, 1074–7.

Haddad H.G., Johnstone F.D., Chambers S.E., Hoskins P.R. & McDicken (1988) Umbilical artery Doppler flow velocity wave form analysis and the outcome of hypertensive pregnancies. *Journal of Obstetrics and Gynaecology*, **9**, 9–13.

Hanretty K.V., Whittle M.J. & Rubin P.C. (1988) Doppler uteroplacental waveforms in pregnancy-induced hypertension: a re-appraisal. *Lancet*, **i**, 850–2.

Huckabee W.E., Metcalfe J., Prystowsky N. & Barron D.H. (1961) Blood flow and oxygen consumption of the pregnant uterus. *American Journal of Physiology*, **200**, 274–8.

Illyes M. & Gati I. (1988) Reverse flow in the human fetal descending aorta as a sign of severe fetal asphyxia preceding intrauterine death. *Journal of Clinical Ultrasound*, **16**, 403–7.

Janbu T., Koss K.S., Nesheim B.I. & Wesche (1985) Blood velocities in the uterine artery in humans during labour. *Acta Physiologica Scandinavica*, **124**, 153–61.

Johnstone F.D., Haddad N.G., Hoskins P., McDicken W., Chambers S. & Muir B. (1988) Umbilical artery Doppler flow velocity waveform: the outcome of pregnancies with absent end diastolic flow. *European Journal of Obstetrics, Gynecology and Reproductive Biology*, **28**, 171–8.

Jouppila P. & Kirkinen P. (1984a) Umbilical vein blood flow as an indicator of fetal hypoxia. *British Journal of Obstetrics and Gynaecology*, **91**, 107–10.

Jouppila P. & Kirkinen P. (1984b) Increased vascular resistance in the descending aorta of the human fetus in hypoxia. *British Journal of Obstetrics and Gynaecology*, **91**, 853–6.

Jouppila P. & Kirkinen P. (1986) Blood velocity waveforms of the fetal aorta in normal and hypertensive pregnancies. *Obstetrics and Gynecology*, **67**, 856–60.

Kaufmann P., Sen D.K. & Schweikhart G. (1979) Classification of human placental villi. I. Histology. *Cell and Tissue Research*, **200**, 409–23.

Kirkinen P., Jouppila P. & Eik-Nes S. (1983) Umbilical vein blood flow in Rhesus-isoimmunization. *British Journal of Obstetrics and Gynaecology*, **90**, 640–4.

Kirkinen P., Muller R., Huch R. & Huch A. (1987) Blood flow velocity waveforms in human fetal intracranial arteries. *Obstetrics and Gynecology*, **70**, 617–21.

Kirschbaum T.H., Lucas W.E., De Haven J.C. & Assali N.S. (1967) The dynamics of placental oxygen transfer. *American Journal of Obstetrics and Gynecology*, **98**, 429–43.

Kjellmer I., Karlsson K., Olsson T. & Rosen K.G. (1974) Cerebral reactions during intrauterine asphyxia in the sheep. I. Circulation and oxygen consumption in the fetal brain. *Paediatric Research*, **8**, 50–7.

Kurjak A., Breyer B., Jurkovic D., Alfirevic Z. & Miljan M. (1987) Color flow mapping in obstetrics. *Journal of Perinatal Medicine*, **15**, 271–81.

Kurjak A. & Rajhvajn B. (1982) Ultrasonic measurements of umbilical blood flow in normal and complicated pregnancies. Review Article. *Journal of Perinatal Medicine*, **10**, 3–10.

Laurin J., Lingman G., Marsal K. & Persson P.H. (1987b) Fetal blood flow in pregnancies complicated by intrauterine growth retardation. *Obstetrics and Gynecology*, **69**, 895–902.

Laurin J., Marsal K., Persson P.H. & Lingman G. (1987a) Ultrasound measurement of fetal blood flow in predicting fetal outcome. *British Journal of Obstetrics and Gynaecology*, **94**, 940–8.

Lingman G. & Marsal K. (1986a) Fetal central blood circulation in the third trimester of normal pregnancy — a longitudinal study. 1. Aortic and umbilical blood flow. *Early Human Development*, **13**, 137–50.

Lingman G. & Marsal K. (1986b) Circulatory effects of fetal heart arrythmia. *Paediatric Cardiology*, **7**, 67–74.

Lunnell N.O., Sarby B., Lavander R. & Nylund L. (1979) Comparison of uteroplacental blood flow in normal and in intrauterine growth-retarded pregnancy. Measurements with indium-113m and a computer-linked gamma camera. *Gynecologic and Obstetric Investigation*, **10**, 106–18.

McCallum W.D. (1977) Thermodilution measurement of human umbilical blood flow at delivery. *American Journal of Obstetrics and Gynecology*, **127**, 491–6.

McCallum W.D., Williams C.S., Napel S. & Daigle R.E. (1978) Fetal blood velocity waveforms. *American Journal of Obstetrics and Gynecology*, **132**, 425–9.

McClure Browne J.C. & Veall N. (1953) The maternal placental blood flow in normotensive and hypertensive women. *Journal of Obstetrics and Gynaecology of the British Empire*, **60**, 141–7.

McCowan L.M., Erskine L.A. & Ritchie K. (1987a) Umbilical artery Doppler blood flow studies in the preterm, small for gestational age fetus. *American Journal of Obstetrics and Gynecology*, **156**, 655–9.

McCowan L.M., Mullen B.M. & Ritchie K. (1987b) Umbilical artery flow velocity waveforms and the placental vascular bed. *American Journal of Obstetrics and Gynecology*, **157**, 900–2.

McCowan L.M., Ritchie K., Mo L.Y., Bascom P.A. & Sherret H. (1988) Uterine artery flow velocity waveforms in normal and growth-retarded pregnancies. *American Journal of Obstetrics and Gynecology*, **158**, 499–504.

McDonald D.A. (1974) *Blood Flow in Arteries*, 2nd edn, Edward Arnold, London.

McParland P. & Pearce J.M. (1988) Review article: Doppler blood flow in pregnancy. *Placenta*, **9**, 427–50.

Makowski E.L., Meschia G., Droegmueller W. & Battaglia F.C. (1968) Distribution of uterine blood flow in the pregnant sheep. *American Journal of Obstetrics and Gynecology*, **101**, 409–12.

Marsal K., Lindblad A., Lingman G. & Eik-Nes S.H. (1984a) Blood flow in the fetal descending aorta; intrinsic factors affecting fetal blood flow, i.e. fetal breathing movements and cardiac arrhythmia. *Ultrasound in Medicine and Biology*, **10**, 339–48.

Marsal K., Lingman G. & Giles W. (1984b) In: *Evaluation of the carotid, aortic and umbilical blood velocity*. Proceedings from Society for the Study of Fetal Physiology. 11th Annual Conference, Oxford (abstract C33).

Marsal K. & Persson P.H. (1988) Ultrasonic measurement of fetal blood velocity wave form as a secondary diagnostic test in screening for intrauterine growth retardation. *Journal of Clinical Ultrasound*, **16**, 239–44.

Mehalek K.E., Berkowitz G.S., Chitkara U., Rosenberg J. & Berkowitz R.L. (1988) Comparison of continuous-wave and pulsed Doppler S/D ratios of umbilical and uterine arteries. *Obstetrics and Gynecology*, **72**, 603–6.

Meschia G., Cotter J.R., Breathnach C.S. & Barron D.H. (1965) The diffusibility of oxygen across the sheep placenta. *Quarterly Journal of Experimental Physiology*, **50**, 466–8.

Metcalfe J., Romney S.L., Swartout J.R., Pitcairn D.M., Lethin A.N. & Barron D.H.

(1959) Uterine blood flow and oxygen consumption in pregnant sheep and goats. *American Journal of Physiology*, **197**, 929–34.

Mires G., Dempster J., Patel N.B. & Crawford J.W. (1987) The effect of fetal heart rate on umbilical artery flow velocity waveforms. *British Journal of Obstetrics and Gynaecology*, **94**, 665–9.

Mulders L.G., Jongsma H.W., Wijn P.F. & Hein P.R. (1988) The uterine artery blood flow velocity waveform in pathological pregnancy. *Early Human Development* (in press).

Mulders L.G.M., Wijn P.F.F., Jongsma H.W. & Hein P.R. (1987) A comparative study of three indices of umbilical blood flow in relation to prediction of growth retardation. *Journal of Perinatal Medicine*, **15**, 3–12.

Neilson J.P., Whitfield C.R. & Aitchison T.C. (1980) Screening for the small-for-dates fetus: A two stage ultrasonic examination schedule. *British Medical Journal*, **280**, 1203–6.

Nicolaides K.H., Bilardo C.M., Soothill P.W. & Campbell S. (1988) Absence of end diastolic frequencies in umbilical artery: a sign of fetal hypoxia and acidosis. *British Medical Journal*, **297**, 1026–7.

Nijhuis J.G., Prechtl H.F., Martin C.B. & Bots R.S. (1982) Are there behavioural states in the human fetus? *Early Human Development*, **6**, 177–95.

Nimrod C., Davies D., Harder J. *et al.* (1987) Doppler ultrasound prediction of fetal outcome in twin pregnancies. *American Journal of Obstetrics and Gynecology*, **156**, 402–6.

Olofsson P., Lingman G., Marsal K. & Sjoberg N.O. (1987) Fetal blood flow in diabetic pregnancy. *Journal of Perinatal Medicine*, **15**, 545–53.

Pearce J.M. (1987) Uteroplacental and fetal blood flow. *Balliere's Clinical Obstetrics and Gynaecology*, **1**, 157–84.

Pearce J.M., Campbell S., Cohen-Overbeek T., Hackett G.A., Hernandez J. & Royston J.P. (1988) References ranges and sources of variation for indices of pulsed Doppler flow velocity waveforms from the uteroplacental and fetal circulation. *British Journal of Obstetrics and Gynaecology*, **95**, 248–56.

Pearce J.M.F. & McParland P. (1988a) Doppler uteroplacental waveforms. *Lancet*, **ii**, 1278.

Pearce J.M.F. & McParland P. (1988b) A comparison of Doppler flow velocity waveforms, amniotic fluid columns and the non-stress test as means of monitoring postdates pregnancies. *American Journal of Obstetrics and Gynecology* (submitted).

Peeters L.L.M., Sheldon R.E., Jones M.D., Makowski D. & Meschia G. (1979) Blood flow to fetal organs as a function of arterial oxygen content. *American Journal of Obstetrics and Gynecology*, **135**, 637–46.

Pourcelot L. (1974) Application clinique de l'examen Doppler transcutane. In *Velocimetrie Ultrasonore*, (Ed. by P. Peronneau), pp. 213–40. Inserm, Paris.

Pretorius D.H., Manchester D., Barkin S., Parker S. & Nelson T.R. (1988) Doppler ultrasound of twin transfusion syndrome. *Journal of Ultrasound in Medicine*, **7**, 117–24.

Reed K.L., Anderson R.D. & Shenker L. (1987) Changes in intracardiac blood flow velocities in fetuses with absent umbilical artery diastolic flow. *American Journal of Obstetrics and Gynecology*, **157**, 774–9.

Reuwer P.J.H.M., Bruinse H.W., Stoutenbeek P. & Haspels A.A. (1984) Doppler assessment of the fetoplacental circulation in normal and growth retarded fetuses. *European Journal of Obstetrics, Gynecology and Reproductive Biology*, **18**, 199–205.

Reuwer P.J.H.M., Sijmons E.A., Rietman G.W., van Tiel M.W.M. & Bruinse H.W. (1987) Intrauterine growth retardation: prediction of perinatal distress by Doppler ultrasound. *Lancet*, **ii**, 415–8.

Rightmire D.A. & Campbell S. (1987) Fetal and maternal Doppler blood flow parameters in postterm pregnancies. *Obstetrics and Gynecology*, **69**, 891–4.

Rightmire D.A., Nicolaides K.M., Rodeck C. & Campbell S. (1986) Fetal blood velocities in Rh isoimmunization: Relationship to gestational age and to fetal haematocrit. *Obstetrics and Gynecology*, **68**, 233–6.

Rochelson B., Schulman H., Farmakides G. *et al.* (1987b) The significance of absent end-diastolic velocity in umbilical artery velocity waveforms. *American Journal of Obstetrics and Gynecology*, **156**, 1213–18.

Rochelson B.L., Schulman H., Fleischer A. *et al.* (1987a) The clinical significance of Doppler umbilical artery velocimetry in the small for gestational age fetus. *American*

*Journal of Obstetrics and Gynecology*, **156**, 1223–6.

Rudelstorfer R., Deutinger J., Katz E. & Bernaschek G. (1988) Vaginosongraphische Stromungsmessungen in der Arteria uterina wahrend der Schwangerschaft — Vorteile der gepulsten Doppler-Methode. *Zeitschrift fur Geburtshilfe und Perinatologie*, **192**, 14–18.

Rudolph A.M. & Heymann M.A. (1967) The circulation of the fetus *in utero*: Methods for studying distribution of blood flow, cardiac output and oxygen flow. *Circulation Research*, **21**, 163–84.

Saldana L.R., Eads M.C. & Schaefer T.R. (1987) Umbilical blood waveforms in fetal surveillance of twins. *American Journal of Obstetrics and Gynecology*, **157**, 712–15.

Schulman H., Ducey J., Farmakides G. *et al.* (1987) Uterine artery Doppler velocimetry: The significance of divergent systolic/diastolic ratios. *American Journal of Obstetrics and Gynecology*, **157**, 1539–42.

Schulman H., Fleischer A., Farmakides G., Bracero L., Rochelson B. & Grunfeld L. (1986) Development of uterine artery compliance in pregnancy as detected by Doppler ultrasound. *American Journal of Obstetrics and Gynecology*, **155**, 1031–6.

Schulman H., Fleischer A., Stern W., Farmakides G., Jagini N. & Blattner P. (1984) Umbilical velocity wave ratios in human pregnancy. *American Journal of Obstetrics and Gynecology*, **148**, 985–90.

Soothill P.W., Nicolaides K.H., Bilardo C.M. & Campbell S. (1986) Relation of fetal hypoxia in growth retardation to mean blood velocity in the fetal aorta. *Lancet*, **ii**, 1118–20.

Steel S.A., Pearce J.M. & Chamberlain G.V. (1988b) Doppler ultrasound of the uteroplacental circulation as a screening test for severe pre-eclampsia with intra-uterine growth retardation. *European Journal of Obstetrics, Gynecology and Reproductive Biology*, **28**, 279–87.

Steel S.A., Pearce J.M., Nash G., Christopher B., Dormandy J. & Bland J.M. (1988a) Maternal blood viscosity and uteroplacental blood flow velocity waveforms in normal and complicated pregnancies. *British Journal of Obstetrics and Gynaecology*, **95**, 747–52.

Steel S.A., Pearce J.M., Nash G., Christopher B., Dormandy J. & Bland J.M. (1989) Correlation between Doppler flow velocity waveforms and cord blood viscosity. (Submitted.)

Stembera Z.K., Hodr J. & Janda J. (1965) Umbilical blood flow in healthy newborn infants during the first minutes after birth. *American Journal of Obstetrics and Gynecology*, **91**, 568–74.

Stuart B., Drumm J., Fitzgerald D.E. & Duignan N.M. (1980) Fetal blood velocity waveforms in normal pregnancy. *British Journal of Obstetrics and Gynaecology*, **87**, 780–5.

Stuart B., Drumm J., Fitzgerald D.E. & Duignan N.M. (1981) Fetal blood velocity waveforms in uncomplicated labour. *British Journal of Obstetrics and Gynaecology*, **88**, 865–9.

Thompson R.S., Trudinger B.J. & Cook C.M. (1986) A comparison of Doppler ultrasound waveform indices in the umbilical artery. 1. Indices derived from the maximum velocity waveform. *Ultrasound in Medicine and Biology*, **12**, 835–44.

Thompson R.S., Trudinger B.J., Cook C.M. & Giles W.B. (1988a) Umbilical artery velocity waveforms: normal reference values for A/B ratio and Pourcelot ratio. *British Journal of Obstetrics and Gynaecology*, **95**, 589–91.

Thompson R.S., Trudinger B.J., Cook C.M. (1988b) Doppler ultrasound waveform indices: A/B ratio, pulsatility index and Pourcelot ratio. *British Journal of Obstetrics and Gynaecology*, **95**, 581–8.

Tonge H.M., Stewart P.A. & Wladimiroff J.W. (1984) Fetal blood flow measurements during fetal cardiac arrythmia. *Early Human Development*, **10**, 23–34.

Tonge H.M., Wladimiroff J.W., Noordam M.J. & Van Kooten C. (1986) Blood flow velocity waveforms in the descending fetal aorta: comparison between normal and growth-retarded pregnancies. *Obstetrics and Gynecology*, **67**, 851–5.

Trudinger B.J., Cook C.M., Giles W.B., Connelly A. & Thompson R.S. (1987) Umbilical artery flow velocity waveforms in high-risk pregnancy — randomised controlled trial. *Lancet*, **i**, 188–90.

Trudinger B.J., Cook C.M., Jones L. & Giles W.B. (1986) A comparison of fetal heart rate monitoring and umbilical artery waveforms in the recognition of fetal compromise. *British Journal of Obstetrics and Gynaecology*, **93**, 171–5.

Trudinger B.J., Giles W.B. & Cook C.M. (1985a) Flow velocity waveforms in the maternal uteroplacental and fetal umbilical placental circulations. *American Journal of Obstetrics and Gynecology*, **152**, 155–63.

Trudinger B.J., Giles W.B. & Cook C.M. (1985b) Uteroplacental blood flow velocity-time waveforms in normal and complicated pregnancy. *British Journal of Obstetrics and Gynaecology*, **92**, 39–45.

Trudinger B.J., Giles W.B., Cook C.M., Bombardieri J. & Collins L. (1985c) Fetal umbilical artery flow velocity waveforms and placental resistance: clinical significance. *British Journal of Obstetrics and Gynaecology*, **92**, 23–30.

Van Eyck J., Wladimiroff J.W., Noordam M.J., Tonge H.M. & Prechtl H.F.R. (1985) The blood flow velocity waveform in the fetal descending aorta; its relationship to fetal behavioural states in normal pregnancy at 37–38 weeks. *Early Human Development*, **12**, 137–43.

Van Eyck J., Wladimiroff J.W., Noordam M.J., Tonge H.M. & Prechtl H.F.R. (1986) The blood flow velocity waveform in the fetal descending aorta; its relationship to behavioural states in the growth retarded fetus at 37–38 weeks of gestation. *Early Human Development*, **14**, 99–107.

Van Eyck J., Wladimiroff J.W., Van Den Wijngaard J.A.G.W., Noordam M.J. & Prechtl H.F.R. (1987) The blood flow velocity waveform in the fetal internal carotid and umbilical artery; its relation to fetal behavioural states in normal pregnancy at 37–38 weeks. *British Journal of Obstetrics and Gynaecology*, **94**, 736–41.

Van Eyck J., Wladimiroff J.W., Noordam M.J., Van Den Wijngaard J.A.G.W. & Prechtl H.F.R. (1988) The blood flow velocity waveform in the fetal internal carotid and umbilical artery: its relation to fetal behavioural states in the growth retarded fetus at 37–38 weeks gestation. *British Journal of Obstetrics and Gynaecology*, **95**, 473–7.

Van Lierde M., Oberweis D. & Thomas K. (1984) Ultrasonic measurement of aortic and umbilical blood flow in the human fetus. *American Journal of Obstetrics and Gynecology*, **63**, 801–5.

Van Vugt J.M.G., Ruissen C.J., Hoogland H.J. & de Haan J. (1987) A prospective study of the umbilical artery waveform in appropriate-for-date and growth-retarded fetuses. *Gynecologic and Obstetric Investigation*, **23**, 217–25.

Van Vugt J.M.G., Ruissen C.J., Nienhuis S.J., Hoogland H.J. & de Haan J. (1988) Comparison of blood velocity waveform indices recorded by pulsed Doppler and continuous wave Doppler in the umbilical artery. *Journal of Clinical Ultrasound*, **16**, 573–6.

Wladimiroff J.W. & McGhie J. (1981) Ultrasonic assessment of cardiovascular geometry and function in the human fetus. *British Journal of Obstetrics and Gynaecology*, **88**, 870–5.

Wladimiroff J.W., Tonge H.M. & Stewart P.A. (1986) Doppler ultrasound assessment of cerebral blood flow in the human fetus. *British Journal of Obstetrics and Gynaecology*, **93**, 471–5.

Wladimiroff J.W., Wiyngaard J.A., Degani S. *et al.* (1987) Cerebral and umbilical arterial blood flow velocity wavesforms in normal and growth retarded pregnancies. *Obstetrics and Gynecology*, **69**, 705–9.

Wolfson M.R. & Blake K.C.H. (1975) Isotopic method using xenon-133 for assessing placental blood flow and for detecting light for dates babies. *South African Medical Journal*, **49**, 117–19.

Woo J.S., Liang S.T. & Lo L.S. (1987a) Significance of an absent or reversed end diastolic flow in Doppler umbilical artery waveforms. *Journal of Ultrasound in Medicine*, **6**, 291–7.

Woo J.S.K., Liang S.T., Lo L.S. & Chan F.Y. (1987b) Middle cerebral artery Doppler flow velocity waveforms. *Obstetrics and Gynecology*, **70**, 613–16.

# 7: Cordocentesis in the investigation of small-for-gestational age fetuses

KYPRIANOS H. NICOLAIDES AND
DEMETRIOS L. ECONOMIDES



Cordocentesis, ultrasound-guided fetal blood sampling from the umbilical cord, has recently been applied in the investigation of severely small-for-gestational age (SGA) fetuses and has provided useful information on fetal karyotype, acid–base status and metabolism. This chapter reviews the data derived from the study of 263 such fetuses at King's College Hospital. The results of blood gases and metabolites of SGA fetuses are compared with reference ranges that were constructed from the study of fetuses that were appropriate-for-gestational age (AGA) at the time of cordocentesis. These latter fetuses were subsequently found to be cytogenetically normal and not to be affected by the genetic disease for which they were investigated.

## Technique of cordocentesis

In our centre cordocentesis is performed as an out-patient procedure, without maternal sedation or fetal paralysis (Nicolaides *et al.* 1986). The site and direction of the umbilical cord at its insertion into the placenta are identified by ultrasound scanning with a curvilinear transducer. With the transducer in one hand, held parallel to the intended course of the needle (Figure 7.1), the chosen site of entry on the maternal abdomen is

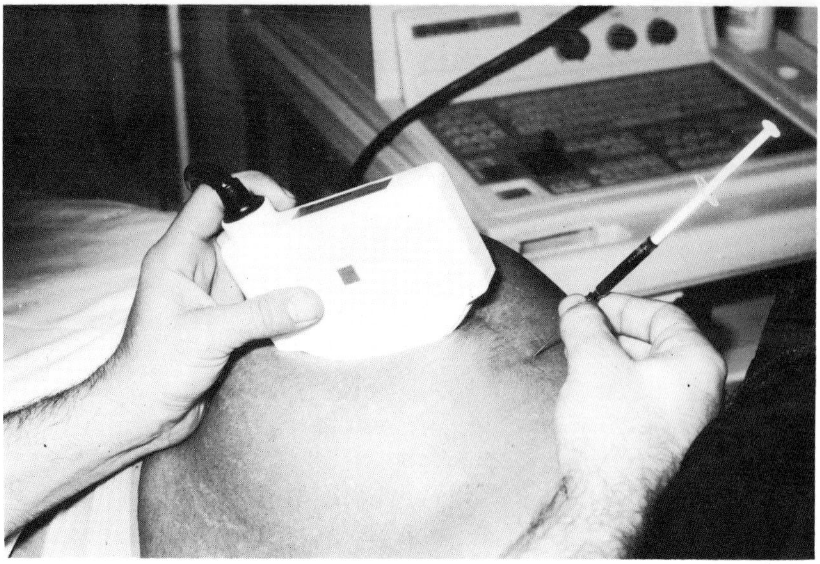

**Fig. 7.1** Cordocentesis: ultrasound-guided fetal blood sampling.

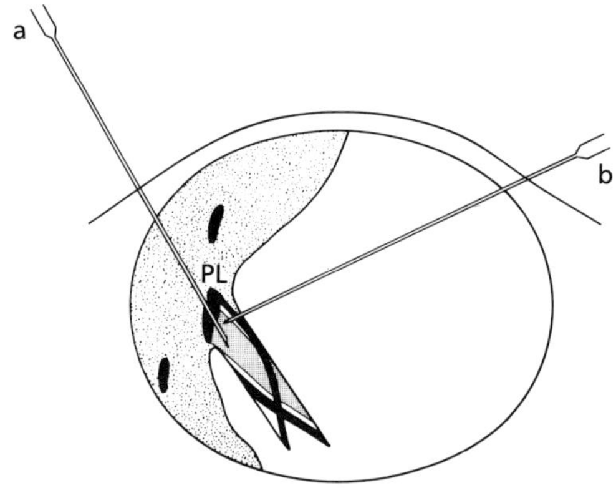


**Fig. 7.2** (a) Transplacental and (b) transamniotic cordocentesis.

cleaned with antiseptic solution and local anaesthetic is infiltrated down to the myometrium. Where the placenta is anterior or lateral, a 20G needle is introduced transplacentally into the umbilical cord. When the placenta is posterior, the needle is introduced transamniotically and the cord punctured close to its placental insertion (Figure 7.2). The umbilical cord vessel sampled is identified as artery or vein by the turbulence seen ultrasonically when sterile saline (200–400 μl) is injected intravascularly through the sampling needle.

## Risks

The risk of fetal death after cordocentesis depends on the indication for sampling and the experience of the operator. In a series of 553 cases sampled for prenatal diagnosis of genetic disease (e.g. thalassaemia), or for karyotyping in cases of minor fetal malformations (e.g. hydronephrosis) the procedure-related fetal loss rate was less than 1 per cent (4 of 469 pregnancies that did not undergo elective abortion). These losses occurred as a result of chorioamnionitis or fetal haemorrhage. Similarly, Daffos *et al.* (1985) in a series of 562 cases, sampled primarily for diagnosis of toxoplasmosis, reported 7 fetal losses.

## Characteristics of small-for-gestational age fetuses

All patients were referred to our centre and were therefore preselected. This is reflected in the extreme degree of fetal smallness and the high incidence of oligohydramnios, abnormal Doppler results, chromosomal defects and intrauterine or neonatal death. The mean gestational age at cordocentesis was 29 (range 17–39) weeks.

### Fetal size

In all cases the fetal abdominal circumference, measured by ultrasonography, was at least 2 standard deviations (range 2–8) below the mean for gestational age of our reference range that was constructed from the study of 1610 normal pregnancies. The amniotic fluid volume was subjectively assessed by ultrasonography to be normal in 94 of the 263 (36 per cent) cases and reduced in 85 (32 per cent) cases. Oligohydramnios, defined by the absence of any pocket of amniotic fluid greater than 1 cm in diameter, was found in 77 (29 per cent) cases.

### Doppler characteristics

In 214 of the 263 pregnancies, Doppler studies of the uterine arteries and fetal circulation were performed. In 133 (62.2 per cent) cases the impedance to flow in the uterine arteries was increased, as demonstrated by the presence of an early diastolic notch (Figure 7.3) or a resistance index above the 97.5th centile of our reference range. These findings presumably reflect the inadequate trophoblastic invasion of the maternal spiral arteries, which may have been the underlying cause of the fetal growth retardation. In 127 (59.3 per cent) cases there were abnormalities in flow velocity waveforms in the umbilical artery (Figure 7.4; absent end-diastolic frequencies or a pulsatility index above the 97.5th centile of our normal range). In 131 of 194 (67.5 per cent) cases there were abnormalities in fetal vessels (absent end-diastolic frequencies in the fetal aorta, decreased velocity of blood in the descending thoracic aorta and increased velocity in the common carotid artery, increased impedance to flow in the aorta or renal arteries and decreased impedance in the common carotid or middle cerebral arteries). These findings presumably reflect the redistribution in the fetal circulation in response to fetal hypoxaemia.

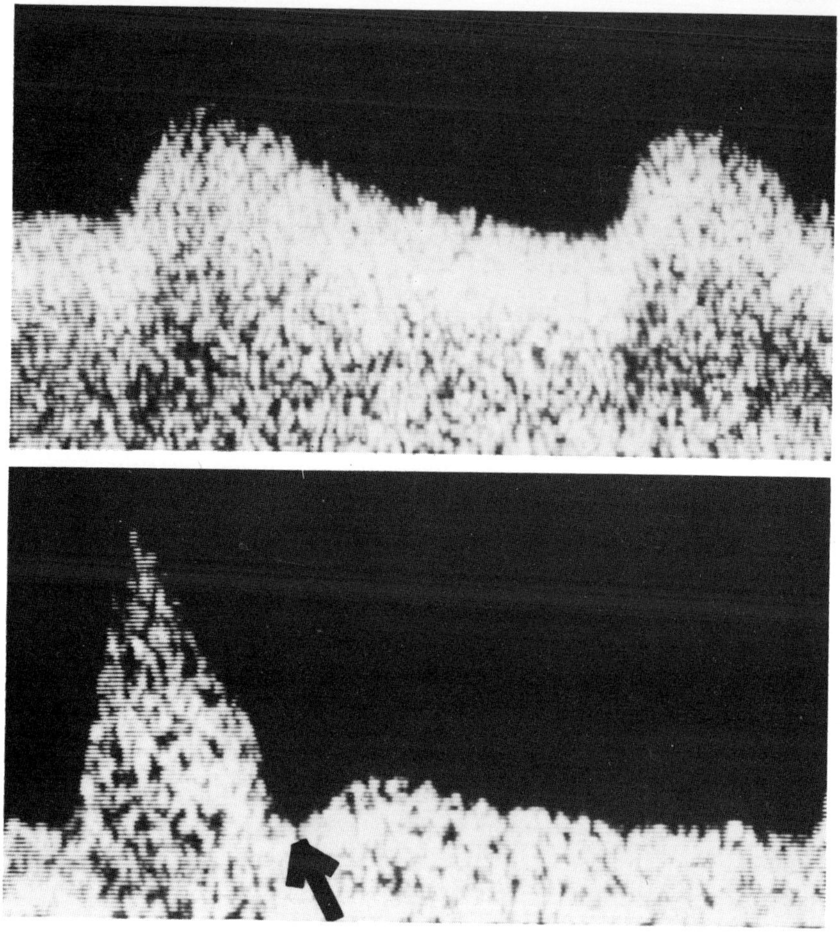

**Fig. 7.3** Normal flow velocity waveforms of uterine artery (top). Early diastolic notch (bottom) is characteristic of high resistance to flow. This is presumably the result of failure of trophoblastic invasion of the spiral arteries.

## Fetal karyotype

Chromosomal abnormalities were found in 42 (16 per cent) of the fetuses. These included triploidy (19 cases), trisomy 21 (2 cases), trisomy 18 (7 cases), trisomy 13 (2 cases), and other aneuploidies, deletions or translocations (12 cases). The triploidies were most commonly encountered in the second trimester while the aneuploidies, deletions and translocations in the third trimester group of fetuses (Figure 7.5). These findings suggest that triploidy is associated with the most severe form of early onset growth retardation and that the majority of affected fetuses die before the third trimester of pregnancy.

It is commonly stated that uteroplacental insufficiency is associated with asymmetrical fetal growth retardation while chromosomal defects result in symmetrical growth retardation. This may well be true for the third trimester of pregnancy but certainly in the second trimester the

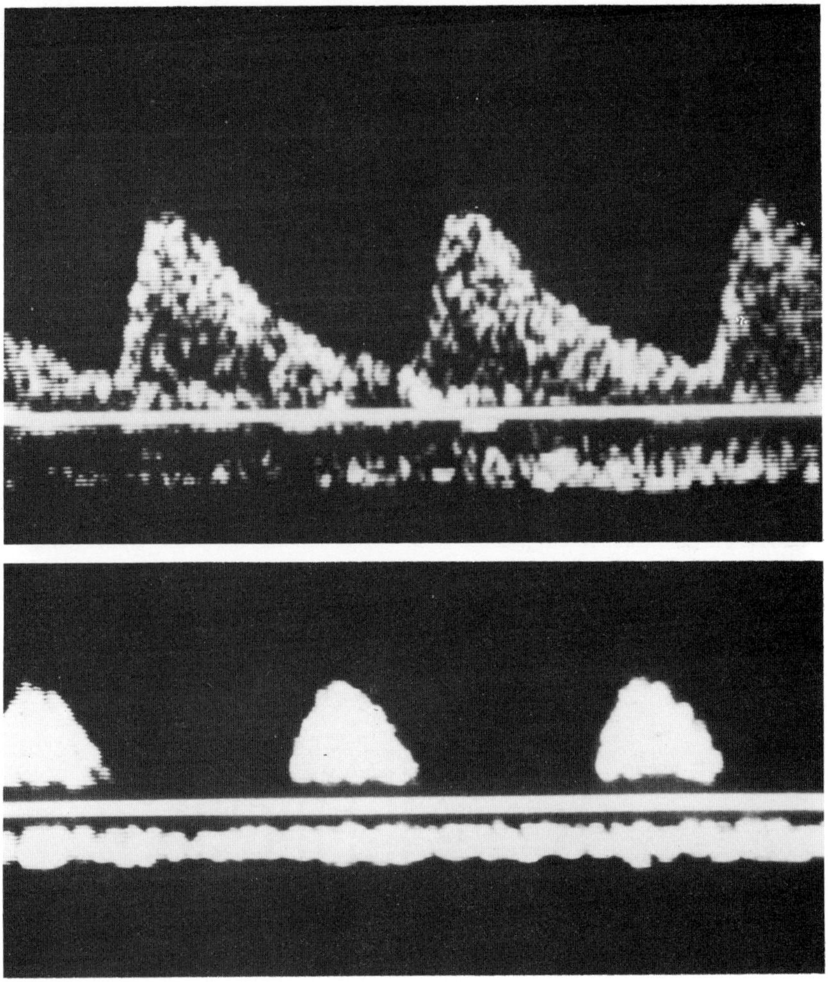

**Fig. 7.4** Normal flow velocity waveforms of umbilical artery (top). Absence of frequencies at the end of diastole (bottom) signifies increased peripheral resistance and is commonly associated with fetal hypoxaemia.

most severely asymmetrically small fetuses are chromosomally abnormal (Figure 7.6).

### Outcome

Of the 263 SGA fetuses 33 (12.5 per cent) were electively aborted because they were either chromosomally abnormal or the severity of growth retardation and hypoxaemia were such that the chances of normal survival were minimal; 43 (16.3 per cent) of the pregnancies resulted in intrauterine and 23 (8.7 per cent) in neonatal deaths; 143 (54 per cent) infants were liveborn and although the majority were very premature preliminary data suggest that development is normal; 21 pregnancies are continuing.

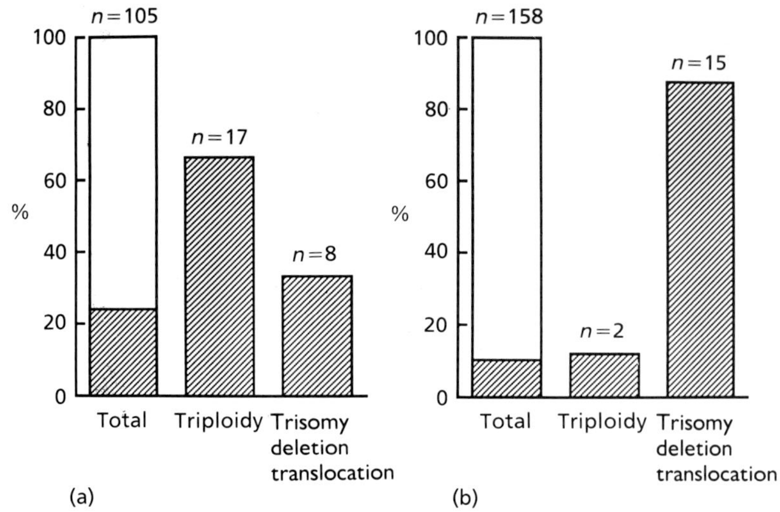


**Fig. 7.5** Chromosomal findings in 263 small-for-gestational age fetuses undergoing cordocentesis. The commonest chromosomal defect in the second trimester severely growth retarded fetus is triploidy. (a) <28 weeks, (b) >28 weeks.

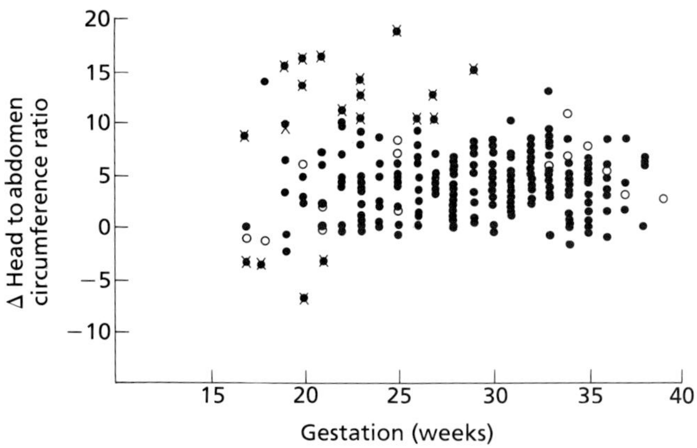


**Fig. 7.6** The head to abdomen ratio in chromosomally normal (●) and abnormal (○) small-for-gestational age fetuses. Triploid fetuses (★) exhibit the most severe degrees of asymmetrical growth retardation; when the placenta is molar there is relative microcephaly and when the placenta appears normal the head to abdomen circumference ratio is increased.

# Blood gases, pH and lactate

## Appropriate-for-gestational age fetuses

The umbilical venous and arterial $PO_2$ and pH decrease with gestational age while $PCO_2$ increases and blood lactate concentration does not change (Figures 7.7–7.10; Soothill *et al.* 1986b; Nicolaides *et al.* 1989). The changes with gestation are compatible with the $PO_2$, $PCO_2$ and pH measurements at hysterotomy in early gestation (Rudolph *et al.* 1971) and at elective Caesarean section at term (Pardi *et al.* 1987).

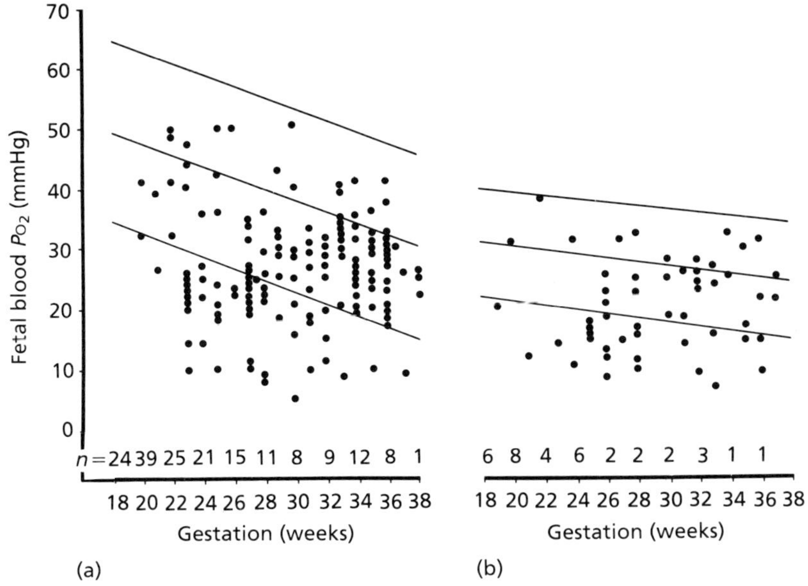


**Fig. 7.7** Reference ranges (mean and individual 95 per cent confidence intervals) for (a) umbilical venous; and (b) arterial blood oxygen tension (mmHg) with gestation in appropriate-for-gestational age fetuses, and the individual values of small-for-gestational age fetuses (●).

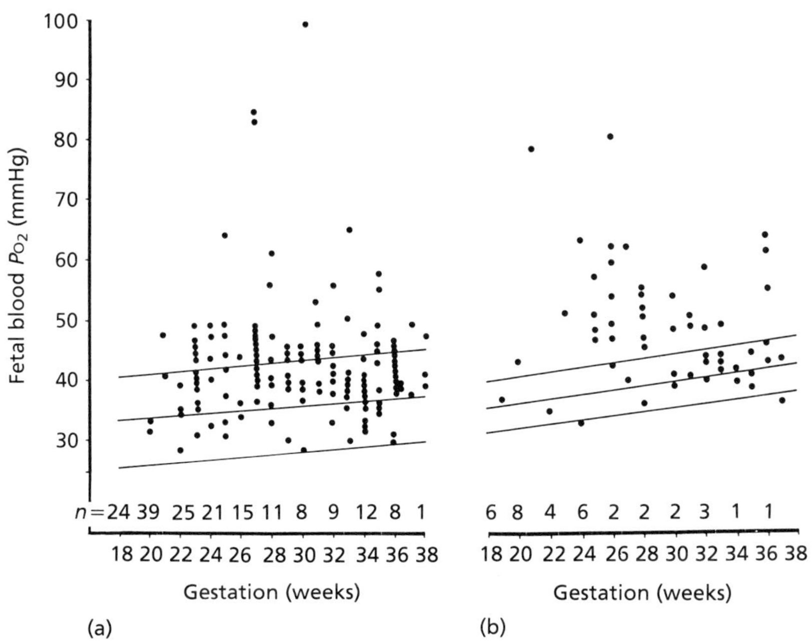


**Fig. 7.8** Reference ranges (mean and individual 95 per cent confidence intervals) for (a) umbilical venous; and (b) arterial blood carbon dioxide tension (mmHg) with gestation in appropriate-for-gestational age fetuses, and the individual values of small-for-gestational age fetuses (●).

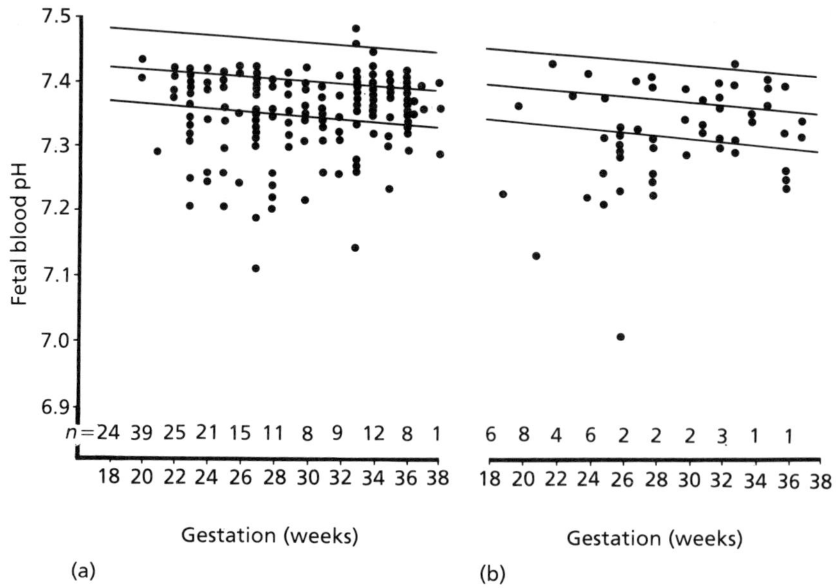


**Fig. 7.9** Reference ranges (mean and individual 95 per cent confidence intervals) for (a) umbilical venous; and (b) arterial blood pH with gestation in appropriate-for-gestational age fetuses, and the individual values of small-for-gestational age fetuses (●).

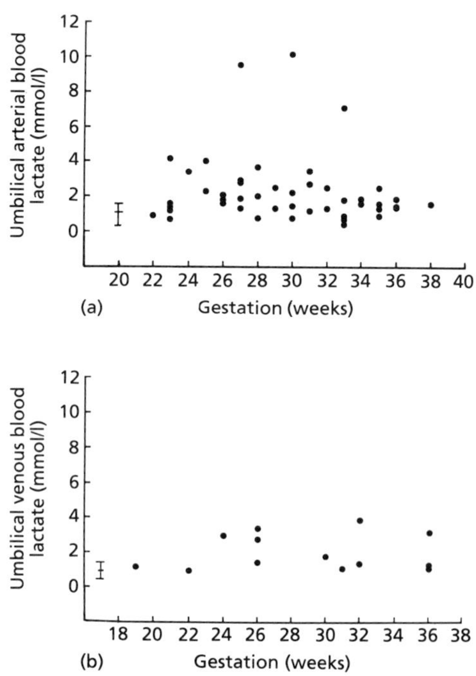


**Fig. 7.10** (a) Umbilical venous; and (b) arterial blood lactate concentration (mmol/l) in small-for-gestational age fetuses. The vertical lines represent the mean and 2 standard deviations in appropriate-for-gestational-age-fetuses.

The oxygen tension in fetal blood is much lower than in maternal blood, and it has been suggested that this is due either to incomplete venous equilibration of uterine and umbilical circulations, or to high placental oxygen consumption. However, the high affinity of fetal haemoglobin for oxygen, together with the high fetal cardiac output in relation to oxygen demand, compensates for the low fetal $Po_2$ (Battaglia & Meschia 1986). The decrease in fetal blood $Po_2$ with gestation is steeper in the umbilical vein than artery (Figure 7.8). Since the uteroplacental blood flow per kilogram remains the same, this decrease must reflect increased placental oxygen consumption with advancing gestation. Indeed, the umbilical arteriovenous oxygen difference decreases with gestation, and since umbilical blood flow per kilogram does not increase (Gerson *et al.* 1987), then umbilical oxygen uptake, and therefore fetal oxygen consumption, is reduced with advancing gestation. Despite the decrease in fetal $Po_2$ with gestational age, the umbilical venous blood oxygen content remains the same because the fetal haemoglobin concentration rises with gestational age (Nicolaides *et al.* 1987a).

Fetal blood lactate concentration does not change with gestation and the values are similar to those in samples obtained at elective Caesarean section at term (Pardi *et al.* 1987). The umbilical venous concentration (mean 0.99, SD 0.32 mmol/l) is higher than the umbilical arterial (mean 0.92, SD 0.21 mmol/l) suggesting that the normoxaemic human fetus is, like the sheep fetus (Burd *et al.* 1975), a net consumer of lactate. Furthermore, the concentration of lactate in umbilical cord blood is higher than in the maternal blood and the two are correlated significantly. This suggests a common source of lactate, which is likely to be the placenta. Indeed, the human placenta has been shown to produce lactate that is secreted into both fetal and maternal circulations (Holzman *et al.* 1979).

## Small-for-gestational age fetuses

Some SGA fetuses were found to be hypoxaemic, hypercapnic, hyperlacticaemic and acidotic (Figures 7.8–7.10; Soothill *et al.* 1987; Nicolaides *et al.* 1989). These findings demonstrate that asphyxia manifested at birth may not be due to the process of birth itself, but rather it may exist antenatally. The degree of acidosis correlates significantly with both hypercapnia and hyperlacticaemia. Furthermore, both respiratory and metabolic acidosis increase with hypoxaemia. The carbon dioxide accumulation is presumably the result of reduced exchange between the uteroplacental and fetal circulations, due to reduced blood flow. Decreased blood velocity in the descending fetal aorta (Soothill *et al.* 1986a) and increased resistance in the umbilical (Nicolaides *et al.* 1988b) and uterine arteries (Soothill *et al.* 1986c) in SGA pregnancies correlate significantly with hypoxaemia, hypercapnia and acidosis.

In umbilical venous blood mild hypoxaemia may be present in the absence of hypercapnia or acidosis, while in umbilical arterial hypoxaemia

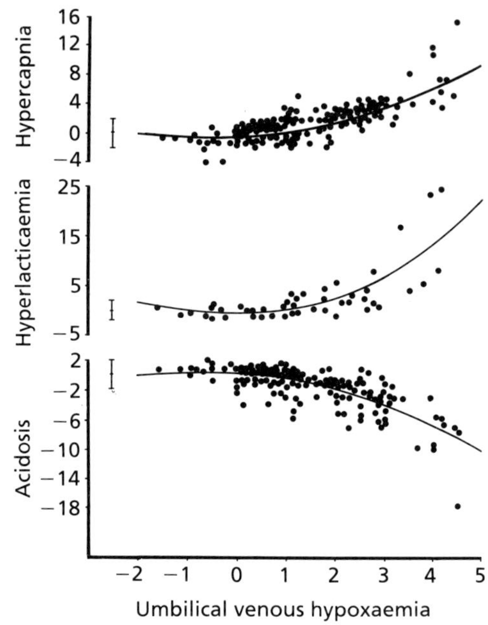


**Fig. 7.11** The correlations between umbilical venous hypoxaemia and hypercapnia, hyperlacticaemia or acidosis in small-for-gestational age fetuses.

there is a linear increase in the degrees of hypercapnia and acidosis (Figures 7.11 and 7.12). Indeed, in the umbilical artery the $P\text{CO}_2$ exceeds the 97.5th centile of the reference range before the development of significant hypoxaemia. Thus, in mild uteroplacental insufficiency the carbon dioxide that accumulates in umbilical arterial blood is cleared by a single passage through the placenta, and this is probably the result of the greater speed of diffusion of carbon dioxide compared to oxygen. In contrast, hyperlacticaemia is present in borderline hypoxaemia and is an early biochemical sign of oxygen deficit. In severe uteroplacental insufficiency the rate of clearance of carbon dioxide is exceeded by the rate of production and umbilical venous hypercapnia and acidosis increase exponentially. Thus the best determinants of uteroplacental insufficiency are umbilical venous hypoxaemia or hyperlacticaemia and umbilical arterial hypercapnia or acidosis.

Some SGA fetuses are hyperlacticaemic. This has also been demonstrated in fetal sheep that were subjected to acute hypoxia (Jones 1977) or that were growth retarded (Robinson *et al.* 1979). When there is inadequate oxygen supply the Krebs cycle is inhibited, and pyruvic acid is converted to lactic acid by the action of lactate dehydrogenase. The correlation between hypoxaemia and hyperlacticaemia supports the concept of reduced oxidative metabolism of lactate. Alternatively, hyperlacticaemia could be the result of impaired fetal gluconeogenesis, resulting in decreased utilization of lactate. Indeed, gluconeogenic substrates are increased in SGA infants (Haymond *et al.* 1974) which also have decreased gluconeogenic ability (Mestyan *et al.* 1974). A third

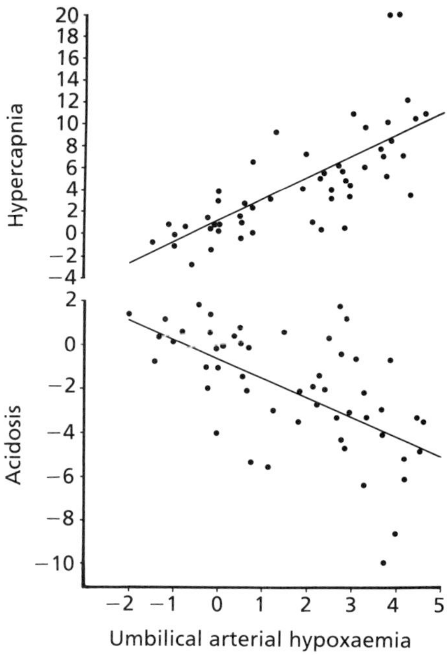


**Fig. 7.12** The correlations between umbilical arterial hypoxaemia and hypercapnia or acidosis in small-for-gestational age fetuses.

possible mechanism producing hyperlacticaemia is increased placental production of lactate. Fetal hypoglycaemia in SGA fetuses is probably caused by a reduction in the supply of glucose to the fetoplacental unit (Economides & Nicolaides 1989). It is possible that there is a compensatory increase in the placental production of lactate, for the fetus to utilize as an alternative energy substrate to glucose. This is supported by studies in the sheep, where experimentally induced growth retarded fetuses show increased consumption and the placenta increased production of lactate (Owens *et al.* 1987). However, since maternal blood lactate is not higher in the SGA than AGA groups, and since there is no correlation between fetal and maternal blood lactate it is unlikely that the high fetal blood lactate is of placental origin.

## Blood glucose and plasma insulin

### Appropriate-for-gestational age fetuses

The mean umbilical venous blood glucose concentration is higher than in the umbilical artery indicating that there is fetal glucose uptake from the placenta (Figure 7.13; Economides & Nicolaides 1989). Similarly, the maternal glucose concentration is higher than the fetal and the levels in the two compartments are significantly correlated, confirming that the major source of fetal glucose is the mother. The umbilical venous plasma insulin concentration and the fetal insulin to glucose ratio increase exponentially with gestation (Figures 7.14 and 7.15; Economides *et al.*

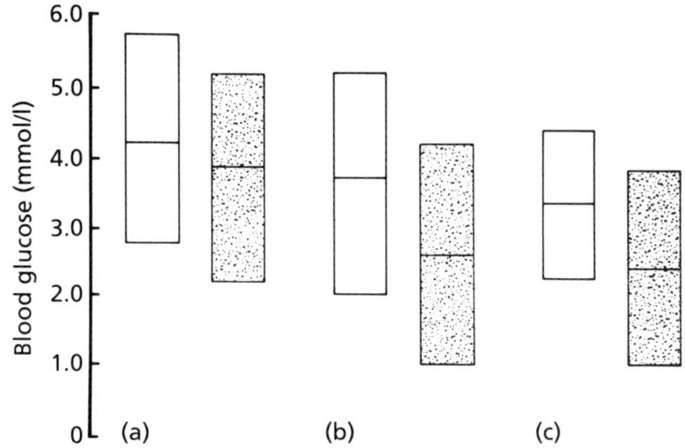


**Fig. 7.13** The (a) maternal, (b) umbilical venous; and (c) umbilical arterial blood glucose concentration (mmol/l) in appropriate and small-for-gestational age pregnancies. (□) AGA, (▨) SGA.

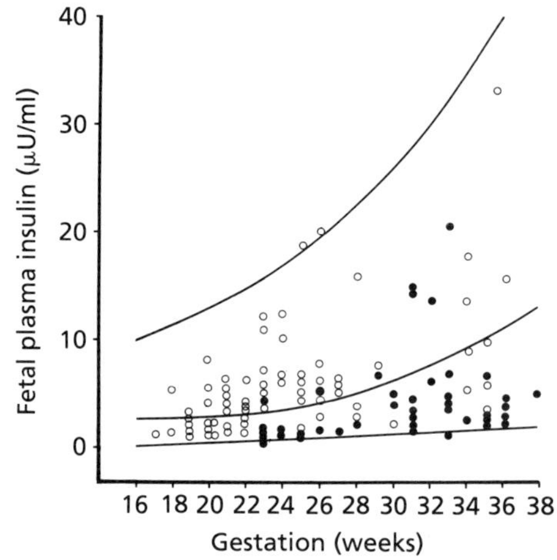


**Fig. 7.14** Reference ranges (mean and individual 95 per cent confidence intervals) of umbilical venous plasma insulin concentration (μU/ml) with gestation. The individual values of appropriate-for-gestational-age (○) and small-for-gestational age (●) fetuses are also shown.

1989b). These findings presumably reflect the progressive maturation of the endocrine activity in the human fetal pancreas.

## Small-for-gestational age fetuses

Some small-for-gestational age babies are at increased risk of hypoglycaemia and it has been suggested that the causes are depletion of liver glycogen stores (Shelley & Neligan 1966) and impaired hepatic gluconeogenesis (Haymond *et al.* 1974). However, hypoglycaemia has also been demonstrated in intrauterine life both in experimental animals (Robinson *et al.* 1979) and in SGA human fetuses (Figure 7.16; Soothill *et al.* 1987).

Possible causes for fetal hypoglycaemia are inadequate maternal

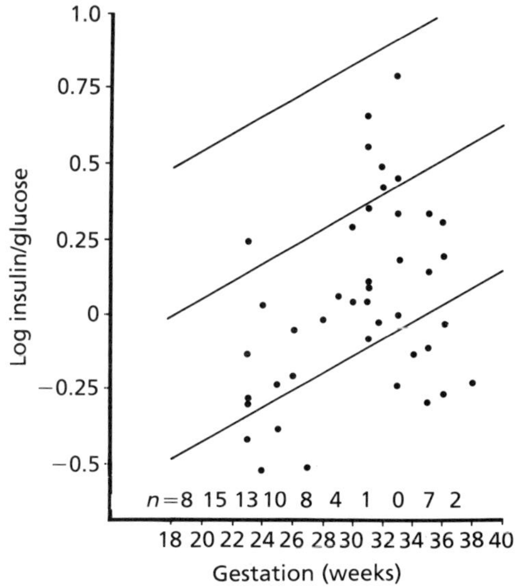


**Fig. 7.15** Reference ranges (mean and individual 95 per cent confidence intervals) in $\log_{10}$ of umbilical venous insulin to glucose ratio with gestation, and the individual values of small-for-gestational age fetuses (●).

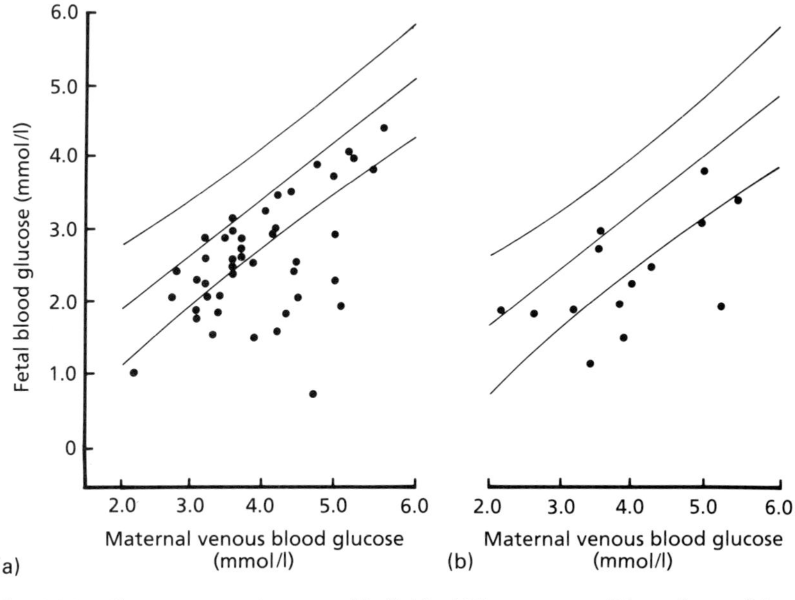


**Fig. 7.16** Reference ranges (mean and individual 95 per cent confidence intervals) of fetal with maternal blood glucose concentration (mmol/l) in pregnancies with appropriate-for-gestational age fetuses, and the individual values in those with small-for-gestational age fetuses (●). (a) Umbilical vein, (b) umbilical artery.

supply of glucose to the fetoplacental unit, either because of decreased maternal glucose concentration or impaired placental perfusion, decreased fetal gluconeogenesis or increased fetal glucose consumption. The maternal blood glucose in the SGA group was significantly lower than the controls (Figure 7.13) and this is thought to be the result of relative hyperinsulinaemia due to decreased placental production of diabetogenic hormones (Khouzami *et al.* 1981). However, the observed decrease in maternal glucose is too small to account for the severity of fetal hypoglycaemia.

In the SGA fetuses, the degree of hypoxaemia correlates with the maternal–fetal glucose gradient in both the umbilical vein and umbilical artery. The two lines describing these correlations are parallel. Therefore, the major cause of fetal hypoglycaemia is unlikely to be decreased endogenous production or increased consumption of glucose. In sheep, restriction of placental growth by removal of endometrial caruncles produces growth retarded fetuses that are also hypoxaemic and hypoglycaemic (Owens *et al.* 1987). However, hypoglycaemia is not due to increased glucose consumption as a result of hypoxaemia, because in experimental fetal growth retardation produced by prolonged maternal hypobaric hypoxia the fetuses are hypoxaemic but not hypoglycaemic (Jacobs *et al.* 1988). Placental transfer of glucose does not require oxygen. Furthermore, placental glucose consumption in experimental growth retardation is not increased (Owens *et al.* 1987). Therefore, it is likely that the major cause of hypoglycaemia in SGA fetuses is reduced glucose supply from the mother and that the maternal–fetal glucose gradient is a measure of impaired placental perfusion.

Some SGA fetuses are hypoinsulinaemic and the degree of hypoinsulinaemia correlates significantly with the degree of fetal hypoglycaemia (Figure 7.14; Economides *et al.* 1989b). Since the major cause of hypoglycaemia in SGA fetuses is reduced uteroplacental blood flow, this suggests that hypoinsulinaemia is the result of reduced glucose supply to the fetus. However, the fetal insulin to glucose ratio is lower in the SGA than the AGA fetuses (Figure 7.15) indicating that fetal hypoinsulinaemia may also be a consequence of pancreatic β-cell dysfunction. This is supported by post-mortem studies of growth retarded infants where the endocrine pancreatic tissue is reduced (Van Assche *et al.* 1977).

Fetal insulin does not correlate with the degree of fetal smallness suggesting that insulin is not the primary determinant of fetal size (Economides *et al.* 1989b). Instead, insulin may influence fetal growth through its action on nutrient uptake and utilization. Hypoinsulinaemia in the fetus will direct nutrients away from the insulin sensitive tissues, such as skeletal muscle, liver and adipose tissue. The result will be decreased glycogen and fat stores and impaired fetal growth.

## Plasma cortisol and ACTH

### Appropriate-for-gestational age fetuses

Plasma cortisol is present in the fetal circulation and the concentration does not change between 18 and 36 weeks' gestation (Figure 7.17;

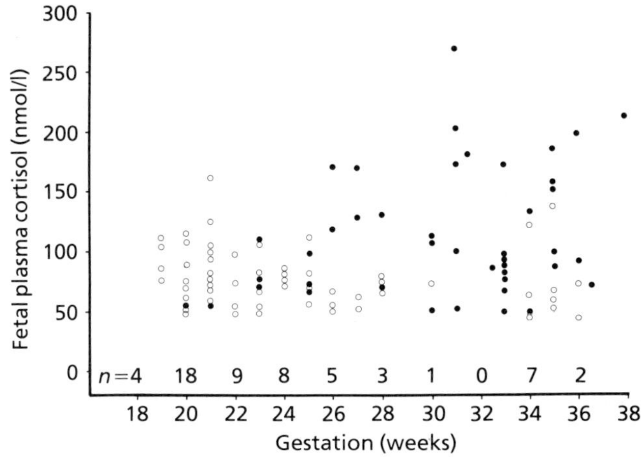


**Fig. 7.17** Plasma cortisol concentration (nmol/l) in appropriate-for-gestational age (○) and small-for-gestational age (●) fetuses.

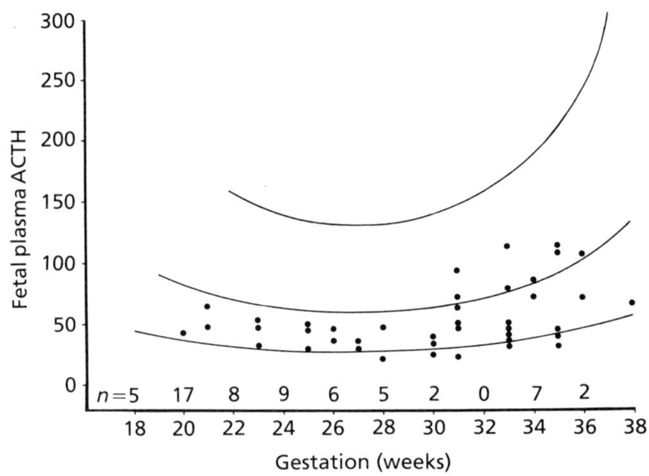


**Fig. 7.18** Reference ranges (mean and individual 95 per cent confidence intervals) of plasma ACTH concentration (pg/ml) with gestation in appropriate-for-gestational age fetuses, and the individual values of small-for-gestational age fetuses (●).

Economides *et al.* 1988b). Fetal plasma ACTH concentration increases with gestation (Figure 7.18) and there is no significant correlation between ACTH and cortisol levels (Economides *et al.* 1988b). This suggests that the fetal pituitary–adrenal axis may be relatively immature. The lack of correlation between cortisol and ACTH has also been shown in the sheep (Robinson *et al.* 1983) where the adrenal becomes sensitive to ACTH stimulation only in very late gestation (Liggins 1976). Alternatively, the findings could be explained if a major source of ACTH is the placenta (Liotta *et al.* 1977); placental secretion of ACTH is insensitive to negative feedback by steroids (Petraglia *et al.* 1987).

### Small-for-gestational age fetuses

In SGA fetuses plasma cortisol concentration is increased, presumably in an effort to combat the accompanying hypoglycaemia (Figure 7.17; Economides *et al.* 1988b). This was also found in experimentally induced growth retarded sheep fetuses, which responded to acute hypoxaemia by increasing both plasma cortisol and ACTH levels (Robinson *et al.* 1983). However, in human SGA fetuses, the plasma ACTH concentration is decreased (Figure 7.18; Economides *et al.* 1988b). Therefore, the most likely explanation for the raised plasma cortisol is increased adrenal blood flow, the consequence of redistribution in fetal circulation in response to hypoxaemia (Peeters *et al.* 1979). The reduced plasma ACTH levels in SGA fetuses may be the result of negative feedback of cortisol on pituitary ACTH secretion or a direct consequence of the reduced placental size and therefore decreased placental production of ACTH, corticotrophin-releasing hormone, or both.

## Plasma lipids

### Appropriate-for-gestational age fetuses

Lipid metabolism is of major importance for fetal cell and organ growth and in late fetal life there are increasing requirements of lipids for special functions in the brain, lung and adipose tissue (Warshaw 1979). Fetal plasma triglyceride concentration decreases exponentially with gestation (Figure 7.19; Economides *et al.* 1989e). This observation is compatible with reported levels in cord blood at the time of delivery. Thus, premature infants of 25–26 weeks had higher cord triglyceride concentration than did those delivered after 27 weeks (Dhanireddy *et al.* 1981). There is no correlation between fetal and maternal triglyceride levels

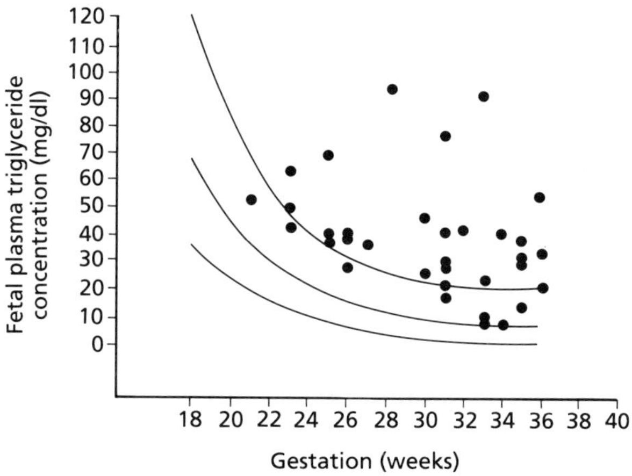


**Fig. 7.19** Reference ranges (mean and individual 95 per cent confidence intervals) of fetal plasma triglyceride concentration (mg/dl) with gestation, and the individual values of small-for-gestational age fetuses (●).

suggesting that there is no significant transplacental transport of these lipids, and that the fetal levels reflect fetal metabolism. Fetal tissues are capable of synthesizing triglyceride from at least 12 weeks' gestation (Vilee & Loring 1961; Yoshioka & Roux 1972). However, deposition of adipose tissue begins after 24 weeks and increases exponentially, so that at 32 weeks the fetal fat content is 3.5 per cent, and at 40 weeks 16 per cent of the body weight (Widdowson 1968). Therefore, the observed decrease in plasma triglyceride concentration with gestation may be the result of increased utilization by the fetus for deposition into adipose tissue.

The plasma non-esterified fatty acids (NEFA) levels, although present in low concentrations in the fetus, correlate significantly with the maternal levels suggesting that there is placental transfer of fatty acids. In contrast, the maternal and fetal glycerol concentrations are not significantly correlated. On the basis of umbilical arteriovenous differences in humans at the time of elective Caesarean section it has also been inferred that NEFA may cross the placenta in significant amounts (Elphick *et al.* 1976). However, studies of the perfused human placenta (Dancis *et al.* 1973) have shown that the rate of NEFA transfer from mother to the fetus was approximately 20 per cent of that required for adipose tissue deposition, and therefore the major source of fetal NEFA is endogenous synthesis. The low fetal NEFA compared to the maternal and the decrease in umbilical venous plasma concentration with gestation may be the result of utilization of NEFA for fat deposition.

### Small-for-gestational age fetuses

In hypoxaemic SGA fetuses the plasma triglyceride concentration is increased (Figure 7.19) and the blood glucose and plasma insulin decreased; plasma NEFA and glycerol levels are not disturbed (Economides *et al.* 1988a). The most likely explanation for the observed hypertriglyceridaemia is decreased utilization of triglycerides, due either to impaired oxidation of lipids or to reduced uptake into adipose tissue. Hypertriglyceridaemia has been associated with perinatal asphyxia (Tsang *et al.* 1974; Cress *et al.* 1977). However, hypoxia is unlikely to be the major cause of hypertriglyceridaemia because although there is a significant correlation between the degree of hypertriglyceridaemia and the degree of hypoxaemia, there is no corresponding elevation in the concentration of NEFA.

The alternative explanation for the observed hypertriglyceridaemia is reduced uptake into adipose tissue. In low birth weight infants and in children with marasmus, lipoprotein lipase and the ability to clear intralipid from the circulation are reduced (Gurson & Saner 1969; Gustafson *et al.* 1972; Shennan *et al.* 1977), suggesting that a critical mass of adipose tissue is necessary for normal metabolism of circulating triglycerides. In AGA fetuses the plasma triglyceride concentration decreases exponentially with gestation and this decrease coincides with increased deposition of fat (Widdowson 1968). Therefore, failure of the normal process of fat deposition will be accompanied by failure of triglyceride levels to decline. Some SGA fetuses are hypoinsulinaemic. Insulin stimulates lipoprotein lipase, augments the activity of hepatic fatty acid synthetase and increases the activity of acetyl-CoA carboxylase in adipose tissue (Warshaw 1979). Therefore, hypoinsulinaemia could result in decreased adipose tissue stores by impairing the uptake of circulating triglycerides as well as by reducing the synthesis of tissue triglycerides.

## Plasma amino acids

### Appropriate-for-gestational age fetuses

The fetal plasma aminogram has been extensively studied in the past from samples obtained at hysterotomy, Caesarean section or vaginal delivery (Lindblad & Baldesten 1967; Young & Prenton 1969; Cockburn *et al.* 1970; Cockburn *et al.* 1971). These studies have shown that the fetal levels are higher than the maternal, providing supporting evidence for active transport across the placenta (Enders *et al.* 1976). In conditions where placental function is impaired fetal amino acid metabolism is disturbed (Young & Prenton 1969) and SGA infants have abnormal amino acid profiles (Lindblad & Zetterstrom 1968; Cetin *et al.* 1988).

Recently, samples obtained by cordocentesis have demonstrated that there is a high correlation between fetal and maternal levels for individual amino acids and that the concentration in the fetus is higher than in the mother (Economides *et al.* 1989c). The fetomaternal amino acid ratio decreases with advancing gestation implying increased consumption by the fetoplacental unit (Economides *et al.* 1989c). This increase in metabolic activity is compatible with the increased oxygen consumption by the fetoplacental unit and the decrease in fetal blood $PO_2$ with advancing gestation (Soothill *et al.* 1986b; Nicolaides *et al.* 1989).

### Small-for-gestational age fetuses

In pregnancies complicated by fetal hypoxaemia and growth retardation there is a disturbance in both maternal and fetal plasma amino acid profiles. Furthermore, there are significant correlations between the change in maternal or fetal plasma amino acid concentrations and the degree of fetal hypoxaemia (Economides *et al.* 1989c).

The maternal plasma concentration of both essential and non-essential amino acids is increased in fetal hypoxaemia (Figure 7.20), and this is compatible with the concept that in uteroplacental insufficiency there is a reduction in both the supply and therefore the consumption of amino acids by the fetoplacental unit.

The fetal plasma concentration and fetomaternal ratio of essential amino acids is decreased (Figure 7.21). These findings could be the result

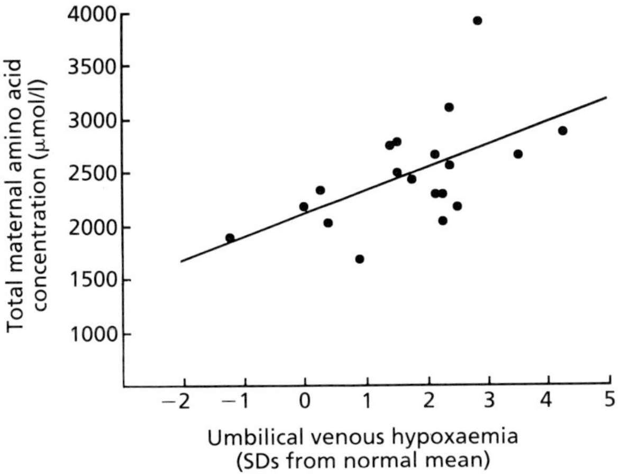


**Fig. 7.20** The correlation between umbilical venous hypoxaemia and the total maternal plasma amino acid concentration (μmol/l).

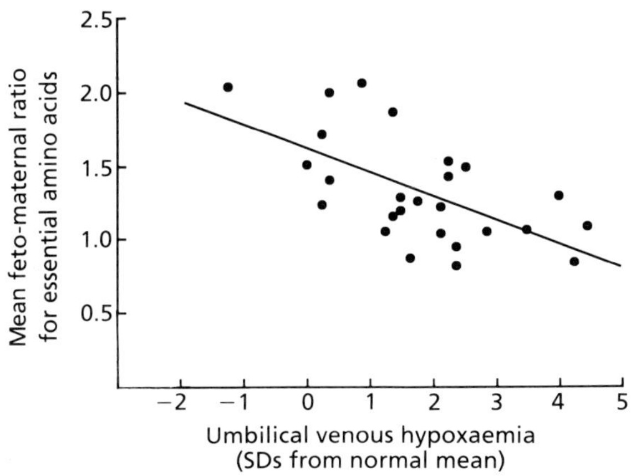


**Fig. 7.21** The correlation between umbilical venous hypoxaemia and the mean fetomaternal ratio of essential amino acids in small-for-gestational age fetuses.

of either increased fetoplacental consumption of these amino acids or reduced perfusion and transport across the placenta. In uteroplacental insufficiency the supply of both oxygen and glucose to the fetoplacental unit is reduced (Economides & Nicolaides 1989). In sheep, removal of endometrial caruncles results in fetal hypoxaemia, hypoglycaemia and growth retardation (Owens *et al.* 1987). In this situation the production of lactate by the placenta is increased, presumably to provide the hypoglycaemic fetus with an alternative substrate for oxidation. It has been suggested that the excess lactate is the result of increased placental consumption of amino acids (Owens *et al.* 1987).

There is a variable response in the fetal plasma concentration of the non-essential amino acids (Figure 7.22). In some cases (serine, tyrosine, taurine and ornithine) both the fetal plasma concentrations and the

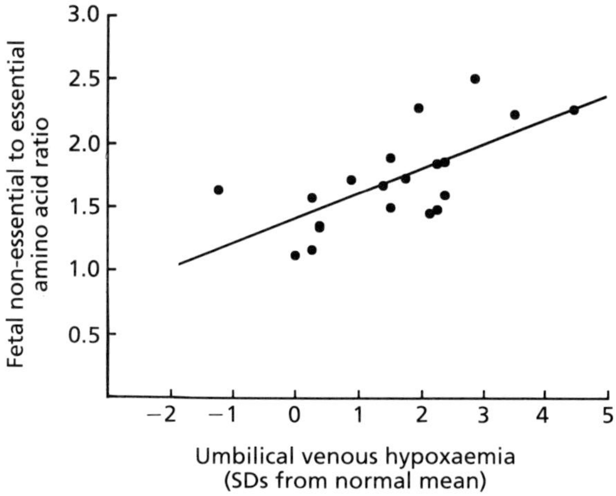


**Fig. 7.22** The correlation between umbilical venous hypoxaemia and the plasma non-essential to essential amino acid ratio in small-for-gestational age fetuses.

fetomaternal ratios are decreased. It is likely that the biosynthetic pathways of these amino acids are not fully established in intrauterine life and therefore they may be considered to be essential for the fetus. Some non-essential amino acids such as glycine (Economides *et al.* 1989d) increase in SGA fetuses and this may be the result of:

**1** Tissue breakdown; during maternal fasting in the sheep, there is a net flow of amino acids away from the fetal hind limb, suggesting that the fetus is capable of diverting amino acids away from areas of tissue growth (Liechty & Lemons 1984).

**2** Decreased utilization for protein synthesis, because of the reduced supply of the essential amino acids. Indeed, this may be the explanation for a similar increase in some non-essential amino acids observed in children with protein malnutrition (Holt *et al.* 1963).

**3** Decreased utilization for oxidation; when fetal sheep are subjected to prolonged hypobaric hypoxia (Jacobs *et al.* 1988), and when human babies are asphyxiated at birth (Schultz *et al.* 1977), the plasma levels of alanine are increased.

**4** Decreased utilization for gluconeogenesis; the gluconeogenic amino acids, such as alanine and glycine are increased in growth retarded babies (Haymond *et al.* 1974) and infusion of alanine in these infants fails to raise the glucose level suggesting impaired gluconeogenesis (Mestyan *et al.* 1974).

## Conclusion

Severe early onset fetal growth retardation is commonly associated with chromosomal abnormalities. Furthermore, some small fetuses are hypoxaemic, hypercapnic, hyperlacticaemic and acidaemic and they have disturbed carbohydrate, lipid and protein metabolism.

# References

Battaglia F.C. & Meschia G. (1986) *An Introduction to Fetal Physiology*, pp. 154–67. Academic Press, London.

Burd L.I., Jones M.D. & Simmons M.A. (1975) Placental production and fetal utilisation of lactate and pyruvate. *Nature*, **254**, 210–11.

Cetin I., Marconi A.M., Bozzetti P. *et al.* (1988) Umbilical amino acid concentrations in appropriate and small for gestational age infants: a biochemical difference present *in utero*. *American Journal of Obstetrics and Gynecology*, **158**, 120–6.

Cockburn F., Blagden A., Michie E.A. & Forfar J.O. (1971) The influence on preeclampsia and diabetes mellitus on plasma free amino acids in maternal umbilical vein and infant blood. *Journal of Obstetrics and Gynaecology of the British Commonwealth*, **78**, 215–31.

Cockburn F., Robins S.P. & Forfar J.O. (1970) Free amino acid concentrations in fetal fluids. *British Medical Journal*, **3**, 747–50.

Cress H.R., Shaher R.M., Laffin R. & Karpowicz K. (1977) Cord blood hyperlipoproteinemia and perinatal stress. *Pediatric Research* **11**, 19–23.

Daffos F., Capela-Pavlovsky M. & Forestier F. (1985) Fetal blood sampling during pregnancy with use of a needle guided by ultrasound: A study of 606 consecutive cases. *American Journal of Obstetrics and Gynecology*, **153**, 655–60.

Dancis J., Jansen V., Kayden H.J., Schneider H. & Levitz M. (1973) Transfer across perfused human placenta II. Free fatty acids. *Pediatric Research* **7**, 192–7.

Dhanireddy R., Hamosh M., Siva K.N., Chowdry P., Scanlon J.W. & Hamosh P. (1981) Postheparin lipolytic activity and Intralipid clearance in very low-birth-weight infants. *Journal of Pediatrics*, **98**, 617–22.

Economides D.L., Crook D. & Nicolaides K.H. (1989e) Hypertriglyceridaemia and hypoxaemia in small for gestational age fetuses. *American Journal of Obstetrics and Gynecology* (in press).

Economides D.L., Crook D. & Nicolaides K.H. (1988a) Investigation of hypertriglyceridaemia in small for gestational age fetuses. *Fetal Therapy*, **3**, 165–72.

Economides D.L. & Nicolaides K.H. (1989a) Blood glucose and oxygen tension in small for gestational age fetuses. *American Journal of Obstetrics and Gynecology*, **160**, 385–9.

Economides D.L., Nicolaides K.H., Gahl W., Bernardini I., Bottoms S.F. & Evans M. (1989d) Cordocentesis in the diagnosis of intrauterine starvation. *American Journal of Obstetrics and Gynecology* (in press).

Economides D.L., Nicolaides K.H., Gahl W., Bernardini I. & Evans M. (1989c) Plasma amino acids in appropriate small for gestational age fetuses. *American Journal of Obstetrics and Gynecology* (in press).

Economides D.L., Nicolaides K.H., Linton E.A., Perry L.A. & Chard T. (1988b) Plasma cortisol and ACTH in appropriate and small for gestational age fetuses. *Fetal Therapy*, **3**, 158–64.

Economides D.L., Proudler A. & Nicolaides K.H. (1989b) Plasma insulin in appropriate and small for gestational age fetuses. *American Journal of Obstetrics and Gynecology*, **160**, 1091–4.

Elphick M.C., Hull D. & Sanders R.R. (1976) Concentration of free fatty acids in maternal and umbilical cord blood during elective Caesarean section. *British Journal of Obstetrics and Gynaecology*, **83**, 539–44.

Enders R.H., Judd R.M., Donohue T.M. & Smith C.H. (1976) Placental amino acid uptake. III. Transport systems for neutral amino acids. *American Journal of Physiology*, **230**, 706–10.

Gerson A.G., Wallace D.A., Stiller R.J., Paul D., Weiner S. & Bolognese R.J. (1987) Doppler evaluation of umbilical venous and arterial blood flow in the second and third trimesters of normal pregnancy. *Obstetrics and Gynecology*, **70**, 622–6.

Gurson C. & Saner G. (1969) Lipoprotein lipase activity in marasmic type of protein calorie malnutrition. *Archives of Disease in Childhood*, **44**, 765–8.

Gustafson A., Kjellmer I., Olegard R. & Victorin L. (1972) Nutrition in low birth weight infants. *Acta Paediatrica Scandinavica*, **61**, 149–58.

Haymond M.W., Karl I.E. & Pagliara A.S. (1974) Increased gluconeogenic substrates in the small-for-gestational age infant. *New England Journal of Medicine* **291**, 322–8.

Holt L.E., Snyderman S.E., Norton P.M., Roitman E. & Finch J. (1963) Plasma

aminogram in Kwashiorkor. *Lancet*, **ii**, 1343–8.
Holzman I.R., Phillips A.F. & Battaglia F.C. (1979) Glucose metabolism, lactate and ammonia production by the human placenta *in vivo*. *Pediatric Research*, **13**, 117–20.
Jacobs R., Owens J.A., Falconer J., Webster M.E.D. & Robinson J.S. (1988) Changes to metabolite concentration in fetal sheep subjected to prolonged hypobaric hypoxia. *Journal of Developmental Physiology*, **10**, 113–21.
Jones C.T. (1977) The development of some metabolic responses to hypoxia in the fetal sheep. *Journal of Physiology*, **265**, 743–62.
Khouzami V.A., Ginsburg D.S., Daikoku N.H. & Johnson J.W. (1981) The glucose tolerance test as a means of identifying intrauterine growth retardation. *American Journal of Obstetrics and Gynecology*, **139**, 423–6.
Liechty E.A. & Lemons J.A. (1984) Changes in ovine fetal hindlimb amino acid metabolism during maternal fasting. *American Journal of Physiology*, **246**, E459–66.
Liggins G.C. (1976) Adrenocortical-related maturational events in the fetus. *American Journal of Obstetrics and Gynecology*, **126**, 931–41.
Lindblad B.S. & Baldesden A. (1967) The normal plasma free amino acid levels of non-pregnant women and of mother and child during delivery. *Acta Paediatrica Scandinavica*, **56**, 37–8.
Lindblad B.S. & Zetterstrom R. (1968) The venous plasma free amino acid levels of mother and child during delivery. II After short gestation and gestation complicated by hypertension with special reference to the 'small for dates' syndrome. *Acta Paediatrica Scandinavica*, **57**, 195–204.
Liotta A.S., Osathanondh R. & Ryan K.J. (1977) Presence of corticotropin in human placenta: demonstration of *in vivo* synthesis. *Endocrinology*, **101**, 1152–8.
Mestyan J., Schultz K. & Horvath M. (1974) Comparative glycemic responses to alanine in normal term and small-for-gestational age infants. *Journal of Pediatrics*, **85**, 276–8.
Nicolaides K.H., Bilardo C.M., Soothill P.W. & Campbell S. (1988b) Absence of end diastolic frequencies in the umbilical artery: a sign of fetal hypoxia and acidosis. *British Medical Journal*, **297**, 1026–7.
Nicolaides K.H., Economides D.L. & Soothill P.W. (1989) Blood gases and pH in appropriate and small for gestational age fetuses. *American Journal of Obstetrics and Gynecology* (in press).
Nicolaides K.H., Soothill P.W., Clewell W.H., Rodeck C.H., Mibashan R.S. & Campbell S. (1988a) Fetal haemoglobin measurement in the assessment of red cell isoimmunisation. *Lancet*, **i**, 1073–5.
Nicolaides K.H., Soothill P.W., Rodeck C.H. & Campbell S. (1986) Ultrasound guided sampling of umbilical cord and placental blood to assess fetal wellbeing. *Lancet*, **i**, 1065–7.
Owens J.A., Falconer J. & Robinson J.S. (1987) Effect of restriction of placental growth on fetal and uteroplacental metabolism. *Journal of Developmental Physiology*, **9**, 225–38.
Pardi G., Buscaglia M., Ferrazzi E., Bozzetti P., Marconi A.M., Cetin I., Battaglia F.C. & Makowski E.L. (1987) Cord sampling for the evaluation of oxygenation and acid–base balance in growth-retarded human fetuses. *American Journal of Obstetrics and Gynecology* **157**, 1221–8.
Peeters L.L.H., Sheldon R.F., Jones M.D., Makowski E.L. & Meschia G. (1979) Blood flow to fetal organs as a function of arterial oxygen content. *American Journal of Obstetrics and Gynecology* **135**, 639–46.
Petraglia F., Sawchenko P.E., Rivier J. & Vale W. (1987) Evidence for local stimulation of ACTH secretion by corticotropin-releasing factor in human placenta. *Nature*, **328**, 717–19.
Robinson J.S., Jones C.T. & Kingston E.J. (1983) Studies on experimental growth retardation in sheep. The effects of maternal hypoxaemia. *Journal of Developmental Physiology*, **5**, 89–100.
Robinson J.S., Kingston E.J., Jones C.T. & Thornburg G.D. (1979) Studies on experimental growth retardation in sheep. The effect of removal of endometrial caruncles on fetal size and metabolism. *Journal of Developmental Physiology*, **1**, 379–98.
Rudolph A.M., Heyman M.A., Teramo K.A.W., Barrett C.T. & Raiha N.C.R. (1971)

Studies on the circulation of the previable human fetus. *Pediatric Research* **5**, 452–65.

Schultz K., Mestyan J. & Soltesz G. (1977) The effect of birth asphyxia on plasma free amino acids in preterm newborn infants. *Acta Paediatrica Academiae Scientiarum Hungaricae*, **18**, 123–30.

Shelley H.J. & Neligan G.A. (1966) Neonatal hypoglycaemia. *British Medical Bulletin*, **22**, 34–9.

Shennan A.T., Bryan M.H. & Angel A. (1977) The effect of gestational age on intralipid tolerance in newborn infants. *Journal of Pediatrics*, **91**, 134–7.

Soothill P.W., Nicolaides K.H., Bilardo C.M. & Campbell S. (1986a) Relation of fetal hypoxia in growth retardation to mean blood velocity in the fetal aorta. *Lancet*, **ii**, 1118–19.

Soothill P.W., Nicolaides K.H., Bilardo C., Hackett G. & Campbell S. (1986c) Utero-placental blood velocity resistance index and umbilical venous $PO_2$, $PCO_2$, pH, lactate and erythroblast count in growth retarded fetuses. *Fetal Therapy*, **1**, 176–9.

Soothill P.W., Nicolaides K.H. & Campbell S. (1987) Prenatal asphyxia, hyperlacticaemia, hypoglycaemia and erythroblastosis in growth retarded fetuses. *British Medical Journal*, **294**, 1051–3.

Soothill P.W., Nicolaides K.H., Rodeck C.H. & Campbell S. (1986b) Effect of gestational age on fetal and intervillous blood gas and acid–base values in human pregnancy. *Fetal Therapy*, **1**, 168–75.

Tsang R., Glueck J., Evans G. & Steiner P.M. (1974) Cord blood hypertriglyceridemia. *American Journal of Diseases of Children*, **127**, 78–82.

Van Assche J.A., De Prins F., Aerts L. & Verjans M. (1977) The endocrine pancreas in small for dates infants. *British Journal of Obstetrics and Gynaecology*, **84**, 751–3.

Vilee C.A. & Loring J.M. (1961) Alternative pathways of carbohydrate metabolism in fetal and adult tissues. *Biochemical Journal*, **81**, 488–94.

Warshaw J.B. (1979) Fatty acid metabolism during development. *Seminars in Perinatology*, **3**, 131–9.

Widdowson E.M. (1968) Growth and composition of the fetus and newborn. In *Biology of Gestation*, (Ed. by N.S. Assali), p. 23. Academic Press, New York.

Yoshioka T. & Roux J.F. (1972) *In vitro* metabolism of palmitic acid in human fetal tissues. *Pediatric Research*, **6**, 675–81.

Young M. & Prenton M.A. (1969) Maternal and fetal plasma amino acid concentrations during gestation and in retarded fetal growth. *Journal of Obstetrics and Gynaecology of the British Commonwealth*, **76**, 333–44.

# 8: What determines fetal heart rate?

PHILIP J. STEER



Considering it is such a basic parameter, there is a surprising amount of mythology about the fetal heart rate. Antenatal mothers are often convinced that the basal fetal heart rate gives a clue to the sex of their baby; midwives and obstetricians say that post-term babies often have a baseline bradycardia. Neither belief is correct.

## Methods

This chapter will review the physiology of fetal heart rate (FHR) control and the clinical variables which influence it. Conclusions will be drawn not only from the published literature but also from a detailed study of cardiotocograph traces carried out in 1984 at St Mary's Hospital in Paddington (Steer *et al.* 1989). During this time, Eigbe performed a detailed analysis of all 1219 deliveries from 1 June to 30 November. Data collected included the baseline FHR of all cardiotocograms performed, either in the antenatal period for women undergoing elective Caesarean section or in labour, assessments being made over the last hour of both the first and second stages. Attempts were made to take umbilical artery blood samples at all deliveries, and this was achieved in 748 cases in which there was also complete heart rate data.

## Physiological control of fetal heart rate

The physiological control of fetal heart rate has been extensively reviewed by Walker (1984). In summary, the heart begins to beat about the 4th week of intrauterine life. Initially it beats at an intrinsic rate of about 180 beats per minute (b.p.m.) but by 15 weeks the rate has fallen to about 150 b.p.m. under the influence of increasing vagal tone. Thereafter, the baseline rate falls slowly to about 135 b.p.m. at the beginning of the third trimester, after which it remains essentially unchanged until labour. The push–pull mechanisms of the autonomic nervous system are the main regulator, with the parasympathetic (vagal) supply slowing the heart while the sympathetic system (the adrenergic nerve supply, and the catecholamines adrenaline and noradrenaline) generally acts to increase the rate and force of cardiac contractions. However, the latter two humoral factors have a complex effect on heart rate which depends upon the physiological background against which they act.

Other major influences include the baroreceptors, sensitive to arterial blood pressure. These are present in the major arteries and in the aorta. They are responsible, for example, for the dramatic bradycardia seen in response to umbilical cord vessel occlusions, when by suddenly increasing peripheral resistance, the blood pressure rises , so stretching the aorta and causing its stretch receptors to fire off.

Chemoreceptors are also functional in the fetus, responding to blood gas tension, particularly to the $PO_2$. Their existence in the aorta is certain, but their presence in the carotid bodies remains unproven, in contrast to the adult.

Fetal sleep state has increasingly been recognized as a strong influence on FHR. Dawes' group in Oxford, studying the fetal sheep, reported changes in FHR associated with the time of day, and more particularly with the presence or absence of fetal breathing movements (Dalton *et al.* 1977). The association between sleep state and fetal breathing, body movement and FHR was subsequently confirmed in the human fetus by Wheeler *et al.* (1980) and by Dawes *et al.* (1981). In summary, the human fetus appears to alternate between periods of quiet sleep, in which there is little or no breathing movement, little body movement, and a decreased FHR, and active sleep, in which the fetus moves its limbs, makes breathing movements and exhibits a rise in FHR. An increase in baseline rate, variability, and the number of accelerations all go hand in hand. The changes in state occur at intervals of 20–40 min. They are largely independent of environmental changes such as mechanical 'shaking the baby' stimulation, glucose infusions or light stimulation, but can be altered by vibroacoustic stimuli (such as a door-buzzer applied to the mother's abdomen) (Romero *et al.* 1988). Thus, shaking the fetus during a non-reactive heart rate episode in order to try and produce reassuring heart rate accelerations is a waste of time (Visser *et al.* 1983). Vibroacoustic stimulation on the other hand produces significant increases in both basal heart rate and accelerations for up to an hour after the stimulus is applied (Gagnon *et al.* 1987b). The changes are probably more a response to the vibration component than to the acoustic component, and may induce a brain state akin to wakefulness in the fetus. Since this state is associated with increased body and breathing movements, it is likely to increase fetal oxygen consumption, and therefore this form of stimulation may prejudice the genuinely compromised fetus whose oxygen supply is already only just adequate; this point remains to be resolved.

The changes in heart rate which occur in spontaneous sleep state cycling are often abrupt and not directly related to fetal movement; rather they appear to represent true changes in the pattern of fetal cerebral activity. The rapid fetal eyeball movements seen on ultrasound during active sleep have lead some workers to suggest that it is equivalent to rapid eye movement (REM) dreaming sleep in the adult, but this remains conjectural. There is increasing evidence that quiet sleep is not a homogeneous state, but can be subdivided into at least four subtypes, depending on the type of fetal activity pattern present (van Woerden *et al.* 1988).

Different heart rate patterns can be distinguished depending on whether there is no fetal activity, somatic movements, breathing movements or sucking movements. Breathing movements are associated with detectable fetal sinus arrythmia (Donchin *et al.* 1984). The development of the two main sleep states, quiet and active, occurs during the middle trimester and is usually well established by 30 weeks gestation (Dawes *et al.* 1981; Gagnon *et al.* 1987a). There is strong evidence that the alternation between states continues during labour, even though the associated drop in $P\text{O}_2$ causes the cessation of fetal breathing movements (Spencer & Johnson 1986).

## Pathological factors affecting fetal heart rate

Maternal thyroid status is known to have a major influence on fetal heart rate, with thyrotoxicosis causing a fetal tachycardia (Robinson *et al.* 1979) and myxoedema a fetal bradycardia (Reginald & Mackinnon 1984).

Structural abnormalities of the fetal heart such as atrial or ventricular septal defects can also disturb the FHR, and can cause either tachycardias or bradycardias due to heart block (Maxwell *et al.* 1988). Disturbances of the conducting tissue, giving rise to conditions such as the Wolff–Parkinson–White syndrome, can also occur *in utero*. If gross disturbances of rate or rhythm are seen antenatally, a detailed cardiac scan of the fetus should always be carried out. The prognosis depends largely on whether there is a major structural defect, and if not, the prognosis for the baby is usually good. Another advantage of scanning is that cardiac failure (due for example to Rhesus isoimmunization) can be diagnosed by detecting the presence of hydrops.

## Clinical factors affecting fetal heart rate

In the St Mary's study the most important influence on baseline fetal heart rate was the duration of the first stage of labour ($R = 0.2$, $P = 0.0005$)

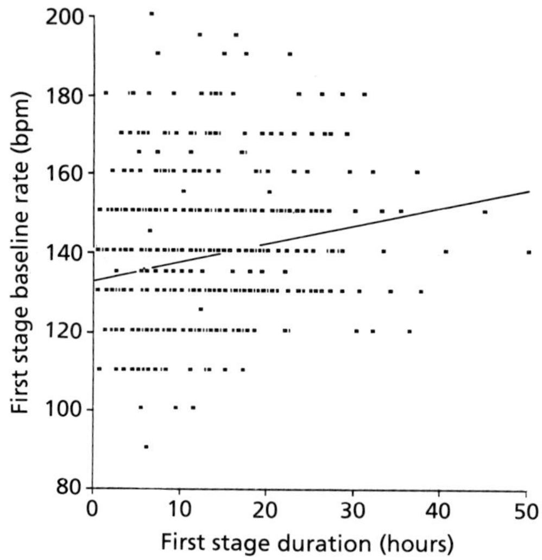


**Fig. 8.1** The relationship between the duration of the first stage of labour in hours, and the baseline fetal heart rate in the last hour of the first stage. (■) First stage baseline rate; (—) simple fit first stage baseline rate.

with the rate rising from 133 b.p.m. at the beginning of labour to 144 b.p.m. after 24 hours as shown in Figure 8.1.

Another major influence was maternal fever. A maternal temperature of 38°C or more occurred in 45 women (3.7 per cent). In these women the mean fetal heart rate was 161 b.p.m. (SD 17) compared with 137 b.p.m. (SD 14) in the non-pyrexial group. In the absence of clinical pyrexia, however, the FHR still rose gradually with time, from 134 b.p.m. at the start of labour to 142 b.p.m. after 24 hours. In contrast, in women with pyrexia, the FHR was already 165 b.p.m. in early labour and continued to be similarly elevated, 160 b.p.m., even after 24 hours. The incidence of pyrexia rose significantly with time, but only in women receiving epidural anaesthesia (Table 8.1). We have reported this phenomenon before (Steer, 1985) and consider that an epidural anaesthetic reduces maternal sweating in the lower half of the body secondary to

**Table 8.1** The incidence of pyrexia in women receiving epidural anaesthesia

| | Epidural | | | No epidural | | | |
|---|---|---|---|---|---|---|---|
| Duration of labour (hours) | Pyrexial | Not pyrexial | Per cent | Pyrexial | Not pyrexial | Per cent | *P* |
| 0–3.9 | 0 | 18 | 0 | 0 | 209 | 0 | NS |
| 4–7.9 | 2 | 63 | 3 | 4 | 294 | 1.3 | NS |
| 8–11.9 | 5 | 59 | 8 | 2 | 161 | 1.2 | 0.02 |
| 12–15.9 | 8 | 54 | 13 | 1 | 83 | 1 | 0.0005 |
| 16+ | 19 | 77 | 20 | 4 | 85 | 4.5 | 0.0002 |

Significance by Fisher's exact test.
Pyrexial = maternal temperature ⩾ 38°C.

autonomic blockade, causing mothers labouring hard in a hot labour ward to develop a positive heat balance. Longitudinal measurements of maternal and fetal temperature using thermocouples have confirmed the effect (Fusi *et al.* 1989). The rise in FHR closely parallels the rise in maternal temperature, and the effect is seen well below 38°C. Thus, if only women not receiving an epidural anaesthetic are considered, the rise in FHR with time was much reduced, being only 4 b.p.m. over 24 hours (from 134 to 138 b.p.m.). In contrast, the rise in women receiving an epidural anaesthetic was three times larger, from 138 b.p.m. at the beginning of labour to 150 b.p.m. at 24 hours.

Because of the effect of the duration of labour, a new variable was created, BaseFHR, from the equation:

$$\text{BaseFHR} = 133.3 + (0.456 \times \text{duration of the first stage})$$

This corrected for the effects of both duration and pyrexia, thus giving an estimate of the true baseline rate for each fetus before the effects of labour.

The sex of the fetus did not correlate with BaseFHR. We found that for males ($n = 545$) the mean BaseFHR was 137 b.p.m. (SD 15) while for the females ($n = 573$) mean BaseFHR was 138.3 b.p.m. (SD 15) ($t = 1.45$, $P =$ NS). Similarly, Table 8.2 shows that gestational age did not correlate. These findings agree with those of Druzin *et al.* (1986), who found no difference in FHR by fetal sex and a significant difference by gestation only before 24 weeks.

There was however a strong correlation between BaseFHR and maternal age shown in Figure 8.2 ($R = 0.136$, $P = 0.0005$). This association remains unexplained; it was not due to intrauterine growth retardation in older mothers as BaseFHR showed no significant correlation with birth weight ($R = 0.032$). There was also a positive association with meconium staining of the liquor, such that if the liquor was meconium stained the BaseFHR was 137 b.p.m. (SD 16), $n = 170$, compared with 133 b.p.m. (SD 15), $n = 1079$, if the liquor was clear ($t = 3.2$, $P < 0.005$). Maternal smoking was associated with a significant reduction in BaseFHR, from 138 b.p.m. (SD 15), $n = 654$, in non-smokers, to 134 b.p.m. (SD 13), $n = 60$, in women smoking more than

**Table 8.2** Mean BaseFHR vs. gestational age

| Gestational age (weeks) | (*n*) | mean BaseFHR (b.p.m.) | SD | Minimum | Maximum |
|---|---|---|---|---|---|
| <37 | (60) | 135.4 | 16 | 107 | 179 |
| 37 | (47) | 135.4 | 17 | 112 | 197 |
| 38 | (144) | 132.1 | 13 | 104 | 167 |
| 39 | (202) | 131.9 | 14 | 96 | 182 |
| 40 | (352) | 133.2 | 14 | 95 | 187 |
| 41 | (177) | 134.2 | 17 | 87 | 189 |
| 42 | (71) | 134.7 | 16 | 105 | 177 |
| 43 | (10) | 135.2 | 15 | 118 | 165 |

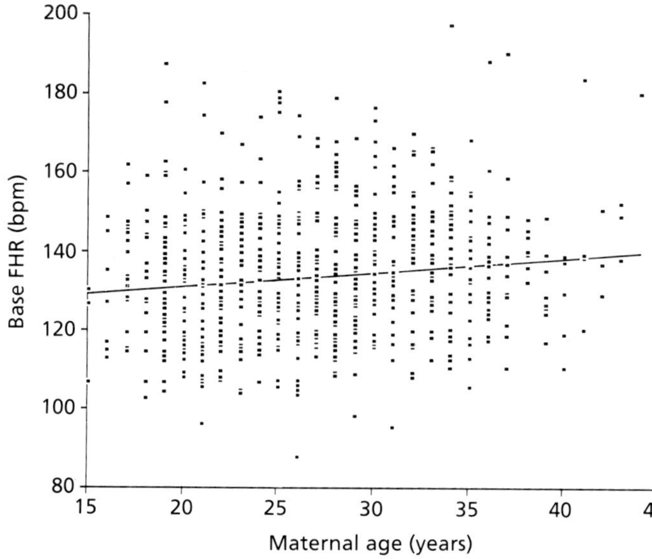


**Fig. 8.2** The relationship between maternal age and baseline fetal heart rate allowing for the effect of labour duration. (□) BaseFHR; (—) simple fit BaseFHR.

20 cigarettes a day ($t = 2.26$, $P < 0.025$). Lighter smokers had intermediate BaseFHRs.

## Fetal heart rate and fetal blood gas and pH values

Despite the fact that cardiotocography has now been in widespread use for twenty years, there is remarkably little unanimity about which aspects of the FHR are most significant in relation to fetal blood gas and pH values. For example, Law and colleagues (1976) considered that the total amount of FHR deceleration in any given period was the best predictor of pH, with baseline rate and variability of relatively little importance. However, they considered these variables independently while Lin *et al.* (1980) suggested that while isolated tachycardia and loss of variability are common, and of little significance by themselves, in combination with decelerations they are more specific. Henson *et al.* (1983) investigated the cord artery pH and base deficit of a series of infants delivered by elective Caesarean section because of an abnormal antenatal cardiotocograph (CTG) and found no evidence of significant acidosis, although nearly all the babies were small-for-gestational age. Their data suggested that disturbances of heart rate can be produced directly by growth retarding processes such as interference with placental blood flow, and that these disturbances may be part of a physiological mechanism to minimize any adverse effect on fetal blood gas status. More recently, Smith *et al.* (1988) have shown that a similar group of babies delivered because of an abnormal antenatal CTG, while not acidotic, were however significantly hypoxic with raised $P\text{CO}_2$ values. Whether it is the hypoxia that causes the CTG abnormality, or whether disturbances of cardiovascular function can precede, and perhaps even cause, blood gas disturbances remains a moot point.

Some of these points were further investigated by interrogating the St Mary's data base. CTG traces were classified by baseline rate, baseline variability (normal >5 b.p.m., reduced <5 b.p.m.), the presence of accelerations (at least two per 15 min) and decelerations (considered significant if late with a lag-time >15 s or early and with an amplitude >40 b.p.m.). These classifications were then compared with umbilical cord artery blood gas and pH values at delivery.

The presence of decelerations in the first stage of labour correlated well with pH ($R = 0.255$, $n = 735$, $P < 0.0005$) and base deficit ($R = 0.235$, $n = 721$, $P < 0.0005$), but less well with $P\text{CO}_2$ ($R = -0.158$, $n = 733$, $P < 0.0005$) and bicarbonate ($R = 0.976$, $n = 720$, $P < 0.004$) and least well with $P\text{O}_2$ ($R = 0.09$, $n = 720$, $P < 0.008$).

Lack of accelerations correlated similarly, although less closely (pH: $R = -0.121$, $n = 736$, $P < 0.001$; base deficit: $R = -0.104$, $n = 722$, $P < 0.003$; bicarbonate: $R = -0.0399$, $n = 721$, $P =$ NS; $P\text{CO}_2$: $R = 0.059$, $n = 734$, $P =$ NS; $P\text{O}_2$: $R = -0.06$, $n = 721$, $P =$ NS). In contrast, baseline rate only correlated significantly with $P\text{O}_2$ ($R = -0.1266$, $n = 721$, $P < 0.0005$), and hardly at all with pH ($R = 0.0012$, $n = 736$, $P =$ NS).

Baseline variability did not correlate significantly with any variable. Similar results were found with second stage traces.

Thus it appeared that decelerations were associated with acidosis whereas baseline rate was associated mainly with $P\text{O}_2$. It was decided to study the physiological relationship between baseline rate and blood gases more closely by analysing the subgroup of fetuses delivered by elective Caesarean section. There were 35 cases in the study with complete data collection, i.e. full records of antenatal CTG classification and cord artery pH measurement. All the antenatal CTGs were classified as clinically normal, without decelerations, although three were non-reactive and in one of these cases variability was also reduced. Baseline rate was within normal limits in all cases (120–160 b.p.m.). The baseline rate was then plotted against cord artery blood gas and pH measurements (Figures 8.3–8.6).

The results show clearly how changes in baseline rate can be associated with changes in $P\text{O}_2$ without changes in pH. A decrease in $P\text{O}_2$ is significantly associated with a rise in FHR (Figure 8.3), possibly as a physiological mechanism to maintain oxygen delivery to the tissues. This rise in FHR and fall in $P\text{O}_2$ is associated with a significant rise in $P\text{CO}_2$ (presumably related to an impedance of placental gas exchange), which is in turn associated with a rise in bicarbonate. Thus the fall in pH which would be expected from the rise in $P\text{CO}_2$ is opposed by the rise in bicarbonate and the potential change in pH is effectively buffered.

In contrast to these findings, in small-for-gestational age fetuses, cordocentesis and fetal blood sampling *in utero* has shown that a significant metabolic acidosis can occur while fetal blood gases remain within the normal range (Pardi *et al.* 1987). In the St Mary's data set, birth weight

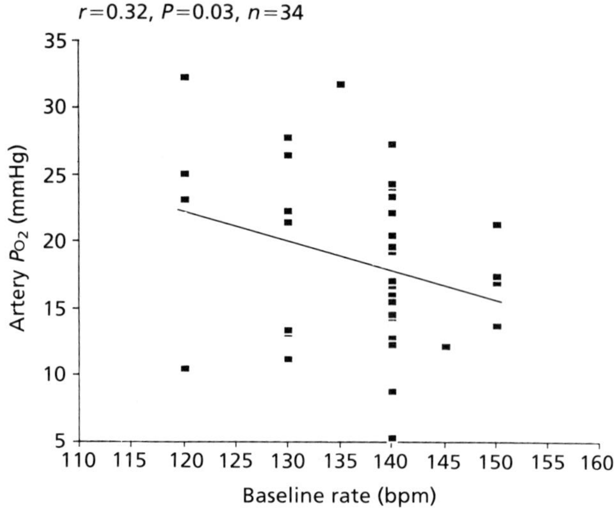


**Fig. 8.3**

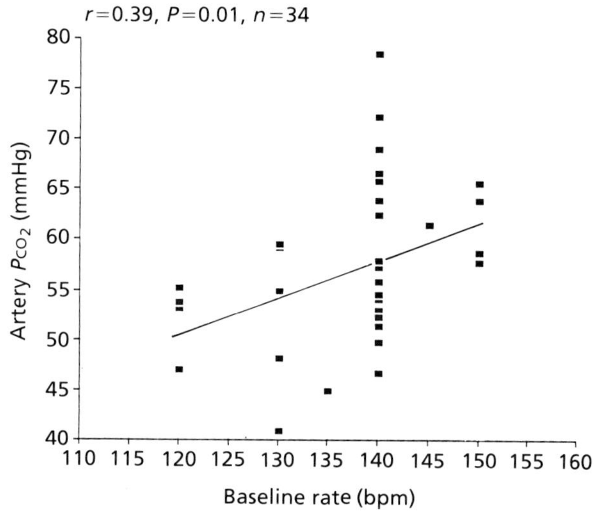


**Fig. 8.4**

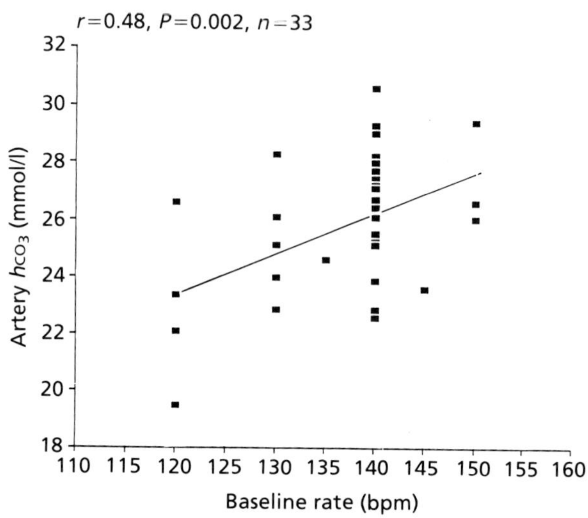


**Fig. 8.5**

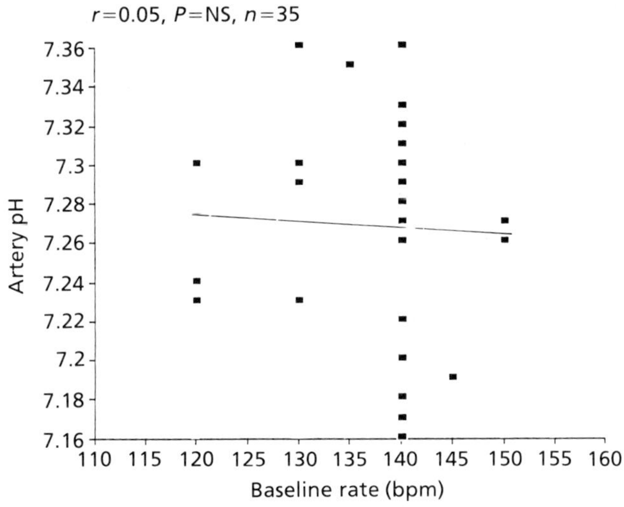


**Figs 8.3–8.6** The relationships between antenatal baseline FHR and umbilical cord artery blood gas and pH measurements at elective Caesarean section. (Note: $PO_2$, $PCO_2$ and bicarbonate measurements were not obtained in 1,1 and 2 cases respectively.) (■) Artery $PO_2$; (—) simple fit artery $PO_2$.

less than the fifth centile, weight for gestational age, resulted in a significantly lower pH at birth compared to better grown fetuses (mean 7.23, SD 0.09, $n$ = 40 vs. mean 7.26, SD 0.09, $n$ = 708, $P < 0.05$). $PO_2$ was not significantly different (mean 21.5 mmHg, SD 9, $n$ = 39 vs. mean 21 mmHg, SD 8, $n$ = 698). In keeping with these results, mean baseline FHR was not significantly different between the two groups (mean 138 b.p.m., SD 14, $n$ = 58 vs. 138 b.p.m., SD 15, $n$ = 1009). There was an increased incidence of variable or late decelerations (17 per cent vs. 10 per cent) which became statistically significant in the second stage of labour (52 per cent vs. 31 per cent). A full account of these results has been published elsewhere (Steer 1989).

Broadly similar results have recently been published by Smith *et al.* (1988). They studied three groups of babies delivered by elective Caesarean section, 30 for mechanical reasons, 20 for maternal disease, and 21 for abnormalities in the antenatal CTG. Babies <10th centile weight for gestational age comprised 3 per cent, 70 per cent and 90 per cent of the groups respectively. The groups will therefore be referred to as AGA, SGA1 and SGA2. In the AGA group, the mean umbilical cord artery pH was 7.27, mean $PO_2$ 13 mmHg and the baseline FHR 132 b.p.m. In the SGA1 group, the pH was almost identical (7.26) but the $PO_2$ was significantly lower at 10 mmHg and accordingly the basal FHR was significantly higher at 140 b.p.m. In the SGA2 group 20/21 of the CTG traces were decelerative and accordingly the pH was lower at 7.23, although because of small numbers this fall was not statistically significant. However, there was a significant further drop in $PO_2$ (6 mmHg) and the basal FHR rose further to 144 b.p.m. Thus these results confirm the close relation between basal FHR and $Po_2$ whereas pH is more closely linked to FHR decelerations. The fact that the SGA babies in this study showed changes in blood gas levels whereas those in the St Mary's study did not may be due to the fact that babies requiring delivery antenatally are beginning to decompensate, whereas those that reach labour without showing signs of compromise are able to maintain relatively normal blood gas levels while still remaining at risk of a metabolically derived acidosis.

## Conclusions

The fetal heart rate is influenced by many physiological and pathological factors and so the rate observed depends on a complex interaction of all of them. Correct clinical deductions about fetal condition depend on a knowledge of these factors. Clinical decisions made without taking into account phenomena such as the dependence of FHR on sleep state of the fetus, and the marked effect of temperature, are likely to be erroneous. Ignorance of the physiology has been one of the major obstacles to the appropriate use of continuous electronic FHR monitoring, both antenatally and in labour. It may be that computer analysis will come to our rescue (Dawes *et al.* 1985) but a preferable alternative would be the proper training of obstetricians.

## References

Dalton K.J., Dawes G.S. & Patrick J.E. (1977) Diurnal, respiratory, and other rhythms of fetal heart rate in lambs. *American Journal of Obstetrics and Gynecology*, **127**, 414–24.

Dawes G.S., Houghton C.R.S., Redman C.W.G. & Visser G.H.A. (1982) Pattern of the normal human fetal heart rate. *British Journal of Obstetrics and Gynaecology*, **89**, 276–84.

Dawes G.S., Redman C.W.G. & Smith J.H. (1985) Improvements in the registration and analysis of fetal heart rate records at the bedside. *British Journal of Obstetrics and Gynaecology*, **92**, 317–25.

Dawes G.S., Visser G.H.A., Goodman J.D.S. & Levine D.H. (1981) Numerical analysis of the human fetal heart rate: Modulation by breathing and movement. *American Journal of Obstetrics and Gynecology*, **140**, 535–44.

Donchin Y., Caton D. & Porges S.W. (1984) Spectral analysis of fetal heart rate in sheep: The occurrence of respiratory sinus arrhythmia. *American Journal of Obstetrics and Gynecology*, **148**, 1130–5.

Druzin M.L., Hutson J.M. & Edersheim T.G. (1986) Relationship of baseline fetal heart rate to gestational age and fetal sex. *American Journal of Obstetrics and Gynecology*, **154**, 1102–3.

Fusi L., Steer P.J., Maresh M.J.A. & Beard R.W. (1989) Maternal pyrexia associated with the use of epidural analgesia in labour. *Lancet*, **i**, 1250–2.

Gagnon R., Campbell K., Hunse C. & Patrick J. (1987a) Patterns of human heart rate accelerations from 26 weeks to term. *American Journal of Obstetrics and Gynecology*, **157**, 743–8.

Gagnon R., Hunse C., Carmichael L., Fellows F. & Patrick J. (1987b) External vibratory acoustic stimulation near term: Fetal heart rate and heart rate variability responses. *American Journal of Obstetrics and Gynecology*, **156**, 323–7.

Henson G.L., Dawes G.S. & Redman C.W.G. (1983) Antenatal heart rate variability in relation to fetal acid–base status at caesarean section. *British Journal of Obstetrics and*

*Gynaecology*, **90**, 516–21.

Lin C.C., Moawad A.H., Rosenow P.J. & River P. (1980) Acid–base characteristics of fetuses with intrauterine growth retardation during labor and delivery. *American Journal of Obstetrics and Gynecology*, **137**, 553–9.

Low J.A., Pancham S.R. & Worthington D. (1976) Fetal heart deceleration patterns in relation to asphyxia and weight–gestational age percentile of the fetus. *Obstetrics and Gynecology*, **47**, 14–20.

Maxwell D.J., Crawford D.C., Curry P.V.M., Tynan M.J. & Allen L.D. (1988) Obstetric importance, diagnosis, and management of fetal tachycardias. *British Medical Journal*, **297**, 107–10.

Pardi G., Buscaglia M., Ferrazzi E., Bozzetti P., Marconi A.M., Cetin I., Battaglia F. & Makowski E.L. (1987) Cord sampling for the evaluation of oxygenation and acid–base balance in growth-retarded human fetuses. *American Journal of Obstetrics and Gynecology*, **157**, 1221–8.

Reginald P.W. & Mackinnon H. (1984) Antenatal baseline fetal bradycardia associated with congenital hypothyroidism. *Journal of Obstetrics and Gynaecology*, **5**, 40–1.

Robinson P.L., O'Mullane N.M. & Alderman B. (1979) Prenatal treatment of fetal thyrotoxicosis. *British Medical Journal*, **1**, 383–4.

Romero R., Mazor M. & Hobbins J.C. (1988) A critical appraisal of fetal acoustic stimulation as an antenatal test for fetal well-being. *Obstetrics and Gynecology*, **71**, 781–6.

Smith J.H., Anand K.J.S., Cotes P.M., Dawes G.S., Harkness R.A., Howlett T.A., Rees L.H. & Redman C.W.G. (1988) Antenatal fetal heart rate variation in relation to the respiratory and metabolic status of the compromised human fetus. *British Journal of Obstetrics and Gynaecology*, **95**, 980–9.

Spencer J.A.D. & Johnson P. (1986) Fetal heart rate variability changes and fetal behavioural cycles during labour. *British Journal of Obstetrics and Gynaecology*, **93**, 314–21.

Steer P.J. (1985) Fetal distress. In *Risks of Labour*, (Ed. by J.W. Crawford), pp. 11–31. John Wiley and Sons, London.

Steer P.J. (1989) Intrapartum monitoring in IUGR. In *Royal College of Obstetricians and Gynaecologists Study Group on Intrauterine Growth Retardation*, (Ed. by P. Howie & R. Fraser). Royal College of Obstetricians and Gynaecologists, London.

Steer P.J., Gigbe F., Lissauer T.J. & Beard R.W. (1989) Interrelationships among abnormal cardiotocograms in labour, meconium staining of the amniotic fluid, arterial cord blood pH, and Apgar scores. *Obstetrics and Gynecology* (in press).

Van Woerden E.E., Van Gejn H.P., Swartjes J.M., Caron F.J.M., Brons J.T.J. & Arts N.F.T. (1988) Fetal heart rhythms during behavioural state 1F. *European Journal of Obstetrics, Gynecology and Reproductive Biology*, **28**, 29–38.

Visser G.H.A., Zeelenberg H.J., De Vries J.I.P. & Dawes G.S. (1983) External physical stimulation of the human fetus during episodes of low heart rate variation. *American Journal of Obstetrics and Gynecology*, **145**, 579–84.

Walker A.M. (1984) Physiological control of the fetal cardiovascular system. In *Fetal Physiology and Medicine*, (Ed. by R.W. Beard & P.W. Nathanielsz), pp. 287–316. Marcel Dekker, Inc., Butterworths, New York, Basel, London.

Wheeler T., Gennser G., Lindvall R. & Murrills A.J. (1980) Changes in the fetal heart rate associated with fetal breathing and fetal movement. *British Journal of Obstetrics and Gynaecology*, **87**, 1068–79.

# 9: Antepartum cardiotocography

JOHN A.D. SPENCER



The fetal heart sounds are identified and used to calculate the fetal heart rate (FHR) which is continuously plotted on a calibrated paper trace. A strain gauge around the maternal abdomen picks up movements of the anterior abdominal wall, especially the forward displacement of the uterus during contractions, and this signal is usually recorded beneath the FHR on the same paper trace. This composite cardiotocograph (CTG) record has become the standard method of fetal assessment in the UK over recent years, both during late pregnancy and in labour (Wheble *et al.* 1989).

The fetal electrocardiogram (FECG) can be readily obtained during labour by direct contact with the fetus once the membranes are ruptured. Fetal monitors calculate instantaneous FHR from consecutive R waves of this signal. It is more difficult to record the fetal heart during pregnancy and techniques include phonocardiography, electrocardiography and Doppler ultrasound. However, only the latter is in common use now for antepartum FHR monitoring.

## Historical aspects

The first sound demonstration of the fetal heartbeats was in 1891 by Pestalozza in Berlin. Subsequently, there were many attempts to record the fetal heart sounds but only after the development of radio and telephone technology was there significant progress (Wulf 1985). The use of continuous FHR records during pregnancy was first made possible when microphone signals were successfully used to trigger a ratemeter (Corner & Stran 1957; Hellmann *et al.* 1958; Hammacher 1962). These early German phonocardiographic studies showed that a reduction in baseline FHR variability and a loss of accelerations were associated with increased perinatal morbidity and mortality (Hammacher *et al.* 1968; Kubli *et al.* 1969b).

The use of the R waves of the FECG to trigger a ratemeter and produce continuous records of FHR was also described at about this time in the USA (Hon & Hess 1957; Swartwout *et al.* 1961). A description of the FECG recorded from the maternal abdomen was first made in 1906 by Cremer but it was not until 1974 that equipment was commercially available to produce FHR records from maternal abdominal electrodes. Problems in obtaining the low voltage ECG signal, especially between 28 and 34 weeks, have prevented this method becoming popular.

The advent of present day antenatal monitoring began with the discovery that the Doppler shifted frequencies produced by fetal heart movements when insonated by ultrasound are, by chance, in the audible range (Callagan *et al.* 1964; Bishop 1966). The envelope of the maximum shifted frequencies of the ultrasound signal was used to identify the heartbeats and, originally, one crystal was used for transmission and another was used to receive the reflected ultrasound. The receptive area was therefore relatively narrow which meant constant repositioning of the transducer. Development of a wide beam or array transducer, with several pairs of transmitting and receiving crystals, reduced the need for repositioning. However, heart wall movements, as well as valve movements, still resulted in jitter which required signal smoothing (such as averaging over 3 heart beats) within the moniter before the rate was displayed on paper. Although this means that FHR values are not instantaneous, the method adequately displays long-term variability.

## Technical aspects

The antepartum FHR monitor has two transducers, one for detection of fetal heartbeat movements by Doppler ultrasound and the other for uterine activity. It is also common practice for the mother to use an event marker to indicate perception of fetal body movements during the recording.

### Signal processing

Modern antepartum FHR monitors use pulsed ultrasound which enables all the crystals in the transducer alternately to transmit and receive. This widens the beam further than is achieved using continuous wave ultrasound and so enhances the pick-up of the fetal heartbeat movements.

The pick-up of extraneous intrauterine movements by the wide beam pulsed Doppler ultrasound transducer is negated by autocorrelation of the signal. This technique compares the signal with itself and thereby cancels out random noise whilst enhancing any repetitive component in the signal.

Modern monitors contain a microprocessor to enable autocorrelation to be performed on-line. The resultant autocorrelation function, which oscillates between a maximum value when consecutive portions of the

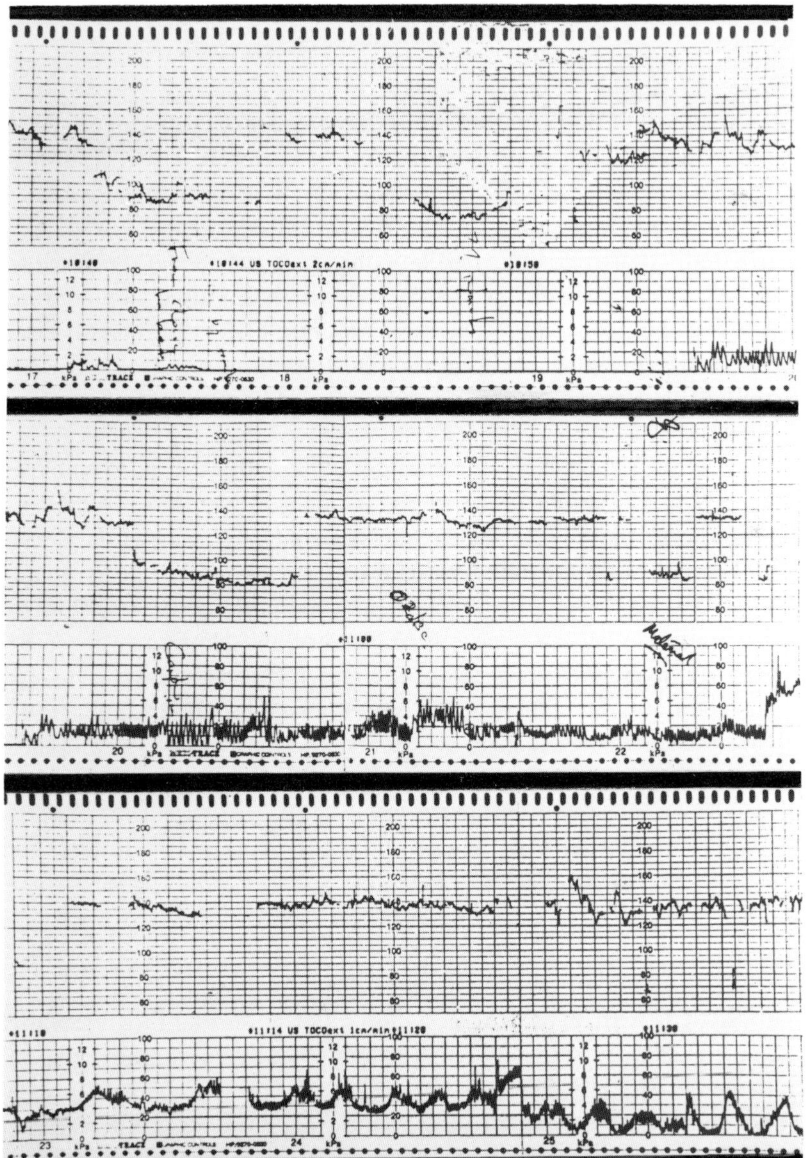

**Fig. 9.1** FHR record (2 cm/min) from a very obese woman showing intermittent spells of maternal heart rate picked up from the maternal aorta following changes in the position of the ultrasound transducer on her abdomen.

signal most closely match, and a minimum value when the signal is least closely matched, has a time period identical to the repetitive component of the signal. Thus a rate identical to that of the heartbeat can be extracted and displayed as a good quality record. One of the problems with autocorrelation is that it may display the maternal heart rate (Figure 9.1) if the transducer is positioned in such a way on the maternal abdomen that it picks up the regular motion of maternal blood pulsing through the major arteries of the pelvis. However, the addition of spurious data to the FHR record (Fukushima *et al.* 1985) is not a major problem in clinical practice.

### Signal loss

Total loss of the FHR signal was found to average 40 per cent in the last trimester using continuous wave ultrasound before the use of autocorrelation. Such signal loss varied considerably without being apparent on the CTG record and did not have significant influence on the accuracy of ultrasound (compared with simultaneous ECG) provided it remained less than 70 per cent (Dawes *et al.* 1981). Nevertheless, pulsed Doppler ultrasound with autocorrelation produces accurate FHR records with a tenfold reduction in signal loss (Lawson *et al.* 1983; Dawes *et al.* 1985) which is still half that achieved by autocorrelation of continuous wave signals (Spencer 1987).

Signal loss is greatest during episodes of high FHR variation which are associated with significant clustering of fetal movements (Wheeler & Guerard 1974; Dawes *et al.* 1982). Loss of signal may also occur as a result of movement of the transducer (Spencer 1987). An accurate estimation of signal loss can be obtained by assessing the number of half-minute or minute intervals which have no FHR record and expressing these as a percentage of the total duration of the record (Spencer 1987). The computer technique developed in Oxford (Wickham *et al.* 1983) identifies signal loss as the percentage of 3.75 second periods without a valid mean pulse interval. Pulsed ultrasound with autocorrelation has improved signal loss to an average of around 2 per cent (Dawes *et al.* 1985) and the FHR thus obtained correlates well with the FHR obtained by simultaneous fetal scalp ECG as assessed by computer (Spencer *et al.* 1987).

## Fetal heart rate changes during normal pregnancy

The FHR falls with advancing gestation and the normal range (mean ± 2SD) after 28 weeks lies between 110 and 150 beats per minute (b.p.m.) (Wheeler & Murrills 1978; FIGO 1987). The fall is maximal up to 30 weeks and is then confined to the FHR during episodes of low variation (Visser *et al.* 1981; Dawes *et al.* 1982).

Accelerations, defined as a rise in FHR above the baseline more than 15 beats, increase steadily in size as pregnancy advances. There is also an increase in the number of accelerations per hour, from around 2 before

28 weeks to between 10 and 14 at 34 weeks and up to 18 at term (Wheeler & Murrills 1978; Visser *et al.* 1981; Dawes *et al.* 1982). The number of decelerations in normal FHR records, defined as a fall in the FHR of 10 or more b.p.m. below the baseline, remains constant throughout pregnancy averaging between 3 and 5 per hour (Dawes *et al.* 1982). Thus after 28 weeks the total area of accelerations exceeds that of decelerations. Decelerations are usually much shorter in duration than accelerations.

FHR variability oscillates at approximately 6 cycles per minute (Hellman *et al.* 1958; Swartwout *et al.* 1961) and has been classified (Figure 9.2) according to the amplitude of the oscillations (Hammacher *et al.* 1968). The usual undulatory variability lies between 10 and 25 b.p.m. amplitude, occupies nearly half of the recording time and does not change with advancing gestation (Wheeler & Murrills 1978). Silent variability, less than 5 b.p.m., is uncommon, occurring for 4 per cent of the recording

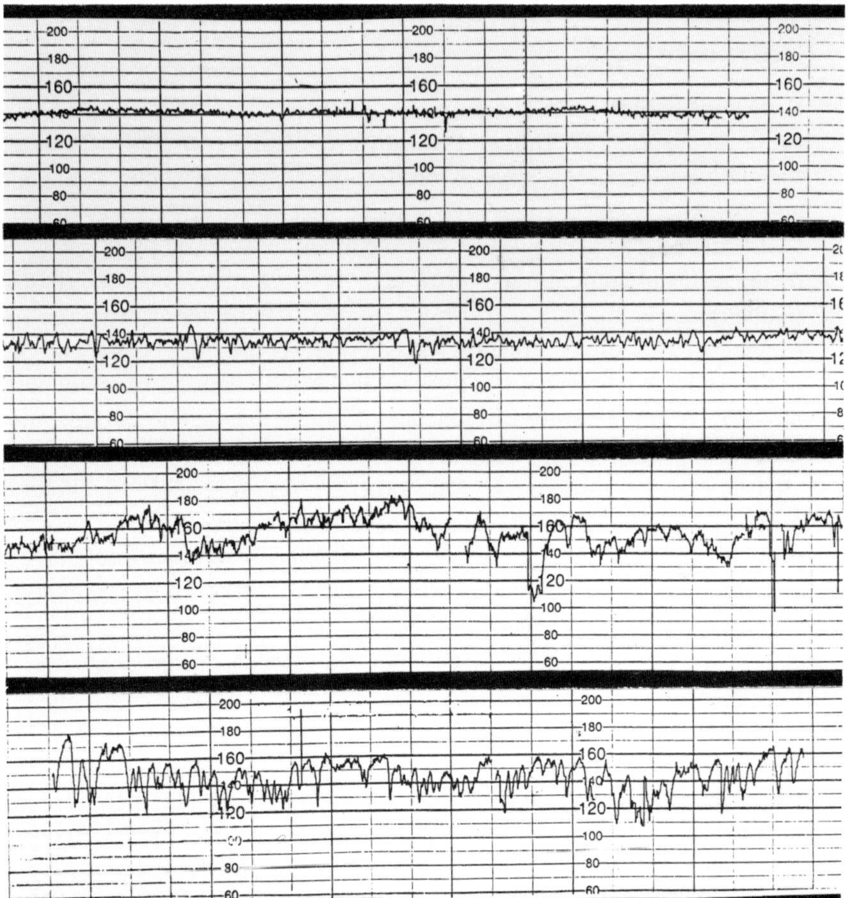

**Fig. 9.2** FHR variability as classified by Hammacher *et al.* (1968). From top to bottom: silent (<5 b.p.m.), narrowed undulatory (5–10 b.p.m.), undulatory (10–25 b.p.m.) and saltatory (>25 b.p.m.). Note that this classification differs from those which talk about baseline variability without including accelerations.

time and similarly does not change with gestation. Overall FHR variability does increase with gestation and this is explained by a significant increase in the proportion of saltatory variability greater than 25 b.p.m. whilst the proportion of narrowed undulatory variability, between 5 and 10 b.p.m. amplitude, decreases (Wheeler & Murrills 1978). Saltatory variability is produced by frequent accelerations of the FHR above the baseline and occurs during episodes of fetal activity (Wheeler & Guerard 1974). Thus after 28 weeks of gestation there are predominantly two patterns of FHR, namely reactive, with high overall variability associated with fetal activity, and non-reactive, with low variability associated with fetal quiescence (Wheeler & Murrills 1978; Visser *et al.* 1981; Dawes *et al.* 1982). These latter episodes average 15 min (Wheeler & Murrills 1978) but may last up to 40 min (Visser *et al.* 1981). Consecutive episodes of low and high FHR variation, associated with the fetal behavioural state rest–activity cycle, are characteristic of the normal antenatal FHR record.

## The antepartum contraction stress test of the fetal heart rate

Early studies of the use of continuous FHR records during labour (Mendez-Bauer *et al.* 1967; Hon and Khazin 1969; Kubli *et al.* 1969a) showed that late decelerations were associated with fetal metabolic acidaemia and low Apgar scores, suggestive of uteroplacental insufficiency. This led to the idea that fetal respiratory reserve might be assessed prior to labour by the artificial induction of uterine activity using an infusion of oxytocin (Kubli *et al.* 1969b; Pose *et al.* 1969). Despite an early report from the UK (Spurrett 1971) the contraction stress test (CST) did not become popular in this country. However, the test rapidly become popular in many parts of the USA and recently the practice of nipple massage to evoke endogenous oxytocin release has been shown to be an effective and simple alternative to an intravenous infusion (Huddleston *et al.* 1984; Lenke & Nemes 1984). Oxytocin infusion is used if this method fails to produce uterine contractions. The risk of preterm delivery following such a test has been shown to be smaller than the general risk in the population (Braly *et al.* 1981).

The CST is performed on patients considered to be at high risk of uteroplacental insufficiency. The oxytocin infusion begins at 0.5 mU per minute and is increased every 10 min to produce contractions every 3 to 4 min. A positive result is the occurrence of recurrent late uniform decelerations of the FHR. A negative result is rarely followed by fetal distress or neonatal asphyxia (Ray *et al.* 1972; Christie & Cudmore 1974; Freeman 1975) even up to one week later (Schifrin *et al.* 1975; Parer & Afonso 1977; Huddleston *et al.* 1979). A false negative result, in which the fetus dies within 7 days of the test, occurs with an incidence of between 0.2 per cent and 1.0 per cent (Evertson *et al.* 1978; Gal *et al.* 1979). However, false positive results are common as between 20 per cent and 60 per cent of subsequent labours show no further evidence of fetal compromise

(Gauthier *et al.* 1979; Huddleston *et al.* 1979; Staisch *et al.* 1980). Thus, although a positive CST in a high risk pregnancy indicates a risk of perinatal death of up to 66 per 1000 (Bissonnette *et al.* 1979), it does not indicate the best mode of delivery. A trial of labour, carefully monitored with fetal pH measurements, seems to be appropriate management (Bhakthavathsalan *et al.* 1976; Bissonnette *et al.* 1979; Gauthier *et al.* 1979; Staisch *et al.* 1980) especially when the FHR record shows reactivity in the form of accelerations despite the late decelerations (Fox *et al.* 1976; Huddleston *et al.* 1979; Grundy *et al.* 1984). A large multi-institutional study has shown the incidence of antenatal fetal death to be eight times greater in the group of women who had a CST compared with the group who had a non-stressed FHR record, or non-stressed test (NST), as the primary method of fetal assessment (Freeman *et al.* 1982b) and others have shown the CST to be more predictive than the NST for both fetal compromise and fetal well-being (Homburg *et al.* 1982). However, in neither of these studies was any attempt made to control the allocation of the test method and so the groups who received each test may well have been quite different. Overall the CST has poor diagnostic accuracy (Thacker & Berkelman 1986).

## Non-stressed antepartum fetal heart rate records

### Antenatal cardiotocography in Germany

Since 1968 in Germany FHR records made in pregnancy were considered the most reliable method of diagnosing impending fetal death (Kubli *et al.* 1972). An increase in the amount of reduced baseline variability (in 83 per cent) and late decelerations (in 91 per cent of such records with contractions) were found to be reliable signs, whereas baseline bradycardia or tachycardia were unusual. The Fischer score became the standard means of assessing antenatal FHR records (Fischer *et al.* 1976) and

**Table 9.1** Fischer score for antepartum FHR records as modified by Meyer-Menk *et al.* (Kubli 1984)

| | Score 0 | Score 1 | Score 2 |
|---|---|---|---|
| Baseline (b.p.m.) | <100, >180 | 100–120 | >120, <160 |
| Variation | | | |
| Amplitude (b.p.m.) | <5, sinusoidal | 5–10, >25 | 10–25 |
| Frequency (cycles/min) | <2, sinusoidal | 2–4 | >4 |
| Accelerations with mvts | None | None | Yes |
| following stimulation | Nonc | Atypical shape | Yes |
| Decelerations with Braxton Hicks uterine contractions | >25% late or severe variable decels | <25% late or mild/moderate variable decels | None, or single mild variable or early decels |

Abnormal score 0–4; suspicious score 5–7; normal score 8–10 (cf. Keirse & Trimbos 1980: abnormal score 0–5; suspicious score 6–7).

is still used in many places although often with slight modification. In a presentation to the 5th European Congress of Perinatal Medicine in Sweden Meyer-Menk *et al.* (1976) suggested that the score be modified by linking FHR accelerations to fetal movements (Kubli 1984) and this scheme is now commonly used in Germany (Table 9.1).

## Antenatal cardiotocography in The Netherlands

FHR monitoring of high risk pregnancies began in The Netherlands in 1969 and two groups soon expressed different opinions regarding the classification of non-stressed FHR records. The group in Groningen described a visual classification of FHR changes associated with severe maternal hypertension and fetal growth retardation (Emmen *et al.* 1975; Visser & Huisjes 1977) which regressed from normal to (decrease in accelerations and FHR variability), decelerative (repeated late decelerations) and then terminal (complete loss of accelerations and variability with recurrent late decelerations, illustrated in Figure 9.3).

This sequence of FHR changes was considered to represent evolving fetal compromise and they showed that the incidence of fetal death, fetal distress, fetal acidaemia, small-for-gestational age and neonatal complications increased as the CTG pattern became worse. They later showed, in conjuction with the unit in Oxford, UK, where FHR monitoring of the high risk fetus during pregnancy began in 1975, that normal FHR variability could differentiate those fetuses with a good prognosis from those who were compromised (Visser *et al.* 1980). A suboptimal or decelerative CTG (Figure 9.4) does not indicate fetal acidaemia but is related to the hypoxia and malnutrition associated with fetal growth retardation (Henson *et al.* 1983; Smith *et al.* 1988). These cases are likely to be

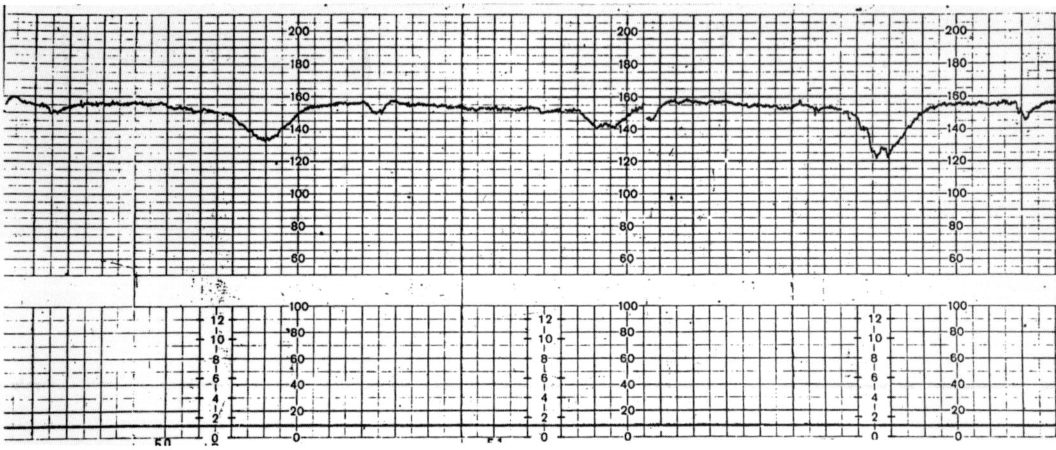

**Fig. 9.3** A terminal (Emmen *et al.* 1975), ominous (Flynn *et al.* 1979) or pathological (FIGO 1987) FHR record (1 cm/min) indicating critical fetal reserve (Beischer *et al.* 1983) from a nulliparous woman with severe proteinuric pregnancy-induced hypertension and IUGR at 33 weeks. Caesarean section resulted in a liveborn SGA infant weighting 780 g whose subsequent outcome was good.

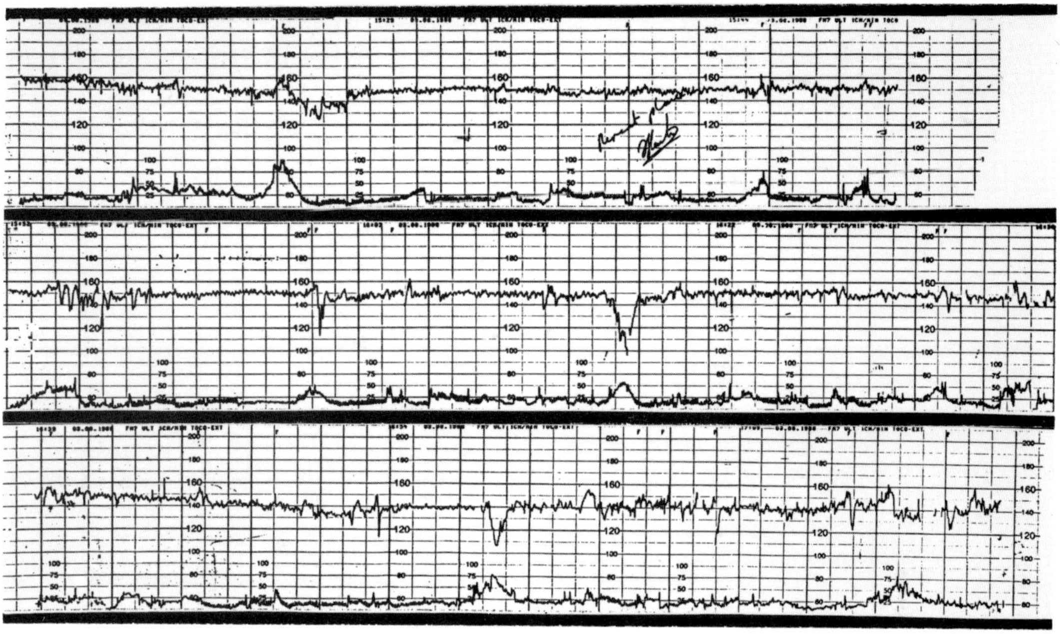

**Fig. 9.4** A decelerative (Visser & Huisjes 1977) or suspicious (Keirse & Trimbos 1980) FHR record (1 cm/min) from a woman aged 43 years with moderate hypertension at 34 weeks in her first pregnancy. Two minutes after the end of the upper trace, which lasted 37 min, the record was continued for a further 90 min. Caesarean section resulted in a healthy infant weighing 1550 g (3rd centile).

delivered by Caesarean section because of the high rate of fetal distress if allowed to labour. A terminal CTG, however, is associated with an increased risk of fetal death prior to delivery, within one week of the recording, and with metabolic acidaemia at birth when delivered by Caesarean section (Visser *et al.* 1980). The high risk of fetal death occurring during a CST if performed when the FHR is terminal (Visser & Huisjes 1977) has been confirmed by others (Langer *et al.* 1982). Elective Caesarean section for these cases, provided the fetus is viable and normally formed, should be considered as the outcome is likely to be good (Lin *et al.* 1981; Beischer *et al.* 1983; Chew *et al.* 1985).

In contrast, the group from Leiden considered the Fischer score to be considerably more reliable than visual assessment with regard to inter- and intra-observer variability (Trimbos & Keirse 1978a). They examined serial antepartum CTGs in normal pregnancies on an out-patient basis as well as high risk in-patients (Trimbos & Keirse 1978b; Keirse & Trimbos 1980; Keirse & Trimbos 1981). The original ten-point Fischer score considered 8–10 as normal, 5–7 suspicious and 0–4 ominous. They found no CTG from normal pregnancies scoring 5 or less but in one-third there was a suspicious trace (redefined as a score of 6 or 7) on at least one occasion with FHR variability less than 10 b.p.m. and an absence of accelerations over the 30 min recording period. In the high risk pregnancies they found that any CTG scoring 5 or less was associated with a poor out-

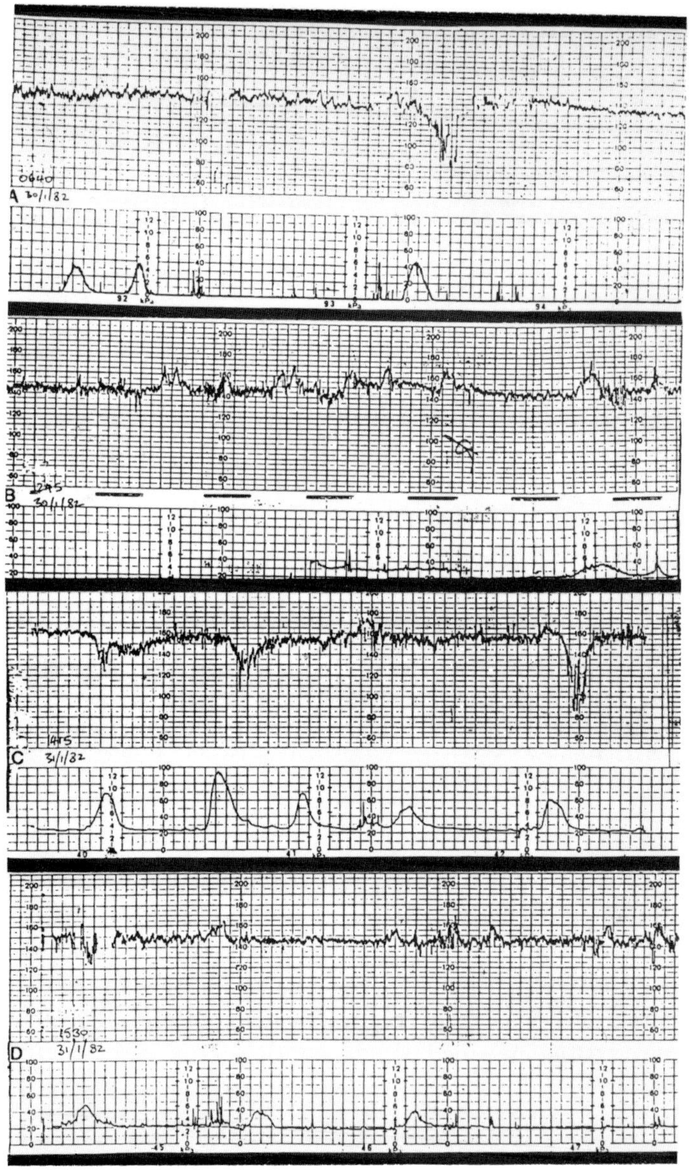

**Fig. 9.5** Four FHR records (1 cm/min) illustrating inconsistency of a decelerative or suspicious FHR from a normotensive nulliparous woman with clinical IUGR at 37 weeks. Traces A and B recorded 6 hours apart on the same day; traces C and D recorded less than 1 hour apart on the following day. Caesarean section resulted in a healthy SGA infant weighing 1700 g.

come and so considered this to be the definition of an ominous trace. Normal scores were reliable predictors of good outcome but the 15 per cent of CTGs which were suspicious, scoring 6 or 7, did not contain enough information to be of clinical value. Suspicious CTGs occurred more often in the high risk pregnancies and repeated traces are required to identify those pregnancies requiring intervention (see Figure 9.5).

## Antenatal cardiotocography in the UK

Soon after the onset of antepartum cardiotocography in the UK (Huntingford & Pendleton 1969; Spurrett 1971) several centres published methods for classification of traces. In Birmingham the use of reactive and non-reactive was based on the presence of at least 4 FHR accelerations greater than 15 b.p.m. in a 20 min period and a normal baseline with variability of 5 or more b.p.m. (Flynn & Kelly 1977). They showed this to correlate better with fetal outcome than did other scoring systems (Flynn *et al.* 1982b). The non-reactive FHR trace was further divided into three subcategories, namely suspect, flat and ominous, and they showed that these related significantly to fetal outcome in pregnancies suspected of fetal growth retardation (Flynn *et al.* 1979). Fetal distress in labour was more common after a flat trace but the only fetal deaths followed an ominous CTG. After their initial experience elective Caesarean section was performed for some cases with an ominous FHR trace and most of these survived and were normal at follow-up.

Following the introduction of antenatal cardiotocography into the unit in Cardiff, Wales, in 1973, for the assessment of fetal well-being, a six-point scoring system was developed which allocated a score of 0–2 each for the baseline, the FHR response to fetal movements and the FHR response to Braxton Hicks contractions (Pearson & Weaver 1978). They also found a steady progression of FHR changes associated with evolving fetal compromise, as assessed by clinical condition at birth. First there was a loss of FHR accelerations with Braxton Hicks contractions followed by a loss of accelerations with fetal movements. Then fetal movements ceased and the baseline often showed a tachycardia. A score of 4 appeared to be the watershed result below which fetal acidosis was more likely.

An extensive visual classification was suggested by Merkur (1979) which had several categories of both normal and abnormal FHR patterns. One of the normal patterns included rest–activity cycles. However, no additional benefit was shown by this extensive subdivision into different FHR groups because only one abnormal subgroup, namely preterminal, had ominous significance and warranted Caesarean section as had been previously described by others using different terminology.

## Evolution of the non-stress test in the USA

In the USA attention was diverted from the CST to non-stress testing following reports that fetal reactivity (accelerations in response to fetal movements) on the CTG (Figure 9.6) appeared to be a reliable indicator of fetal well-being (Lee *et al.* 1975, 1976; Rochard *et al.* 1976; Trierweiler *et al.* 1976; Rayburn *et al.* 1978). It was soon shown that a CST was not necessary following a normal NST and the false negative rate of the NST was found to be very low (Phelan *et al.* 1982). However, the number of accelerations required for a normal result has varied between different

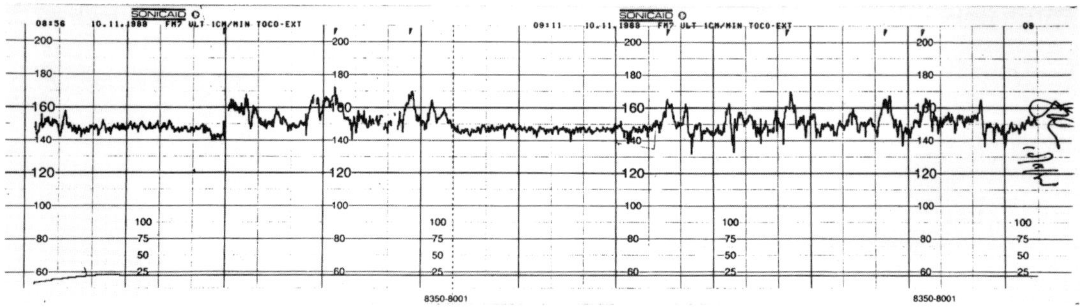

**Fig. 9.6** A normal (FIGO 1987), reactive, FHR record (1 cm/min) showing FHR accelerations associated with fetal movements as perceived by the mother and indicated by the event marker.

centres: 5 in 20 min, extended to 40 min if non-reactive (Evertson *et al.* 1979), 5 in 30 min (Krebs & Petres 1978; Bishop 1981), 3 in 20 min (Lee *et al.* 1976), 3 in 30 min (Devoe 1980), 2 in 20 min (Keegan & Paul 1980), 1 in 20 min (Rayburn *et al.* 1978), 1 in 30 min (Mendenhall *et al.* 1980). Early signs of fetal compromise were again confirmed to be progressive loss of baseline variability and decreased frequency of accelerations (Weingold *et al.* 1980). However, the results of a large multi-centre prospective study suggested that late decelerations on a CST were an earlier warning of fetal compromise than loss of reactivity on a NST (Freeman *et al.* 1982a).

In the USA two modified versions of the Fischer scoring system have been published. One was similar to the Meyer-Menk proposal and suggested that four accelerations in 20 min were required to obtain the maximum 2 points (Lyons *et al.* 1979). Using the original division of the score into normal (8–10), intermediate (5–7) and low (0–4) they showed that perinatal mortality rates correlated strongly, being 5, 70 and 433 per 1000 respectively. The other scheme added fetal movements to the original Fischer scheme thereby increasing the potential score to 12 if five or more movements were present in 30 min (Krebs & Petres 1978). Of these reactive CTGs 99.5 per cent had a score of 9 or more and fetal morbidity was 6 per cent. Non-reactive traces had lower scores and increased fetal morbidity (44 per cent) and mortality (8 per cent), especially with scores less than 6. A few non-reactive traces scored above 9 and the outcome was normal.

The results of antepartum testing of high risk pregnancies in the USA show that about 85 per cent of tests are normal (Phelan 1981; Freeman *et al.* 1982a). The false negative rate of a reactive FHR is low with a negative predictive value of greater than 96 per cent in most studies (Weingold *et al.* 1980; Devoe *et al.* 1985). It is still normal practice to further evaluate a non-reactive NST by performing a CST (Barrett *et al.* 1981; Phelan 1981). A non-reactive NST followed by a positive CST is frequently associated with fetal growth retardation (Slomka & Phelan 1981) and such cases form the majority of those who subsequently exhibit fetal distress in

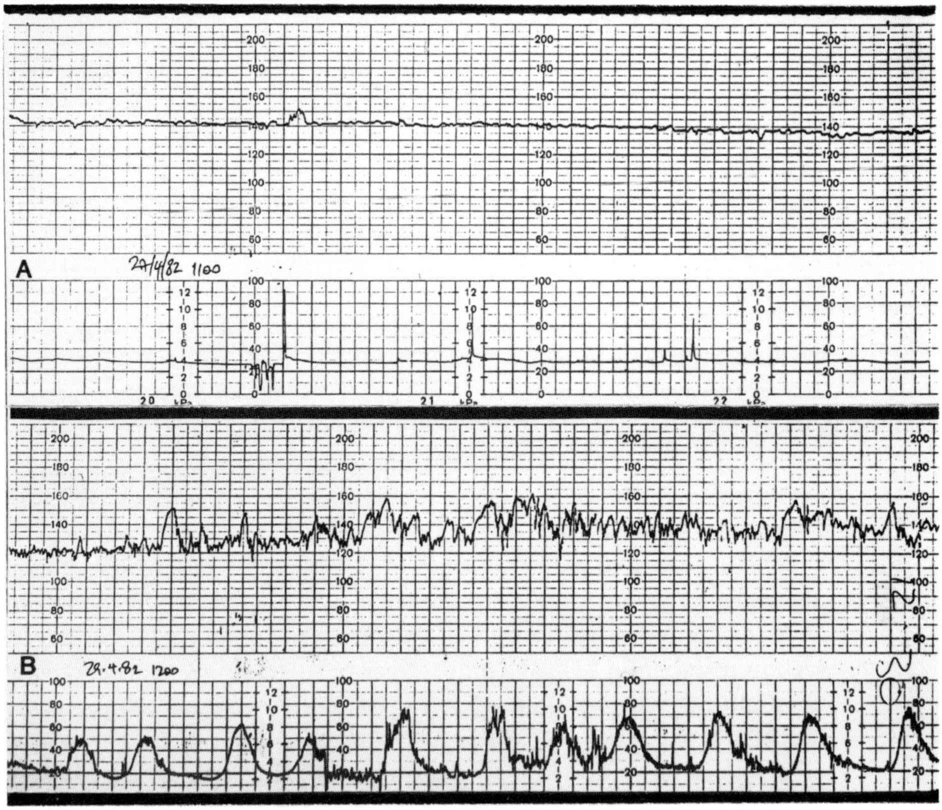

**Fig. 9.7** Upper trace (A): a suboptimal (Visser & Huisjes 1977), suspicious (Keirse & Trimbos 1980), flat (Flynn *et al.* 1979), non-reactive FHR record (1 cm/min) indicating reduced fetal reserve (Beischer *et al.* 1983) from a nulliparous woman with reduced fetal movements at 37 weeks. Lower trace (B): a normal FHR record from the same fetus two days later following administration of prostaglandin for induction of labour which proceeded to a normal vaginal delivery of a healthy infant weighing 2785 g.

labour. Liberal use of Caesarean section, especially when the cervix is unfavourable for induction or when FHR changes are seen in labour, assures a good outcome (Lin *et al.* 1981). Reports of the positive predictive value of a non-reactive NST have varied between 11 and 53 per cent (Devoe *et al.* 1985) which indicates the large number of false positive traces (Figure 9.7) that do not contain enough information to reassure the clinician. In one study a positive predictive value of 85.5 per cent was obtained by performing the NST for up to 2 hours (Brown & Patrick 1981).

## Antenatal cardiotocography in Australia

Assessment of high risk pregnancies using antenatal FHR records began in Melbourne in 1973 (Beischer *et al.* 1983) and two units have recently reported large audits. In one, the traces were classified as normal (if reactive), suspicious, ominous or unsatisfactory (Humphrey *et al.* 1987).

**Table 9.2** Assessment of antepartum fetal reserve (Oats *et al.* 1987)

| | Critical | Reduced | Satisfactory |
|---|---|---|---|
| FHR variability (b.p.m.) | <7 | 5–7 | 7+ |
| FHR accelerations (*n*/20 min) | <5 | <5 | 5+ |
| FHR late decelerations | Present | Absent | Absent |

The other used a different classification which, according to the degree of fetal reserve indicated by FHR reactivity, was satisfactory, reduced or critical (Beischer *et al.* 1983; Oats *et al.* 1987). Both systems were visual and unscored. The assessment of critical reserve used only the presence of variability, accelerations and late decelerations for classification of the CTG, as shown in Table 9.2. CTGs were requested on 32 per cent of just over 31 000 women over the 6 year period between 1981 and 1986 and 91 per cent of these were satisfactory.

The incidence of perinatal death in this group, excluding lethal fetal malformations, was 3 per 1000 (Oats *et al.* 1987). Increased incidences of SGA (rising from 8 per cent to 11 per cent and 30 per cent), Caesarean section (rising from 16 per cent to 27 per cent and 62 per cent) and perinatal mortality (rising from 0.8 per cent to 4 per cent and 20 per cent) occurred in the 8 per cent with reduced and 1 per cent with critical fetal reserve. The latter, terminal, traces indicated delivery by Caesarean section because the outcome was good (Beischer *et al.* 1983) unless associated with fetal malformation as occurred in 18 per cent of such traces (Chew *et al.* 1985). The other unit reported a 1.7 per cent incidence of ominous traces over a three year period during which 3000 women (42 per cent of the total) were tested (Humphrey *et al.* 1987). The rate of ominous traces fell markedly with gestation, there being 5.5 per cent before 30 weeks, 3 per cent between 30 and 32 weeks, 1.6 per cent between 33 and 36 weeks, 0.7 per cent between 37 and 41 weeks and none after that. In half of the cases with an ominous trace this was the first record made.

## Recent developments with cardiotocograph classification and analysis

In Finland, an analysis of the components of the Fischer FHR score with respect to differences between normal and high risk pregnancy, particularly with fetal growth retardation, showed that the FHR baseline was not significantly different. It has therefore been suggested that baseline be excluded from the scoring system (Kaar 1980). Fetal movements were included and the various parameters were weighted according to their ability to predict fetal outcome. Late decelerations carried the most weight and were scored 0–3 whereas oscillation frequency of the variability was only scored 0–1 (Table 9.3). A score of 8 was close to the 5th percentile of the normal range, which agrees with the normal range of the original Fischer score.

**Table 9.3** Kaar score (1980) for antepartum cardiotocograms

| | Score 0 | Score 1 | Score 2 | Score 3 |
|---|---|---|---|---|
| Variability | | | | |
| Amplitude (b.p.m.) | <5 | 5–9 | 10+ | |
| Frequency (cycles/min) | <3 | >3 | | |
| Accelerations (*n*/30 min) | 0 | 1–4 | 5+ | |
| Decelerations | Recurrent Late | Occasional Late | Variable | Early/ none |
| Fetal movements (*n*/30 min) | 0 | 1–4 | 5+ | |

Abnormal score 0–7; normal score 8–10.

A comparison between the visual system of Visser & Huisjes (1977), the Fischer score (Fischer *et al.* 1976) and a new visual method, which entailed a close look at a 1-min window, showed that the intra-observer variability of five experienced clinicians was high for all three classification systems (Lotgering *et al.* 1982). However inter-observer variability was low for all three methods. The development in Oxford of a computerized analysis system for antepartum FHR records (now commerically available from Oxford Sonicaid Ltd, Chichester, UK) has shown the feasibility of uniform interpretation of the numerical data derived from the fetal monitor (Dawes *et al.* 1985). Normal limits have been derived from many thousands of records and are used to indicate whether a given CTG is normal or abnormal. Although undoubtedly able to give a uniform interpretation of the CTG the value of the system will need to be proven by clinical trials.

## The present status of fetal heart rate reactivity and fetal stimulation

The majority of reports in the literature now talk about reactive and non-reactive FHR traces, although there is no consensus regarding the number of accelerations required. One of the problems with antepartum FHR recording in the USA was the time constraint placed upon it by early definitions of the record as a non-stress test. Many papers refer to manual stimulation of the maternal abdomen in order to arouse the fetus and alter its state from quiescence to activity (Keegan & Paul 1980; Mendenhall *et al.* 1980; Barrett *et al.* 1981; Bishop 1981) and some also used a ringing bell (Rayburn *et al.* 1978; Weingold *et al.* 1980). Recognition that the fetal rest–activity cycle may produce periods of fetal quiescence with low FHR variability and few accelerations for up to 40 min (Wheeler & Guerard 1974; Timor-Tritsch *et al.* 1978) resulted in some advocates of the NST extending the duration of the FHR record until spontaneous transition from quiet to active state by the fetus (Evertson *et al.* 1979; Brown & Patrick 1981). This remains the practice in the UK (Figure 9.8) and 40 min seems to be the time by which at least 95 per cent of normal

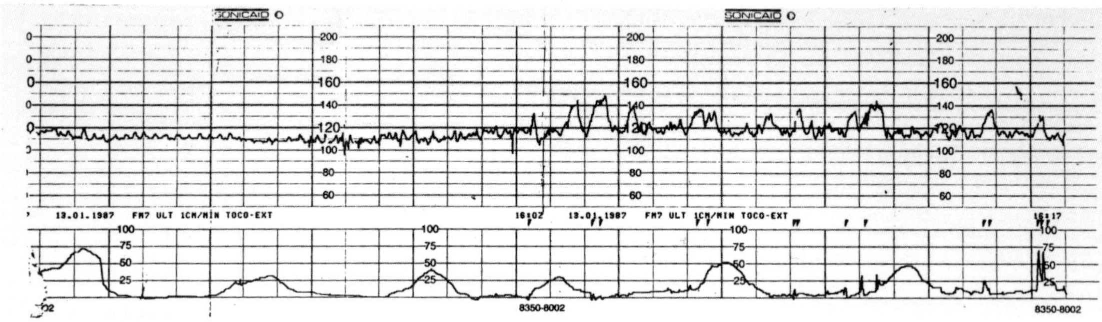


**Fig. 9.8** A normal FHR record (1 cm/min) showing the effect of a spontaneous change in fetal behavioural state from quiescence to activity. Note that the duration of the record is necessarily governed by the time spent in the quiet state before FHR reactivity in the active state provides evidence of fetal well-being.

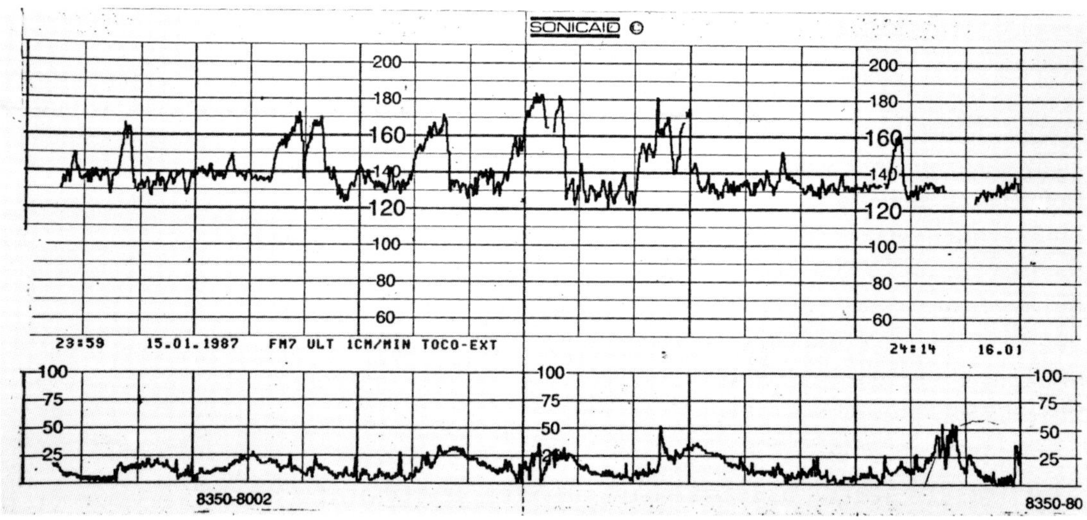


**Fig. 9.9** A normal FHR record (1 cm/min) of 18 min duration showing 6 accelerations of approximately 30 b.p.m. during the first 10 min.

fetuses will exhibit FHR accelerations (Brown & Patrick 1981; Devoe *et al.* 1985). The mean duration of monitoring required to obtain three accelerations in a 10 min period was found to be 18.5 min when the initial record was good but was 39 min when the initial record was uncertain (Odendaal & Basson 1979). It would not seem necessary to extend the duration of the FHR record once fetal activity and FHR reactivity occur (Figure 9.9).

As has been mentioned, in the presence of a non-reactive FHR trace manual manipulation has been used to try and alter the fetal state from quiescence to activity. However, prospective studies showed that this was ineffective (Richardson *et al.* 1981; Issel 1983; Visser *et al.* 1983; Druzin *et al.* 1985). Sound (Goodlin & Schmidt 1972; Read & Miller 1977; Trudinger & Boylan 1980) and vibroacoustic (Gagnon *et al.* 1986; Ohel *et al.*

1986) stimulation applied to the maternal abdomen have been shown to be effective in changing the fetal state to one of activity thereby reducing the rate of false positive, non-reactive, FHR records (Smith *et al.* 1986). This technique also significantly shortens the testing time (Smith *et al.* 1986) and has become accepted practice in many centres, especially in the USA. The crucial question of whether stimulation is necessary has not yet been answered and the practice has not been accepted in the UK.

## Routine antepartum fetal heart rate testing

Four randomized controlled trials have been performed in an attempt to establish the potential value of routine antenatal FHR testing in high risk pregnancies. Of the three British studies, the first to be published was from Birmingham (Flynn *et al.* 1982a) where the visual classification of reactive or non-reactive was used. Brown *et al.* (1982) modified the Cardiff scoring system to take account of basal heart rate and FHR response to fetal movements only whilst Kidd *et al.* (1985) used the original Cardiff scoring system. The trial from Melbourne used visual analysis of the baseline, variability, reactivity and decelerations (Lumley *et al.* 1983). CTGs were performed weekly (Brown *et al.* 1982; Lumley *et al.* 1983) or daily (Kidd *et al.* 1985) but only the last one from each patient was used for the correlation with outcome. Significant differences in birth weight and gestation at delivery between the low and high scoring CTGs were seen whether or not the CTGs was revealed to the clinician (Brown *et al.* 1982) suggesting that other factors, present in both groups, were influential in dictating management. The availability of routine antenatal CTG in high risk pregnancy had no effect on perinatal morbidity or mortality and did not significantly influence the timing or mode of delivery in these small studies. However, the availability of the CTG report resulted in significantly more women being allowed to continue their pregnancy as an out-patient (Flynn *et al.* 1982a). In Melbourne the use of antenatal FHR testing increased 16 times after their study ended.

Women whose pregnancy continues beyond two weeks past the estimated date of delivery are increasingly being managed on an out-patient basis with routine weekly (Keegan *et al.* 1980; Phelan *et al.* 1984) or thrice-weekly (Cario 1984) non-stress antepartum FHR traces. However, others consider that the CST is a better method (Freeman *et al.* 1981), particularly for unmasking potential cord compression (Miyazaki & Miyazaki 1981). The rate of intervention based on either method seems to be 1 in 20 (Freeman *et al.* 1981; Cario 1984).

## Indications for antepartum fetal heart rate testing

The reported indications for antepartum cardiotocography are listed in Table 9.4 where it can be seen that post-dates and hypertension in pregnancy are the commonest reasons. Not many studies have reported the

**Table 9.4** Main indications for antepartum cardiotocography

| | Post-dates | BP | IUGR | Diab | Decr FM | APH | Rh |
|---|---|---|---|---|---|---|---|
| Flynn & Kelly (1977) | 39 | 13 | 33 | 1.3 | — | 3 | 3 |
| Rayburn *et al.* (1978) | 39 | 25 | 3 | 18 | — | 2 | 4 |
| Keegan & Paul (1980) | 52 | 6 | 14 | 10 | 35 | — | 2 |
| Keirse & Trimbos (1980) | 32 | 26 | 10 | <5 | <5 | <5 | 6 |
| Mendenhall *et al.* (1980) | 38 | 28 | 13 | 10 | — | 1 | — |
| Barrett *et al.* (1981) | 27 | 15 | 13 | 10 | 12 | 1 | 1 |
| Bishop (1981) | 19 | 36 | 10 | 12 | — | — | — |
| Phelan (1981) | 35 | 13 | 21 | 8 | 7 | — | 0.4 |
| Freeman *et al.* (1982a) | 39 | 27 | 8 | 14 | — | — | 2 |
| Homburg *et al.* (1982) | 66 | 12 | 1 | 11 | 3 | — | 1 |
| Humphrey *et al.* (1987) | 10 | 19 | 16 | 5 | 19 | 8 | 1 |
| Oats *et al.* (1987) | 18 | 28 | 18 | 6 | 9 | 4 | 0.5 |
| Average | 35 | 20 | 13 | 9 | 9 | 3 | 1.5 |

All values are percentages.
IUGR = intrauterine growth retardation; BP = hypertension in pregnancy (including pre-eclampsia); Diab = diabetes; Decr FM = decreased or no fetal movements; APH = antepartum haemorrhage; and Rh = Rhesus isoimmunization.

**Table 9.5** The incidence of abnormal antenatal FHR traces according to the reason for request

| | Post-dates | BP | IUGR | Decr FM | APH | Rh |
|---|---|---|---|---|---|---|
| Non-reactive: | | | | | | |
| Flynn & Kelly (1977) (4 accels/20 min) | 19 | 10 | 18 | — | 33 | 56 |
| Mendenhall *et al.* (1980) (1 accel/30 min) | 10 | 31 | 20 | — | 33 | — |
| Reduced reserve: | | | | | | |
| Oats *et al.* (1987) | 6 | 10 | 13 | 5 | 8 | 0 |
| Critical reserve or ominous: | | | | | | |
| Oats *et al.* (1987) | 0.1 | 1.3 | 1.7 | 0.2 | 1.7 | 2 |
| Humphrey *et al.* (1987) | 0.3 | 2 | 4 | 1.5 | 2 | 9 |

All values are percentages. IUGR = intrauterine growth retardation; BP = hypertension in pregnancy (including pre-eclampsia); Decr FM = decreased or no fetal movements; APH = antepartum haemorrhage; Rh = Rhesus isoimmunization.

incidence of abnormal traces according to the reason for request but Table 9.5 shows the results from four studies. The overall incidence of critical reserve or ominous traces is between 0.9 per cent (Oats *et al.* 1987) and 1.7 per cent (Humphrey *et al.* 1987). Suspicious CTGs indicating reduced reserve are found in 8 to 15 per cent of tested high risk pregnancies (Keirse & Trimbos 1980; Oats *et al.* 1987) but adequate follow-up of such cases with repeat CTGs will usually allow those pregnancies requiring intervention to be identified adequately (Keirse & Trimbos 1981).

## The FIGO guidelines

In 1985 a workshop of experts was organized in Zurich by the Perinatal Medicine Standards subcommittee of the International Federation of Gynaecology and Obstetrics (FIGO). The aim was to draw up a set of guidelines for the use of fetal monitoring and these were subsequently published (FIGO 1987). They state that antepartum cardiotocography should only be performed for clinical indications and should not be interpreted in isolation. When indicated it should be started 2 weeks before there is a reasonable chance of extrauterine survival. The main objective is to detect chronic placental dysfunction which usually evolves slowly unless placental separation or uterine contractions intervene. Weekly tests may be sufficient for a higher risk pregnancy managed as an outpatient but in-patients with increased risk for fetal distress should be monitored at least daily.

The recommended classification of antepartum FHR records is normal, suspicious or pathological. The criteria for these groups is shown in Table 9.6. The guidelines do not mention scoring systems or refer to reactive and non-reactive traces. A reactive FHR, therefore, is to be called normal and requires at least two accelerations in a 10 min period. A non-reactive FHR without accelerations for more than 40 min but also without recurrent decelerations is termed suspicious. A pathological pattern is one which has been described previously as abnormal, ominous, critical or terminal. No recommendation is made regarding the duration of the antepartum FHR record but the recommended paper speed is 1 cm/min. The FHR trace is part of the case record and should be filed as such.

**Table 9.6** FIGO criteria for classification of antenatal FHR records

| | Pathological | Suspicious | Normal |
|---|---|---|---|
| Baseline (b.p.m.) | <100 or >170 | 100–110 or 150–170 | 110–150 |
| Variability (b.p.m.) | <5 >40 min or sinusoidal | 5–10 >40 min or >25 | 5–25 |
| Accelerations (*n*/10 min) | Absent | Absent >40 min | 2+ |
| Decelerations | Any recurrent or large, long or late | Ocasional Small | Absent |

## Summary

Until recently there were no generally agreed recommendations regarding the use of antepartum cardiotocography and so a number of methods for the interpretation of traces has evolved. The practice of antepartum FHR monitoring has become established in many countries despite the cost and despite the fact that no prospective study has shown it to be of value. In Europe and Australia the non-stressed FHR record continues to be the method of choice and the duration of the test is governed by the time taken for a normal or reactive trace to be obtained. In the USA, however, there seems to be an increasing tendency to use vibroacoustic stimulation if the FHR is not normal within the initial 10–20 min and a persistently non-reactive NST is usually considered an indication for a CST. There would seem to be no place for CTGs to be performed as an out-patient procedure except, possibly, as part of the management of the post-term pregnancy.

There is little doubt about the diagnostic value of antepartum FHR records when used as part of the management of certain pregnancy complications. Following antepartum haemorrhage the presence of decelerations indicates probable abruption and the need for prompt delivery by Caesarean section. If this is delayed then perinatal death is likely (Figure 9.10). With fetal growth retardation the sequence of changes in the FHR which have been shown to accompany increasing fetal hypoxia and metabolic acidaemia mean that the FHR is particularly useful when it

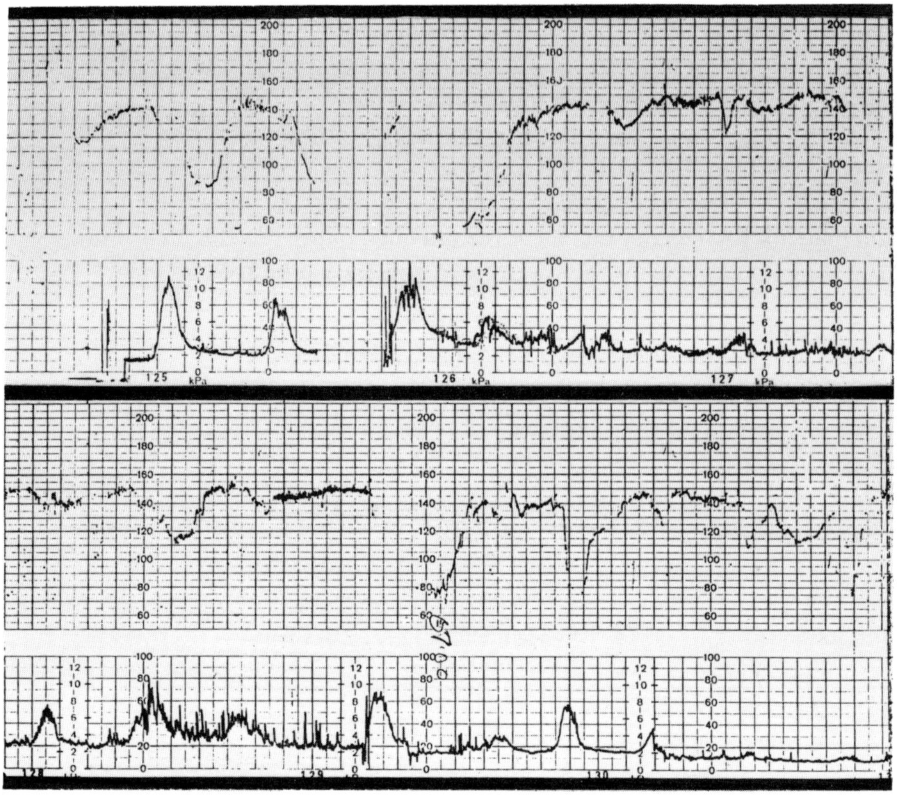

**Fig. 9.10** A terminal, or pathological, FHR record (1 cm/min) from a woman presenting with an antepartum haemorrhage at 34 weeks. After a period of deliberation a Caesarean section was performed which confirmed a moderate placental abruption. An AGA infant weighing 1830 g was delivered in poor condition (Apgar scores 1 at 1 min and 3 at 5 min) and died in the neonatal period. Appropriate management, indicated by the FHR record, would have been immediate Caesarean section as uneventful recovery is likely if the episode of asphyxia, despite its severity, is short.

comes to the timing of delivery. Such practice is now so well established that it is probably impossible to test the use of the CTG in this situation. Nevertheless, the limits of FHR testing need to be remembered in order to avoid an unnecessary waste of time and money by performing FHR monitoring in situations where it has not been shown to be helpful (Thacker & Berkelman 1986).

## References

Barrett J.M., Salyuer S.L. & Boehm F.H. (1981) The nonstress test: an evaluation of 1000 patients. *American Journal of Obstetrics and Gynecology*, **141**, 153–7.

Beischer N.A., Drew J.H., Ashton P.W., Oats J.N., Gaudry E., Chew F.T.K. & Parkinson P. (1983) Quality of survival of infants with critical fetal reserve detected by antenatal cardiotocography. *American Journal of Obstetrics and Gynecology*, **146**, 662–70.

Bhakthavathsalan A., Mann L.I., Tejani N.A. & Weiss R.R. (1976) Correlation of the oxytocin challenge test with perinatal outcome. *Obstetrics and Gynecology*, **48**, 552–6.

Bishop E.H. (1966) The Doppler ultrasonic motion sensor. *Obstetrics and Gynecology*, **28**, 712–13.

Bishop E.H. (1981) Fetal acceleration test. *American Journal of Obstetrics and Gynecology*, **141**, 905–9.

Bissonnette J.M., Johnson K. & Toomey C. (1979) The role of a trial of labor with a positive contraction stress test. *American Journal of Obstetrics and Gynecology*, **135**, 292–6.

Braly P.S., Freeman R.K., Garite T.J., Anderson G.G. & Dorchester W. (1981) Incidence of premature delivery following the oxytocin challenge test. *American Journal of Obstetrics and Gynecology*, **141**, 5–8.

Brown R. & Patrick J. (1981) The nonstress test: How long is enough? *American Journal of Obstetrics and Gynecology*, **141**, 646–51.

Brown V.A., Sawer R.S., Parson R.J., Duncan S.L.B. & Cooke I.D. (1982) The value of antenatal cardiotocography in the management of high-risk pregnancy: a randomized controlled trial. *British Journal of Obstetrics and Gynaecology*, **89**, 716–22.

Callagan D.A., Rowland T.C. & Goldman D.E. (1964) Ultrasonic Doppler observation of the fetal heart. *Obstetrics and Gynecology*, **23**, 637.

Cario G.M. (1984) Conservative management of prolonged pregnancy using fetal heart rate monitoring only: a prospective study. *British Journal of Obstetrics and Gynaecology*, **91**, 23–30.

Chew F.T., Drew J.H., Oats J.N., Riley S.F. & Beischer N.A. (1985) Nonstressed antepartum cardiotocography in patients undergoing elective cesarean section — fetal outcome. *American Journal of Obstetrics and Gynecology*, **151**, 318–21.

Christie G.B. & Cudmore D.W. (1974) The oxytocin challenge test. *American Journal of Obstetrics and Gynecology*, **118**, 327–30.

Corner G.W. & Stran H.M. (1957) A fetal heart ratemeter. *American Journal of Obstetrics and Gynecology*, **73**, 190–3.

Dawes G.S., Houghton C.R.S, Redman C.W.G. & Visser G.H.A. (1982) Pattern of the normal human fetal heart rate. *British Journal of Obstetrics and Gynaecology*, **89**, 276–84.

Dawes G.S., Redman C.W.G. & Smith J.H. (1985) Improvements in the registration and analysis of fetal heart rate records at the bedside. *British Journal of Obstetrics and Gynaecology*, **92**, 317–25.

Dawes G.S., Visser G.H.A., Goodman J.D.S. & Redman C.W.G. (1981) Numerical analysis of the human fetal heart rate: The quality of ultrasound records. *American Journal of Obstetrics and Gynecology*, **141**, 43–52.

Devoe L.D. (1980). Clinical implications of prospective antepartum fetal heart rate testing. *American Journal of Obstetrics and Gynecology*, **137**, 983–90.

Devoe L.D., McKenzie J., Searle N. & Sherline D.M. (1985) Nonstress test: Dimensions of normal reactivity. *Obstetrics and Gynecology*, **66**, 617–20.

Druzin M.L., Gratacos J., Paul R.H., Broussard P., McCart D. & Smith M. (1985) Antepartum fetal heart rate testing. XII. The effect of manual manipulation of the fetus on the nonstress test. *American Journal of Obstetrics and Gynecology*, **151**, 61–4.

Emmen L., Huisjes H.J., Aarnoudse J.G., Visser G.H.A. & Okken A. (1975) Antepartum diagnosis of the 'terminal' fetal state by cardiotocography. *British Journal of Obstetrics and Gynaecology*, **82**, 353–9.

Evertson L.R., Gauthier R.J. & Collea J.V. (1978) Fetal demise following negative contraction stress tests. *Obstetrics and Gynecology*, **51**, 671–3.

Evertson L.R., Gauthier R.J., Schifrin B.S. & Paul R.H. (1979) Antepartum fetal heart rate testing. I. Evolution of the nonstress test. *American Journal of Obstetrics and Gynecology*, **133**, 29–33.

FIGO News (1987) Guidelines for the use of fetal monitoring. *International Journal of Gynaecology and Obstetrics*, **25**, 159–67.

Fischer W.M., Stude I. & Brandt H. (1976) A suggestion for the evaluation of the antepartal cardiotocogram. *Zeitschrift für Geburtshilfe und Perinatologie*, **180**, 117–23.

Flynn A.M. & Kelly J. (1977) Evaluation of fetal wellbeing by antepartum fetal heart monitoring. *British Medical Journal*, **1**, 936–9.

Flynn A.M., Kelly J., Mansfield H., Needham P., O'Conor M. & Viegas O. (1982a) A randomized controlled trial of non-stress antepartum cardiotocography. *British Journal of Obstetrics and Gynaecology*, **89**, 427–33.

Flynn A.M., Kelly J., Matthews K., O'Conor M. & Viegas O. (1982b) Predictive value of, and observer variability in, several ways of reporting antepartum cardiotocographs. *British Journal of Obstetrics and Gynaecology*, **89**, 434–40.

Flynn A.M., Kelly J. & O'Conor M. (1979) Unstressed antepartum cardiotocography in the management of the fetus suspected of growth retardation. *British Journal of Obstetrics and Gynaecology*, **86**, 106–10.

Fox H.E., Steinbrecher M. & Ripton B. (1976) Antepartum fetal heart rate and uterine activity studies. 1 Preliminary report of accelerations and the oxytocin challenge test. *American Journal of Obstetrics and Gynecology*, **126**, 61–9.

Freeman R.K. (1975) The use of the oxytocin challenge test for antepartum clinical evaluation of uteroplacental respiratory function. *American Journal of Obstetrics and Gynecology*, **121**, 481–9.

Freeman R.K., Anderson G. & Dorchester W. (1982a) A prospective multi-institutional study of antepartum fetal heart rate monitoring. I. Risks of perinatal mortality and morbidity according to antepartum fetal heart rate test results. *American Journal of Obstetrics and Gynecology*, **143**, 771–7.

Freeman R.K., Anderson G. & Dorchester W. (1982b) A prospective multi-institutional study of antepartum fetal heart rate monitoring. II. Contraction stress test versus nonstress test for primary surveillance. *American Journal of Obstetrics and Gynecology*, **143**, 778–81.

Freeman R.K., Garite T.J., Modanlou H., Dorchester W., Rommal C. & Devaney M. (1981) Postdate pregnancy: Utilization of contraction stress testing for primary fetal surveillance. *American Journal of Obstetrics and Gynecology*, **140**, 128–34.

Fukushima T., Flores C.A., Hon E.H. & Davidson E.C. (1985) Limitations of autocorrelation in fetal heart rate monitoring. *American Journal of Obstetrics and Gynecology*, **153**, 685–92.

Gal D., Neuhoff S., Lilling M.I. & Tanger M.L. (1979) False negative oxytocin challenge test: report of three cases. *American Journal of Obstetrics and Gynecology*, **133**, 111–13.

Gagnon, R., Hunse C., Carmichael L., Fellows F. & Patrick J. (1986) Effects of vibratory acoustic stimulation on human fetal breathing and gross fetal body movements near term. *American Journal of Obstetrics and Gynecology*, **155**, 1227–30.

Gauthier R.J., Evertson L.R. & Paul R.H. (1979) Antenatal fetal heart rate testing. II. Intrapartum fetal heart rate observation and newborn outcome following a positive contraction stress test. *American Journal of Obstetrics and Gynecology*, **133**, 34–9.

Goodlin, R.C. & Schmidt W. (1972) Human fetal arousal levels as indicated by heart rate recordings. *American Journal of Obstetrics and Gynecology*, **114**, 613–21.

Grundy H., Freeman R.K., Lederman S. & Dorchester W. (1984) Nonreactive contraction stress test: clinical significance. *Obstetrics and Gynecology*, **64**, 337–42.

Hammacher K. (1962) Neue methoden zur selektiven registrierung der fetalen herzschlagfrequenz. *Geburtshilfe und Frauenheilkunde*, **22**, 1542–3.

Hammacher K., Huter K.A., Bokelmann J. & Werners P.H. (1968) Foetal heart frequency and perinatal condition of the foetus and newborn. *Gynaecologia*, **166**, 349–60.

Hellmann L.M., Schiffer M.A., Kohl S.G. & Tolles W.E. (1958) Studies in fetal well-being: variations in fetal heart rate. *American Journal of Obstetrics and Gynecology*, **76**, 998–1010.

Henson G., Dawes G.S. & Redman C.W.G. (1983) Antenatal fetal heart-rate variability in relation to fetal acid–base status at caesarean section. *British Journal of Obstetrics and Gynaecology*, **90**, 516–21.

Homburg R., Ben-David M. & Zakut H. (1982) Oxytocin-stressed and unstressed cardiotocograms for the prediction of fetal compromise. *British Journal of Obstetrics and Gynaecology*, **89**, 516–19.

Hon E.H. & Hess O.W. (1957) Instrumentation of fetal electrocardiography. *Science*, **125**, 553–4.

Hon E.H. & Khazin A.F. (1969) Observations on fetal heart rate and fetal biochemistry. I. Base deficit. *American Journal of Obstetrics and Gynecology*, **105**, 721–9.

Huddleston J.F., Sutliff G., Carney F.E. & Flowers C.E. (1979) Oxytocin challenge test for antepartum fetal assessment. Report of clinical experience. *American Journal of Obstetrics and Gynecology*, **135**, 609–14.

Huddleston J.F., Sutliff G. & Robinson D. (1984) Contraction stress test by intermittent nipple stimulation. *Obstetrics and Gynecology*, **63**, 669–73.

Humphrey M.D., Dossor S.L., Trickey D.J., Gumley S.J., Webb L.A., Bishop A.K., Davis C.M. & Crook S.L. (1987) The relevance of antenatal cardiotocography. *Australian and New Zealand Journal of Obstetrics and Gynaecology*, **27**, 87–9.

Huntingford P.J. & Pendleton H.J. (1969) The clinical application of cardiotocography. *Journal of Obstetrics and Gynaecology of the British Commonwealth*, **76**, 586–95.

Issel E.P. (1983) Fetal response to external mechanical stimuli. *Journal of Perinatal Medicine*, **11**, 232–42.

Kaar K. (1980) Antepartal cardiotocography in the assessment of fetal outcome. *Acta Obstetricia et Gynecologica Scandinavica*, Supplement 94.

Keegan K.A. & Paul R.H. (1980) Antepartum fetal heart rate testing. IV. The nonstress test as a primary approach. *American Journal of Obstetrics and Gynecology*, **136**, 75–80.

Keegan K.A., Paul R.H., Broussard P.M., McCart D. & Smith M.A. (1980) Antepartum fetal heart rate testing. V. The nonstress test — an outpatient approach. *American Journal of Obstetrics and Gynecology*, **136**, 81–3.

Keirse M.J.N.C. & Trimbos J.B. (1980) Assessment of antepartum cardiotocograms in high-risk pregnancy. *British Journal of Obstetrics and Gynaecology*, **87**, 261–9.

Keirse M.J.N.C. & Trimbos J.B. (1981) Clinical significance of suspicious antepartum cardiotocograms: a study of normal and high-risk pregnancies. *British Journal of Obstetrics and Gynaecology*, **88**, 739–46.

Kidd L.C., Patel N.B. & Smith R. (1985) Non-stress antenatal cardiotocography — a prospective randomized clinical trial. *British Journal of Obstetrics and Gynaecology*, **92**, 1156–9.

Krebs H.-B. & Petres R.E. (1978) Clinical application of a scoring system for evaluation of antepartum fetal heart rate monitoring. *American Journal of Obstetrics and Gynecology*, **130**, 765–72.

Kubli K. (1984) Antepartum monitoring of the fetal heart rate. In *Fetal Physiology and Medicine*, (Ed. by R.W. Beard & P.W. Nathanielsz), pp. 655–77. Butterworths, London.

Kubli F.W., Hon E.H., Khazin A.F. & Takemura H. (1969a) Observations on heart rate and pH in the human fetus during labour. *American Journal of Obstetrics and Gynecology*, **104**, 1190–206.

Kubli F., Kaeser O. & Hinselmann M. (1969b) Diagnostic management of chronic placental insufficiency. In *The Foetoplacental Unit*, (Ed. by A. Pecile & C. Finci). pp. 323–39. Exerpta Medica, Amsterdam.

Kubli F., Ruttgers H., Haller U., Bogdan C. & Ramzin M. (1972) Antepartum fetal heart rate. II. Baseline levels, baseline irregularity and decelerations with antepartum fetal death. *Zeitschrift fur Geburtshilfe und Perinatologie*, **176**, 309–23.

Langer O., Sonnendecker E.W.W. & Jacobson M.J. (1982) Categorization of terminal fetal heart-rate patterns in antepartum cardiotocography. *British Journal of Obstetrics and Gynaecology*, **89**, 179–85.

Lawson G.W., Belcher R., Dawes G.S. & Redman C.W.G. (1983) A comparison of ultrasound (with autocorrelation) and direct electrocardiogram fetal heart rate detector systems. *American Journal of Obstetrics and Gynecology*, **147**, 721–2.

Lee C.Y., DiLoreto P.C. & Logrand (1976) Fetal activity acceleration determination for the evaluation of fetal reserve. *Obstetrics and Gynecology*, **48**, 19–26.

Lee C.Y., DiLoreto P.C. & O'Lane J.M. (1975) A study of fetal heart rate acceleration patterns. *Obstetrics and Gynecology*, **45**, 142–6.

Lenke R.R. & Nemes J.M. (1984) Use of nipple stimulation to obtain contraction stress test. *Obstetrics and Gynecology*, **63**, 345–8.

Lin C.C., Devoe L.D., River P. & Moawad A.H. (1981) Oxytocin challenge test and intrauterine growth retardation. *American Journal of Obstetrics and Gynecology*, **140**, 282–8.

Lotgering F.K., Wallenburg H.C.S. & Schouten H.J.A. (1982) Interobserver and intra-observer variation in the assessment of antepartum cardiotocograms. *American Journal of Obstetrics and Gynecology*, **144**, 701–5.

Lumley J., Lester A., Anderson I., Renou P. & Wood C. (1983) A randomized trial of weekly cardiotocography in high-risk obstetric patients. *British Journal of Obstetrics and Gynaecology*, **90**, 1018–26.

Lyons E.R., Bylsma-Howell M., Shamsi S. & Towell M.E. (1979) A scoring system for nonstressed antepartum fetal heart rate monitoring. *American Journal of Obstetrics and Gynecology*, **133**, 242–46.

Mendenhall H.W., O'Leary J.A. & Phillips K.O. (1980) The nonstress test: the value of a single acceleration in evaluation of the fetus at risk. *American Journal of Obstetrics and Gynecology*, **136**, 87–91.

Mendez-Bauer C., Arnt I.C., Gulin L., Escarcena L. & Caleyro-Barcia R. (1967) Relationship between blood pH and heart rate in the human fetus during labor. *American Journal of Obstetrics and Gynecology*, **97**, 530–45.

Merkur H. (1979) Normal and abnormal antenatal ultrasonic cardiotocographic patterns. *British Journal of Obstetrics and Gynaecology*, **86**, 533–9.

Miyazaki F.S. & Miyazaki B.A. (1981) False positive nonstress tests in postterm pregnancies. *American Journal of Obstetrics and Gynecology*, **140**, 269–76.

Oats J.N., Chew F.T.K. & Rarren V.J. (1987) Antepartum cardiotocography — an audit. *Australian and New Zealand Journal of Obstetrics and Gynaecology*, **27**, 82–6.

Odendaal H.J. & Basson J.P.H. (1979) Combined (stressed and non-stressed) antenatal fetal heart rate monitoring. *European Journal of Obstetrics, Gynecology and Reproductive Biology*, **9**, 351–60.

Ohel G., Birkenfeld A., Rabinowitz R. & Sadovsky E. (1986) Fetal response to vibratory acoustic stimulation in periods of low heart rate reactivity and low activity. *American Journal of Obstetrics and Gynecology*, **154**, 619–21.

Parer J.T. & Afonso J.F. (1977) Validity of the weekly interval between oxytocin challenge tests. *American Journal of Obstetrics and Gynecology*, **127**, 204–5.

Pearson J.F. & Weaver J.B. (1978) A six-point scoring system for antenatal cardiotocograms. *British Journal of Obstetrics and Gynaecology*, **85**, 321–7.

Phelan J.P. (1981) The nonstress test: a review of 3000 tests. *American Journal of Obstetrics and Gynecology*, **139**, 7–10.

Phelan J.P., Cromartie A.D. & Smith C.V. (1982) The nonstress test: the false negative test. *American Journal of Obstetrics and Gynecology*, **142**, 293–6.

Phelan J.P., Platt L.D., Yeh S.-Y., Trujillo M. & Paul R.H. (1984) Continuing role of the nonstress test in the management of postdates pregnancy. *Obstetrics and Gynecology*, **64**, 624–8.

Pose S.V., Castillo, J.B., Mora-Rojas E.O., Soto-Yances A & Caldeyro-Barcia R. (1969) Test of fetal tolerance to induced uterine contractions for the diagnosis of chronic distress. *Pan American Health Organisation Scientific Publication*, **185**, 96–104.

Ray M., Freeman R., Pine S. & Hesselgesser R. (1972) Clinical experience with the oxytocin challenge test. *American Journal of Obstetrics and Gynecology*, **114**, 1–9.

Rayburn W.F., Duhring J.L. & Donaldson M. (1978) A study of fetal acceleration tests. *American Journal of Obstetrics and Gynecology*, **132**, 33–5.

Read J.A. & Miller F.C. (1977) Fetal heart rate acceleration in response to acoustic stimulation as a measure of fetal well-being. *American Journal of Obstetrics and Gynecology*, **129**, 512–17.

Richardson B., Campbell K., Carmichael L. & Patrick J. (1981) Effects of external physical stimulation on fetuses near term. *American Journal of Obstetrics and Gynecology*, **139**, 344–52.

Rochard F., Schifrin B.S., Goupil F., Legrand H., Blottiere J. & Sureau C. (1976) Non-stressed fetal heart rate monitoring in the antepartum period. *American Journal of Obstetrics and Gynecology*, **126**, 699–706.

Schifrin B.S., Lapidus M., Doctor G.S. & Leviton A. (1975) Contraction stress test for antepartum fetal evaluation. *Obstetrics and Gynecology*, **45**, 433–8.

Slomka C. & Phelan J.P. (1981) Pregnancy outcome in the patient with a nonreactive nonstress test and a positive contraction stress test. *American Journal of Obstetrics and Gynecology*, **139**, 11–15.

Smith C.V., Phelan J.P., Platt L.D., Broussard P. & Paul R.H. (1986) Fetal acoustic stimulation testing. II. A randomized clinical comparison with the nonstress test. *American Journal of Obstetrics and Gynecology*, **155**, 131–4.

Smith J.H., Anand K.J.S., Cotes P.M., Dawes G.S., Harkness R.A., Howlett T.A., Rees L.H. & Redman C.W.G. (1988) Antenatal fetal heart rate variation in relation to the respiratory and metabolic status of the compromised human fetus. *British Journal of Obstetrics and Gynaecology*, **95**, 980–9.

Spencer J.A.D. (1987) The quality of ultrasound telemetry fetal heart rate records. *Journal of Obstetrics and Gynaecology*, **8**, 12–15.

Spencer J.A.D., Belcher R. & Dawes G.S. (1987) The influence of signal loss on the comparison between computer analyses of the fetal heart rate in labour using pulsed Doppler ultrasound (with autocorrelation) and simultaneous scalp electrocardiogram. *European Journal of Obstetrics, Gynecology and Reproductive Biology*, **25**, 29–34.

Spurrett B. (1971) Stressed cardiotocography in late pregnancy. *Journal of Obstetrics and Gynaecology of the British Commonwealth*, **78**, 894–900.

Staisch K.J., Westlake J.R. & Bashore R.A. (1980) Blind oxytocin challenge test and perinatal outcome. *American Journal of Obstetrics and Gynecology*, **138**, 399–403.

Swartwout J.R., Campbell W.E. & Williams L.G. (1961) Observations on the fetal heart rate. *American Journal of Obstetrics and Gynecology*, **82**, 301–3.

Thacker S.B. & Berkelman R.L. (1986) Assessing the diagnostic accuracy and efficacy of selected antepartum fetal surveillance techniques. *Obstetrical and Gynecological Survey*, **41**, 121–41.

Timor-Tritsch I.E., Dierker L.J., Hertz R.H., Deagan N.C. & Rosen M.G. (1978) Studies of antepartum behavioral state in the human fetus at term. *American Journal of Obstetrics and Gynecology*, **132**, 524–8.

Trierweiler M.W., Freeman R.K. & James J. (1976) Baseline fetal heart rate characteristics as an indicator of fetal status during the antepartum period. *American Journal of Obstetrics and Gynecology*, **125**, 618–23.

Trimbos J.B. & Keirse M.J.N.C. (1978a) Observer variability in assessment of antepartum cardiotocograms. *British Journal of Obstetrics and Gynaecology*, **85**, 900–6.

Trimbos J.B. & Keirse M.J.N.C. (1978b) Significance of antepartum cardiotocography in normal pregnancy. *British Journal of Obstetrics and Gynaecology*, **85**, 907–13.

Trudinger B.J. & Boylan P. (1980) Antepartum fetal heart rate monitoring: value of sound stimulation. *Obstetrics and Gynecology*, **55**, 265–8.

Visser G.H.A., Dawes G.S. & Redman C.W.G. (1981) Numerical analysis of the normal human antenatal fetal heart rate. *British Journal of Obstetrics and Gynaecology*, **88**, 792–802.

Visser G.H.A. & Huisjes H.J. (1977) Diagnostic value of the unstressed antepartum cardiotocogram. *British Journal of Obstetrics and Gynaecology*, **84**, 321–6.

Visser G.H.A, Redman C.W.G., Huisjes H.J. & Turnbull A.C. (1980) Nonstressed antepartum heart rate monitoring: implications of decelerations after spontaneous contractions. *American Journal of Obstetrics and Gynecology*,**138**, 429–35.

Visser G.H.A., Zeelenberg H.J., de Vries J.I.P. & Dawes G.S. (1983) External physical stimulation of the human fetus during episodes of low heart rate variation. *American Journal of Obstetrics and Gynecology*, **145**, 579–84.

Weingold A.B., Yonekura M.L. & O'Kieffe J. (1980) Nonstress tesing. *American Journal of Obstetrics and Gynecology*, **138**, 195–202.

Wheble AM, Gillmer M.D.G., Spencer J.A.D. & Sykes G.S. (1989) Changes in fetal monitoring practice in the UK: 1977–1984. *British Journal of Obstetrics and Gynaecology*, **96**, 1140–7.

Wheeler T. & Guerard P. (1974) Fetal heart rate during late pregnancy. *Journal of Obstetrics and Gynaecology of the British Commonwealth*, **84**, 348–56.

Wheeler T. & Murrills A. (1978) Patterns of fetal heart rate during normal pregnancy. *British Journal of Obstetrics and Gynaecology*, **85**, 18–27.
Wickham P.J.D., Dawes G.S. & Belcher R. (1983) Development of methods for quantitative analysis of the fetal heart rate. *Journal of Biomedical Engineering*, **5**, 302–8.
Wulf K.H. (1985) History of fetal heart rate monitoring. In *Fetal Heart Rate Monitoring*, (Ed. by W. Kunzel), pp. 3–15. Springer-Verlag, Berlin.

# 10: Fetal electrocardiography

HOWARD M.L. JENKINS



The first demonstration of a fetal electrocardiogram (FECG) was published by Cremer in 1906 when he used an abdominal electrode combined with either a vaginal or a rectal electrode. Work by other authors over the next fifty years was concerned mainly with the display of better quality recordings, and because of the technical difficulties, changes in waveform patterns were not defined. This period was comprehensively reviewed by Symonds (1971).

The first tentative steps in the interpretation of the FECG were taken in 1954 by Enhorning & Westin. Pre-viable fetuses, which had been delivered vaginally or by hysterotomy, were studied. With increasing asphyxia it was noted that there was increasing bradycardia, a prolonged P–R interval, and inversion of T waves. In 1957, Southern carried out a study of the antenatal FECG, recorded with abdominal electrodes, in an attempt to identify fetal anoxia. In 96 cases, the FECG was compared to the fetal condition, as assessed by arterial oxygen concentration at birth. In cases of fetal distress, there was a lengthening of P–R interval from 60 ms to 120 ms, lengthening of QRS complex, depression of ST segments and T wave inversion. Southern felt that the earliest changes in the FECG during anoxia occurred in the ST segments and T waves. Kaplan & Toyama (1958) used similar apparatus to Southern and found wide variation in the FECG conduction intervals in normal cases, even in the absence of fetal distress, and found no change in the FECG during the course of labour. They also noted a considerable improvement in the FECG signal when using an electrode inserted into the intrauterine cavity after rupture of the membranes (as first described by Smyth in 1953), and suggested that further work was required before accurate diagnoses of fetal distress from FECG tracings could be made.

## Techniques for signal improvement

Hon & Hess (1957) reviewed the technical difficulties of obtaining abdominal FECG recordings and proposed a system which discriminated signal from noise. In addition, they pointed out that a data reduction system should be used if the whole labour were to be recorded. In 1960, Hon & Hess suggested that the abdominal FECG was useful for monitoring fetal heart rate (FHR) but of very limited value in the diagnosis of fetal distress. Larks and his colleagues, however, felt that they were able to demonstrate FECG changes in different clinical situations (Larks & Anderson 1962; Larks & Longo 1962; Larks 1963). They stated that in cases of fetal distress, widening of the QRS complex occurred, with or without notching of the waves. Elevation or depression of the ST segment took place in some of these cases, and apparent arrhythmias and gross QRS distortion were also demonstrated. Retrospectively, it is extremely doubtful whether such detailed observations can be made from the tracings presented, in view of the poor signal quality.

Hunter *et al.* (1960), recognizing the difficulties caused by high levels of electrical noise when recording the abdominal FECG, described the use of a direct lead clipped onto the fetal scalp after rupture of the membranes. A second lead was clipped to the maternal perineum, and an indifferent grounding lead was attached to the maternal leg. A differential amplifier was used, and it was found that marked attenuation of the maternal ECG signs was obtained with this lead configuration. As the maternal ECG signals were normally a major component in simple abdominal recordings of the FECG, this technique represented a considerable advance. The tracings presented by Hunter *et al.* showed well-defined QRS complexes, but P and T waves remained obscured by low amplitude noise.

Hon (1963) described his results using a rather more practical electrode based on a surgical skin clip. The clip was applied to the fetal presenting part and an electrical lead was attached. A second lead was arranged to lie nearby in the cervical and vaginal secretions, thus replacing Hunter's perineal lead. The two leads were fixed to a terminal block mounted on an earthing plate resting on the maternal thigh. Hon demonstrated that this arrangement proved superior in noise rejection than the method using a perineal lead, particularly when the mother was moving or pushing with contractions. The FECG signal obtained was filtered and used principally as a means of plotting a continuous record of FHR.

Vasicka *et al.* (1963) noted that although these new methods of direct fetal recording reduced the problem of extraneous electrical interference, when compared to abdominal recording, the problem remained when the membranes were intact. They described their experience with intra-amniotic platinum electrodes inserted by transabdominal amniocentesis.

(This method had been originally proposed by Caldeyro-Barcia and his group in Uruguay.) FECG tracings of good quality were obtained, but the main purpose was to assess fetal rate changes. Needless to say, the trans-abdominal, intra-amniotic electrode never became a popular method of human fetal cardiac monitoring. The risks of such a technique were never considered justifiable.

The use of the direct clip method of recording was endorsed by Stander *et al.* (1963), who described an instrument complex for monitoring fetal heart rate with changes in maternal blood pressure, heart rate and intra-amniotic pressure. An Australian group (Mayes *et al.* 1963) also devised an advanced system for monitoring the FHR and FECG. They used vaginal (direct) fetal electrodes and also abdominal electrodes. They did not find consistent FECG waveform changes in cases of fetal hypoxia and thought that such changes were of dubious value in the prediction of fetal distress, and considered that the observation of FHR was of prime clinical importance. Hon & Lee (1963a) also found inconsistency in the changes of FECG configuration in 22 fetuses which died during the recording period. They noted that without techniques of signal-to-noise enhancement, interference by extraneous noise (e.g. maternal ECG) gave spurious changes such as apparent ST segment elevation or depression. They also found insufficient consistency in FECG configuration changes to be of clinical value, although changes in P wave shape were fairly consistent as was shortening of the P–R interval.

In order to overcome the problems inherent in the poor signal-to-noise ratio of the FECG, Hon & Lee (1963b) devised an averaging technique using a digital computer (a Computer of Averaged Transients). It was found that by averaging groups of 10 to 20 FECG complexes, the signal-to-noise ratio improved dramatically and allowed the recovery of obscured P and T waves. In 1964, Hon & Lee showed that this method allowed the definition of precise turning points in the FECG complex but they noted that very short-term changes in the FECG configuration would be missed by the group averaging method. However, the method permitted a continuous observation of the FECG, thus improving the chances of detecting significant transient changes in the complex. Such changes were found in the QRS complex during cord manipulation but they thought the significance of these was very dubious since animal and adult work in conditions of hypoxia showed no such changes (Lee & Hon 1965). Again, a degree of disenchantment about the value of the FECG as an early indication of fetal hypoxia was expressed by these authors.

Shenker, in 1966, reviewed the progress in fetal electrocardiography to that date. He found that the method of direct, continuous recording of the FECG had provided much understanding of fetal heart rate patterns which would have been unobtainable by auscultation alone. He considered that the monitoring of fetal heart rate in labour by these methods would become routine practice. The value of the FECG itself, however, remained in much doubt in the diagnosis of fetal cardiac disease or fetal hypoxia. It was concluded that despite much work purporting to demonstrate FECG changes in these conditions, a good deal was suspect due to technical considerations, and that even the normal FECG had yet to be classified.

Millican *et al.* (1966) also reviewed the value of fetal electrocardiography and compared it with phonocardiography and heart rate monitoring. With the techniques available, P and T waves were obliterated, and QRS complex distortion occurred. This was due to the electrical filters used to suppress extraneous electrical noise. No electrocardiographic abnormalities could be correlated with clinically proven fetal distress, but the instantaneous FHR derived from the (direct) FECG correlated well with obstetrical and fetal events. As no abnormalities could be recognized with the use of phonocardiography, Millican *et al.* accordingly strongly favoured the use of instantaneous heart rate, rather than the other methods, for intrapartum monitoring.

## The fetal cardiac axis

Despite the doubts of others, Larks and his group continued to be optimistic about the value of the fetal electrocardiogram. In 1965, Larks introduced a new method of assessment of the FECG: the estimation of the electrical axis of the fetal heart. The sum of the positive and negative deflections of the abdominal FECG complex was projected, using the Einthoven triangle, to estimate the electrical axis of the fetal heart. Larks had already shown that the abdominal FECG resembled standard lead II in the case of vertex presentations (Larks 1964). Projections on lead II were mathematically related to the electrical axis vector times the sine of the angle which the electrical axis formed with the 150° line. Lead II projections were sensitive to changes in the electrical axis in the vicinity of 150°. The normal electrical axis of the fetal heart was found to fall between +90° to +180°, with a mean of +134°. Negative values were found in breech presentations. Several papers from Larks and his group, concerning the electrical axis of the fetal heart, followed this original publication. Larks & Larks (1965) presented 11 cases, from a series of 2500, where right axis deviation had occurred. In each case, there was some evidence of fetal asphyxia at birth, and other obstetric problems such as postmaturity, cord problems, and pre-eclamptic toxaemia. The authors suggested that right axis deviation represented chronic hypoxia, and noted the analogous situation of infants born at high altitudes who also had persistent right axis deviation.

Later, Larks & Larks (1966a) published quantitative data comparing the estimation of the cardiac electrical axis of the fetus with the electrical axis of lead II in the neonate. The fetal axis *in utero* was calculated to have a mean value of 135.7 compared with a mean value of 134.9 in the same cases as neonates. However, it should be noted that the standard deviations were high, at 46.4 and 40.0 respectively, and that the number of cases was not stated. Nevertheless, the authors felt that, clinically, these findings were consistent with right ventricular prominence and muscularity, and with relatively high right ventricular and pulmonary arterial pressures. A similar quantitative paper (Larks & Larks 1966b) presented the results from 1606 cases, comprising consecutive recordings of the fetal and neonatal ECG. The cases were divided into normal and abnormal categories, although consignment to the abnormal group was not necessarily on grounds of hypoxia. In the normal group there was a fairly good correlation between the electrical axis of the fetus and the neonate, with a coefficient of linear regression ($r$) of 0.60. In the abnormal group the $r$ value was 0.39, a statistically significant difference. No explanation was offered for this, other than the fact that 'greater variability and birth process changes were indicated' in this group.

In 1967, Larks *et al.* proposed that the Apgar score at birth could be predicted using a complex equation derived from multiple linear regression analyses of data from 1906 cases. The equation included measured amplitudes of R and S waves of the FECG (but not expressed as the cardiac axis) and these components were the most significant variables studied. The same process of multiple linear regression of the data was applied to 2028 cases in a paper presented in 1968 by the same authors. In twin pregnancies the mean fetal cardiac axis was found to be 103.8 (standard deviation was 74.6) but the mean neonatal cardiac axis in the same cases was 78.5 (standard deviation 68.4). Again, no explanation was offered. It is also interesting to note that the mean values of the singleton cases in this paper were 123.4 and 121.2 respectively, which are lower figures than the previous values published by Larks *et al.*, but this may have been so because breech presentations were included. The paper also demonstrated that there was a statistically significant degree of right rotation of the electrical axis of male fetus and neonate when compared with the female. It was suggested that this reflected greater right ventricular development in the male.

The electrical axis of breech presentations was examined by Larks *et al.* in 1969. This study confirmed earlier work that the complex was inverted in breech presentation, thus resulting in a much lower figure (mean 123.5) for the mean fetal electrical axis. The authors also put forward an interesting argument that rotation from breech to cephalic presentation in early pregnancy 'takes place under the influence of an optimal endocrine environment.' This theory was based on the differences of neonatal S wave amplitudes, and has not subsequently been substantiated.

Hon and his colleagues have never published any data on the fetal cardiac axis. Most of their papers on fetal electrocardiography at this time were devoted to the technical problems of capturing and presenting the FECG. Hon & Lee in 1965 presented charts displaying group averages of 64 complexes. This method was found successfully to demonstrate transient changes in the FECG complex and two cases, where P wave flattening occurred during an episode of bradycardia, were presented. The authors commented that group averaging may mask transitory changes in the FECG and that the use of weighted and running averages would tend to minimize this problem.

## Transmission pathways of the fetal electrocardiogram

Roche & Hon in 1965 published an important paper which considered the transmission pathways of FECG. The conventional view of volume conductor theory did not adequately explain the transmission characteristics of the fetal signal since the known high impedance of the fetal skin would have attenuated the FECG to the extent that no signal would have reached the maternal skin directly. The authors compared waveforms obtained by abdominal recording, direct recording and also in the immediate neonatal period. The complex shape appeared similar in all three instances in vertex presentations. When there was a breech presentation the waveform polarity was reversed in the abdominal and vaginal recordings compared to that of the neonate, but the complex shape was similar when this was taken into account. The configuration of the abdominal FECG appeared to change little or not at all from varying electrode positions on the maternal abdominal wall, nor was it altered during labour or delivery. If the maternal tissues had been acting as a simple volume conductor for the radiating FECG, it would have been expected that configuration changes would have taken place. Similarly, no change in waveform shape was noted in direct recording when the electrode was placed at different points on the presenting part. When leads were attached to the umbilical cord of the neonate, the configuration and the ECG was similar to the abdominal (indirect) and vaginal (direct) FECG. The authors concluded that since there must have been a low-impedance pathway in order to detect the FECG, then the most likely pathway was via the umbilical cord and placenta. There was also some evidence that mucus-lined passages of the fetus (i.e. nasopharynx and oropharynx) were pathways.

## The problem of extreme tachycardia

Hon and his group did not publish any further significant papers on the FECG complex and eventually used it merely as a trigger for FHR monitoring. By 1970, general disenchantment with the potential of the FECG as a predictor of fetal distress was fairly universal, and the use of FHR monitoring appeared to be simpler and equally effective.

The case for the FECG was not improved by the publication of two papers which appear, retrospectively, to contain absurdities. Talledo & Zuspan (1963) described four cases where an FECG of apparently extremely high rate (200–700 b.p.m.) was recorded from a macerated fetus. They considered that their recordings showed that electrical activity of the fetal heart was still present even when the fetus had been dead for some time and that the rapid rate was due to continued auricular fibrillation of the fetal heart. A similar publication from Caughey & Krohn (1963) showed a recording of FECG of live fetus with an apparent rate of 500–700 b.p.m. This provoked a vigorous reply by Teteris (1964) who pointed out that such a rate was physiologically unlikely, and parasitic oscillation in the amplifier system was the most likely explanation. Caughey & Krohn (1964) did not accept this and remained convinced that the recording was not artefactual.

Whitfield (1966) investigated the matter in a careful study of abdominal FECG recordings. It was found that a series of rapid electrical impulses, similar to those described by the previous authors, were present in 12 out of 22 recordings from 7 patients. These were normally of short duration and usually started spontaneously but in some cases could be initiated when the mother contracted her abdominal muscles. Whitfield felt that a fetal origin of such impulses from a macerated fetus seemed far-fetched, but demonstrated that the impulses he had recorded were not due to parasitic oscillations. The most likely explanation, therefore, appeared to be that these impulses originated in motor units in the maternal abdominal muscles. The previous authors appeared to have made a clinical misinterpretation of the recordings. In mitigation it should be stressed that the quality of recordings obtained at this time were generally poor, as has been previously mentioned concerning the early work of Larks.

## Later work using direct recording and signal enhancement

Direct recording using the new type of vaginal electrode originally described by Hon (1967) improved the signal quality considerably. Davidsen (1971) presented FECG recordings where all the components of the complex could be clearly seen. However, interfering signals (e.g. maternal ECG) were still present and contributed to the distortion of the FECG. For this reason, successive complexes were not identical, although this was not noted by the author. No clearly defined differences were found by Davidsen between the recordings in normal cases and those from asphyxiated cases, and it was again concluded that 'compared with the FHR, the FECG was a poor indication of fetal welfare during labour'.

Symonds (1971) also used a direct fetal electrode and obtained recordings of good quality. In a study of 102 cases where the fetus was considered to be at risk, the FECG was analysed in relation to maternal and fetal acid–base status and plasma electrolytes. Some 600 hours of paper chart FECG recordings were obtained and these were measured manually. Symonds' study overcame the disadvantages of earlier attempts to assess the FECG, since the majority of earlier reports had assessed fetal condition on clinical grounds alone. It was found that increasing fetal acidosis was associated with a prolonged Q–T interval, and this trend became statistically significant when the latter was corrected for fetal heart rate. A significant relationship was also found between fetal plasma potassium levels and cord arterial and venous pH levels. It should be noted that, in this study, short sections only of the FECG were measured, usually between contractions, although hundreds of individual measurements were made. Using the method, Symonds was unable to show that

FECG measurements gave a more accurate method of predicting fetal outcome than scalp blood pH measurements.

In a further paper in 1972, Symonds applied the method of measurements of fetal cardiac axis proposed by Larks. Of course, Larks had used abdominal recordings exclusively, and Symonds used direct (scalp) recordings exclusively. The latter was able to confirm the resemblance of the scalp FECG with the neonatal lead II, and, more interestingly, found that fetal cardiac axis measurements from the scalp FECG gave similar results in normal cases to those from the abdominal FECG reported by Larks.

Although the work of Symonds could be judged the first modern scientific study of the FECG, the methodology was severely limited by the lack of continuous evaluation of the FECG, and in particular the behaviour of FECG parameters during contractions was not examined. Roemer *et al.* (1972) made an attempt to correlate changes in FECG parameters with contractions. They found that the P–Q interval decreased at the beginning of FHR decelerations of variable types; at the same time P wave amplitude decreased markedly. It was suggested that this was due to a wandering pacemaker. The authors also demonstrated ST segment and T wave changes in severe variable and late FHR decelerations and stated that these were signs of acute hypoxia. In the case of what they termed *chronic severe fetal acidosis*, these changes were not always found. In regard to the fetal cardiac axis, the authors found increasing R wave amplitudes (left-axis shift) when there was decreased fetal $P\text{O}_2$ or increased fetal $P\text{CO}_2$. However, this data not well documented, and the paper also suffers from the total lack of information on the technical methodology. This does not apply to the paper of Lee & Blackwell (1974), who used similar methods to Symonds, except that the principal method of assessment of the infant at birth was by Apgar scoring. During FHR decelerations, the authors found shortening of the P–R and corrected Q–T intervals, and also left deviation of the cardiac axis. Interestingly, in the case of tachycardia, the cardiac axis deviated to the right, although P–R and corrected Q–T intervals were again shortened. The authors also found that notching of the P and R waves bore no relationship to fetal outcome, neither did the presence of fetal extrasystoles.

The results of Lee & Blackwell agree with Symonds (1972) but disagree with Larks & Larks (1965) concerning the deviation of the cardiac axis in the presence of fetal distress. However, Symonds (1972) found lengthening of the corrected Q–T interval when there was fetal acidosis; Lee & Blackwell found the reverse when there was fetal bradycardia (and assumed fetal distress). There is similar conflict with regard to notching of the components of the FECG complex. Lee & Blackwell found that to be of no significance although Larks & Anderson (1962) had previously reported otherwise.

In 1974, Pardi *et al.* used a group averaging technique in the analysis of the direct FECG in 234 labours. It was found that during severe variable decelerations, the P–Q interval became progressively shorter and then the P wave became biphasic or absent. In late decelerations P wave amplitude also decreased and the P–Q interval increased or decreased. Changes in ST segment and T wave were observed in 17 out of 35 cases of late decelerations, but no definite relationship was found between the onset of those changes and the biochemical state of the fetus determined by scalp blood sampling. It was noted that 12 of the 17 babies had an Apgar score of less than 7 at one minute and 13 had an umbilical artery blood pH less than 7.20. However, there was no significant difference of these values and those of cases with late decelerations without FECG changes. The authors clearly demonstrated the value of averaging a small number of FECG complexes and presented waveforms as the easily defined components. Using this method, transient changes of FECG morphology could be detected. Nevertheless, the method was still restricted to sampling short segments of the FECG and could not provide continuous evaluation.

Hioki (1975) also used a group averaging method. In his study, fetal distress was diagnosed purely on the grounds of FHR patterns. In cases where fetal distress was thought to be present, P wave amplitude was reduced during periods of bradycardia and increased in periods of tachycardia. In these cases, Hioki also found depressed ST segments, reduced R/S amplitude ratio, reduced ventricular activation time, reduced T wave duration, shortened corrected Q–T interval and shortened P–Q interval. It can be seen that these results are at variance with each of the previous authors for one component, but in agreement with the same author for another. The principal problem with the paper of Hioki is that the reliability of FHR patterns alone in the diagnosis of fetal hypoxia is limited, and there may not have been fetal asphyxia in every case of abnormal FHR pattern.

Several authors have used direct FECG recordings to diagnose fetal cardiac arrhythmias. Abinader *et al.* (1976) presented three cases of atrial premature beats, ventricular premature beats, and conduction defect respectively. In each case, the diagnosis of the arrhythmias made the interpretation of FHR patterns possible. Schneider *et al.* (1977) presented a case of trigeminal rhythm. They thought that the appearance of a fetal arrhythmia without evidence of fetal hypoxia did not constitute an indication for therapy, and should be managed expectantly. Young *et al.* (1979) were of the same view. They presented 15 cases where the outcome was normal and in 9 of these cases, when the acid–base status was measured, there was no indication for drug treatment of arrhythmias *in utero* and were not convinced that previous claims to the contrary had been proven to be advantageous.

Marvell *et al.* (1980) described the use of a real-time computer system which continuously monitored the FECG during labour. Data was presented from 37 cases which were defined as normal by strict clinical and biochemical criteria. When an assessment of FECG complex shape was made, it was found that variations in waveform shape occurred quite commonly. Some of these changes, for example notching of waveform components, had been reported by previous workers as characteristic of fetal distress. The major advance presented by the authors was the continuous measurement of time intervals of the FECG throughout labour. When the short-term and long-term behaviour of these intervals was analysed, it was found that the P–R interval was up to 10 per cent shorter during contractions towards the end of labour and there was a long-term trend for the P–R interval to fall by 7 per cent. The P wave amplitude fell by 30 per cent over the last hour. These trends were statistically significant. The QRS complex was found to lengthen slightly towards the end of labour, but the R–T interval and ST segment displacement displayed no significant changes.

Averaging techniques were also applied to the abdominal FECG by Brambati & Pardi (1980). Patients were placed in a completely shielded room to avoid external electrical interferences, and five electrodes were placed on the maternal abdomen. It is not clear whether the processing system was of the hard-wired type or whether a software method was used, but the detection of a maternal R wave triggered the suppression of the relevant maternal QRS complex. Thereafter, 50 FECG complexes were averaged. The system did not display P and T waves clearly, but the QRS complexes were well defined. The duration of these complexes was measured in 421 pregnancies between 17 and 41 weeks gestation. A close relationship was found between QRS duration and maturity of the fetus, ranging from a mean of 28.7 ms at 17 weeks to a mean of 53.0 ms at 41 weeks. There was also a highly significant relationship between the QRS duration and weight at birth; it was suggested that this measurement could be used as a method of predicting birth weight.

Brambati & Pardi (1981) also used their system in the study of 88 pregnancies complicated by Rhesus isoimmunization. A clear correlation between QRS duration and infant haemoglobin levels at birth was observed; the lower the haemoglobin value, the longer the duration of the QRS complex. Following an intrauterine transfusion, the QRS duration decreased. The authors suggested that QRS duration increased because hypertrophy of the fetal cardiac muscle had taken place as a result of chronic anaemia. It was also noted that notching of the QRS complex occurred in 30 per cent of all cases, and in 50 per cent of cases where intrauterine death occurred. The authors concluded that notching of the QRS complex indicated a grave prognosis and suggested that myocardial infarctions may have been the cause.

## Fetal electrocardiogram studies in experimental animals

Despite the reduction of interest in the human FECG, there has been an increasing number of publications concerned with the animal FECG. With improved techniques, later work has demonstrated changes in the animal FECG with experimental hypoxia. As in the human, however, initial work was confined to the problems of recording. Jackson *et al.*

(1960) demonstrated good quality recordings obtained from fetal rabbits, using direct leads which were attached to the fetal limbs by inserting electrodes through the uterine wall, without performing a hysterotomy. Previous workers had exteriorized the fetus and had admitted that this may have significantly altered fetal–maternal relationships and that some fetal hypoxia may have resulted. Jackson *et al.* were able to demonstrate all components of the waveform without resorting to enhancement methods. Some changes to the ST segment and T waves were seen when the uterus was excessively manipulated. When the uterine arteries and veins were clamped, bradycardia and T wave flattening occurred; on release there was tachycardia and elevation of T waves.

Gelli & Gyulai (1969) also made direct recordings, from fetal rabbits, but these had been delivered prematurely by laparotomy. Limb leads were attached and lead I configuration recorded, and the fetuses were divided into two groups: those whose mothers had had a glucose infusion prior to delivery and those whose mothers had not. In both groups, increasing anoxia initially increased the conduction times of P–Q and Q–T, and also ST segment depression and T wave inversion occurred. The onset of these changes was significantly later in the glucose infused group than the controls and the authors demonstrated that the former group had a higher glycogen content in the fetal heart muscle.

In 1972, Myers published a comprehensive study on perinatal brain damage in monkeys under conditions of sudden total asphyxia and serial episodes of partial asphyxia. In the partial asphyxia group the patterns of damage were similar to those seen in humans, but those of total asphyxia were not. Type II dips in fetal heart rate were found in the presence of partial asphyxia, but Myers found that changes in the configuration of the FECG were variable and depended partly on the degree of asphyxia and partly on lead placement. When such changes did occur, however, they usually consisted of ST segment elevation and T wave inversion. Because of the inconsistency of these changes, Myers questioned the validity of depending upon FECG configuration for monitoring purposes, and thought that only those changes taking place during the continuous monitoring of a single fetus, through the same lead placement, would provide a firm basis for the diagnosis of fetal asphyxia.

Yeh *et al.* (1975) studied the effect of cord occlusion on baboon fetuses. In all cases, sinus bradycardia occurred after occlusion, the P–R interval lengthened first, and then second degree heart block developed. When atropine was given, the fetal bardycardia still occurred, but no heart block developed. The authors made no comments on the configuration of the FECG during occlusion, but the tracings presented clearly show ST segment elevation with marked increase in T wave height.

Since 1975 a Swedish group, based in Göteborg, has published a series of papers documenting their findings when hypoxia was induced in animal fetuses. In the first paper (Rosen & Kjellmer 1975), hypoxia was induced in the mother to render the fetus hypoxic, rather than by doing so by cord occlusion. In some cases the vagal nerves of the fetus were divided. There was no evidence of any vagal component in fetal hypoxic bradycardia, and the authors concluded that bradycardia was therefore a sign of myocardial hypoxia and failing fetal circulation. When the FECG waveform was examined, it was noted that elevation of the ST segment with increased T wave amplitude was a constant finding during hypoxia. When there was only a moderate degree of hypoxia, no bradycardia occurred in spite of marked changes in the ST segment; with a further degree of hypoxia, the ST segment changes occurred earlier than the onset of fetal bradycardia. Further examination of the FECG confirmed the findings of Yeh *et al.* that the bradycardia was due to second degree atrioventricular (AV) block.

When the changes in the FECG were compared with glycogen levels in the various fetal organs (Rosen & Isaksson 1976), there was found to be a strong linear correlation between an ECG scoring system, which took ST segment and T wave (ST–T) changes into account, and the depletion of cardiac glycogen and creatine phospate. Adenosine triphosphate (ATP) levels in the fetal heart remained constant until glycogen levels were severely depleted, and then AV block occurred. The authors considered that this demonstrated the dependency of fetal myocardial metabolism, during hypoxia, on the anaerobic utilization of glycogen. Because the depletion of glycogen was well correlated to the severity of ST–T changes, it was postulated that these changes closely reflected myocardial glycolysis, and could be regarded as the earliest sign of fetal hypoxic stress.

To improve quantification of T wave changes, Rosen *et al.* (1976a) introduced the concept of comparing the height of the T wave with another component of the waveform. In this paper the ratio of the T and S wave amplitude was measured in lamb fetuses, since it was found that S wave amplitude was not affected by hypoxia; changes in the T/S ratio thus reflected changes in T wave amplitude. When changes in the T/S ratio were compared to somatosensory-evoked electroencephalogram responses (SER), there was found to be a good correlation between deterioration of the electrical performance of the brain and an increasing T/S ratio. Deterioration in SER also correlated with the ECG scoring system previously described by Rosen & Isaksson (1976). A strong correlation was obtained between T/S ratio and fetal pH and lactate levels. The authors therefore concluded that ST–T changes not only reflected anaerobic glycolysis in the fetal heart, but also similar metabolic events in the fetal brain.

Although the terminal phases of hypoxia in the experiments with lamb fetuses had been associated with a failing circulation, it was important to determine whether the ECG changes were associated with haemodynamic alterations compatible with an efficient circulation or compatible with a failing circulation. Rosen *et al.* (1976b) correlated ECG changes with cardiovascular function measured by heart rate, mean arterial pressure, end-diastolic pressure, and combined cardiac output. It was found that alterations in the ECG pattern consistently preceded signs of failing cardiovascular function and this was thought to confirm that ECG changes reflected myocardial metabolism rather than performance. Almost as a postscript in this paper the authors noted that small doses of the beta-receptor stimulating agent, isoprenaline, initiated the typical pattern of changes already noted in the FECG during hypoxia, but this was not fully documented until a later paper (Hokegard *et al.* 1979). Again, acutely exteriorized lamb fetuses were used and it was confirmed that small doses of isoprenaline given during normoxia could elicit the FECG changes previously recorded during hypoxia; the dose required appeared to be equivalent to the levels of catecholamines secreted naturally during hypoxia. When small doses of a beta-adrenoceptor blocking agent (propranolol) were given it was found that the FECG changes were abolished when caused by isoprenaline or mild hypoxia, but in more severe hypoxia, beta-blockade had no influence on the ECG changes. These findings raised the question as to whether the increase in T wave amplitude in hypoxia was induced by the augmentation of myocardial glycogenolysis, or by a direct effect of catecholamines on the function of the myocardial cell membrane. The authors argued in favour of the former hypothesis and concluded that mild hypoxia initiated the ECG changes via an activation of beta-adrenoceptors whilst severe hypoxia induced ECG changes through a direct effect.

A change in the quantification of T wave height was made by the Swedish group in 1978 (Hokegard *et al.* 1978), when it was compared with the overall height of the QRS complex, rather than S wave height alone as previously. In this paper, the ECG waveforms of (human) babies were studied using the T/QRS ratio and the previously described ECG scoring system; the infants were divided into three groups based on (i) normal, (ii) moderately abnormal, and (iii) severely abnormal cardiotocograms recorded during labour. Babies in the abnormal groups had lower 1-min Apgar scores and significantly elevated T/QRS ratios, and babies with the lowest Apgar scores had more severe changes in the ST–T waveform as measured by the scoring system.

The work of Rosen, Hokegard and their colleagues has been characterized by the use of the acutely exteriorized fetal lamb preparation with recordings made from bipolar (usually precordial) leads. In the human, of course, it is not possible to apply precordial leads to the fetus, other than by a transabdominal amniocentesis, and in current clinical practice the FECG is obtained by the use of a unipolar lead attached to the presenting part (usually the scalp). Hokegard & Rosen (1980) investigated the use of a unipolar scalp electrode in the acutely exteriorized fetal lamb. It was found that the unipolar scalp lead gave an ECG waveform with an unstable baseline, smaller QRS complexes, and generally of inferior technical quality. When the scoring system was applied, there was not a good correlaton of ECG changes with fetal hypoxia and acidosis, but T/QRS ratios were better correlated, particularly when the fetuses were both hypoxic and acidotic. Overall, it was concluded that the unipolar scalp electrode gave less information which was more difficult to interpret, and that this might explain the controversy over the value of the FECG in the detection of fetal hypoxia during labour in the human. The authors suggested that a bipolar scalp lead might have been an improvement, but did not test this idea.

The question as to whether the method of acutely exteriorizing the fetal lambs may have affected the results of the Swedish group was examined by Greene *et al.* (1982). Since the animals were also anaesthetized, factors may have been introduced other than hypoxaemia. Greene *et al.* therefore examined chronically instrumented fetal lambs which were maintained *in utero*, no experiment being carried out before the fifth postoperative day. The ST waveform was enhanced by computer based averaging system which was triggered by the R or S wave of the ECG. The data obtained complemented the experiments on the acutely exteriorized fetal lambs and confirmed the elevation of the ST segment and an increase in T/QRS ratio when hypoxia was induced; these changes reverted to normal when normoxia was restored. The changes in the ECG waveform were accompanied by an increase in plasma lactate levels and a fall in pH during hypoxia, again reverting to normal when normoxia was restored. The authors felt that these findings confirmed the ECG changes occurred when the fetal myocardium switched to anaerobic metabolism and suggested that ECG changes in the human fetus might discriminate various changes in fetal heart rate.

## Continuous intrapartum fetal electrocardiography

In summary, it may be stated that, until recently, the conventional view of the FECG was that observation of the waveform was of little value for the assessment of the fetus in labour. The reasons for this are clear. In early work, there was too much subjective interpretation of waveforms which, however, may have been of insufficient quality to be useful. It was also felt by Hon, whose views were highly regarded for he was virtually the founder of modern clinical fetal monitoring, that fetal heart rate changes always preceded any changes which may occur in the FECG waveform. Later work on the FECG, using computer techniques, overcame the technical difficulties experienced by earlier workers. Unfortunately, the findings were contradictory. Part of the reason lay in the different methods of assessment of the fetus at birth, and in some cases the reliance on FHR patterns for definition of fetal condition. There was also insufficient attention paid to any distortion in the waveform introduced during computer processing, and in most studies only short segments of waveform were investigated.

Current practice, therefore, has been to use the FECG signal purely as a trigger for FHR monitoring. Although the data of the FECG waveform is passing down the lead from the fetal electrode, this has been studiously ignored. Nevertheless, there has been a slowly growing number of publications concerning changes in the FECG waveform in animal fetuses when subjected to experimental asphyxia. In later reports, there is evi-

**Table 10.1** Electrical noise sources affecting FECG

| | |
|---|---|
| 1 | Fetal electroencephalogram |
| 2 | Fetal electromyogram |
| 3 | Maternal electrocardiogram |
| 4 | Maternal electromyogram (striated) |
| 5 | Maternal electromyogram (smooth) |
| 6 | Interface noise of fetal electrode in skin |
| 7 | Mains interference |
| 8 | Miscellaneous interference |

dence that these changes are consistent and reproducible, and many precede any changes in fetal heart rate. If such changes could be demonstrated in the human fetus, active monitoring of the FECG in labour would be an important adjunct to FHR monitoring, and would have the potential for overcoming the present difficulties and uncertainties when monitoring by FHR alone.

The problem of clear definition of the morphology of the human FECG is that the signal-to-noise ratio of the waveform is poor. The FECG signal is immersed in a sea of extraneous electrical noise which arises from many sources (Table 10.1). The electrical noise considerably distorts the waveform as a whole, and may completely submerge smaller components such as P wave and T wave. Even in a high quality FECG tracing, when all of the waveform components are visible in one complex, these smaller components may be lost in the immediate succeeding complex (Figure 10.1). Whilst improvements in biological signal amplifiers made many of the earlier studies possible, no research group previously had been able to devise a method of continuously enhancing the FECG signal from noise to permit analysis of the human FECG waveform for a prolonged period of time.

The development of a digital computer-based system for monitoring the FECG in labour has been proceeding for some time at the University of Nottingham. The purpose of the work has been to develop a system with the capability for continuous real-time analysis of the FECG throughout the whole labour. In order to achieve this goal, solutions to several

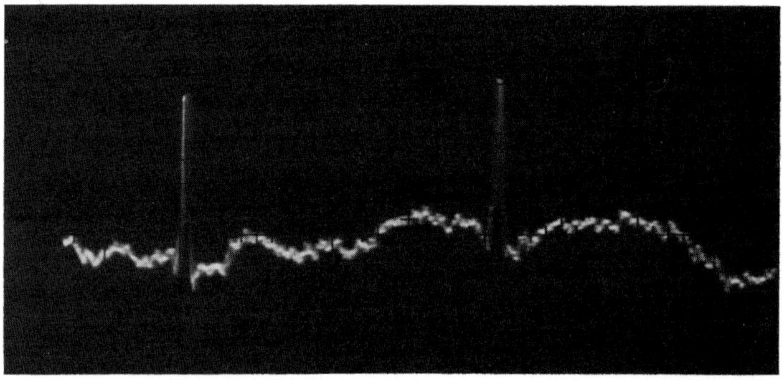

**Fig. 10.1** Unprocessed FECG signal.

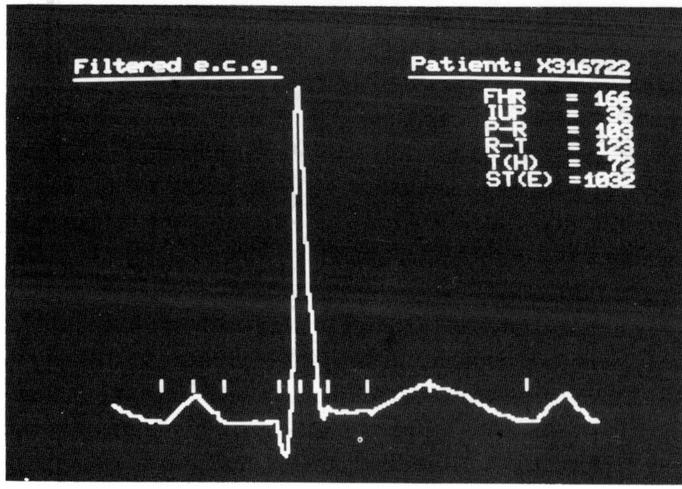


**Fig. 10.2** Computer-enhanced FECG waveform from a baby born in normal conditions. (From Jenkins *et al.* 1986, by permission.)

fundamental problems in FECG processing were required. Firstly, the hardware and software components required rigorous design and careful frequency control to ensure that no waveform distortion occurred due to the signal processing. Secondly, a method of signal enhancement was required which could operate continuously and not be limited to short segments of signal. Finally, since the computer system generated large amounts of data, a method of data reduction was required which could display clinically interpretable patterns.

A method of signal enhancement using a moving window averaging process was implemented as a software digital filter (Sheild & Kirk 1981) and subsequently refined (Kirk & Smith 1986). The FECG waveform produced was of sufficient quality (Figure 10.2) to allow measurements to be made of time constants and shape every 15 s during the course of a whole labour (Jenkins 1982). Unfortunately, this generated a very large amount of data since, on average, there are 72 000 FECG complexes in an eight hour labour. Methods of data reduction using graphical display were developed. Marvell *et al.* in 1980 described a method of producing labour profiles which portrayed long and short-term variations of each waveform component (Figure 10.3), but these were not found appropriate for clinical use and so a method of computer-generated graphics was adopted.

Initial clinical studies with the computer system were carried out by recording and processing the FECG waveform continuously during 66 labours (Jenkins 1984). The trends in behaviour of the components of the FECG were examined in the short term and in the long term. Short-term changes were found to be few; the only component which consistently showed such changes was the P–R interval. When the long-term changes were examined it was found that an increase in P wave amplitude occurred in fetal acidosis, and that a P–R interval of 92 ms or less was

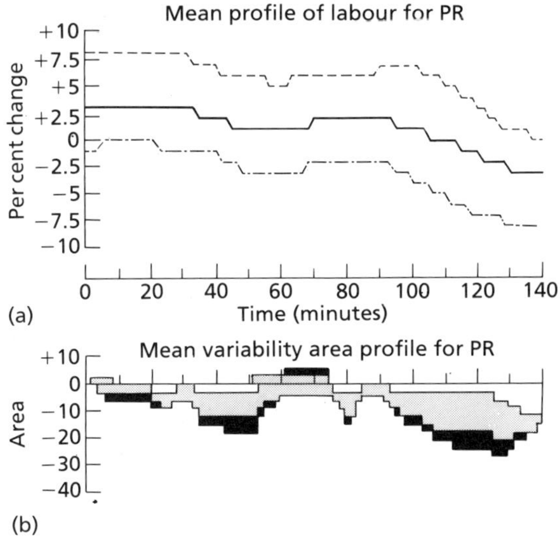


**Fig. 10.3** Averaged profiles of labour for P–R interval in 37 patients with normal outcome. The charts represent the last 140 min of labour. (a) The long-term changes in P–R interval from averaged values earlier in labour ± 1SD. (b) Short-term changes occurring between contractions (▭, Type 0), during contractions (▨, Type 1), or up to 90 s after contractions (■, Type 2). (From Marvell *et al.* 1980, by permission.)

associated with a low Apgar score. The principal finding, however, was a highly significant correlation between both a long-term increase in ST segment elevation and T wave height and fetal acidosis.

The behaviour of these waveform components in 14 fetuses with normal outcomes were compared with ten cases where the babies were acidotic at birth (Jenkins *et al.* 1986). The total duration of FECG analysis made in these cases was 124 hours and 50 minutes. The patients were

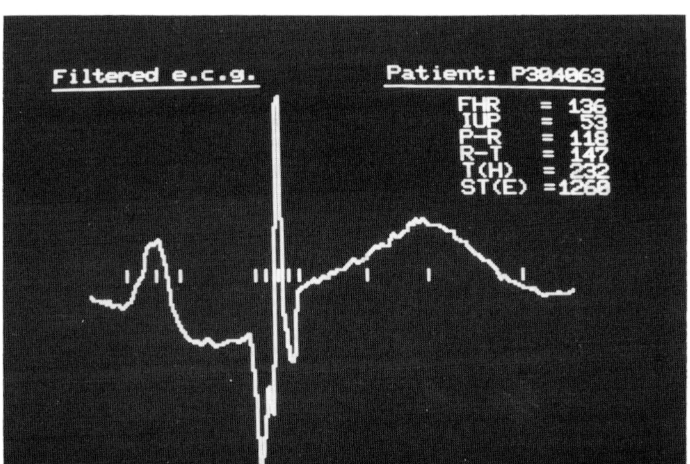


**Fig. 10.4** Computer-enhanced FECG waveform from a baby born in an acidotic condition. (From Jenkins *et al.* 1986, by permission.)

divided into two groups according to the outcome of labour assessed by clinical neonatal condition (Apgar score) and biochemical condition (cord blood pH and gas values). Of these, it was considered that the cord artery pH values would give the best objective assessment of hypoxia in labour. The infants with normal outcome were placed in Group 1; in each of these, the cord artery pH was 7.25 or greater and the 1-min Apgar score was 8 or better. In the acidotic group (Group 2), the cord artery pH was less than 7.20 and the Apgar score was less than 7 in six of the ten babies. The normal shape of the FECG waveform (Figure 10.2) was confirmed as being similar to standard lead II. The principle features were found to be a small P wave, a small Q wave, a large R wave, a variably sized S wave, an essentially isoelectric ST segment, and a small or absent T wave. In contrast, an example of a waveform from a fetus in the acidotic group is

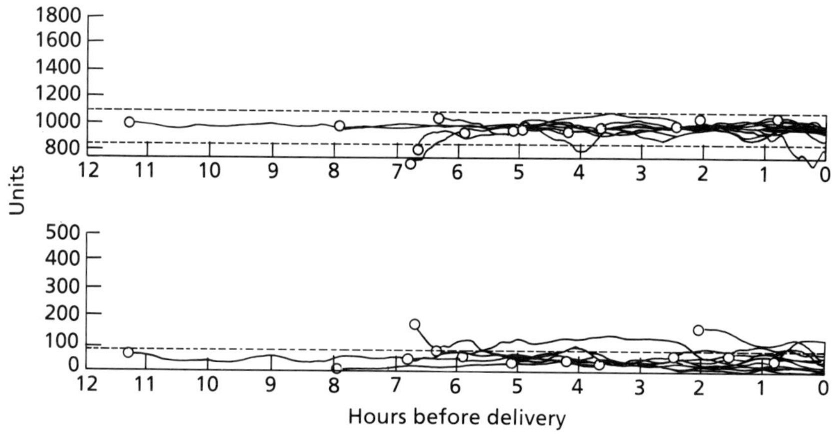


**Fig. 10.5** (a) Long-term trends (profile of means) of ST segment elevation; and (b) T wave height for all patients in Group 1: normal babies. (From Jenkins *et al.* 1986, with permission.)

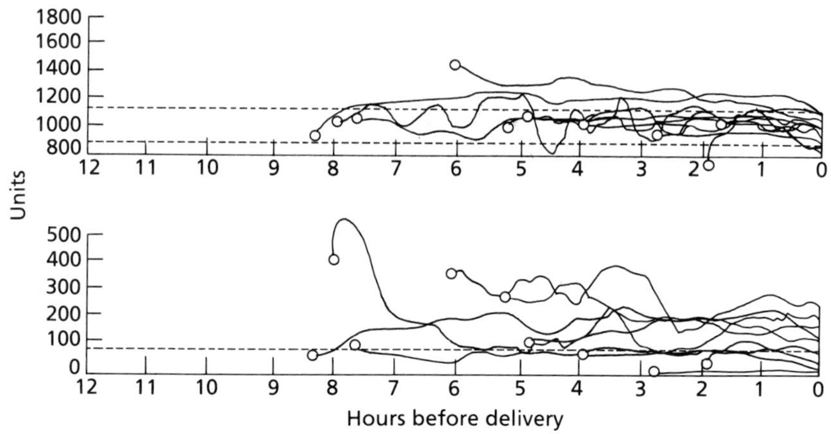


**Fig. 10.6** (a) Long-term trends (profile of means) of ST segment elevation; and (b) T wave height for all patients in Group 2: acidotic babies. (From Jenkins *et al.* 1986, with permission.)

shown in Figure 10.4; in this case there was a large Q wave, an elevated ST segment, and a large T wave. The trends in behaviour of these components were plotted graphically in both groups (Figures 10.5 and 10.6). When the ST segment was considered, there was little variation about the isoelectric line in the normal group. In the acidotic group, the ST segment was elevated above the defined normal range for periods greater than 30 min in all except two, and the elevation was more marked in those with a low Apgar score. When T wave height was considered, only two patients in the normal group consistently exceeded the normal range, and ST segment elevation was normal in both of them. In the acidotic group, eight of the ten exceeded the normal range of T wave height. In one of the remaining two, the ST segment was elevated; in only one was there no deviation from the normal range in either ST segment elevation or T wave height.

## The conduction index

The most recent studies in Nottingham have been devoted to expanding the number of cases monitored and also exploring the P–R interval. As noted previously, many earlier workers had shown changes in the configuration of the P wave and alterations in the P–R interval. The ability to observe the latter component continuously has added a new dimension to the interpretation of these changes, both in assessing actual alterations and in correlating them with other variables. The relationship between the P–R interval and umbilical vein adrenaline levels has now been found to have a highly significant negative correlation in the human fetus; the shorter the P–R interval, the higher the adrenaline concentration (Symonds 1987). Moreover, Murray (1986) has observed a positive correlation between P–R and R–R intervals (a negative correlation between P–R and FHR). This correlation was highly significant in the healthy fetus (pH greater than 7.24 at delivery). The close relationship between P–R interval and R–R interval appeared to alter as the fetal pH and base excess began to fall. A negative correlation, where the R–R interval was seen to increase despite the shortened P–R interval, indicated umbilical artery pH values of 7.17 to 7.29, and these values were found to be statistically significantly different from fetuses with positively correlated P–R to R–R intervals.

The P–R interval is a measure of atrioventricular conduction time and in view of the correlations outlined above it was felt appropriate to use the term conduction index to describe the correlation that exists between the P–R interval and fetal heart rate (which is normally negative). Further work with the conduction index has shown that fetuses showing ST segment changes occurring in the presence of a positive index (P–R positively correlated with FHR) were more severely acidotic than those fetuses with a positive conduction index alone, and the longer the duration of the ST segment changes, the more severe the acidosis (Figure 10.7).

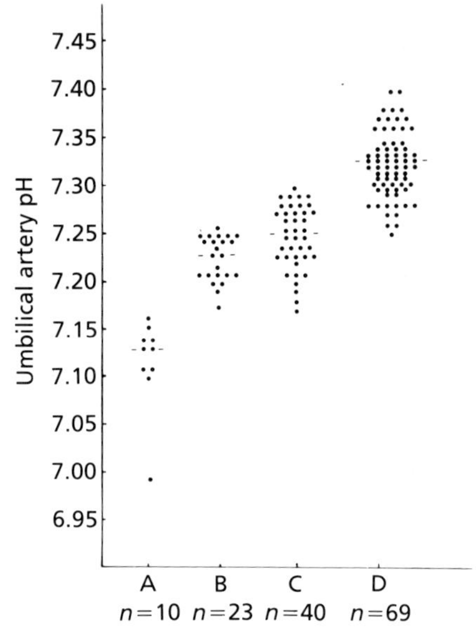


**Fig. 10.7** Changes within the FECG complex correlated against umbilical artery pH at delivery. Population A includes all cases with a positive conduction index associated with a change in ST segment level of >5 per cent of R wave height persisting for longer than 5 min. Population B includes those cases with a positive conduction index associated with a similar change in ST segment, but persisting less than 5 min. Population C includes those cases with a positive conduction index only. Population D includes cases with a normal, negative, conduction index. The difference between the pH values for each group is highly significant: $\chi^2 = 100.8$, $P < 0.001$. (Based on Murray 1986, with permission.)

## Conclusions

It is very difficult to derive consistently a fetal electrocardiogram with sufficient clarity to enable the performance of detailed clinical studies. Unfortunately, many conflicting results were obtained by early workers who perhaps based their conclusions on waveforms of a sufficient quality. In the end, the subject fell into disrepute, particularly with respect to the monitoring of fetal condition during labour. In any event, the use of the FECG complex to provide a trigger for FHR measurements was technically much more straightforward and FHR recording seemed clinically more useful.

The conventional view of the fetal electrocardiogram became that the observation of the waveform was of little value for the assessment of fetal condition during labour. This view has meant that information concerning the waveform, available from all fetal electrodes, is studiously ignored. However, modern observations of FECG morphology and time intervals (Murray 1986) and a comprehensive review of the subject (Greene 1987) have both shown that detailed studies of the FECG waveform have certainly improved our understanding of fetal physiology in labour, and that it may no longer be appropriate to ignore the FECG. The only problem that remains, from the conceptual point of view (but not of course from the technological point of view), is whether it would be worthwhile clinically to perform fetal electrocardiography routinely in labour.

It is certainly very satisfactory that the consistent strands throughout all studies over the years — P–R interval changes, with or without an association with FHR changes, and ST segment changes — now seem to be near clear definition. The conduction index seems to offer a sensitive discriminator for differentiating between FHR changes due to fetal asphyxia and those arising from other factors, and thus permit a more accurate diagnosis of fetal condition during labour. When combined with persistent changes in ST segment, the prediction of a significantly low fetal pH seems possible. These findings indicate that intrapartum fetal electrocardiography may have great promise for the future. Clearly, however, there are many technical problems to be overcome before machines are routinely available at the bedside, and, more importantly, the clinical basis of the subject needs to be defined in even more detail. Whilst there is no doubt that there is a need for much greater precision in the diagnosis of fetal acidosis in the modern labour ward, the last thing that is needed at the present time is a premature introduction of machines whose observations are poorly understood, as happened with cardiotocography. Notwithstanding any of this, the evidence is that fetal electrocardiography has come of age, and that its potential for overcoming many of our current difficulties in intrapartum fetal monitoring should no longer be ignored.

## References

Abinader E.G., Klein A., Eibschitz, B., Zilberman A., Pezeshk B. & Sharf M. (1976) The significance of fetal electrocardiography in the diagnosis of intrauterine bradycardia. *American Journal of Obstetrics and Gynecology*, **126**, 266–70.

Brambati B. & Pardi G. (1980) The intraventricular conduction time of fetal heart in uncomplicated pregnancies. *British Journal of Obstetrics and Gynaecology*, **87**, 941–8.

Brambati B. & Pardi G. (1981) The intraventricular conduction time of fetal heart in pregnancy complicated by rhesus haemolytic disease. *British Journal of Obstetrics and Gynaecology*, **88**, 1233–40.

Caughey A.F. & Krohn L.H. (1963) Variation in the fetal electrocardiogram with period of gestation. *American Journal of Obstetrics and Gynecology*, **87**, 525–8.

Caughey A.F. & Krohn L.H. (1964) Reply to 'variations in fetal electrocardiogram' (letter). *American Journal of Obstetrics and Gynecology*, **88**, 983.

Cremer M. (1906) Ueber die direkte Ableitung der Aktionsstrome des menschlichen Herzens vom Oesophagus und uber das Electrokardiogram des fotus. *Muenchener Medizinische Wochenschrift*, **53**, 811–13.

Davidsen P.C.B. (1971) The significance of the foetal electrocardiogram during labour with detailed report of one case. *Acta Obstetricia et Gynecologica Scandinavica*, **50**, 45–9.

Enhorning G. & Westin B. (1954) Experimental studies of the human fetus in prolonged asphyxia. *Acta Physiologica Scandinavica*, **31**, 359–75.

Gelli M.G. & Gyulai F. (1969) Effect of glucose infusion in the mother before delivery on the ECG of rabbit foetuses under anoxia. *Acta Obstetricia et Gynecologica Scandinavica*, **48**, 56–63.

Greene K.R. (1987) The ECG waveform. In *Clinical Obstetrics and Gynaecology, Vol. 1, No. 1: Fetal Monitoring* (Ed. by M.J. Whittle), pp. 131–55. Baillière, Tindall, London.

Greene K.R., Dawes G.S., Lilja H. & Rosen K.G. (1982) Changes in the ST waveform of the fetal lamb electrocardiogram with hypoxia. *American Journal of Obstetrics and*

*Gynecology*, **144**, 950–8.

Hioki T. (1975) Averaged fetal electrocardiogram obtained by direct lead in fetal distress diagnosed by fetal heart rate pattern. *Acta Obstetricia et Gynecologica Japonica*, **22**, 162–74.

Hokegard K.H., Karlsson K., Kjellmer I. & Rosen K.G. (1979) ECG changes in the fetal lamb during asphyxia in relation to beta-adrenoceptor stimulation and blockade. *Acta Physiologica Scandinavica*, **105**, 195–203.

Hokegard K.H., Karlsson K., Lilja H. & Rosen K.G. (1978) Neonatal electrocardiographic changes in relation to cardiotocographic changes. *British Journal of Obstetrics and Gynaecology*, **85**, 165–70.

Hokegard K.H. & Rosen K.G. (1980) Alterations in the electrocardiogram of the fetal lamb as a sign of fetal asphyxia. A comparison between the scalp lead and the precordial lead. *Acta Obstetricia et Gynecologica Scandinavica*, **59**, 411–15.

Hon E.H. (1963) Instrumentation of fetal heart rate and fetal electrocardiography. II. A vaginal electrode. *American Journal of Obstetrics and Gynecology*, **86**, 772–84.

Hon E.H. (1967) Instrumentation of fetal heart rate and fetal electrocardiography. III. Fetal ECG electrodes; further observations. *Obstetrics and Gynecology*, **30**, 281–6.

Hon E.H. & Hess O.W. (1957) Instrumentation of fetal electrocardiography. *Science*, **125**, 553–4.

Hon E.H. & Hess O.W. (1960) The clinical value of fetal electrocardiography. *American Journal of Obstetrics and Gynecology*, **79**, 1012–23.

Hon E.H. & Lee S.T. (1963a) The fetal electrocardiogram. I. The electrocardiogram of the dying fetus. *American Journal of Obstetrics and Gynecology*, **87**, 804–13.

Hon E.H. & Lee S.T. (1963b) Noise reduction in fetal electrocardiography. II. Averaging techniques. *American Journal of Obstetrics and Gynecology*, **87**, 1086–96.

Hon E.H. & Lee S.T. (1964) The fetal electrocardiogram. II. Measuring technics. *Obstetrics and Gynecology*, **24**, 6–11.

Hon E.H. & Lee S.T. (1965) The fetal electrocardiogram. III. Display techniques. *American Journal of Obstetrics and Gynecology*, **91**, 56–60.

Hunter C.A., Lansford K.G., Knoebel S.B. & Braunline R.J. (1960) A technic for recording fetal ECG during labor and delivery. *Obstetrics and Gynecology*, **16**, 567–70.

Jackson B.T., Clarke J.P. & Egdahl R.H. (1960) Direct lead fetal electrocardiography with undisturbed fetal–maternal relationships. *Surgery, Gynecology and Obstetrics*, **110**, 687–92.

Jenkins H.M.L. (1982) Continuous intrapartum fetal electrocardiography using a real-time computer. *Lecture Notes in Medical Informatics*, **16**, 136–42.

Jenkins H.M.L. (1984) *A study of the intrapartum fetal electrocardiogram using a real-time computer*. DM thesis, University of Nottingham.

Jenkins H.M.L., Symonds E.M., Kirk D.L. & Smith P.R. (1986) Can fetal electrocardiography improve the prediction of intrapartum fetal acidosis? *British Journal of Obstetrics and Gynaecology*, **93**, 6–12.

Kaplan, S. & Toyama S. (1958) Fetal electrocardiography (utilising abdominal and intrauterine leads). *Obstetrics and Gynecology*, **11**, 391–7.

Kirk D.L. & Smith P.R. (1986) Techniques for the routine on-line processing of the fetal electrocardiogram. *Journal of Perinatal Medicine*, **14**, 391–7.

Larks S.D. (1963) The abnormal fetal electrocardiogram: intrauterine fetal difficulty and fetal distress. *Obstetrics and Gynecology*, **22**, 427–32.

Larks S.D. (1964) Resemblance of the fetal ECG complex to the standard lead II QRS of the newborn. *Obstetrics and Gynecology*, **24**, 1–5.

Larks S.D. (1965) Estimation of the electrical axis of the fetal heart. *American Journal of Obstetrics and Gynecology*, **91**, 46–55.

Larks S.D. & Anderson G.V. (1962) The abnormal fetal electrocardiogram. *American Journal of Obstetrics and Gynecology*, **84**, 1893–9.

Larks S.D. & Larks G.G. (1965) The electrical axis of the fetal heart: a new criterion for fetal well-being or distress. *American Journal of Obstetrics and Gynecology*, **93**, 975–83.

Larks S.D. & Larks G.G. (1966a) Comparative aspects of the fetal and newborn electrocardiograms. *American Journal of Obstetrics and Gynecology*, **96**, 553–5.

Larks S.D. & Larks G.G. (1966b) Components of the fetal electrocardiogram and intrauterine electrical axis: quantitative data. *Biologia Neonatorum*, **10**, 140–52.

Larks S.D. & Longo L.D. (1962) Electrocardiographic studies of the fetal heart during delivery. *Obstetrics and Gynecology*, **19**, 740–7.

Larks S.D., Webster A. & Larks G.G. (1967) Quantitative studies in fetal electrocardiography. I. Prenatal prediction of the condition of the infant at birth. *American Journal of Obstetrics and Gynecology*, **98**, 52–5.

Larks S.D., Webster A. & Larks G.G. (1968) Quantitative studies in fetal electrocardiography. II. Distribution of basic data, twin and sex differences. *American Journal of Obstetrics and Gynecology*, **100**, 1135–8.

Larks S.D., Webster A. & Larks G.G. (1969) Quantitative studies in fetal electrocardiography. III. Comparison of breech and cephalic presentation data; endocrine basis for fetal rotation, a hypothesis. *American Journal of Obstetrics and Gynecology*, **103**, 282–9.

Lee K.H. & Blackwell R. (1974) Observations on the configuration of the fetal electrocardiogram before and during labour. *Journal of Obstetrics and Gynaecology of the British Commonwealth*, **81**, 61–9.

Lee S.T. & Hon E.H. (1965) The fetal electrocardiogram. IV. Unusual variations in the QRS complex during labour. *American Journal of Obstetrics and Gynecology*, **92**, 1140–8.

Marvell C.J., Kirk D.L., Jenkins H.M.L. & Symonds E.M. (1980) The normal condition of the fetal electrocardiogram during labour. *British Journal of Obstetrics and Gynaecology*, **87**, 786–96.

Mayes B.T., Bradfield A. & Smyth E.J. (1963) Clinical experience in foetal electrocardiography. *Medical Journal of Australia*, **22**, 905–12.

Millican E., Urbach J.R., Carrington E.R. & Lambert R.L. (1966) The clinical value of fetal electrocardiography, phonocardiography, and heart rate monitoring. *American Journal of Obstetrics and Gynecology*, **96**, 565–75.

Murray H.G. (1986) The fetal electrocardiogram: current clinical developments in Nottingham. *Journal of Perinatal Medicine*, **14**, 399–404.

Myers R.E. (1972) Two patterns of perinatal brain damage and their conditions of occurrence. *American Journal of Obstetrics and Gynecology*, **112**, 246–76.

Pardi G., Tucci E., Uderzo A. & Zanini D. (1974) Fetal electrocardiogram changes in relation to fetal heart rate patterns during labour. *American Journal of Obstetrics and Gynecology*, **118**, 243–50.

Roche J.B. & Hon E.H. (1965) The fetal electrocardiogram. V. Comparison of lead systems. *American Journal of Obstetrics and Gynecology*, **92**, 1149–59.

Roemer V.M., Ruppin E. & Bartschi R. (1972) Direct foetal electrocardiography in management of high risk pregnancies. Proceedings of the International Symposium on the Treatment of Foetal Risks, Baden, Austria, pp. 28–32.

Rosen K.G., Hokegard K.H. & Kjellmer I. (1976b) A study of the relationship between the electrocardiogram and hemodynamics in the fetal lamb during asphyxia. *Acta Physiologica Scandinavica*, **98**, 275–84.

Rosen K.G., Hrbek A., Karlsson K., Kjellmer I., Olsson T. & Riha M. (1976a) Changes in the ECG and somato-sensory evoked EEG responses during intrauterine asphyxia in the sheep. *Biologia Neonatorum*, **30**, 95–101.

Rosen K.G. & Isaksson O. (1976) Alterations in fetal heart rate and ECG correlated to glycogen, creatine phosphate and ATP levels during graded hypoxia. *Biologia Neonatorum*, **30**, 17–24.

Rosen K.G. & Kjellmer I. (1975) Changes in the fetal heart rate and ECG during hypoxia. *Acta Physiologica Scandinavica*, **93**, 59–66.

Schneider H., Weinstein H.M. & Young B.K. (1977) Fetal trigeminal rhythm. *Obstetrics and Gynecology*, **50**, 58s–61s.

Sheild J.E.A. & Kirk D.L. (1981) The use of digital filters in enhancing the fetal electrocardiogram. *Journal of Biomedical Engineering*, **3**, 44–8.

Shenker L. (1966) Review: Fetal electrocardiography. *Obstetrical and Gynaecological Survey*, **21**, 367–88.

Smyth C.N. (1953) Experimental electrocardiography of the foetus. *Lancet*, **i**, 1124–6.

Southern E.M. (1957) Fetal anoxia and its possible relation to changes in the prenatal fetal electrocardiogram. *American Journal of Obstetrics and Gynecology*, **73**, 233–47.

Stander R.W., Barden T.P. & Braunlin R.J. (1963) Instrument complex for intrapartum investigation of human fetal cardiac function. *Obstetrics and Gynecology*, **22**, 265–70.

Symonds E.M. (1971) *Fetal acid–base status and fetal electrocardiography*. MD thesis, University of Adelaide.

Symonds E.M. (1972) Vectorcardiography and acid–base balance in the human fetus.

*Journal of Obstetrics and Gynaecology of the British Commonwealth*, **79**, 416–23.

Symonds E.M. (1987) On-line processing of the fetal electrocardiogram. A new direction for fetal monitoring. *Journal of Reproductive Medicine*, **32**, 509–12.

Talledo E. & Zuspan F.P. (1963) When is the fetus dead? *Journal of the American Medical Association*, **186**, 926–8.

Teteris N.J. (1964) Variation in fetal electrocardiogram (letter). *American Journal of Obstetrics and Gynecology*, **88**, 982–3.

Vasicka A., Hutchinson H.T., Rylander W.J. & Murray C. (1963) Simultaneous monitoring of uterine contractility and fetal heart rate using an intra-amniotic platinum electrode. *Obstetrics and Gynecology*, **22**, 271–7.

Whitfield C.R. (1966) A source of diagnostic error in fetal electrocardiography. *American Journal of Obstetrics and Gynecology*, **95**, 669–75.

Yeh M.-N., Morishima H.O., Niemann W.H. & James L.S. (1975) Myocardial conduction defects in association with compression of the umblical cord. *American Journal of Obstetrics and Gynecology*, **121**, 951–7.

Young B.K., Katz M. & Klein S. (1979) Intrapartum fetal cardiac arrhythmias. *Obstetrics and Gynecology*, **54**, 427–32.

# 11: Bacterial infections of the fetus and newborn

GEOFFREY L. RIDGWAY



Accurate figures on the incidence of bacterial infection, or on the influence of such infection on the fetus are not available. The importance of bacterial infection is almost certainly underestimated. Pryse-Davis & Hurley (1979) found that infection (predominantly bacterial) was the primary cause of death in 3.8 per cent of 835 fetal and neonatal necropsies. However, evidence of pneumonia as a secondary feature was found in 19.2 per cent, with mild secondary meningitis in a further 0.6 per cent. In addition, 29.1 per cent of placentas examined revealed histological evidence of chorioamnionitis; a condition increasingly suspected of a key role in fetal wastage, prematurity and low birth weight (Hillier *et al.* 1988).

The pattern of bacterial infection is continuously changing. The predominating organism associated with perinatal sepsis was the Group A haemolytic streptococcus until the late 1940s. During the next decade, certain phage types of *Staphylococcus aureus* predominated, to be replaced in the 1960s by aerobic Gram-negative rods (e.g. *Escherichia coli*). Today, the predominating organisms are the aerobic Gram-negative rods, and the Group B haemolytic streptococcus. Already one can detect change from this general picture, with the emergence of multiply-resistant aerobic Gram-negative rods (e.g. *Enterobacter* spp.). A further factor to be considered is the problem of separating colonization with bacteria, which may have little consequence to the newborn from infection. The routine sampling of various sites from the newborn will certainly give a picture of the organisms colonizing the baby, but whether the results will provide useful information on imminent infection is another matter (Fox *et al.* 1988). The detection of environmental marker organisms (e.g. *Pseudomonas aeruginosa*) may play a useful role in monitoring the stand-

**Table 11.1** Periods of infection risk

| |
|---|
| Maternal antenatal infection |
| Intrapartum — from cervix and vagina |
| Intrapartum — secondary to procedures |
| Perinatal and postnatal hygiene |

ard of hygiene in the nurseries and neonatal unit, but results should not be confused with attempts to diagnose *infection* in an individual baby.

The time of onset of bacterial infections of the fetus and newborn can be broadly divided into four periods (Table 11.1). The literature on fetal and neonatal infection is extensive, and fragmented. It is not possible to comprehensively review all aspects, and this discussion is primarily restricted to a personal view of the importance of infections during the antenatal and intrapartum periods. Infections secondary to therapeutic procedures and those acquired postnatally will generally be with nosocomial organisms, and reflect failures or lapses in aseptic technique. Such infections are all too common, and yet are almost completely preventable. The importance of these infections must not be underestimated.

## Antenatal infection

Table 11.2 lists the important infections to be considered under this heading. They underline the fact that at this time the mother and fetus should be considered as a single unit. Any infection acquired by the mother will potentially have an effect on the fetus.

### Maternal systemic infection

In the developed world, florid maternal septicaemias with aerobic Gram-negative organisms are rare. Acute bacterial infections are usually

**Table 11.2** Bacterial infections of the fetus and newborn

| |
|---|
| *Antenatal infection* |
| Systemic |
| Urinary tract |
| Syphilis |
| Listeriosis |
| |
| *Antenatal or intrapartum infection* |
| Mycoplasmal |
| |
| *Intrapartum* |
| Group B streptococcal |
|   Chlamydial |
|   Gonococcal |
| Other |
|   Staphylococcal |
|   Coliform |
|   *Gardnerella vaginalis* |

promptly recognized, and specific antibacterial treatment given early. Infection resolves without adverse effect on the fetus. Chorioamnionitis as a secondary infection may result in some abortions, but the incidence is unknown. In general, involvement of the fetus is via ascending infection from the lower genital tract of the mother. Specific infections such as *Brucella abortus, Campylobacter fetus,* and *Salmonella typhi* may reach the fetus by the transplacental route. In contrast, cholera leads to maternal prostration, with consequent fetal loss or premature delivery. *Brucella abortus* although well known to cause abortion in animals, rarely causes abortion in humans. Pregnancy may increase the severity of acute infection, but it is no more likely to do this in brucellosis than in any other acute systemic infection.

## Urinary tract infection

Urinary tract infection will occur in 3–8 per cent of pregnant women (Kass & Zinner 1973); that is the same rate as for the non-pregnant woman of the same age, activity and social class. One-third of those with asymptomatic infection will ultimately develop symptoms. The possible consequences of urinary tract infection are an increase in preterm birth, intrauterine growth retardation and stillbirth. These effects are commoner in lower socioeconomic groups, and there remains some controversy as to role of socioeconomic status *per se.*

The majority of infections will be with Gram-negative aerobic organisms, and the main complication in the mother is acute pyelonephritis. Previously, this complication resulted in fetal loss in between 16 and 30 per cent of cases. The condition is now rare owing to early diagnosis and treatment. Most antenatal clinics carry out routine screening of women for asymptomatic bacteriuria, and although this practice has recently been questioned (Campbell-Brown *et al.* 1987), until further evidence is available it would seem prudent and economic to continue.

## Syphilis

In the UK, syphilis in pregnancy is now rare. The reported incidence of congenital syphilis is of the order of 8 cases per year in children under 2 years of age (Adler 1984). It is considered mandatory to screen all pregnant women for the disease at some stage of the pregnancy. Historically, this reflects attitudes to sexually transmitted diseases and individual freedom of times past. Such a requirement would be unlikely to be tolerated today, as has been well demonstrated by the controversy surrounding the routine screening of pregnant women for carriage of the human immunodeficiency virus (Report 1987).

An excellent account of congenital syphilis is to be found in King *et al.* (1980). The effect of maternal infection on the fetus will depend on the duration of the mother's infection. Recently acquired maternal infection is likely to result in death of the fetus. At the other extreme, pro-

**Table 11.3** Outcome of pregnancy in syphilis

| Stage | Fetus affected (per cent) |
|---|---|
| Primary or secondary | 100 |
| Early latent | 80 |
| Late latent | 30 |
| Treated (adequate) | 0 |

**Table 11.4** Interpretation of serological tests for syphilis

| | Reagin | TPHA | FTA-ABS |
|---|---|---|---|
| Early primary infection | − | − | +/− |
| Late primary | +/− | + or − | + |
| Secondary | ++ | + | + |
| Latent | ++ or + | + | + |
| Late latent | +/− | + | + |
| Treated | +/− or + | + | + |
| Treated yaws, etc. | + or +/− | + | + |
| Biological false positive | + | − | − |

longed maternal infection may have little or no effect on the fetus (Table 11.3).

There is no primary stage in syphilis of the newborn. The baby will be born healthy, and lesions appear over the following weeks. A wide variety of rashes is found, mainly maculo-papular. The lesions may be hypertrophic, presenting as condylomata lata and mimic condylomata acuminata. A bullous eruption (syphilitic pemphigus), with large (>3 cm) lesions may occur particularly on the palms and soles of the feet. Rhinitis, snuffles, wrinkled skin, rhagades, mucous patches and choroidoretinitis are other stigmata found early in the neonatal period. A rubbery lymphadenitis, and hepatosplenomegaly will develop. Thus the presenting features of syphilis in the newborn are essentially the manifestations of secondary syphilis as seen in the adult. Other lesions will occur after 6 months, for example osteochondritis; or be delayed for some years, such as gummata, as the disease progresses to an accelerated tertiary stage.

Antenatal screening involves the use of one or more of the tests shown in Table 11.4. There is little advantage in using a combination of the *Treponema pallidum* haemagglutination test (TPHA) and a reagin test (e.g. venereal disease reference laboratory test (VDRL) or rapid plasma reagin test (RPR)) over the TPHA alone. Further, the reagin tests are subject to biological false positive reactions, of which pregnancy is itself one. A positive test will need confirmation with the other two tests, and the examination of a further specimen of serum. It is important to request an absorbed fluorescent antibody test (FTA-ABS) if the patient is suspected of primary infection (in addition to dark ground microscopy of the lesion if appropriate), as this may be the only positive test at this stage of the disease. Examination of neonatal serum requires all tests, along with a maternal serum for comparison. The FTA-ABS IgM test is a useful adjunct in the diagnosis of congenital infection. It is important to note that these tests cannot differentiate syphilis from the non-venereal trepanematoses (e.g. yaws or pinta). The differentiation is clinical, and important, as there is no evidence for placental passage of the organisms causing yaws and pinta. Successful treatment of syphilis (preferably with intramuscular penicillin) at any stage of the pregnancy will result in an unaffected infant.

### Listeriosis

*Listeria monocytogenes* is a small Gram-positive rod morphologically resembling the diphtheroids. It has a wide growth temperature range, and is ubiquitous in its environmental distribution. The organism can be serotyped, and types 1/2a, 4a and 4b are responsible for over 90 per cent of human infections (Kerr & Lacey 1988). In the UK, type 4b is responsible for the majority of reported infections. Because these serotypes occur in both human and animal infections, it had been assumed that listeriosis was a zoonosis. However, the organism is widely distributed in soil, and is a frequent contaminant of food. It survives and multiplies at 4°C, and therefore contaminated food will not be protected at this temperature. There is also evidence that the organism survives inadequate pasteurization (Kerr & Lacey 1988). Reports of human infection were unusual before 1950, but the number of microbiologically confirmed cases has shown a marked increase in recent years, and outbreaks associated with milk, chicken, coleslaw and cheese described. Human faeces may be an important reservoir. Kampelmacher & Van Noorle Jansen (1972) reported an incidence of 12 per cent in healthy people, but 44 per cent in a cohort of pregnant women studied. Although much infection is asymptomatic, people with decreased host resistance are particularly susceptible, and this may include pregnancy. A further study by Kampelmacher *et al.* (1972) followed the pregnant women to term. All of the 60 women were delivered of normal babies. It is therefore not possible to use stool isolation to predict the outcome of pregnancy in carriers.

Perinatal listeriosis is currently estimated to affect one in 20 000 births in the UK (Spencer 1987). Relier (1979) provides a useful review of the disease in pregnancy and in the newborn. Seventy-five cases of suspected maternal listeriosis are described. Three patterns of maternal infection were seen. Twelve women (16 per cent) had a biphasic illness. The first episode (diagnosed retrospectively) was characterized by fever, headache, backache, pharyngitis, conjunctivitis and diarrhoea (essentially 'flu-like symptoms) up to three weeks before delivery. The second episode occurred 10–15 days after delivery, and was thought to reflect reinfection from the infected placenta. In 33 cases (44 per cent) the mother was febrile on or a few days before the day of delivery. The remaining 30 mothers (40 per cent) were apparently asymptomatic. The overall neonatal mortality was 22.6 per cent, but was higher (34 per cent) in those with a gestational age less than 37 weeks. No deaths occurred in babies over 36 weeks gestation, although the author comments that some of these infants were severely ill. A series of 69 affected babies reported by Poirier (1978) demonstrated the relationship between outcome of infection and gestational age (Table 11.5).

The predominant features of neonatal infection are listed in Table 11.6. It should be appreciated that infection may occur transplacentally during pregnancy, or occur during parturition. This latter infection will lead to late onset disease (from 5–7 days post-partum), characterized by meningitis. Babies infected during the pregnancy are ill at birth or within hours. Symptoms are non-specific, with respiratory problems often requiring assisted ventilation, in over 90 per cent. A papular rash occurs in some 30 per cent, but focal cutaneous granulomata are unusual. Haematological investigation is not helpful, as both leucocytosis and leucopenia may be found.

*L.monocytogenes* may be cultured from a variety of sites from the mother and fetus. Failure to isolate the organism does not exclude the infection. Routine examination of the placenta both macroscopically and, if indicated, microscopically and microbiologically is to be encouraged. The characteristic pathological feature of listeriosis is the formation of miliary granulomata with focal necrosis in tissue. These will be seen as white nodules on the cut surface of the placenta or as small abscesses on

**Table 11.5** Prognosis for fetal listeriosis

| Gestational age (weeks) | Mortality (per cent) |
|---|---|
| <28 | 100 |
| 28–30 | 90 |
| 31–35 | 41 |
| 36–37 | 14 |
| Term | 0 |

**Table 11.6** Neonatal listeriosis

| | |
|---|---|
| Respiratory distress<br>Bradycardia or apnoea<br>Cyanosis | 90% |
| Hepatosplenomegaly | 40% |
| Early onset jaundice | 50% |
| Neurological complications | 40% |
| Skin rashes | 30% |
| Conjunctivitis | 10% |

**Table 11.7** Pathology of listeriosis

| |
|---|
| *Placenta* |
| White nodules on slices |
| Abscesses on maternal surface |
| Disruption of trophoblasts and villi by cellular infiltrates |
| |
| *Fetus* |
| Miliary granulomata |
| Focal necrosis and suppuration |
| Meningo-encephalitis (mononuclear and glial cell reaction) |

the maternal surface (Table 11.7). Culture of placental samples has a high yield of the organism. Necropsy of the newborn reveals severe pulmonary and cerebral damage, with intracranial bleeding; signs in themselves consistent with prematurity. Miliary granulomata are found throughout the viscera, particularly the liver, adrenal glands and lungs. Cases with neurological involvement will show involvement not only of the meninges, but also foci of necrosis within the brain.

*L.monocytogenes* is susceptible to many antibiotics. Optimal therapy would appear to be the use of a combination of ampicillin or amoxycillin with an aminoglycoside such as gentamicin. However, prompt therapy is essential if outcome in the newborn is to be improved. Maternal prophylaxis is unlikely to be effective owing to a high chance of recolonization. The role of *L.monocytogenes* in recurrent abortion remains conjectural.

## Antenatal or intrapartum infection

### Mycoplasmal infection

*Mycoplasma hominis* and *Ureaplasma urealyticum* are common commensal flora of the genital tract in both sexes. *M.hominis* will be present in 10 per cent of women attending an antenatal clinic, and *U.urealyticum* in up to 75 per cent. Table 11.8 (Taylor-Robinson & McCormack 1980a)

**Table 11.8** Relation of sexual experience to colonization with genital mycoplasmas in vaginal specimens from healthy young women (after Taylor-Robinson & McCormack 1980)

| | *U.urealyticum* isolated (per cent) | *M.hominis* isolated (per cent) |
|---|---|---|
| No genital contact | 6 | 1 |
| Genital contact without vaginal penetration | 27 | 0 |
| Sexual intercourse | | |
| 1 partner | 38 | 9 |
| 2 partners | 55 | 9 |
| 3 partners or more | 75 | 17 |

**Table 11.9** Fetal and neonatal infection by genital mycoplasmas

| | Evidence for causation | |
|---|---|---|
| Condition | *M.hominis* | *U.urealyticum* |
| Recurrent spontaneous abortion | +/− | + |
| Chorioamnionitis | +/− | ++ |
| Low birth weight | − | ++ |
| Pneumonia or bacteraemia | +/− | − |
| Meningitis | + | + |

shows the relation between sexual experience and colonization by mycoplasmas. Against this background, the difficulty in proving a causal role for these organisms can be appreciated. Table 11.9 summarizes the present position. Both organisms may be isolated from the amniotic fluid from 16 weeks of gestation (Cassell *et al.* 1983). *U.urealyticum* would seem to be a cause of chorioamnionitis, prematurity and recurrent abortion. Shurin *et al.* (1975) recovered *U.urealyticum* from the placentas of 37.5 per cent of women with histological evidence of chorioamnionitis, compared to 19 per cent of controls. A recent study by Hillier *et al.* (1988) recovered *U.urealyticum* from 47 per cent of women delivered prematurely. Naessens *et al.* (1988) found an association between *U.urealyticum* serotype 4 and recurrent abortion.

*M.hominis* has been associated with prolonged delivery, spontaneous rupture of membranes and spontaneous abortion, but the evidence is largely anecdotal. The organism is a cause of post-partum pyrexia, which usually follows a benign course. Isolated incidents of maternal bacteraemia with positive amniotic fluid cultures, followed by death of the newborn from respiratory distress have also been reported.

The difficulty of separating colonization from infection is no clearer in the newborn. Infection may occur either *in utero* or at delivery. *M.hominis* has been isolated from the lungs of 8–10 per cent of spontaneously aborted fetuses, but the association may be casual. Some 5 per cent of babies will colonize with *M.hominis* after birth, and 30 per cent with *U.urealyticum*. Carriage is usually transient. There seems little doubt that *U.urealyticum* is associated with low birth weight (Taylor-Robinson & McCormack 1980b). Kundsin *et al.* (1984) investigated the role of ureaplasmas and other organisms in perinatal mortality and morbidity. Their data showed a strong correlation between the presence of *U.urealyticum* and low birth weight, and they further concluded that the presence of the organism in the placenta was consistent with transcervical spread.

The incidence of respiratory infection caused by genital mycoplasmas in the newborn is unknown. There are a few reports implicating *M.hominis*, for example Unsworth *et al.* (1985). They describe a full-term baby who acquired fever, respiratory distress and pneumonia within 20 hours of birth. The organism was isolated from blood culture, and a serum antibody rise was demonstrated. Recent reports concerning a role for ureaplasmas in chronic lung disease of premature babies are of interest. Cassell *et al.* (1988) studied 200 low birth weight children with signs of respiratory disease. *U.urealyticum* was the commonest organism isolated from endotracheal aspirates, and its presence correlated with the development of chronic lung disease in babies with a birth weight of <1000 g. Fourteen per cent of the isolates were from babies born by Caesarean section, indicating intrauterine infection. Similar findings are reported by Wang *et al.* (1988) and Sanchez & Regan (1988). An interesting additional finding in the study by Cassell *et al.* (1988) was an association between a birth weight of <1000 g, the presence of ureaplasmas and the probability of neonatal death. Cassell's group have also drawn attention to a possible role for the genital mycoplasmas in central nervous system infection of the preterm infant (Waites *et al.* 1988). *U.urealyticum* was isolated from the CSF of 8 per cent, and *M.hominis* from the CSF of 5 per cent, of 100 predominantly preterm babies under investigation for suspected sepsis or treatment of hydrocephalus. All of these studies require further work in different centres to verify the findings.

The genital mycoplasmas require special media for reliable isolation in the laboratory. However, the routine screening of antenatal patients for the presence of the organisms cannot at present be justified until more is known of the role and circumstances of genital mycoplasma infection in both the mother and the baby. Should antimicrobial therapy be indicated, the best available antibiotic is a tetracycline. However, caution will be necessary before using this group of antibiotics in the pregnant woman, lactating mother or newborn. Alternative therapy is less satisfactory. Erythromycin is effective against *U.urealyticum*, but not against *M.hominis*, whilst the reverse is the case with clindamycin.

## Intrapartum infection

### Group B streptococcal infection

Puerperal sepsis caused by infection with the group B haemolytic streptococcus has been known for over 50 years. There has however been a steady increase in the number of reports of neonatal and maternal infection over the last 20 years, until the organism now ranks among the commonest causes of severe neonatal sepsis.

The organism is carried in the genital tract, in the rectum and on the perineal skin. Rates of carriage in women vary between 4.5 and 36 per cent (Parker 1979). Swabbing of the vagina in late pregnancy is poorly predictive of the likelihood of neonatal infection, as only a small proportion of babies born to colonized mothers will become unwell. Further, the importance of rectal and perineal carriage is probably underestimated. Between 28 and 72 per cent of babies born to colonized mothers acquire group B streptococci (Ancona *et al.* 1980), yet the incidence of neonatal septicaemia is variously estimated at between 0.3 and 3.7 cases per 1000 live births (Leading Article 1984).

**Table 11.10** Features of fetal and neonatal Group B streptococcal infection

| |
|---|
| *Early onset* |
| Septicaemic and meningitic |
| Prolonged rupture of membranes |
| Low birth weight |
| High mortality |
| Organism in mother's vagina or rectum |
| *Late onset* |
| Meningitic |
| Previously healthy infant |
| Normal labour |
| Good prognosis |
| Relation to maternal colonization? |
| Cross infection? |

Group B streptococcal disease in babies is usefully divided into two categories (Table 11.10). Late onset disease is often caused by nosocomial infection, and is predominantly meningitic. Providing diagnosis and therapy is prompt, the prognosis is good. The disease is also preventable by strict observance of hygiene practices (Easmon *et al.* 1981). Instances of transmission of streptococcal infection on, for example, neonatal resuscitation equipment are not unknown (Mehtar *et al.* 1986).

Early onset disease follows infection at birth. Risk factors can be identified, and should alert the clinician to the diagnosis even in the absence of prior positive cultures from the mother. The major factors are prolonged rupture of membranes, vaginal intervention during labour, and low birth weight. The baby becomes acutely unwell within 24 hours of birth, showing signs of respiratory distress similar to hyaline membrane disease. Fever may be absent, and hypothermia was frequent in one series (Gamsu 1979). Leucopenia with neutropenia may be seen. Mortality is often as high as 60–75 per cent despite early diagnosis and specific therapy. At post-mortem, consolidation of the lungs is a striking feature.

There have been a number of approaches to the prevention of postpartum Group B infection. Swabbing of the vagina during the antenatal period and treating carriers is unlikely to succeed. Not all carriers will have been identified, and patients will recolonize from other sites or from their partners. The chemotherapy of the carrier state is not reliably effective. Conventional bacteriological techniques cannot give rapid enough results on swabs obtained at delivery, and antigen detection tests are not yet sensitive enough for routine use. Unselective prophylaxis is likely to be counterproductive. Boyer & Gotoff (1986) selected women known to be colonized with Group B streptococci, who presented with premature labour or prolonged rupture of membranes. They were given intrapartum ampicillin (2 g intravenously followed by 1 g 4 hourly until delivery). Colonization of the babies was significantly reduced, and there was a trend to reduction in bacteraemia. A simpler regime of 500 mg ampicillin given to all carriers of the organism at delivery had earlier been shown by Yow *et al.* (1979) to effectively reduce neonatal colonization. The administration of penicillin to high risk babies at delivery has also been studied, with conflicting results. Siegel *et al.* (1982) reported an extensive study on early single does penicillin prophylaxis in babies. The incidence of Group B streptococcal infection was reduced in the treated group. The authors commented that the regime was unlikely to be effective against infection acquired *in utero*. A later study by Pyati *et al.* (1983), also involving a large number of babies concluded that early penicillin prophylaxis was not effective, as in their study the majority of infections were well established before the first hour of postnatal life.

Preliminary studies with a vaccine directed against type III Group B streptococci are encouraging. Baker *et al.* (1988) vaccinated a cohort of women at a mean gestation of 31 weeks. Evidence of an antibody response was found in 63 per cent, with transmission of protection to the newborn. Clearly improvement is necessary before routine vaccination can be advised. For the present, recognition of the problem is the best course, with specific therapy if indicated. The best antimicrobial therapy is with ampicillin or amoxycillin plus an aminoglycoside, e.g. gentamicin. However, unless therapy is given early, the prognosis remains poor.

## Chlamydial infection

*Chlamydia trachomatis* infection has been known to cause non-gonococcal ophthalmia neonatorum for over 80 years. However, it was not until the development of cell culture techniques suitable for routine diagnostic use in the early 1970s that the extent of neonatal chlamydial infection was appreciated.

*C.trachomatis* is the commonest bacterial cause of sexually transmitted infection in the western world. It is an important cause of non-gonococcal urethritis and epididymitis in men, and a major cause of pelvic inflammatory disease in women. Conjunctivitis (paratrachoma) occurs in both sexes, and in non-trachomatous areas is caused by the same serotypes as cause genital infection (Ridgway 1986). Infection of the cervix is frequently asymptomatic. Mucopurulent cervicitis is an important, but non-specific clue to possible chlamydial infection.

The incidence of chlamydial infection in antenatal clinic attenders is of the order of 4 per cent. This compares with similar findings for gynaecology and family planning clinics. In contrast, isolation rates of up to 16 per cent have been reported in women attending for termination of pregnancy, and between 12 and 31 per cent for women attending clinics for sexually transmitted diseases (Oriel & Ridgway 1982).

Mårdh (1987) reviewed chlamydial pelvic inflammatory disease, and emphasized the relationship with tubal factor infertility and ectopic pregnancy. The effects of chlamydial infection on fetal outcome are less clear. Martin *et al.* (1982) reported a ten-fold increase in neonatal death or stillbirth between cervically infected women and matched controls. They also found an association between chlamydial infection and low birth weight. In contrast, Heggie *et al.* (1981) and Sweet *et al.* (1987) found no statistical difference for prematurity, premature rupture of membranes, spontaneous abortion, stillbirth or neonatal death between infected women and uninfected controls. In addition, Sweet *et al.* (1987) found no increase in the incidence of low birth weight in the infected group. Chlamydial infection of the fetus is in general not acquired from ascending spread of the organism. Chlamydial infection in babies born by Caesarean section with intact membranes is rare. Bell (1988) recently reported a case of chlamydial infection of the conjunctiva, pharynx and rectum of one of a pair of dizygotic twins delivered by Caesarean section. The membranes were intact at delivery and the mode of infection is unknown.

The transmission rate of *C.trachomatis* from mother to infant at birth is approximately 50 per cent (Hammerschlag 1987). The major syndromes associated with neonatal chlamydial infection are conjunctivitis and pneumonitis (Table 11.11).

Chlamydial conjunctivitis is at least five times as common as gonococcal ophthalmia. Onset is from 4 to 14 days after birth, and the condition may vary in severity from a mild sticky eye to a florid ophthalmia indistinguishable from gonococcal ophthalmia. A copious mucopurulent discharge with periorbital oedema and chemosis may occur. Conjunctivitis will usually involve both eyes eventually. Prophylaxis with silver nitrate drops is ineffective against chlamydial ophthalmia. In the UK, chlamydial and gonococcal ophthalmia are sufficiently uncommon that ocular prophylaxis in the newborn is not justified. There is no ideal agent, and topical prophylaxis will not prevent chlamydial pneumonia.

Beem & Saxon (1977) described a distinctive pneumonia syndrome. It is an afebrile and relatively non-toxic illness presenting between the 4th and 12th weeks of life. Partial nasal obstruction and otitis media may occur, but the predominating features are tachypnoea and a distinctive staccato cough. Chest radiography shows hyperexpansion, with bilateral symmetrical diffuse interstitial and patchy alveolar infiltrates. The disease is self-limiting after a protracted course. The possibility of long-term respiratory damage has not been entirely excluded. Infection of the other sites listed in Table 11.11 may be asymptomatic or not. *C.trachomatis* is an established cause of early onset otitis media, but the extent of its involvement is not clear. Colonization of the gastrointestinal

**Table 11.11** Sites of chlamydial infection in the newborn

| Site |
|---|
| Conjunctiva |
| Nasopharynx |
| Middle ear |
| Lungs |
| Vagina |
| Rectum |

tract is not uncommon, but there is no evidence as yet to relate this to subsequent disease.

Chlamydial infections are best diagnosed by isolation of the organism in cell culture. Where such facilities are not available, modern antigen detection methods using immunofluorescence or enzyme immunoassay may be employed. The interpretation of these tests, particularly in the low risk antenatal patient requires caution (Ridgway 1986). The tests should not be used for diagnosing chlamydial pneumonia until they have been properly evaluated in this area. Antibody tests are even less precise, but specific tests for chlamydial IgM are of value in diagnosing pneumonia in the newborn. A specimen of maternal serum should always be tested in parallel.

The antibiotics of choice for treating chlamydial infections are tetracyclines and erythromycin. The former should be avoided in pregnancy and in the newborn. Chlamydial ophthalmia is best treated with systemic erythromycin (50 mg/kg/day for 3 weeks); local therapy is not required. The routine use of topical chloramphenicol for sticky eyes should be avoided, as not only will chlamydial ophthalmia simply be suppressed, with a high rate of relapse, but subsequent attempts to isolate the organism will be unlikely to succeed. Neomycin provides a better alternative for undiagnosed ophthalmia, having first excluded gonococcal infection. Pneumonia is treated with erythromycin as for ophthalmia. It is important to contact trace both parents, to avoid reinfection, which may compromise subsequent pregnancies.

## Gonococcal infection

Once the commonest cause of blindness in children, gonococcal ophthalmia is now uncommon. Providing diagnosis and treatment are prompt, the sight will not be compromised. The incubation period is 1–5 days in general, but may be longer. A severe purulent conjunctivitis affecting one or both eyes occurs, with swollen lids. Septicaemic infection may occur, with all the features of adult disseminated infection, including skin rashes, arthritis and meningitis. Antenatal infection is not associated with prematurity or fetal wastage, except as a non-specific response to disseminated gonococcal infection. The condition is readily diagnosed by Gram stain of the conjunctival discharge. Culture should also be carried out to confirm the diagnosis and determine the sensitivities of the organism. Treatment is with systemic antibiotics. Other than local conjunctival toilet, topical therapy is not indicated. The antibiotic of choice is benzyl penicillin (50 000 units; 30 mg/kg/day), although in areas where the incidence of β-lactamase producing strains of *Neisseria gonorrhoeae* is high, cefotaxime or gentamicin should be used. Concurrent chlamydial infection occurs in 50 per cent of women with gonorrhoea, and this will be reflected in the dual incidence of gonococcal and chlamydial ophthalmia. Penicillin will not reliably eradicate *C.trachomatis*, and tests for this organism should be carried out before commencing penicillin therapy in each case. Sequential therapy for gonococcal and chlamydial infection will be required if both organisms are identified. As is the case for chlamydial infection, contact tracing of both parents is essential.

### Other bacterial infections

Almost any bacterium has the potential to infect the fetus and newborn. It is not the purpose of this review to examine in detail infections of the newborn, other than those conditions associated with birth. Staphylococcal septicaemia is no longer common, and usually postnatally acquired. It remains a potential problem of increased intervention in labour, particularly when the principles of hygiene are overlooked. The application of 0.33 per cent hexachlorophane powder to the *umbilicus* is still to be recommended. The emerging problem of infection in the neonatal unit with coagulase-negative staphylococci (e.g. *Staphylococcus epidermidis*) and the methicillin-resistant *Staph. aureus* should be borne in mind, along with the ever present risk of infection with coliforms and other Gram-negative aerobic organisms.

The potential for organisms carried in the mother's genital tract to cause infection is well illustrated by a report by Berardi-Grassias *et al.* (1988). They describe a case of neonatal meningitis thought to be caused by *Gardnerella vaginalis.* Unfortunately, although the organism was isolated from the baby's CSF, cultures from the mother's vagina were negative for this organism. Hillier *et al.* (1988) found that *G.vaginalis,* along with *U.urealyticum,* correlated with chorioamnionitis, and they postulate a possible role for this organism as a cause of premature birth in some circumstances.

Patterns of infection are continually changing. The discovery of new organisms, and the reappraisal of known organisms, leads to changing thoughts on the effect of bacterial infection on the fetus and newborn. Knowledge of these changes is essential if the most favourable conditions for fetal development and childbirth are to be attained.

## References

Adler M. (1984) Pregnancy and the neonate. *British Medical Journal,* **288**, 624–7.

Ancona R.J., Ferrieri P. & Williams P.P. (1980) Maternal factors that enhance acquisition of group B streptococci by newborn infants. *Journal of Medical Microbiology,* **13**, 273–80.

Backer C.J., Rench M.A., Edwards M.S., Carpenter R.J., Hays B.M. & Kasper D.L. (1988) Immunization of pregnant women with a polysaccharide vaccine of group B streptococcus. *New England Journal of Medicine,* **319**, 1180–5.

Beem M.O. & Saxon E.M. (1977) Respiratory tract colonisation and a distinctive pneumonia syndrome in infants infected with *C.trachomatis. New England Journal of Medicine,* **296**, 306–10.

Bell T.A. (1988) *Chlamydia trachomatis* infection in dizygotic twins delivered by caesarian section. *Genitourinary Medicine,* **64**, 347–8.

Berardi-Grassias L., Roy O., Berardi J.C. & Furioloi J. (1988) Neonatal meningitis due to *Gardnerella vaginalis. European Journal of Microbiology and Infectious Disease,* **7**, 406–7.

Boyer K.M. & Gotoff S.P. (1986) Prevention of early onset group B streptococcal disease with selective intrapartum chemoprophylaxis. *New England Journal of Medicine*, **314**, 1665–9.

Campbell-Brown M., McFayden I.R., Seal D.V. & Stephenson M.L. (1987) Is screening for bacteriuria in pregnancy worth while? *British Medical Journal*, **294**, 1579–82.

Cassell G.H., Davis, R.O., Waites K.H., Brown M.B., Marriott P.A., Stagno S. & Davis J.K. (1983) Isolation of *M.hominis* and *U.urealyticum* from amniotic fluid at 16–20 weeks gestation: potential effect on pregnancy outcome. *Sexually Transmitted Diseases*, **10**, 294–302.

Cassell G.H., Waites K.B., Crouse D.T., Rudd P.T., Canupp K.C., Stagno S. & Cutter G. (1988) Association of *U.urealyticum* infection of the lower respiratory tract with chronic lung disease and death in very-low-birth-weight infants. *Lancet*, **i**, 241–4.

Easmon C.S.F., Hastings M.J.G., Clare A.J., Bloxham B., Marwood R., Rivers R. & Stringer J. (1981) Nosocomial transmission of group B streptococci. *British Medical Journal*, **283**, 459–61.

Fox G.P., Clarke T.A. & Mattews T.G. (1988) Are routine superficial cultures worthwhile in neonatal practice? *British Medical Journal*, **296**, 1443.

Gamsu H.R. (1979) Clinical experience of group B streptococcal infection of the newborn. *Journal of Antimicrobial Chemotherapy*, **5** (suppl. A), 45–9.

Hammerschlag M.R. (1987) *Chlamydia trachomatis* infections and pregnancy. In *Chlamydial Infection*, (Ed. by P. Reeves) pp. 57–71. Springer-Verlag, Berlin.

Heggie A.D., Lumicao G., Stuart L.A. & Gyves M.T. (1981) *Chlamydia trachomatis* infections mothers and infants. *American Journal of Diseases of Children*, **135**, 507–11.

Hillier S.L., Martius J., Krohne M., Kiviat N., Holmes K.K. & Eschenbach D. (1988) A case controlled study of chorioamnion infection and histologic chorioamnionitis in prematurity. *New England Journal of Medicine*, **319**, 972–8.

Kampelmacher E.H., Huysinga L. & Van Noorle Jansen L. (1972) The presence of *L.monocytogenes* in faeces of pregnant women and neonates. *Zentralblatt für Bakteriologie, Parasitenkunde, Infektionskrankheiten und Hygiene (Abteilung I)*, **222**, 258–62.

Kampelmacher E.H. & Van Noorle Jansen L. (1972) Further studies on the isolation of *L.monocytogenes* in clinically healthy individuals. *Zentralblatt für Bakteriologie, Parasitenkunde, Infektionskrankheiten und Hygiene (Abteilung I)*, **221**, 70–7.

Kass E.H. & Zinner S.H. (1973) Bacteriuria and pyelonephritis in pregnancy. In *Obstetric and Perinatal Infections*, (Ed. by D. Charles & M. Finland), pp. 407–46. Lea & Febiger, Philadelphia.

Kerr K.G. & Lacey R.W. (1988) Listeriosis: new problems with an old pathogen. *Journal of Hospital Infection*, **12**, 247–50.

King A., Nicol C. & Rodin P. (1980) *Venereal Diseases*, 4th edn, pp. 104–32. Baillère, Tindall, London.

Kundsin R.B. Driscott S.G., Monson R.R., Yeh C., Biano S.A. & Cochran W.D. (1984) Association of *Ureaplasma urealyticum* in the placenta with perinatal morbidity and mortality. *New England Journal of Medicine*, **310**, 941–5.

Leading Article (1984) Prevention of early onset group B streptococcal infection in the newborn. *Lancet* **i**, 1056–7.

Mårdh P-A. (1987) Chlamydial pelvic inflammatory disease. In *Chlamydial Infection*, (Ed. by P. Reeves), pp. 45–56. Springer-Verlag, Berlin.

Martin D.H., Koutsky L., Eschenbach D.A., Daling J.R., Alexander E.R., Bendetti J.K. & Holmes K.K. (1982) Prematority and perinatal mortality in pregnancies complicated by maternal *C. trachomatis* infections. *Journal of the American Medical Association*, **247**, 1585–8.

Mehtar S., Drabu Y.J., Vijeratnam S. & Mayet F. (1986) Cross infection with *Streptococcus pneumoniae* through a Resuscitaire. *British Medical Journal*, **292**, 25–6.

Naessens A., Foulon W., Breynaert J. & Lauwers S. (1988) Serotypes of *U.urealyticum* isolated from normal pregnant women and patients with pregnancy complications. *Journal of Clinical Microbiology*, **26**, 319–22.

Oriel J.D. & Ridgway G.L. (1982) *Genital Infection by Chlamydia trachomatis*, pp. 53–77. Edward Arnold, London.

Parker M.T. (1979) Infections with group-B streptococci. *Journal of Antimicrobial Chemotherapy*, **5** (suppl. A), 21–6.

Poirier M. (1978) *Analyse de l'epidemie de listeriose survenue en Anjou en 1975–1976*. These de Medecine (Angers).

Pryse-Davis J. & Hurley R. (1979) Infection and perinatal mortality. *Journal of Antimicrobial Chemotherapy*, **5** (suppl. A), 59–70.

Pyati, S.P., Pildes R.S., Jacobs N.M., Ramamurthy R.S., Yeh, T.F., Raval D.S., Lilien L.D., Amma P. & Metzger W.I. (1983) Penicillin in infants weighing two kilograms or less with early onset group B streptococcal disease. *New England Journal of Medicine*, **308**, 1383–9.

Relier J.P. (1979) Listeriosis. *Journal of Antimicrobial Chemotherapy*, **5** (suppl. A), 51–7.

Report (1987) *Report of the RCOG sub-committee on problems associated with AIDS in relation to obstetrics and gynaecology*. The Royal College of Obstetricians and Gynaeocologists, London.

Ridgway G. (1986) Chlamydial infections in man. *Postgraduate Medical Journal*, **62**, 249–53.

Sanches P.J. & Regan (1988) *Ureaplasma urealyticum* colonisation and chronic lung disease in low birthweight infants. *Paediatric Infections Diseases Journal*, **7**, 542–6.

Shurin P.A., Alpert S., Rosner B., Criscoll S.H., Lee Y-H., McCormack W.M., Santamarina B.A.G. & Kass E.H. (1975) Chorioamnionitis and colonization of the newborn infant with genital mycoplasmas. *New England Journal of Medicine*, **293**, 5–8.

Siegel J.D., McCracken G.H., Threlkeld N., DePasse B.M. & Rosenfield C.R. (1982) Single dose prophylaxis of neonatal group B disease. *Lancet*, **i**, 1426–30.

Spencer A.D. (1987) Perinatal listeriosis. *British Medical Journal*, **295**, 349.

Sweet R.L., Landers D.V., Walker C. & Schachter J. (1987) *Chlamydia trachomatis* infection and pregnancy outcome. *American Journal of Obstetrics and Gynecology*, **156**, 824–31.

Taylor-Robinson D. & McCormack W. (1980a) The genital mycoplasmas. *New England Journal of Medicine*, **302**, 1003–10.

Taylor-Robinson D. & McCormack W. (1980b) The genital mycoplasmas. *New England Journal of Medicine*, **302**, 1063–7.

Unsworth P.F., Taylor-Robinson D., Shoo E.E. & Furr P.M. (1985) Neonatal mycoplasmaemia: *M.hominis* as a significant cause of disease? *Journal of Infection*, **10**, 163–8.

Waites K.B., Rudd P., Crouse D.T., Canupp K.C., Nelson K.G., Ramsey C. & Cassell G.H. (1988) Chronic *U.urealyticum* and *M.hominis* infections of central nervous system in preterm infants. *Lancet*, **i**, 17–21.

Wang E.E.C., Frayha H., Watts J., Hammerberg O., Cherneskey M., Mahony J.B. & Cassell, G.H. (1988) Role of *Ureaplasma urealyticum* and other pathogens in the development of chronic lung disease of prematurity. *Paediatric Inflections Diseases Journal*, **7**, 547–51.

Yow M.D., Mason E. O., Leeds L.J., Thompson P.K., Clark D.J. & Gardner S.E. (1979) Ampicillin prevents intrapartum transmission of group B streptococci. *Journal of the American Medical Association*, **241**, 1245–7.

# 12: Viral infections in pregnancy

STUART LOGAN



Viral infections of the newborn may be acquired *in utero* (congenital infection), at the time of birth (natal infection), or during the neonatal period (postnatal infection). Maternal viraemia may be associated with placental infection and transplacental spread to the fetus. The fetus may also be infected *in utero* by ascending infection from the genital tract. During delivery infection may result from contact with infected genital secretions, blood or faeces (Figure 12.1).

There has been considerable difficulty in elucidating the effects of congenital viral infections. The majority of maternal viral infections that may infect the fetus are mild or asymptomatic, and therefore unlikely to be diagnosed. Many infected infants are apparently well at the time of birth, with no stigmata of infection, but may manifest or develop signs of damage after months or years (Peckham 1972). Large prospective studies monitoring women during pregnancy for signs of infection, and following their infants for prolonged periods after birth, are required to elucidate possible causal relationships between infection and adverse outcome for the fetus or newborn. For infections that are uncommon in pregnancy, the numbers required for such studies may be impracticably large, forcing reliance on case reports. Unfortunately, even serological or virological evidence of infection in a damaged infant cannot establish a causal relationship, though it may raise strong suspicions, particularly if the pattern of damage is unusual and constant for a particular agent. In clinical practice, damage appearing after the neonatal period is often incorrectly ascribed to congenital infection on the basis of past infection

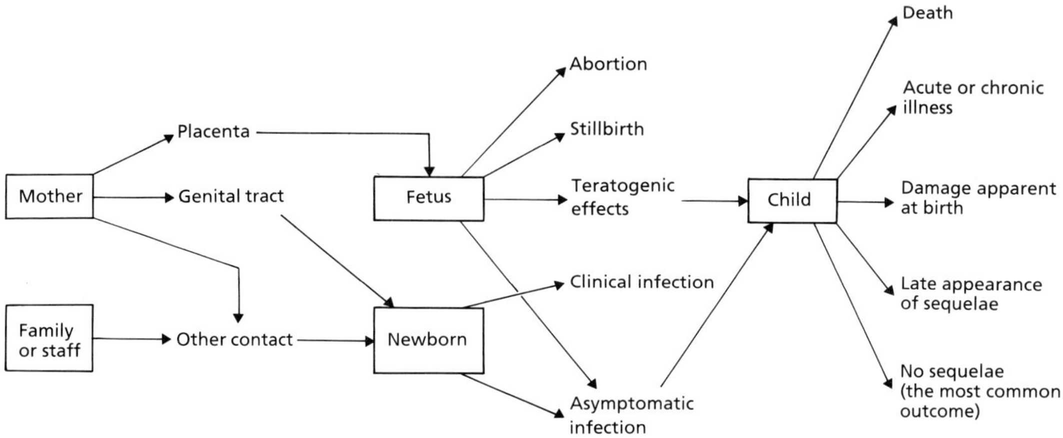


**Fig. 12.1** Pathogenesis of viral infections of the fetus and newborn. (Adapted from Overall 1981.)

with an agent known to cause damage compatible with that seen in the child. Unfortunately, it is seldom possible to differentiate in such cases between congenital and postnatally acquired infection.

A number of viral infections have been implicated in the pathogenesis of illness and damage in the fetus and newborn (Tables 12.1 and 12.2). There is little information available on the frequency of such viral infections in the fetus or newborn infant, though a cumulative frequency of 6–8 per cent of all live births has been suggested (Overall 1981). In this review common and important viral infections that can have an

**Table 12.1** Congenitally acquired viral infections causing illness or damage

| Established causes | Suggested causes |
|---|---|
| Cytomegalovirus | Echovirus |
| Rubella | Coxsackie B virus |
| HIV | Polio virus |
| Varicella-zoster* | Mumps |
| Hepatitis B virus* | Vaccinia |
| Herpes simplex* | Influenza |
| | Epstein–Barr virus |

* Rare.

**Table 12.2** Natally and postnatally acquired viral infections causing illness or damage

| Established causes | Suggested causes |
|---|---|
| Herpes simplex | HIV |
| Hepatitis B virus | Echovirus |
| Varicella zoster | Coxsackie B |
| Cytomegalovirus* | |

* Illness rare except in very premature infants.

adverse effect on the fetus are discussed; rubella and human immunodeficiency virus, however, will not be discussed as these are dealt with in separate chapters.

## Cytomegalovirus infection

Cytomegalovirus (CMV) is a ubiquitous agent which infects most individuals at some time in their lives. The infection is usually asymptomatic or mild, although in immunocompromised individuals and in very premature infants it may be life-threatening. CMV is a herpes group virus, and like others of this family (herpes simplex types 1 and 2, varicella and Epstein–Barr virus), it persists in the body in a latent form after the initial infection. Recurrences, which are usually asymptomatic, may occur at intervals throughout an individual's lifetime, and the virus may be intermittently isolated from various bodily fluids.

### Congenital CMV

CMV is now the commonest agent causing congenital infection in the developed world, occurring in approximately 1 in 300 births in the UK (Stern 1977; Macdonald & Tobin 1978), and even more frequently in the USA (Stagno *et al.* 1983). Worldwide, rates from 0.2 to 2.2 per cent have been reported (Stagno *et al.* 1983).

Early studies, based largely on infants identified because of the presence of symptoms, suggested a high prevalence of defects associated with congenital infection. However, more recent prospective studies of infants identified by systematic screening at birth have suggested considerably lower rates of handicap (Peckham *et al.* 1983; Ahlfors *et al.* 1984; Stagno *et al.* 1986).

In the UK some 50 per cent of women of child-bearing age are seronegative for CMV (Peckham *et al.* 1983), while in some populations virtually 100 per cent of adults show evidence of past infection (Schopfer *et al.* 1978). Past infection does not, however, protect against fetal infection; unlike congenital rubella, intrauterine transmission may follow a recurrent infection in the mother, even in the presence of humoral immunity. Damage compatible with congenital CMV infection has been reported in infected infants of women known to be seropositive before pregnancy (Ahlfors *et al.* 1981; Rutter *et al.* 1985), but it has been suggested that the risk of damage is lower in congenital infection following recurrence of CMV during pregnancy than in that following primary infection (Stagno *et al.* 1982).

Prospective studies suggest that 5–10 per cent of congenitally infected children will have signs or symptoms of CMV infection in the neonatal period. These clinical manifestations include hepatosplenomegaly, intrauterine growth retardation, microcephaly, thrombocytopenia, petechiae, prolonged neonatal jaundice and pneumonitis. Periventricular intracranial calcifications have also been described but are very rare. Virtually all symptomatic babies will develop major handicaps, including cerebral palsy, epilepsy, mental retardation, microcephaly, chorioretinitis, optic atrophy, delayed psychomotor development and sensorineural deafness (Pass *et al.* 1980; Williamson *et al.* 1982). The mortality rate in this group is high. Of the children who are asymptomatic at birth, a further 5–10 per cent manifest disabilities, most commonly sensorineural hearing loss, later in childhood (Peckham *et al.* 1983; Ahlfors *et al.* 1984; Stagno *et al.* 1986). In a large prospective study of 35 000 pregnancies in London, in which 103 congenitally infected infants were identified, four children showed signs of congenital CMV infection in the neonatal period, and overall less than 10 per cent have discernible handicap by the age of five (Logan and Peckham, unpublished data). There have been a few reports of progressive hearing loss in children with congenital CMV (Dahle 1979; Williamson *et al.* 1982), but damage does not appear to develop in children who are normal at the age of one year.

It has been suggested that apparently asymptomatic children may have subtle intellectual damage (Hanshaw *et al.* 1976) but recent studies have shown no difference in IQ scores between congenitally infected children without neurological abnormality and matched controls (Conboy *et al.* 1986; Pearl *et al.* 1986). It appears, therefore, that about 90 per cent of children with congenital CMV will be neurologically and developmentally normal. The risk of transmission of infection to the fetus after a primary maternal infection during pregnancy is of the order of 40 per cent. This suggests that the risk of damage after a primary maternal infection is about 1 in 25. The risk of damage in a congenitally infected infant does not appear to be related to the gestational age at which infection occurs as damage has been described following late gestational infection. In view of the low risk of damage to the fetus, routine termination because of documented primary infection in the mother is not justified, though parents should be given this option after suitable counselling. Routine serological screening in pregnancy with a view to identifying primary infection and offering termination is clearly not appropriate. In the study reported by Preece *et al.* (1984), a policy of screening in pregnancy and offering women termination if this occurred would have resulted in the termination of a number of normal fetuses without preventing any handicap.

Although the risk of handicap in an infected infant exposed to maternal CMV infection is low, because this is such a common infection during pregnancy the number of affected fetuses is considerable. Assuming an annual number of births in England and Wales of 680 000 and a rate of congenital CMV infection of 3–4 per 1000 live births, between 2000 and 2700 infants are born with congenital infection each year. If 10 per cent of these children have significant handicaps, this would amount to between 200 and 270 children with handicaps resulting from congenital CMV infection.

The minimum incubation period of CMV is about 3 weeks. Because both natal and early postnatal infection are common, congenital infection can only be reliably diagnosed if the virus is isolated from urine or saliva within the first 3 weeks of life, or if CMV-specific IgM can be detected in blood taken at or shortly after birth. In children presenting after this period with problems compatible with congenital CMV infection, congenital and postnatally acquired infection cannot be distinguished.

Although there have been isolated case reports of women who have had children with congenital CMV infection giving birth to second infected children, there have been no reports of damage in the second child. There is clearly a theoretical risk of damage occurring in such children, but the risk appears to be exceedingly low, and parents of children with CMV-related handicap can be reassured about the low risk of damage in subsequent pregnancies.

### Postnatally acquired infection

Infants of seropositive mothers commonly acquire CMV infection from their mothers during the first year of life. Approximately 10 per cent of seropositive women shed the virus into the genital tract around the time of delivery (Reynolds *et al.* 1980; Dworsky *et al.* 1983), and about 40 per cent of their infants will acquire infection at the time of birth from this source (Reynolds *et al.* 1980). Virus has been isolated from breast milk in between 20 per cent (Peckham *et al.* 1987) and 32 per cent (Dworsky *et al.* 1983) of seropositive women. In the study by Dworsky *et al.* (1983), 39 per cent of infants breast fed for over one month by seropositive mothers acquired CMV infection. In countries with high rates of maternal seropositivity and widespread breast feeding, mothers are likely to be the most common source of infection for their infants. Infection may also be acquired from blood transfusion from seropositive donors (Yeager *et al.* 1981; Adler 1983; Logan *et al.* 1988). Infection acquired natally or postnatally is seldom symptomatic, though it has been associated with pneumonitis (Stagno *et al.* 1981) and, in very low birth weight babies infected following transfusion, with acute illness and even death (Yeager *et al.* 1981; Logan *et al.* 1988). Most neonatal intensive care units now use only blood products which have been screened for the presence of CMV antibodies, for children born at less than 32 weeks gestation.

## Herpes simplex virus (types I and II)

During the late 1970s and early 1980s, there has been an apparent large increase in the incidence of genital herpes simplex (HSV) infection. The number of new cases of HSV infection reported by sexually transmitted disease clinics has risen from 9576 in 1979 to 20 315 in 1987 (Communicable Disease Surveillance Centre, unpublished 1988). It is unclear whether this represents a real increase in incidence or of increased attention being focused on the disease by the public and professionals.

Parallel with this apparent increase in genital herpes has been increasing concern about neonatal HSV infection. Although population-based figures are sparse, the incidence of neonatal herpes varies widely in different populations. Nahmias *et al.* (1983) estimate an incidence of up to 1/2000 deliveries in the USA. In England, Scotland and Northern Ireland, 136 cases were notified between 1976 and 1985 to the PHLS (Communicable Disease Surveillance Centre, unpublished). This is a rate of 2 to 3 per 100 000 births. In an active monthly reporting system paediatricians in the UK reported 23 confirmed cases over a 24 month period, 1986–1988 (British Paediatric Surveillance Unit, unpublished). These figures are likely to be an underestimate since less severe and subclinical infection is likely to go unreported, and children presenting with disseminated disease without skin involvement may go undetected (Arvin *et al.* 1982).

### Infections in women

Both HSV I and HSV II typically establish latent infection in the dorsal root ganglion after primary infection. They may reactivate periodically to produce either overt lesions or asymptomatic shedding of virus. Traditionally it was said that HSV I produced lesions of the face, lips and eyes, while HSV II produced lesions of the genitalia. It is probable that either type can produce lesions at either site (Anon. 1981).

HSV I is an extremely common infection, with nearly 100 per cent of the population acquiring the infection. Infection with HSV II is less common and varies widely amongst different ethnic groups. A recent study of pregnant women in London (Ades *et al.* 1989) found seroprevalence rates varying from 3.4 per cent in Asian women to 7.2 per cent in white UK-born women to 36.5 per cent in black women born in Africa. There have been a number of studies in the USA of asymptomatic shedding of virus during pregnancy. Overall it has been estimated that 1 in 1000 pregnant women shed HSV asymptomatically during pregnancy. However, rates of shedding range from less than 1 in 1000 to as high as 4 per 100 (Ng *et al.* 1970; Bolognese *et al.* 1976; Harger *et al.* 1983), with the highest rates amongst women from the most socially deprived groups. Amongst women with a history of current genital herpes, reported rates of asymptomatic viral shedding during pregnancy range from 0.66 to 2.4 per cent (Vontver *et al.* 1972; Harger *et al.* 1983; Yeager 1984). Figures on viral shedding during pregnancy are not available from the UK.

### Transplacental infection

Transplacental infection is rare. There are, however, isolated case reports linking primary maternal infection with congenital abnormalities (Florman *et al.* 1973; Komorous *et al.* 1977). The evidence is inconclusive, and early primary infection is not an indication for termination of pregnancy.

Nahmias *et al.* (1971) have suggested that HSV infection is associated with an increase in spontaneous abortion and premature delivery. Brown *et al.* (1987) reported that 1 of 5 women with primary infection in the first trimester had a spontaneous abortion. Examination of the fetal membranes showed features consistent with herpetic chorioamnionitis. Of the 5 women who had primary infection during the second trimester, all gave birth to non-infected infants, 4 at term and 1 at 32 weeks gestation. Of the 5 women with primary infection in the last trimester, 4 went into premature labour within 2 to 3 weeks of infection, although in 2 of these cases this subsided with conservative management. These findings provide some evidence for the possible role of herpes simplex infection in causing abortion and premature labour, but further research will be required to clarify the position.

### Neonatal infection

Neonatal HSV infection is associated with a substantial morbidity and mortality (Nahmias *et al.* 1983). The infection may present as a disseminated disease with or without CNS involvement, or may be localized to the CNS, skin or oral cavity. About 80 per cent of the children with disseminated disease will die, and half of the survivors will have long-term sequelae. Localized CNS disease has a similarly poor prognosis, but other forms of localized disease are far less likely to result in death or long-term sequelae. Asymptomatic neonatal infection is considered rare, but this conclusion is not based on screening populations and infants. It has been suggested that infection with HSV I leads to less serious long-term sequelae than that with HSV II (Corey *et al.* 1988) but this remains to be confirmed.

Infection with HSV is most commonly acquired by contact with genital secretions during delivery (Corey & Spear 1980). Ascending infection, particularly in the presence of prolonged rupture of membranes or with the use of fetal scalp monitoring may also occur. Non-genital contact with herpes infections of the mother, other family members or even nursery staff, has also been postulated as a source of viral infection although is at most a rare source of infection.

The highest risk of neonatal HSV infection is amongst infants of women who have primary genital infections at the time of delivery. The attack rate in this group is estimated to be 50 per cent (Nahmias *et al.* 1983). The risk appears to be much lower in women with recurrent overt genital infection or with asymptomatic viral shedding at the time of delivery. Prober *et al.* (1987) have studied 34 infants born by vaginal delivery to women with a history of recurrent genital herpes who were shedding virus at the time of delivery. None of the infants was infected. Based on the 95 per cent confidence limits, this suggests a theoretical maximum likely risk of infection in this situation of 8 per cent. All of these infants had demonstrable neutralizing antibody. The lower risk of attack in the presence of recurrent infection may be due to the less frequent involvement of the cervix in a recurrent infection, lower titres of virus in the genital tract, and possibly a protective effect of transplacentally acquired antibody.

Although the risk of neonatal infection amongst infants of women with recurrent overt or asymptomatic genital herpes appears to be low, it does account for at least some cases. Visintine *et al.* (1981) reported that of 400 mothers of infants with HSV infection, 10 per cent had no signs or symptoms of disease. Of these, 13 per cent gave a history of genital HSV and 20 per cent reported infections in their sexual partners.

There is unfortunately no general agreement on the management of women with genital herpes during pregnancy. There is agreement that delivery by Caesarean section should be offered to women with primary HSV infections near term, with membranes which are either intact or ruptured for less than 4 hours. Most obstetricians would extend this recommendation to women with recurrent genital herpes with overt lesions at the time of delivery. In the USA it has been further recommended that women with a history of genital herpes should have repeated viral cultures from 32 weeks gestation to detect asymptomatic viral shedding with the intention of performing Caesarean sections on those women in whom viral cultures are positive at the time of delivery. Even with the relatively high prevalence of neonatal infection in the USA this policy may lead to many unnecessary Caesarean sections. Binkin *et al.* (1984) have used decision and cost-benefit analysis to compare the effects of this recommended screening policy with weekly history and examination. They conclude that the screening would prevent 30.6 cases of neonatal HSV infection per year at a cost of $1.8 million per case. They also estimate that 5700 unnecessary Caesarean sections would be performed, leading to 3.3 maternal deaths.

On the basis of present evidence, women with clinical evidence of genital HSV infection at the time of delivery, either primary or recurrent disease, should be delivered by Caesarean section. Routine viral culture in women with a history of genital herpes is, however, not justified.

## Hepatitis B virus (HBV)

It has been estimated that there are 200 million people in the world chronically infected with hepatitis B virus (Beasley 1978). In parts of Africa, the Far East and South East Asia, carrier rates in the population of up to 35 per cent have been reported (Tong *et al.* 1971; Stevens *et al.* 1975). In adults the major routes of transmission are associated with contaminated blood products or needles and sexual transmission. In areas of high indemnicity, however, vertical transmission is of major importance.

### Transplacental infection

Teratogenic effects have not been reported either after acute hepatitis B infection during pregnancy, or related to chronic HBsAg carriage during pregnancy. Transplacental spread has, however, been reported in a few cases (Stevens *et al.* 1984). In one series of 140 children born to HBsAg carrier mothers, 3 children were judged to have acquired infection *in utero* on the basis of either the presence of IgM anti-HBc presence in cord blood or the presence of HBsAg in a third day sample (Wong *et al.* 1984). This is an uncommon route of infection.

### Perinatal transmission

Although the exact mechanism of transmission remains unclear, perinatal acquisition of virus has been widely reported (Crumpacker 1983). The probability of vertical transmission from a woman who is a chronic carrier of HBsAg to her infant varies greatly in different ethnic groups independently of the country of residence (Derso *et al.* 1978; Logan & Nicol, 1989). Rates of vertical transmission appear to be very low (0–5 per cent) amongst European and North American Caucasians, and very high (40–90 per cent) amongst ethnic Chinese, with intermediate rates amongst other Asians. These differences appear to be closely related to HBeAg and HBe antibody status. Women who are HBeAg positive and HBe-antibody negative are at the highest risk of transmitting the virus perinatally (Okada *et al.* 1976) (Table 12.3).

The majority of infants who acquire HBV in the perinatal period are clinically well. Some may develop neonatal hepatitis, but this is generally transient although acute fulminant hepatitis may occur (Duprey *et al.* 1975). Many infants will, however, remain chronic carriers of HBsAg. Although apparently well, they may have raised transaminase levels and signs of chronic hepatitis on biopsy. In addition to chronic liver disease it has been suggested that neonatal HBV infection may play a major role in the development of primary hepatocellular carcinoma (Szmuness 1978). It has been estimated that 25 per cent of infants who become chronic carriers of HBV will die from primary hepatocellular carcinoma or sclerosis of the liver (Beasley & Hwang 1984).

It has been estimated that infants born to mothers positive for HBsAg and HBeAg have a 70–90 per cent chance of acquiring perinatal HBV infection, and that 85–90 per cent of the infected infants will become chronic HBV carriers (Stevens *et al.* 1975; Stevens *et al.* 1985). Both passive immunization with hepatitis B immunoglobulin (HBIG), and active immunization with hepatitis B vaccine (HB vaccine) in the neo-

**Table 12.3** Risk of perinatal HBV transmission according to maternal HBe antigen and antibody status

| Maternal e antibody and e antigen status | Risk group |
|---|---|
| HBeAg −ve, HBeAb +ve | Low risk |
| HBeAg +ve, HBeAb −ve | High risk |
| HBeAg −ve, HBeAb −ve | Intermediate risk |

natal period have been shown to decrease the rates of vertical transmission. Combined active and passive immunization has been shown to be 85–95 per cent effective in preventing the development of chronic HBV carriage (Wong 1983; Stevens *et al.* 1985). The American Immunization Practices Advisory Committee (ACIP) (MMWR 1984) recommend that all infants of women HBsAg positive during pregnancy should receive combined therapy at birth. Further doses of HB vaccine should be given at 1 and 6 months. The effectiveness of this therapy should be monitored by testing the infants at the age of 12 months for HBsAg and anti-HBs. In some countries, the infants of women who are HBe-antibody positive are not given immunoprophylaxis, as they are considered to be at low risk of infection. Shiraki *et al.* (1980) have, however, reported 2 infants of HBe-antibody positive mothers who developed acute hepatitis in the neonatal period.

The ACIP suggest that in countries with a high prevalence of HBsAg carriage, where screening may be difficult, resources should be devoted to giving HB vaccine to all newborns. This policy has been implemented in Alaska, American Samoa and in parts of Taiwan and the People's Republic of China (Anon. 1988).

Lee *et al.* (1988) have recently suggested that the efficacy of combined immunoprophylaxis in infants of mothers with HBe antigen could be increased by the performance of Ceasarean section. At present this suggestion remains controversial, and cannot be recommended without further evidence.

## Parvovirus B19

The human parvovirus B19 was discovered in 1975 by Cossart *et al.* It has been associated with erythema infectuosum (fifth disease) (Anderson *et al.* 1983), with aplastic crises in patients with haemolytic anaemia (Serjeant *et al.* 1981) and acute arthritis (White *et al.* 1985).

Parvovirus infection in animals is known to be associated with fetal death and congenital malformations. A number of case reports have linked maternal parvovirus infection with spontaneous abortion and stillbirth (Anderson 1987); the detection of parvovirus B19 DNA in fetal tissue supported a causal association. Weiland *et al.* (1987) reported abnormalities including damage to the eyes, mild carditis and generalized myositis in a fetus aborted therapeutically at 11 weeks in a woman who had an acute parvovirus infection at 4 weeks gestation. Abnormalities have not been reported in liveborn infants of women known to have had parvovirus infection during pregnancy. A number of aborted or stillborn fetuses of women with parvovirus infection have had hydrops fetalis (Burton 1986; Anand *et al.* 1987). It has been suggested (Gray *et al.* 1987) that this may be the result of severe fetal anaemia due to the inhibition or the multiplication of erythroid progenitor cells.

There is little prospective data about the effects of parvovirus B19 infection in pregnancy. The PHLS working party on fifth disease have reported on the outcome of 134 pregnancies in women with proven parvovirus infection (PHLS 1987). Twenty (15 per cent) of the pregnancies ended in spontaneous abortions. This suggests a small increased risk of spontaneous abortion, though confirmation by matched controlled studies is required. No obvious congenital abnormalities were detected in the survivors.

It seems likely that parvovirus B19 infection may increase the risk of spontaneous abortion and stillbirth, but it is not an indication for termination of pregnancy.

## Varicella-zoster (VZ)

Chickenpox is a common and highly contagious disease, which is usually acquired during childhood. Relatively few adults are susceptible, so chickenpox during pregnancy is uncommon. Data from collaborative prospective studies of viral infection in pregnancy in the USA (Enders 1985) suggests an incidence of varicella-zoster (VZ) infection in pregnancy of between 1.3 and 7 cases per 10 000 pregnancies. Much of the information about the effects on the fetus are inevitably based on case reports. Two distinct patterns of fetal disease arise, according to the timing of maternal infection.

### Congenital varicella syndrome (early congenital chickenpox)

In 1947 LaForet & Lynch described an association between maternal varicella in early pregnancy and congenital anomalies in the infant. Alkalay *et al.* (1987) have reviewed the case reports in English language literature. They summarize the findings in 22 cases where there was evidence of maternal VZ infection, and skin lesions corresponding to a dermatome distribution in the infant, which they judge to be the minimum criteria for diagnosis of congenital varicella syndrome. Other findings in these children include neurologic, eye and skeletal anomalies. Approximately one-third of the children died in early infancy.

Although the evidence from these case reports strongly suggests a causal link, a number of prospective studies (Siegel 1973; Bradford-Hill *et al.* 1978; Paryani & Arvin 1986) have demonstrated no excess of abnormalities amongst the offspring of mothers with VZ infection during pregnancy. This suggests either that the association is not causal, or that congenital varicella syndrome is a rare outcome of maternal VZ infection.

Higa *et al.* (1987) have suggested that the lesions of congenital varicella syndrome may be a result of intrauterine herpes-zoster. This is an elegant hypothesis which would help to account for both the rarity of abnormalities amongst infants of women with VZ infection during pregnancy, and also the segmental distribution of abnormalities. Fetal anomalies have also been reported rarely after maternal herpes-zoster infection. The association, however, remains controversial. It seems likely, from evidence available, that fetal anomalies may occur in infants of women with VZ infection early in pregnancy. This is undoubtedly a very rare consequence of infection and therefore no numerical estimate of frequency is available. Maternal VZ infection is not an indication for termination of pregnancy.

## Late congenital chickenpox

When a susceptible woman acquires chickenpox in the last weeks of pregnancy the virus may cross the placenta and infect the fetus. The attack rate is of the order of 20 per cent (Enders 1985). The clinical course of the infection in the newborn is largely determined by the time of onset of maternal infection (Table 12.4). If the maternal rash appears 5–21 days before delivery, the infant is usually mildly infected. If it occurs more than 21 days before delivery, it is extremely unusual for the infant to show signs of infection. If, however, the onset of rash is from 4 days before to 2 days after delivery, the course in the newborn is likely to be severe, with an untreated case fatality rate as high as 30 per cent (Enders 1985). Severely affected infants have widespread cutaneous and visceral lesions, which may be haemorrhagic, and usually have a severe pneumonitis. The mild course of the disease in infants born to mothers whose onset of infection was 5 or more days before delivery is thought to be due to the protective effect of maternally derived antibody.

Despite the lack of any controlled trials, it is believed that the administration of zoster-immune globulin (ZIG) modifies the course of chickenpox infection in the newborn. Miller *et al.* (1986) report that of 74 infants of mothers with onset of chickenpox rash between 5 days before and 7 days after delivery who received ZIG, 46 were infected of whom 9 had a moderately severe clinical illness and 2 died. This suggests that ZIG is effective in modifying the course of neonatal chickenpox and it is recommended for all neonates whose mothers develop chickenpox around the time of delivery. It is also recommended for the protection of pregnant women who come into contact with chickenpox and have no history of previous infection.

## Postnatal infection

In congenital varicella the interval between the onset of rash in the mother and the onset in the fetus or newborn is usually 9 to 15 days,

**Table 12.4** Clinical course of late congenital chickenpox in relation to time of onest of maternal rash

| Day of onset of maternal rash | Clinical course in the newborn |
|---|---|
| 5–21 days antepartum | Mild |
| 4 days antepartum to 2 days post-partum | Severe |

with an average of 11 days. Children in whom the rash appears after this time are regarded as having acquired the infection postnatally. Postnatal VZ infection is generally mild. Rubin *et al.* (1986) reviewed 13 case reports of infants with onset of VZ infection 11–28 days after birth and four had severe or fatal disease. Although two of these might conceivably have represented intrauterine infection, two were undoubtedly acquired postnatally. As mild cases are unlikely to be reported, this gives no indication of the spectrum of severity of the disease. However, it must raise questions about the benign nature of the illness. Although offical recommendations both in the UK and the USA do not recommend the use of ZIG in this group, some infectious disease paediatricians (Wurzel *et al.* 1987) would recommend its use in children less than a week of age, particularly if there is no past history of maternal infection. This requires further evaluation.

## Rubella and human immunodeficiency virus infections

These are considered separately in Chapters 13 and 14, respectively.

## Conclusions

A number of other viruses have been implicated in the pathogenesis of fetal damage but for most the link is tenuous and based on case reports. However, many children with congenital disabilities have no obvious cause for their problems and it is possible that in some, other, yet to be discovered, agents may be responsible. When a link between a pathogen and congenital damage is suspected, careful investigation is required to establish causation and the extent of the problem before embarking on clinical intervention. It is important that where such associations are suggested, careful investigations are performed before clinical intervention begins. For example, prospective studies have shown that the proposal (Anon. 1977) that pregnant women should be screened for CMV, and offered terminations if they had acquired infection in the first trimester, would have resulted in the termination of numbers of unaffected fetuses and prevented only a small proportion of CMV-related handicap.

Although case reports may provide valuable clues, an estimation of risk and the spectrum of disease can only be made from prospective studies. Without this information it is not possible to evaluate the benefits and risks associated with changes in treatment or intervention.

## References

Ades A.E., Peckham C.S., Dale G.E., Best J.M. and Jeansson S. (1989) Prevalence of antibodies to Herpes Simplex virus types 1 and 2 in pregnant women, and estimated rates of infection. *Journal of Epidemiology and Community Health*, **43**, 53–60.

Adler S.P. (1983) Transfusion-associated cytomegalovirus infections. *Reviews of Infec-*

*tious Diseases*, **5**, 977–93.

Ahlfors K., Harris S., Ivarsson S. & Svanberg L. (1981) Secondary maternal cytomegalovirus infection causing symptomatic congenital infection. *New England Journal of Medicine*, **305**, 284.

Ahlfors, K., Ivarsson S.A., Harris S., Svanberg L., Holmquist R., Lernmark R. & Theander G. (1984) Congenital cytomegalovirus infection and disease in Sweden and the relative importance of primary and secondary maternal infections: preliminary findings from a prospective study. *Scandinavian Journal of Infectious Disease*, **16**, 129–37.

Alkalay A.L., Pomerance J.J. & Rimoin D.L. (1987) Fetal varicella syndrome. *Journal of Pediatrics*, **III(3)**, 320–3.

Anand A., Gray E.S., Brown T., Clewley J.P. & Cohen B.J. (1987) Human parvovirus infection in pregnancy and hydrops fetalis. *New England Journal of Medicine*, **316**, 183–6.

Anderson L.J. (1987) Role of parvovirus in human disease. *Pediatric Infectious Disease Journal*, **6**, 711–18.

Anderson L.J., Jones S.E., Fisher-Hoch S.P., Lewis E., Paul S.M., Barlett C.C.R., Cohen B.J., Martin P.P. & Perbira M.S. (1983) Human parvovirus, the cause of erethema infectiosum (Fifth disease)? *Lancet*, **i**, 1378.

Anon. (1977) Cytomegalovirus in adults. Editorial. *Lancet*, **ii**, 541.

Anon. (1981) Herpes simplex — changing patterns. Editorial. *Lancet*, **ii**, 1025–6.

Anon. (1988) Prevention of perinatal transmission of hepatitis B virus: prenatal screening of all pregnant women for hepatitis B surface antigen *Morbidity and Mortality Weekly Report*, **37**, 341–7.

Arvin A.M., Yeager A.S., Bruhn F.W. & Grossman M. (1982) Neonatal herpes simplex infection in the absence of mucocutaneous lesions. *Journal of Pediatrics*, **100**, 715–21.

Beasley R.P. (1978) Hepatitis B virus as the aetiologic agent in hepato-cellular carcinoma — epidemiologic considerations. *Hepatology*, **2** (suppl.), 21S–26S.

Beasley R.P. & Hwang L-Y. (1984) Epidemiology of hepatocellular carcimona In *Viral Hepatitis and Liver Disease*, (Ed. by G.M. Vyas, J.L. Dienstag & K.H. Hoonagle), pp. 209–24. Grune and Stratton, Orlando.

Binkin N.J., Koplan J.P. & Cates W. (1984) Preventing neonatal herpes: the value of weekly viral cultures in pregnant women with recurrent genital herpes. *Journal of the American Medical Association*, **251**, 2816–21.

Bolognese R.J., Corson S.L., Fuccillo D.A., Traub R., Moder F. & Sever J.L. (1976) The natural history of herpes simplex virus infection of mother and newborn. *Pediatrics*, **66**, 489–94.

Bradford Hill A., Doll R., Galloway T.M. & Hughes J.P. (1978) Virus diseases in pregnancy and congenital defects. *British Journal of Preventive and Social Medicine*, **12**, 1–17.

Brown Z.A., Vontver L.A., Benedetti J., Critchlow C.W., Sells C.J., Berry S. & Corey L. (1987) Effects on infants of a first episode of genital herpes during pregnancy *New England Journal of Medicine*, **317**, 1246–51.

Burton P.A. (1986) Intranuclear inclusions in marrow of a hydropic foetus due to parvovirus infection. *Lancet*, **ii**, 1155.

Conboy T.J., Pass R.F., Stagno S. & Britt W.J. (1986) Intellectual development in school-aged children with asymptomatic congenital cytomegalovirus infection. *Pediatrics*, **77**, 801–6.

Corey L. & Spear P.G. (1986) Infections with herpes simplex viruses. *New England Journal of Medicine*, **314**, 686–91, 749–57.

Corey L., Whitley R.J., Stone E.F. & Mohan K. (1988) Difference between Herpes Simplex Virus type 1 and type 2 neonatal encephalitis in neurological outcome. *Lancet*, **i**, 1–4.

Cossart Y.E., Field A.M., Cant B. & Widows D. (1975) Parvovirus-like particles in human sera. *Lancet*, **i**, 72–3.

Crumpacker C.S. (1983) Hepatitis. In *Infectious Diseases of the Foetus and Newborn Infant*, (Ed. by J.S. Remington & K.O. Klein), pp. 591–698. W.B. Saunders, Philadelphia.

Dahle A.J., McCollister F.P., Stagno S., Reynolds D.W. & Hoffman H.E. (1979) Progressive hearing impairment in children with congenital cytomegalovirus infection. *Journal of Speech and Hearing Disorders*, **44**, 220–9.

Derso A., Vauxhall E.H., Tarlow N.J. & Fluewett T.H. (1978) Transmission of HBsAG from mother to infant in 4 ethnic groups. *British Medical Journal*, **1**, 949–52.

Duprey K.M., Frommel B. & Alagilie D. (1975) Severe viral hepatits type B in infancy. *Lancet*, **i**, 191–9.

Dworsky M.E., Yow M., Stagno S., Pass R.F. & Alford C.A. (1983) Cytomegalovirus infection of breast milk and transmission in infancy. *Pediatrics*, **72**, 295–9.

Enders G. (1985) Varicella zoster virus infection in pregnancy, *Progress in Medical Virology*, **29**, 166–96.

Florman A.L., Gershon A.A., Blackett P.R. & Nahmias A.J. (1973) Intrauterine infection with herpes simplex virus: resultant congenital malformations. *Journal of the American Medical Association* , **225**, 129–32.

Gray E.S., Davidson R.J. & Anand A. (1987) Human parvorius and fetal anaemia. *Lancet*, **i**, 1144.

Hanshaw J.B., Scheiner A.P., Moxley A.W., Gaev L., Avel V. & Scheiner B. (1976) School failure and deafness after 'silent' congenital cytomegalovirus infection. *New England Journal of Medicine*, **295**, 468–70.

Harger J.H., Pazin G.J., Armstong J.A. & Breinig M.C. (1983) Characteristics and management of pregnancy in women with genital herpes simplex virus infection. *American Journal of Obstetrics and Gynecology*, **145**, 784–91.

Higa K., Dan K. & Manabe H. (1987) Varicella-Zoster virus infections during pregnancy; hypothesis concerning the mechanisms of congenital malformations. *Obstetrics and Gynecology*, **69**, 214–22.

Komorous J.M., Wheeler C.E. & Briggamann R.A. (1977) Intrauterine herpes simplex infections. *Archives of Dermatology*, **113**, 918–22.

Laforet E.G. & Lynch C.L. (1947) Multiple congenital defects following maternal varicella: report of a case. *New England Journal of Medicine*, **236**, 534–7.

Lee S-D., Lo K-J., Tsai Y-T., Woo J-C., Woo T-C., Yang Z-L. and Ng H-T. (1988) Role of Caesarean section in prevention of mother–infant transmission of hepatitis B virus. *Lancet*, **i**, 833–4.

Logan S., Barbara J. & Kovar I. (1988) Cytomegalovirus screened blood for neonatal intensive care units. *Archives of Disease in Childhood*, **63**, 753–5.

Logan S. & Nicol A. (1989) Viral infections in pregnancy and childhood. In *Ethnic Factors in Disease*, (Ed. by J.K. Cruikshank). Butterworth, London.

MacDonald H & Tobin J. O'H. (1978) Congenital cytomegalovirus infection: a collaborative study on epidemiological, clinical and laboratory findings. *Developmental Medicine and Child Neurology*, **20**, 471–82.

Miller E., Hopkison W.M., Craddock-Watson J.E. & Ridehalgh M.K.S. (1986) Use of varicellar-zoster immunoglobulin for the prevention of chickenpox in neonates and pregnant women. CDR 86/14.

MMWR (1988) Prevention of perinatal transmission of Lepatitis B virus: prenatal screening of all pregnant women for Lepatitis B surface antigen. *Morbidity and Mortality Weekly Report*, **37**, 341–7.

Nahmias A.J., Alford C.A. & Korones S.B. (1971) Infections of the newborn with herpesvirus hominis. *Advances in Pediatrics*, **17**, 185–226.

Nahmias A.J., Keyserling H.H. & Kerick G. (1983) Herpes simplex. In *Infectious Diseases of the Fetus and Newborn Infant*, (Ed. by J.S. Remington & J.O. Klein), pp. 636–78. W.B. Saunders, Philadelphia.

Ng A.B., Reagan Y.W. & Yen S.S.C. (1970) Herpes genitalis. *Obstetrics and Gynecology*, **36**, 645–51.

Okada M., Miyakawa Y. & Mayumi M. (1976) E. antigen in mothers serum as an indicator of vertical transmission of HBV. *New England Journal of Medicine*, **292**, 746.

Overall J.C. (1981) Viral infections of the fetus and newborn. In *Textbook of Pediatric Infectious Disease*, (Ed. by R.D. Feigin & J.D. Cherry), pp. 684–721. W.B. Saunders, Philadelphia.

Paryani S.G. & Arvin A.M. (1986) Intrauterine infection with Varicella-Zoster virus after maternal varicella. *New England Journal of Medicine*, **314**, 1542–6.

Pass R.F., Stagno S., Myers G.J. & Alford C.A. (1980) Outcome of symptomatic congenital cytomegalovirus infection: results of long-term longitudinal follow-up. *Pediatrics*, **66**, 758–62.

Pearl K.N., Preece P.M., Ades A. & Peckham C.S. (1986) Neurodevelopmental assessment after congenital cytomegalovirus infection. *Archives of Disease in Childhood*, **61**,

323–6.

Peckham C.S. (1972) A clinical and laboratory study of children exposed *in utero* to maternal rubella. *Archives of Disease in Childhood*, **47**, 571–7.

Peckham C.S., Coleman J.C., Hurley R., Chin K.S. & Henderson K. (1983) Cytomegalovirus infection in pregnancy: preliminary finding from a prospective study. *Lancet*, **i**, 1352–6.

Peckham C.S., Johnson C., Ades A.E., Pearl K. & Chin K.S. (1987) The early acquisition of cytomegalovirus infection. *Archives of Disease in Childhood*, **62**, 780–5.

PHLS report (1986) Sexually transmitted disease surveillance in Britain — 1984. *British Medical Journal*, **293**, 942–3.

PHLS Report (1987) PHLS working party on Fifth Disease: Study of human Parvovirus (B19) infection in pregnancy. CDR 87/20.

Preece P., Pearl K & Peckham C.S. (1984) Congenital cytomegalovirus. *Archives of Disease in Childhood*, **59**, 1120–6.

Prober C.G., Sullender W.M., Yasukawa L.L., Av D.S., Yeager A. & Arvin A.M. (1987) Low risk of herpes simplex virus infections in neonates exposed to the virus at the time of vaginal delivery to mothers with recurrent genital herpes simplex virus infection. *New England Journal of Medicine*, **316**, 240–4.

Reynolds D.W., Stagno S. & Hosty T.S. (1980) Maternal cytomegalovirus excretion and perinatal infection. *New England Journal of Medicine*, **302**, 1073–6.

Rubin L.G., Leggiadro R., Elie T. & Lipsitz P. (1986) Disseminated varicella in a neonate: implications for immunoprophylaxis in neonates post-natally exposed to varicella. *Pediatric Infectious Disease*, **5**, 100–2.

Rutter D., Griffiths P.D. & Trompeter R.S. (1985) Cytomegalic inclusion disease after recurrent maternal infection. *Lancet*, **ii**, 1182.

Schopfer K., Lauber E. & Krech U. (1978) Congenital cytomegalovirus infection in newborn infants of mothers infected before pregnancy. *Archives of Disease in Childhood*, **53**, 536–9.

Serjeant G.R., Topley J.M., Mason K., Serjeant B.E., Pattison J.R., Jones S.E. & Mahommed R. (1981) Outbreak of aplastic crises in sickle cell anaemia associated with parvovirus-like agent. *Lancet*, **ii**, 595–7.

Shiraki K., Yoshihara N., Sakyurai M., Eto T. & Kawana T. (1980) Acute hepatitis B in infants born to carrier mothers with the antibody to hepatits B e antigen. *Journal of* Pediatrics, **97**, 768–70.

Siegel M. (1973) Congenital malformations following chickenpox, measles, mumps and hepatitis. *Journal of the American Medical Association*, **226**, 1521–4.

South M.A., Tompkins W.A.F., Morris C.R. & Rawls W.E. (1969) Congenital malformations of the central nervous system associated with genital type (type 2) herpes virus. *Journal of Pediatrics*, **75**, 13–18.

Stagno S., Brasfield D.M. & Brown M.B. (1981) Infant pneumonitis associated with cytomegalovirus, chlamydia, pneumocystis and ureaplasma — A prospective study. *Pediatrics*, **68**, 322–9.

Stagno S., Pass, R., Cloud G., Britt W.J., Henderson R.E., Walton P.D., Veren D.A., Page F. & Alford C.A. (1986) Primary cytomegalovirus infection in pregnancy. *Journal of the American Medical Association*, **256**, 1904–8.

Stagno S., Pass, R.F. & Dworsky M.E. (1982) Congenital cytomegalovirus infection: the relative importance of primary and recurrent maternal infection. *New England Journal of Medicine*, **306**, 945–9.

Stagno S., Pass R.F., Dworsky M.E. & Alford C.A. (1983) Congenital and perinatal cytomegalovirus infections. *Seminars in Perinatology*, **7**, 31–42.

Stern H. (1977) Cytomegalovirus infection in the neonate and its prevention. *Postgraduate Medical Journal*, **55**, 588–91.

Stevens C.E., Beasley R.P., Tsui J. & Lee W-C. (1975) Vertical transmission from hepatitis B antigen in Taiwan. *New England Journal of Medicine*, **292**, 771–4.

Stevens C.E., Taylor T.E. & Tong N.J. (1984) Hepatitis B vaccine: an overview. In *Viral Hepatitis and Liver Disease*, (Ed. by G.M. Vyas, J.L. Dienstag & J.H. Hoofnagle), pp. 275–92. Grune and Stratton, New York.

Stevens C.E., Toy P.T., Tong N.J., Taylor P.E., Vyas G.N., Nair P.V., Guduvalli M. & Krugman S. (1985) Perinatal Hepatitis B virus transmission in the United States: prevention by passive–active immunization. *Journal of the American Medical Association*, **253**, 174–5.

Szmuness W., Stevens L.E., Ikram H., Much M.I. & Harley E.J. (1978) Prevalence of Hepatitis B virus infection and hepatocellular cancer in Chinese – Americans. *Journal of Infectious Disease*, **137(6)**, 822–9.

Tong N.J., Sun S.C.M., Shaefer B.T., Chang H-K., Lo K-J. & Peters R.L. (1971) Hepatitis-associated antigen and hepato-cellular carcinoma in Taiwan. *Annals of Internal Medicine*, **75**, 687–91.

Visintine A.M., Nahmias A.J., Whitley R.J. & Alford C.A. (1981) The natural history and epidemiology of neonatal herpes simplex virus infection. In *The Human Herpes Viruses*, (Ed. by A.J. Nahmias, W.R. Dowdle & R.F. Schinazi), pp. 599–600. Elsevier, New York.

Vontver L.A., Hickok D.E., Brown Z.A., Reid L. & Corey L.J. (1982) Recurrent genital herpes simplex virus infection in pregnancy: infant outcome and frequency of asymptomatic recurrence. *American Journal of Obstetrics and Gynecology*, **142**, 75.

Weiland H.T., Verney-Keers C.H.R., Salimans M.M.M., Fleuren G.J. & Verwey R.A. (1987) Parvovirus B19 associated with foetal abnormality. *Lancet*, **i**, 682–3.

White D.G., Woolf A.D., Mortimer P.P., Cohen B.J., Blake D.R. & Bacon P.A. (1985) Human parvovirus arthropathy. *Lancet*, **i**, 419–21.

Williamson W.D., Desmond M.M., LaFevers N., Taber L.H., Catlin F.I. & Weaver T.G. (1982) Symptomatic congenital cytomegalovirus: disorders of language learning and hearing. *American Journal of Diseases in Children*, **136**, 902–5.

Wong V.C.W., Ip H.M.H., Reesink H.W., Nco Lelie P., Reesink-Brongers E.E., Yeung C.Y. & Ma H.K. (1984) Prevention of the HBsAg carrier state in newborn infants of mothers who are chronic carriers of the HBsAg and HBeAg by administration of hepatitis B vaccine and hepatitis B immunoglobulin. *Lancet*, **ii**, 1099–1102.

Wurzel C.L., Rubin L.G. & Krilov L.R. (1987) Varicella-zoster immunoglobulin after post-natal exposure to varicella: survey of experts. *Pediatric Infectious Disease*, **6**, 466–8.

Yeager A.S. (1984) Genital herpes simplex infection: effect of asymptomatic shedding and latency on management of infections in pregnant women and neonates. *Journal of Investigative Dermatology*, **83**, 53s–56s.

Yeager A.S., Arvin A.M., Urbani L.J. & Kemp J.A. (1980) Relationship of antibody to outcome in neonatal herpes simplex virus infections. *Journal of Infectious Immunology*, **29**, 532–8.

Yeager A.S., Grumet F.C., Hafleigh E.B., Arvin A.M. & Bradley J.S. (1981) Prevention of transfusion-acquired cytomegalovirus infection in newborn infants. *Journal of Pediatrics*, **98**, 281–7.

# 13: Rubella infection in pregnancy

ELIZABETH MILLER



Rubella infection in pregnancy can have devastating consequences for the fetus. Congenital cataracts following early gestational infection were first described in 1941 by an Australian ophthalmologist, Norman Gregg, who noted an increased referral of such cases in the wake of a rubella outbreak (Gregg 1941). Enquiry to fellow Australian ophthalmologists revealed a similar increase and identified other ocular and cardiac defects occurring in association with congenital cataracts. In most cases there was a maternal history of German measles in early pregnancy. The suggestion that a mild virus infection could cause major fetal malformations was at first treated with scepticism, since it challenged the then-accepted faulty germ plasm theory as the cause of congenital defects. However, reports from other countries of a similar association established the causal connection and Gregg was subsequently knighted for his historic contribution to medicine. The full spectrum of congenital rubella defects, including sensorineural deafness, mental retardation, microcephaly and growth retardation was subsequently established by epidemiological studies in USA and UK during rubella epidemics in the 1960s and 1970s (Peckham 1972; Cooper 1975; Miller *et al.* 1982).

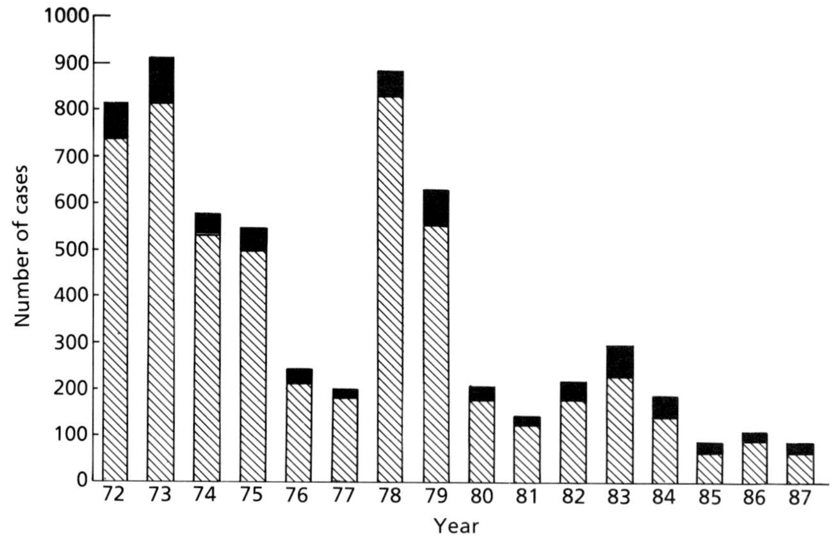


**Fig. 13.1** Number of congenital rubella cases and therapeutic abortions for rubella in pregnancy reported in England and Wales 1972–1987. (▧) Rubella abortions; (■) congenital rubella cases.

Until rubella vaccine became available in 1969, the only way of preventing congenital rubella was by offering termination of pregnancy when maternal infection was diagnosed. Unfortunately, the availability of a safe and effective vaccine has not solved the problem. Almost 1000 children with congenital rubella are known to have been born in the UK since the introduction of the national rubella vaccination programme 18 years ago (Holzel *et al.* 1987); about 400 of them have multiple defects. These cases represent only a fraction of the morbidity attributable to rubella in pregnancy since for every reported case of congenital rubella syndrome (CRS) there are about 10 rubella associated terminations of pregnancy (Figure 13.1). Unfortunately, the UK experience is not unique and no country has yet succeeded in eliminating congenital rubella. The diagnosis, management and future prevention of rubella infection in pregnancy is therefore a topic which remains of considerable importance to the obstetrician.

This chapter reviews current evidence on the risk to the fetus of maternal infection at successive stages of pregnancy, including the outcome following maternal reinfection. The laboratory diagnosis of congenital rubella and the prospects for prenatal diagnosis of fetal infection are discussed together with the problems of distinguishing primary rubella from reinfection. The various strategies for the prevention of congenital rubella by vaccination are evaluated.

## Epidemiology of rubella

Evidence of rubella virus infection has been found in every country where serological studies have been undertaken. The problem of con-

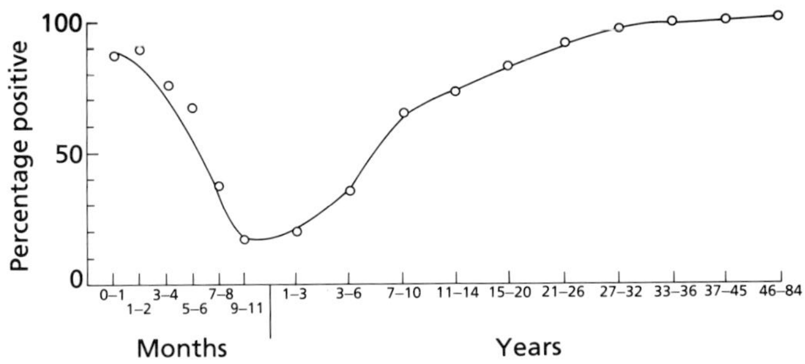


**Fig. 13.2** Rubella antibody status by age. West Germany, 1967. (Reproduced with permission from Professor Gisela Enders.)

genital rubella must therefore be worldwide although, without appropriate surveillance, the occurrence of such cases may not be detected among the background of congenital malformations that arise from non-preventable causes. Serological surveys conducted in different countries show that the average age of infection varies, being lower in densely populated areas than in isolated communities where there is little opportunity for mixing. Figure 13.2 shows a typical age-dependent serological profile from a European country without a rubella vaccination programme. Although infection is common in childhood, 10–20 per cent of the population nevertheless reach adult life still susceptible to rubella. Thereafter, susceptibility continues to decline with age reflecting the risk of acquiring rubella during adult life.

In temperate climates, rubella is endemic with seasonal peaks in the spring and early summer. Before the advent of mass rubella vaccination, epidemics occurred at intervals of about 4–5 years in Europe, and 6–9 years in the USA (Assaad & Ljungars-Esteves 1985). For the susceptible woman who is unfortunate enough to be pregnant during an epidemic year, the risk of infection may be 10-fold higher than during a non-epidemic period (Miller 1986). The epidemic pattern of rubella in tropical areas is less well documented although serological studies have identified outbreaks in African communities with their ensuing toll of congenital rubella cases (Assaad & Ljungars-Esteves 1985).

## Incidence of congenital rubella

Figures for the incidence of congenital rubella in the pre-vaccine era are scarce. One follow-up study of babies born in the USA following a major epidemic in 1964 showed an incidence of congenital rubella of 2 per cent among live births; this represents some 20 000 infants born with a major handicap as a result of that one epidemic alone. In non-epidemic periods the incidence among live births was under 0.1 per cent (Assaad & Ljungars-Esteves 1985). Serological surveys of handicapped children in the UK suggest that congenital rubella accounted for about 16 per cent of cases of moderate to severe deafness and about 2 per cent of cases of congenital heart defect among English children before the introduction of rubella vaccination (Peckham 1985). This represents some 200–300 children born with rubella defects in England and Wales during a non-epidemic year, an incidence of about 1 per 2000 births. A similar rate has been estimated for the non-epidemic incidence of rubella defects among births in Australia during the pre-vaccine era (Menser *et al.* 1985).

## Laboratory diagnosis of acquired and congenital infection

The original studies of Gregg and others relied on clinical diagnoses of rubella in the mother and congenital infection in the infant. However, with the isolation of rubella virus in 1962, laboratory confirmation became possible. The duration of virus excretion in acquired and congenital cases, and the nature of the antibody responses, were intensively studied. With these documented, laboratory methods for the confirmation of suspected clinical cases could then be established using virus isolation and serological techniques.

### Acquired infection

The rubella-specific IgG and IgM serum antibody responses that accompany a primary infection are shown in Figure 13.3. IgM antibody is usually detectable within 5 days of onset of symptoms and persists for at least one month. Thereafter the IgM antibody level declines and in most cases becomes undetectable within 2–3 months. Detection of rubella-specific IgM is therefore evidence of recent infection. IgG antibody rises somewhat later but persists throughout the life of the individual. By itself, therefore, the detection of rubella-specific IgG antibody simply shows that the individual has experienced rubella some time in the past. However, IgG antibody tests on paired sera with the first taken before antibody appears, or while levels are still low, can confirm recent infec-

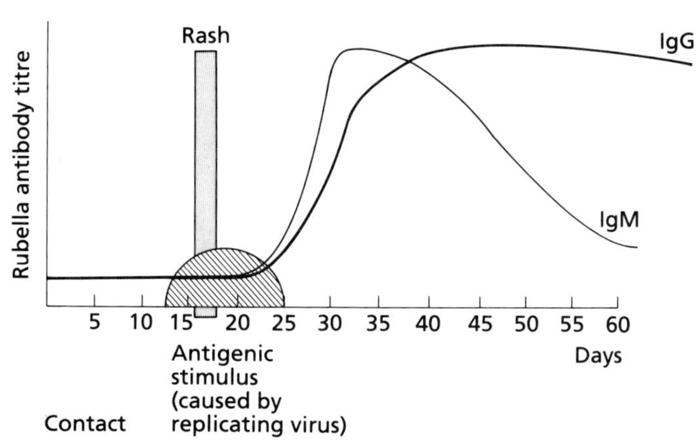


**Fig. 13.3** IgM and IgG responses in a primary rubella virus infection.

tion if a fourfold or greater rise in titre is demonstrated. Isolation of the virus from the nasopharynx is also evidence of recent infection although it is rarely used as a diagnostic test. First, the slow growth of the virus in tissue culture means a delay of several weeks before results are available. Second, the period of virus excretion is short and a negative result may be obtained if the nasopharyngeal swab is taken more than 3 days after onset of rash. Virus can also be isolated from blood but samples have to be taken during the prodromal phase of the illness since viraemia ends with the onset of rash (Plotkin 1969).

Close contact with rubella virus in an individual who has been infected or vaccinated in the past can occasionally result in reinfection. Diagnosis is made by the detection of a fourfold or greater rise in rubella antibody titre in an individual with pre-existing antibody. Unlike primary rubella, reinfection rarely results in rash or other symptoms and in most cases it is thought that virus replication, if it occurs at all, is restricted to the nasopharynx. However, a low level IgM response may be detected (Morgan-Capner *et al.* 1985a) making the differentiation between asymptomatic primary rubella and rubella reinfection difficult. Unless earlier sera from the patient are available for IgG antibody testing a definitive diagnosis may not be possible. Basing the diagnosis of reinfection solely on a documented history of vaccination or a single laboratory record of previous immunity is risky because of the possibility of vaccine failure, or earlier technical or clerical error.

## Congenital infection

Unlike acquired infection, congenital infection can result in chronic virus excretion. This appears to be largely confined to infants infected during the first 4 months of pregnancy (Cradock-Watson *et al.* 1989). Diagnosis of congenital infection can be made in such cases by isolating virus from urine, nasopharyngeal swabs or other body tissues. The period of virus excretion persists for up to 6 months after birth with the consequent risk of such infants infecting susceptible contacts (Cooper & Krugman 1967).

A diagnosis of congenital infection can also be made serologically by the demonstration of rubella-specific IgM antibody in cord blood. Unlike IgG antibody, maternal IgM does not cross the placenta and its presence in cord blood therefore indicates fetal infection. IgM antibody only begins to appear in fetal blood at about 20 weeks gestation even when infection occurs early in pregnancy. However, it persists after birth and is usually detectable up to 6 months of age (Chantler *et al.* 1982). Detection of rubella-specific IgG antibody between 10–12 months of age is also indicative of congenital infection since passively-acquired maternal antibody disappears by this age (see Figure 13.2). Diagnosis of congenital rubella after the first year of life by the detection of IgG antibody is less reliable since an increasing proportion of children will have rubella antibody from an acquired infection. Lymphocyte transformation testing for cell-mediated immunity (CMI) to rubella virus may be of help in distinguishing acquired from congenital rubella in older children since a significant reduction in CMI has been demonstrated in children infected *in utero* during the first trimester (Iuorio *et al.* 1984).

## Fetal outcome following rubella in pregnancy

The management of cases of rubella in pregnancy requires accurate information on the risk to the fetus in relation to the timing of the maternal infection. Such information can only come from the prospective follow-up of pregnancies in which maternal infection has been confirmed serologically and the date of onset of rash or seroconversion in relation to the date of the last menstrual period (LMP) is known. Follow-up of cases in which the diagnosis has been made solely on clinical grounds will inevitably lead to an underestimate of risk since only a proportion of such cases are likely to be attributable to rubella. The risk will also be underestimated if infants are not followed up after birth since defects such as deafness may not be apparent initially.

### Primary symptomatic rubella in pregnancy

The consequences for the fetus of confirmed symptomatic maternal rubella at successive stages of pregnancy were assessed in a large prospective study carried out in England and Wales by the Public Health Laboratory Service (PHLS) during 1976–1978 (Miller *et al.* 1982). Over a 1000 pregnant women in whom the dates of LMP and rash were known were followed up; two-thirds of the women were parous. More than 90 per cent of those infected during the first trimester, and half of those infected between 13–16 weeks, chose to have a therapeutic abortion. Termination of pregnancy was carried out in some women infected as late as 20–24 weeks. Among the 407 pregnancies that continued to term there were 9 stillbirths (2 per cent). Without a matched control group it is uncertain whether this is higher than expected although in comparison with national figures it is about twice the expected number. In 4 cases the cause of stillbirth was unexplained, the remainder being due to congenital defects unrelated to rubella (4 cases) or intrapartum haemorrhage (1 case). There were 5 neonatal deaths among the 398 live births (1 per cent), about the expected number. From the results of this study, therefore, maternal rubella does not appear to cause a major increase in perinatal mortality.

Among the infants who survived, congenital infection was diagnosed by the detection of rubella-specific IgM antibody at birth or the persistence of IgG antibody at a year. The frequency of congenital infection after maternal rubella with a rash was found to be 81 per cent in the first 12 weeks; the only infants to escape infection were those where maternal rash occurred within 2 weeks of LMP or between 11–12 weeks

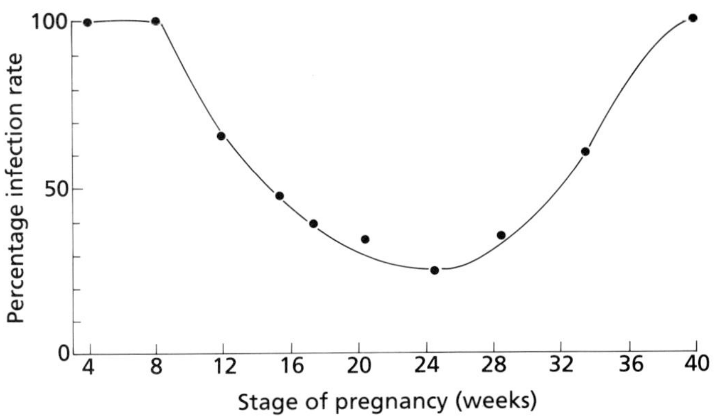


**Fig. 13.4** Congenital infection rate following symptomatic maternal rubella at successive stages of pregnancy.

after. These findings confirm the results of an earlier study in which rubella virus was isolated from 15 of 17 fetuses obtained by therapeutic abortion following first trimester rubella (Thompson & Tobin 1970). At 13–16 weeks the congenital infection rate had fallen to 54 per cent, and to 25 per cent at the end of the second trimester. The infection rate rose again to a high figure in the last month of pregnancy (Figure 13.4). The reason for this U-shaped relationship between fetal infection rate and gestational stage of maternal rubella remains unexplained.

The likelihood and severity of defects in congenitally infected infants is critically dependent on the timing of the maternal infection. Few infected infants escape damage following infection in the first 10 weeks after LMP (Table 13.1). Among 20 such infants followed up by the author only 2 were found to be free of rubella defects at 2 years of age. Infants infected in the first 6–8 weeks usually have multiple defects involving heart, ear and eye; hepatosplenomegaly, purpuric rash and intrauterine growth retardation may also be evident at birth. Additional defects include cerebral palsy and microcephaly, although the latter is not necessarily associated with mental retardation; over half the children with microcephaly reported to the National Congenital Rubella Surveillance Registry were reported to be of normal intelligence at follow-up (Munro *et al.* 1987). The risk of fetal damage declines progressively after the 10th week (Table 13.1) and sensorineural deafness is frequently the only manifestation (Miller *et al.* 1982; Munro *et al.* 1987). However, this is likely to be bilateral and sufficiently severe for the child to require attendance at a special school (Munro *et al.* 1987). In some cases hearing loss is progressive hence the importance of continued follow-up of congenitally infected infants despite an apparently normal auditory response during the first year of life. Intrauterine growth retardation also occurs following infection between 11 and 16 weeks but there appears to be little correlation between this type of damage and the subsequent development of deafness (Miller *et al.* 1982). Parents whose congenitally

**Table 13.1** Risk of congenital rubella defects following confirmed maternal rubella at successive stages of pregnancy*

| Stage of pregnancy (completed weeks from LMP) | Risk of defect† if infant infected: Followed up no. | Defect present: no. | Defect present: Per cent | Overall risk of pregnancy resulting in infant with rubella defect (per cent) |
|---|---|---|---|---|
| 2–10 | 20 | 18 | 90 | 90 |
| 11–12 | 12 | 6 | 50 | 34 |
| 13–16 | 36 | 12 | 33 | 17 |
| 17–18 | 15 | 1 | 7 | 3 |
| >19 | 58 | 0 | — | — |

* Overall risk of defect = Fetal infection rate (from Figure 13.4) × Risk of defect if infected

† All infants had sensorineural deafness; 8 infants infected before 8 weeks also had congenital heart disease. Data from Miller *et al.* (1982), Enders *et al.* (1988) and Communicable Disease Surveillance Centre (unpublished).

infected infant has evidence of growth retardation can therefore be reassured that his or her risk of deafness is not necessarily increased. After 16 weeks, the likelihood of severe sensorineural deafness is remote (Miller *et al.* 1982; Munro *et al.* 1987); the one child with a defect infected at 17–18 weeks in Table 13.1 had mild sensorineural deafness only. No other congenital abnormalities attributable to congenital infection after 16 weeks have been demonstrated although intrauterine growth retardation may occur. This does not persist after birth and by 2 years of age height and head circumference of such children are not significantly lower than those of control children (Miller *et al.* 1982).

## Primary asymptomatic rubella in pregnancy

The consequences for the fetus of primary rubella in which the mother remains symptom-free are less well established because of the difficulty of diagnosing such cases at the time of maternal infection. Only by investigating pregnant women who report contact with rubella can such cases be identified but, under these circumstances, it may be difficult to distinguish between an asymptomatic primary infection and a rubella reinfection. One prospective study in the UK identified 6 cases of asymptomatic primary infection in pregnancy (Cradock-Watson *et al.* 1981); in 5 cases stored sera taken some time before contact were shown to be seronegative, and in the 6th case the woman was bled 14 days after contact before rubella antibody had appeared. Three of the six women gave birth to congenitally infected infants. The finding that in over half the cases of congenital rubella reported in the UK there is no history of maternal rash is further evidence that asymptomatic infection is a significant risk to the fetus (Smithells *et al.* 1985). Clearly, when primary asymptomatic rubella is diagnosed it must be assumed that the risk to the fetus is similar to that following rubella with a rash.

## Rubella reinfection in pregnancy

Although viraemia is not thought to be a feature of reinfection, there have nevertheless been a number of published reports attributing congenital rubella to maternal reinfection in pregnancy (Morgan-Capner 1986). The most convincing of these are cases where pre-exisiting immunity in the mother has been vaccine-induced. Although such case reports demonstrate that maternal reinfection may occasionally result in fetal infection, they give no idea of the risk. The largest prospective study of the outcome of asymptomatic reinfection found no cases of serologically confirmed fetal infection among 34 pregnancies that contined to term (Cradock-Watson *et al.* 1981). Maternal reinfection was diagnosed by the detection of IgG antibody in serum samples taken before or within a few days of contact and a subsequent fourfold or greater rise in titre. Although only one of the 34 women had IgM antibody detected initially, later testing with a more sensitive IgM assay showed a low level IgM antibody response in a further 8 cases (Cradock-Watson 1985). A subsequent study of the outcome of 7 asymptomatic maternal reinfections, all of which were accompanied by an IgM response, also found no cases of intrauterine infection (Morgan-Capner *et al.* 1985a). On the available evidence therefore it is reasonable to assume that asymptomatic reinfection in pregnancy rarely gives rise to fetal infection. The absence of any documented cases of CRS in siblings other than twins supports this conclusion. However, precise information on the degree of risk is still lacking particularly on the outcome in women whose initial immunity results from vaccination; only 5 of the 41 cases described above were in confirmed vaccinees.

The occurrence of clinically apparent reinfection has been documented in pregnancy (Morgan-Capner 1986) and, although there has been no prospective study of the outcome of such cases, rash probably indicates viraemia and it is likely therefore that the fetus is at significant risk.

## Maternal rubella just before pregnancy

There have been isolated reports of possible congenital rubella following maternal infection some months before conception. However, in none of these cases was the maternal or fetal infection confirmed by adequate laboratory methods. The only prospective study of the outcome of confirmed periconceptional maternal rubella reported to date (Enders *et al.* 1988) suggests that the risk of fetal infection starts around the time of conception. Rubella before LMP does not appear to present a risk to the fetus (Figure 13.5). The earliest time after LMP that maternal rubella has been shown to result in fetal infection is 11 days (Brokelmann *et al.*

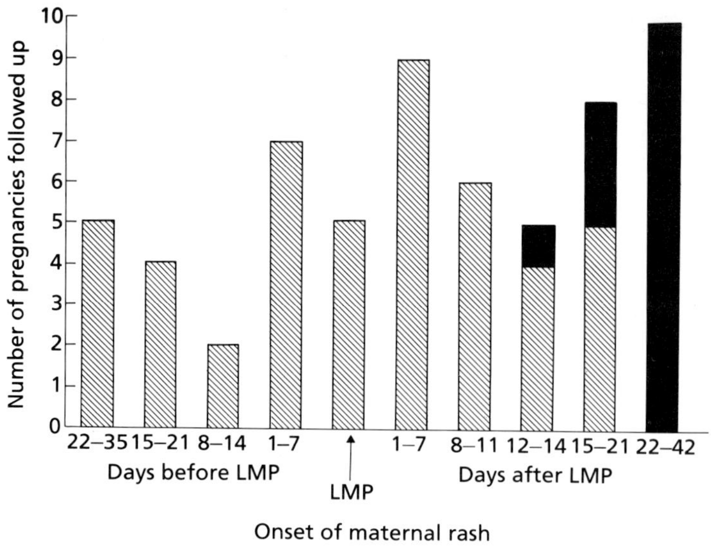


**Fig. 13.5** Outcome of confirmed symptomatic periconceptional maternal rubella. (▧) No evidence of fetal infection; (■) evidence of fetal infection.

1974). However, because of individual differences in the duration of the menstrual cycle, and in the onset of viraemia in relation to onset of rash, the possibility of fetal infection resulting from maternal rubella at shorter intervals after LMP cannot be excluded.

## Management of rash or rubella contact in pregnancy

Achieving a correct diagnosis of recent rubella or susceptibility to infection is of critical importance in deciding the management of pregnant women who present with a history of rash or contact with rubella. Because a diagnosis based on clinical evidence alone is often inaccurate, laboratory investigation of all such women is essential.

### Women presenting with a rash

Rubella-like illnesses may be caused by various agents other than rubella, for example enteroviruses and human parvovirus B19. Infections due to the latter may be particularly difficult to distinguish from rubella since they not only induce a similar rash but frequently cause arthralgia as the rash is clearing, a clinical feature which is also common to adult rubella. Serological investigation of all pregnant women presenting with a rubella-like rash is therefore essential, however typical the symptoms and signs; a study in one Public Health Laboratory showed that less than 50 per cent of such women actually had rubella (Cradock-Watson *et al.* 1973).

Some women who develop a rubella-like illness may have been screened for rubella antibody previously and reported immune. Full serological investigation is nevertheless required because of the possibility of earlier error. Among nearly 1000 pregnant women with confirmed symptomatic rubella reported to the Communicable Disease Surveillance Centre during the period 1983–87, 23 (2 per cent) had a record of immunity in their notes; 9 congenitally infected infants were identified among the 15 pregnancies that continued to term. In some cases technical or clerical errors were discovered retrospectively. However, in most cases no error was identified and it is possible that the earlier test result was a so-called false positive; this is more likely with the older haemagglutination inhibition method than with the newer method of single radial haemolysis (SRH). Where the woman has been screened more than once in the past by SRH and reported immune the possibility of earlier error or false positive result is remote. Nevertheless, it is still recommended that such women are investigated for rubella-like illnesses because of the possibility of clinically apparent rubella reinfection. Only one of the above 23 women with confirmed clinical rubella and a record of previous immunity had been tested more than once in the past. Her serological results suggested reinfection at 25 weeks gestation. Pregnancy continued to term and IgM antibody was detected in the infant.

When a pregnant woman presents with a rash, an initial blood sample should be taken as soon as possible after onset. In order for the laboratory to carry out the appropriate tests it is essential to make it clear on the request form that a diagnostic investigation is required, otherwise the usual immune status screening test may be done. Where this is SRH the result will not be quantitative and would not therefore detect a fourfold rise in titre. Also, IgM antibody detection requires special tests which are not routinely done on sera unless identified as coming from suspected rubella cases. The importance of providing adequate clinical information is demonstrated by the finding that, of 118 mothers known to have given birth to an infant with congenital rubella following the 1978/79 outbreak in England, 21 (18 per cent) had a serum sample sent to a laboratory because of rash but with insufficient information to identify the need for a diagnostic investigation. As a result only an immune status screen was done. The patient was reported to have rubella antibody present and it was assumed that she had had rubella in the past (Marshall *et al.* 1983).

The need for follow-up sera will depend on the timing of the initial sample in relation to onset of rash and on the approach taken by the virologist to the diagnosis of rubella in pregnancy. It is therefore essential to provide precise information on the date of onset of symptoms and to seek advice from the laboratory about appropriate follow-up samples. If the rash is due to rubella and the initial sample has been taken more than 5 days after onset it will usually be IgM antibody positive. Nevertheless, the virologist will often request a second sample in order to independently confirm the diagnosis by demonstrating a fourfold rise in titre. Doing this ensures that the decision to terminate a pregnancy does not rest solely on the results of a single sample. An IgM negative sample taken as late as 10 days after onset of rash does not necessarily exclude recent rubella as in some cases IgM does not appear until after the 10th day. Under these circumstances a further sample must be tested.

Occasionally a patient does not present until some weeks or months after the onset of rash; this is particularly likely if symptoms develop within a few weeks of LMP before the patient is aware that she is pregnant. Here the virologist is faced with the problem of making a retrospective diagnosis based solely on the presence or absence of rubella-specific IgM antibody; there is no particular titre of IgG antibody which can be considered diagnostic of recent infection. While the detection of IgM antibody is evidence of recent rubella, a false positive result occasionally occurs. Distinguishing between this and a low level of IgM antibody from rubella some weeks previously can be difficult. Repeat testing by alternative IgM tests and by a different laboratory is usually undertaken before a definitive diagnosis is made, again because of the knowledge that termination of pregnancy is the likely consequence of a positive laboratory report. Excluding a diagnosis of recent infection on the basis of failure to detect rubella-specific IgM antibody is hazardous if the only sample available was taken more than one month after onset of rash. While in most cases IgM antibody persists for 2–3 months, it does not do so in all; a patient who is IgG antibody positive but IgM antibody negative 6–8 weeks after a rash may well have had rubella. Unless the patient has been tested in the past, there will be no way of knowing how long the IgG antibody has been present. This circumstance will be one of the few where the decision to terminate a pregnancy may have to be made on the basis of a clinical diagnosis alone. Recently, however, it has been reported that there are qualitative differences between recently acquired and long-standing IgG antibody. Assays which measure specific IgG subclasses and the avidity of specific IgG have shown a distinction but have not been fully validated in use (Thomas & Morgan-Capner 1988).

### Women exposed to rubella-like illness during pregnancy

Clearly, contacts who claim to have had rubella in the past, even if diagnosed by a physician, cannot be reassured of their immunity without appropriate serological testing being undertaken. Those who have a documented history of previous rubella vaccination must also be investigated because of the possibility of vaccine failure which will occur in a small proportion (2–5 per cent). For the reasons described above, women who have been tested only once in the past and reported immune should also be investigated. Women previously screened on two or more occasions and found to be antibody positive by SRH can be reassured and only investigated in the event of a rash or other rubella-like symptoms developing. However, some virologists recommend investigation of all such women even if one of the earlier tests was carried out by their own laboratory in the current pregnancy, because the possibility of error can never be entirely ruled out. Given the serious clinical and medico-legal consequences that could arise in the event of an error, such a cautious approach is understandable.

An initial blood sample should be taken as soon as possible after contact. On the request form it is essential to report that the patient has been exposed to rubella otherwise the sample may be treated inadvertently as a routine immune status screen and only an SRH test performed. The patient may be inappropriately reassured that she has had rubella in the past, but unless an IgM test is performed it is not possible to exclude current asymptomatic infection. Of the 118 mothers of infants with congenital rubella described above, 6 (5 per cent) were investigated following contact but the diagnosis of asymptomatic rubella missed because inadequate clinical information was provided to suggest the need for an IgM test (Marshall *et al.* 1983). Precise information on date, duration and type of contact (e.g. casual or prolonged household contact) together with the patient's rubella vaccination history and the results of any previous rubella tests, must be given in order for the virologist to reliably interpret the test results.

If the initial sample has been taken within 10 days of a defined single contact (for example, a visit to a house where a child has rubella) it will be tested for IgG antibody and, if positive, the patient can be reassured that she has had rubella in the past. However, many virologists will also test this sample for IgM antibody, or ask for a second to exclude a fourfold rise in titre. This is in case there has been an earlier unknown contact and the IgG antibody originates from a current asymptomatic infection. Clearly, when questioning a pregnant woman who presents with a history of recent contact it is essential to establish whether there may have been an earlier exposure, particularly when rubella is known to be prevalent in the community. Testing for IgM antibody, or testing of paired sera, would always be carried out if the initial sample has been taken more than 10 days after a defined contact, or where there has been continuous exposure, for example in the home. If the patient is found to be IgG antibody negative, she must be followed up serologically for a month after the last date of exposure. Anxiety during this time may be allayed by serological investigation of the contact since his or her illness may be shown not to be due to rubella. Prophylaxis with normal human immunoglobulin is not recommended as it does not prevent infection, although it does reduce the likelihood of a rash (Anon. 1968). This may falsely reassure the woman and thereby cause a delay in obtaining follow-up samples. Patients who remain seronegative should be offered rubella vaccine post-partum.

Inevitably the investigation of pregnant contacts will identify some cases of asymptomatic reinfection, particularly in those who have been vaccinated or reported immune in the past and experience home contact with rubella. Deciding on a course of action should asymptomatic reinfection in early pregnancy be diagnosed poses considerable problems since the degree of risk, although low, is not precisely known. Also, the serological evidence may not be so clear cut that the virologist can state with absolute certainty that the patient has had a reinfection and not primary asymptomatic rubella. If the initial sample is IgG antibody negative this is consistent with a primary infection. If the initial sample is IgG antibody positive and a fourfold rise in titre is demonstrated with a low or negative IgM response, this is consistent with a reinfection. However, if the initial sample already has a good level of IgG antibody and is IgM positive this could be consistent with either a recent asymptomatic primary infection or a reinfection which produces an IgM response. Information on the amount of IgM antibody present, the time since contact, the patient's rubella vaccination history and results of any previous tests can help decide whether primary rubella or reinfection is likely but inevitably the final diagnosis will made by balancing probabilities. The anxiety generated for clinician, virologist and patient under these circumstances can be considerable. This should be borne in mind when deciding whether to investigate an asymptomatic contact who has been reported immune by a reliable test two or more times in the past, given that the real risk of repeated laboratory or clerical error must be remote.

## Prenatal diagnosis of congenital infection

Because of the high risk of fetal damage associated with early gestational primary rubella, most women choose to have a therapeutic abortion. However, when the circumstances of the maternal infection are such that there is a good chance that the fetus may escape unharmed, prenatal diagnosis of congenital infection would be of considerable help. This situation can arise when it is uncertain whether the mother has had a primary asymptomatic infection or a reinfection in early pregnancy, or when maternal rubella occurs between 12 and 16 weeks of gestation, although in the latter case, diagnosis of congenital infection does not necessarily mean a damaged baby (Table 13.1). Three methods of prenatal diagnosis have been tried: examination of amniotic fluid for rubella virus, testing of fetal blood for specific IgM antibody and examination of samples of chorionic villi for virus.

### Amniotic fluid testing

It is uncertain whether rubella virus is invariably present in the amniotic fluid of infected fetuses. The largest study to be reported (Hayes *et al.* 1982) found virus in 6 of 10 fluids from pregnancies in which primary rubella had occurred. Fetal infection was subsequently confirmed in all 6 cases by isolating virus from the products of conception or by detecting specific IgM antibody at term. There was no evidence of fetal infection in the 4 cases with rubella-negative amniotic fluid. However, in a subsequent study, virus was isolated from only 1 of 3 fluids from pregnancies where the fetus was shown to be infected (Morgan-Capner *et al.* 1985b). Whether this represents failure of the laboratory methods or genuine absence of virus in the amniotic fluid of infected fetuses is uncertain. For practical purposes, it means that deciding to continue with a pregnancy on the basis of a negative culture result is hazardous. Even when rubella virus is isolated, it may take as long as 6 weeks to grow in tissue culture by which time pregnancy will be well advanced necessitating a late termination. The practical value of amniotic fluid testing would therefore be improved by the use of a more rapid and reliable method for detecting rubella virus. The recently developed technique of nucleic acid hybridization for rubella antigen detection (Cradock-Watson *et al.* 1989), could reawaken interest in amniotic fluid testing as a means of antenatal diagnosis. Nucleic acid hybridization is both specific and rapid, and is potentially highly sensitive if augmented by the technique of polymerase chain reaction (PCR). The results of studies using these methods on amniotic fluid samples have yet to be reported.

### Fetal blood testing

Although the fetus is capable of responding to intrauterine infection by the production of specific IgM antibody, it may not appear in fetal blood until mid-gestation. This inevitably limits the practical value of this technique as a method of antenatal diagnosis. Also, it is essential to avoid contamination of the fetal sample with maternal blood otherwise a false positive result will be obtained if the mother still has IgM antibody present. The first study to be reported (Daffos *et al.* 1984) found specific IgM antibody in blood samples from 12 of 18 fetuses whose mothers' had rubella before the 18th week of pregnancy; fetal blood samples were obtained between 20–26 weeks gestation. However, one of the 6 IgM negative fetuses, bled at 20 weeks, was IgM positive at birth showing that a negative result is not reliable if sampling is carried out at this stage of pregnancy. A subsequent study showed the fetal blood samples taken as late as 23 weeks can be negative for specific IgM antibody in infants with confirmed CRS (Enders & Jonatha 1987).

### Chorionic villus sampling

The technique of chorionic villus sampling together with RNA hybridization has been used to diagnose congenital infection as early as 15 weeks gestation (Terry *et al.* 1986), and could in theory be used as early as 8–10 weeks. At present, however, there is insufficient experience with this technique to know whether infection of chorionic and fetal tissues invariably occur together. There is evidence that placental infection can occur without fetal infection from early studies on abortion material using virus isolation methods (Alford *et al.* 1964). More recently, the relationship has been studied using nucleic acid hybridization (Cradock-Watson *et al.* 1989); the results obtained are shown in Table 13.2. It is uncertain whether the disparity found in 3 of the 6 cases is genuine or arises from lack of sensitivity of the technique unless augmented by PCR.

**Table 13.2** Detection of rubella virus by nucleic acid hybridization in placentae and corresponding fetal organs obtained from 6 abortions after confirmed maternal rubella

| Weeks after LMP of maternal rubella infection | Placenta | Fetal organs |
|---|---|---|
| 4 | + | + |
| 11 | + | + |
| 17 | + | + |
| 11 | + | − |
| 19 | + | − |
| 18 | − | + |

Data from Cradock-Watson *et al.* (1989).

If the former, then chorionic villus testing could give a false positive as well as a false negative indication of fetal infection.

In summary, it is clear that no single method of prenatal diagnosis is sufficiently reliable to allow a negative result to be interpreted with confidence. A combination of methods might improve reliability, for example using chorionic villus testing as an initial screen, with subsequent amniotic fluid or fetal blood testing for those with a negative result who elect to continue with their pregnancy. However, the possibility of a false positive result with chorionic villus testing limits its value as an initial screening method. Further validation is therefore required before the results with this method alone are used to manage a pregnancy.

## Prevention of congenital rubella by vaccination

### Vaccination strategies

The objective of rubella vaccination is clear — to prevent infection during pregnancy. However, when the vaccine became available in 1969, opinions differed about the best way of achieving this. Either the vaccine could be given selectively to women to prevent them entering pregnancy susceptible to rubella, or it could be given to both sexes in early childhood to interrupt circulation of the virus and so protect susceptible pregnant women from exposure.

In the UK, the more cautious approach of selective vaccination was adopted largely because of uncertainty about the duration of vaccine-induced immunity and whether females vaccinated in the second year of life would still be protected 20–30 years later. Ideally, in a selective programme, vaccination should be delayed until just before childbearing age so that the majority of women can acquire natural immunity. However, because rubella vaccine contains live attenuated virus, there were fears about its potential teratogenicity and the consequences of inadvertent vaccination in pregnancy. It was therefore decided to vaccinate school girls aged 12–14 years; at this age about one in three are still susceptible. Since wild virus would continue to circulate freely in a selective vaccination programme, it was envisaged that boosting by natural exposure would be useful in maintaining antibody levels between school and childbearing years. It was realized that this policy would take at least 10 years before a reduction in CRS could be achieved, and vaccination of susceptible adult women was therefore introduced in 1972 in order to obtain a more rapid effect. The rationale of pre-vaccination antibody testing was to reduce the number of adult women vaccinated and therefore the number who might have to be offered an abortion if subsequently found to be pregnant.

In America, the more ambitious approach of universal vaccination was chosen largely as a result of experiencing the devastating epidemic of 1964. The epidemiology of rubella was well understood and another major epidemic was expected in the 1970s. It was realized that prevention of such an epidemic could only be achieved by vaccinating the pool of susceptible young children in the population. However, this policy was not without risk since the long-term effects of vaccination on individual immunity and on the epidemiology of the disease were unknown.

Clearly, had information been available in 1969 about the persistence of vaccine-induced immunity, the safety of the vaccine and the epidemiological effects of universal vaccination, it would have been possible to devise the most effective strategy at the outset. However, it is only through the experience gained during the last 20 years that we have learned the answers to these important questions.

## Duration of vaccine-induced immunity

Three types of rubella vaccine (HPV-77, Cendehill and RA27/3) have been used in Europe and North America, each developed from strains of virus grown in different tissue culture systems. RA27/3 is considered to be the best vaccine since the antibody responses it evokes in the serum and nasal secretions are closely similar to those produced by natural infection (Plotkin 1988). HPV-77, which was widely used in North America in the early 1970s and Cendehill, which was initially used in the UK, have now both been replaced by RA27/3.

The best evidence of the persistence of vaccine-induced immunity comes from a study in Hawaii in which antibody was detected in over 96 per cent of 1290 individuals vaccinated 16 years previously. These results are particularly encouraging for two reasons: first the vaccines used were HPV-77 and Cendehill which are considered to be less immunogenic than RA27/3 and second, the population studied lived on an island where there had been no opportunity for boosting of antibody levels by exposure to wild rubella virus since vaccination (Chu *et al.* 1988). Smaller studies in Switzerland and the UK have confirmed the persistence of vaccine-induced antibody 15–18 years after vaccination with each of the three virus strains (O'Shea *et al.* 1984; Just *et al.* 1985).

Although rubella antibody was detected in over 96 per cent of individuals in these studies, in a small proportion the concentration was below the International Unit (IU) level regarded as protective; this is taken to be 15 IU/ml in the UK and 10 IU/ml in the USA. While it is likely that low levels of vaccine-induced antibody will prevent viraemia (O'Shea *et al.* 1983), a conservative approach is often taken and revaccination recommended for those with levels below the cut-off. Inevitably there is some variation between tests, and women with levels around the cut-off who have been screened for rubella antibody several times may be reported as having antibody present on some occasions and not on others. This does not mean that the patient is immune on some occasions and susceptible on others. The fact that many such women are repeatedly vaccinated and still remain around the cut-off demonstrates that they are immune since their antibody level cannot be boosted. For this reason many virologists now report patients to be positive if a low level of rubella antibody is detected by two independent assays (PHLS 1987).

## Risk of rubella vaccination in pregnancy

Although vaccine virus can be recovered from the nasopharynx between 1 and 3 weeks after administration, there has never been any evidence that it can be transmitted to susceptible contacts (Plotkin 1988). It was clearly important to establish lack of transmissability before introducing universal vaccination of children otherwise infection of susceptible pregnant contacts might result. While this aspect of vaccine safety was quickly established, reports of a rubella-like rash in some vaccinees suggested that viraemia could occur in the second week after vaccination. It was subsequently shown that vaccine virus could be cultured from the blood between 7 and 11 days post-inoculation (Balfour *et al.* 1981). This bolstered fears that vaccination in pregnancy could lead to fetal infection and possibly congenital rubella defects.

The results of three prospective studies (Banatvala & Best 1990) in which a total of 449 seronegative women, vaccinated shortly before or after LMP, were followed up are summarized in Table 13.3. About one-third of the women were vaccinated between 1 week before to 4 weeks

**Table 13.3** Pregnancy outcome in susceptible women going to term following rubella vaccination during pregnancy or within one month before conception

| Country | Abnormalities compatible with congenital rubella | Evidence of fetal infection |
|---|---|---|
| USA | 0/267 | 6/167 (3.0%) |
| Federal Republic of Germany | 0/139 | 2/139 (1.4%) |
| UK | 0/38 | 1/32 (3.1%) |
| Sweden | 0/5 | 0/4 — |
| Total | 0/449 | 9/372 (2.4%) |

Data from Banatvala & Best (1989).

after the estimated time of conception, thereby giving rise to vaccine-induced viraemia at a stage which would coincide with the period of greatest fetal risk in the case of natural rubella. Although 2.4 per cent of infants had serological evidence of intrauterine infection, none had abnormalities compatible with congenital rubella. It is reassuring that more than half the women in these studies received RA27/3 vaccine, the strain which evokes antibody responses most similar to those produced by wild rubella virus. These results, together with the fact that there are no reports of CRS resulting from rubella vaccine despite its widespread use in women of childbearing age in many countries since 1970, show that if there is a risk of damage from the vaccine, it is so small as to be negligible. Inadvertent vaccination in pregnancy should not therefore be treated as grounds for termination. Nevertheless, as with all live vaccines, immunization of pregnant women should be avoided. It is also recommended that pregnancy is avoided for one month after rubella vaccination (DHSS 1988), to ensure that any vaccine-induced viraemia is over before LMP. Formerly, the recommended interval in the UK was 3 months but this has now been reduced because of the reassuring data on the safety of the vaccine, and the recent evidence that natural rubella before LMP does not present a risk to the fetus (Enders *et al.* 1988). However, it is important that studies continue in order to obtain further evidence of the safety of RA27/3 vaccine when given shortly after conception. Obstetricians in the UK should therefore still report cases of inadvertent vaccination before or during pregnancy to the National Congenital Rubella Surveillance Programme.

Although vaccination in pregnancy is no longer grounds for termination, screening adult women before vaccination is still recommended in the UK (DHSS 1988) since, in addition to reducing the amount of vaccine used, it also provides valuable information on the immune status of the individual woman and of the childbearing population as a whole. However, if a clinician considers that carrying out an antibody test before vaccination is likely to interfere with delivery of the vaccine (for example, the patient is unlikely to return for the result) then vaccination should be done without prior screening (DHSS 1988).

## Effect of vaccination on the epidemiology of rubella

The objective of universal vaccination is to interrupt transmission of wild rubella virus by replacing naturally-acquired with vaccine-induced immunity. Clearly, the success of this policy depends on vaccinating most of the population before the age at which they would normally get rubella. The earliest age at which vaccination can be done is 12–15 months since the presence of passively-acquired maternal antibody during the first year of life interferes with seroconversion. The rubella vaccination programme in the USA was therefore targeted at children in the second year of life and, where this opportunity was missed, at preschool children. Uptake rates in excess of 80 per cent by 5 years of age were achieved and as a result there was a substantial reduction in the incidence of natural rubella; this was most marked in the 1–4 year age group. The epidemic cycle was broken and there has been no major epidemic since universal vaccination was introduced (Bart *et al.* 1985). This alone has prevented thousands of CRS cases in the USA.

However, cases of rubella continued to occur in older age groups with outbreaks reported in colleges, military establishments and other institutions where there was a concentration of young adults. Serological surveys showed that 20–30 per cent of young adults were susceptible to rubella, an increase from the pre-vaccine era (Bart *et al.* 1985). These were individuals who were too young to have been offered rubella vaccine at the start of the programme and who then escaped natural infection because circulation of the virus had been reduced by vaccination. As a result, some cases of CRS continued to occur.

The opposite epidemiological effects were produced by selective vaccination in the UK. Vaccination of adolescent girls (of whom two-thirds were already immune) had no measurable effect on circulation of the virus in the rest of the population and rubella outbreaks continued to occur at 4–5 yearly intervals (Figure 13.6). Serological surveys showed that, although susceptibility in the antenatal population had been reduced from about 10 per cent in the pre-vaccine era to about 2–3 per cent by the mid 1980s, the number of infections in pregnancy was still unacceptably high, particularly during epidemic years (Figure 13.6) (Miller *et al.* 1985). The risk for the susceptible parous woman was shown to be especially great since her own children frequently act as a source of infection. This underlines the importance of post-partum vaccination in the prevention of rubella in pregnancy. In areas of the UK where post-partum

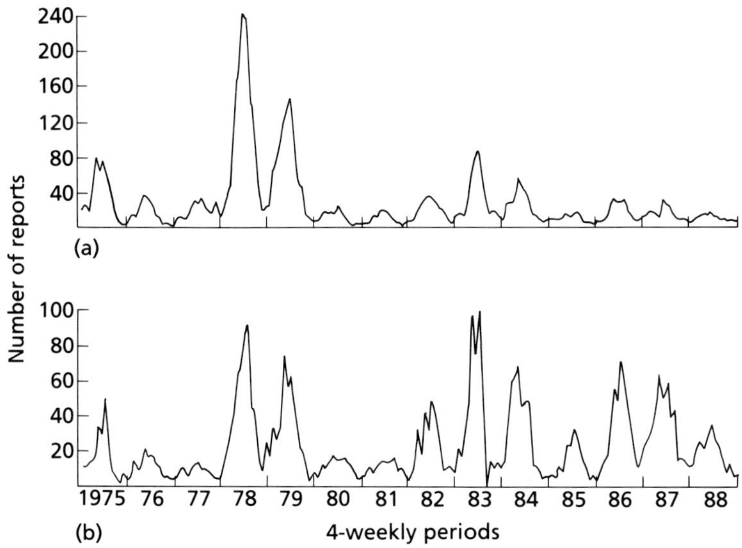


**Fig. 13.6** PHLS reports of rubella January 1975 to December 1988. (a) Pregnant women; and (b) children under 15 years.

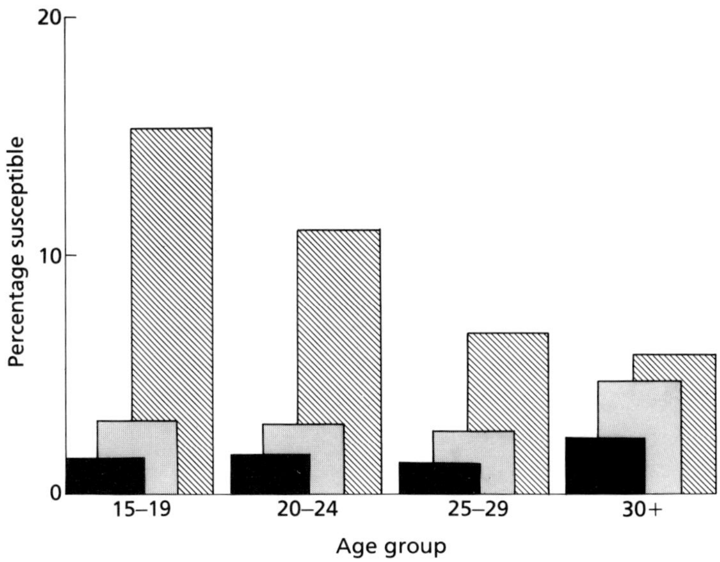


**Fig. 13.7** Rubella susceptibility in males and pregnant women according to parity. Eight public health laboratories 1985–1986. (■) Parous; (□) nulliparous; (▧) males.

vaccination is successful, susceptibility in parous women in substantially lower than in nulliparous women of the same age (Figure 13.7). Unfortunately, implementation of post-partum vaccination is variable and in some areas fewer than 5 per cent of susceptible women are vaccinated before discharge (Miller *et al.* 1985). Obstetricians who do not place a high priority on post-partum vaccination may not be aware that as many as one in 20 susceptible parous women are likely to have a confirmed rubella infection during their next pregnancy (Miller *et al.* 1985, 1987).

While there is undoubtedly room for improvement in vaccine uptake in the UK, it is now accepted that a selective vaccination programme will inevitably leave 1–2 per cent of women at risk, either because they have not been offered or have refused vaccine, or have failed to seroconvert. This means the continuing occurrence of several hundred rubella infections in pregnancy each year. The considerable anxiety and laboratory workload caused by investigation of pregnant contacts during rubella outbreaks is another inevitable consequence of leaving circulation of the virus uncontrolled.

## Achieving elimination of congenital rubella

Since it is now established that rubella vaccine is safe and produces a long-lasting immunity, it can be used with confidence and in either a selective or a universal vaccination programme. It is also established that, despite their different methods, both types of programme can produce a substantial reduction in CRS. For countries currently considering the introduction of rubella vaccination, the choice of strategy will therefore largely depend on factors such as cost of the vaccine, accessibility of the target population and facilities for appropriate epidemiological surveillance. Where there may be difficulty in achieving high vaccine uptake in young children, or in monitoring the effect of the programme, selective vaccination is the wisest choice. The single most cost-effective measure is undoubtedly the introduction of post-partum vaccination.

However, experience over the last 20 years has also shown that in order to achieve elimination of CRS, which must be the long-term objective, a combination of selective and universal vaccination is required. This was recognized early in the USA where, in 1978, the universal vaccination programme was augmented by the selective vaccination of women. Elimination targets for both acquired and congenital rubella were set and are now thought to be within reach (Bart *et al.* 1985).

More recently, the UK has followed suit with the introduction of a combined measles, mumps and rubella (MMR) vaccine for children of both sexes in place of single antigen measles vaccine in the second year of life. For the first few years of the programme, MMR vaccine is also being given to preschool children aged 4–5 years, irrespective of previous measles vaccination. This will ensure that children currently entering school have a high level of immunity to rubella and do not give rise to a susceptible cohort of young adults as happened in the USA. Where the opportunity presents itself, older children should also be given MMR vaccine although, because a higher proportion have experienced natural infection by this age (Morgan-Capner *et al.* 1988), the resulting reduction in virus circulation will be limited. This component of the programme may nevertheless be essential for the elimination of measles, mumps and rubella, which together with CRS, is now the objective in the UK. In practice, MMR vaccine should never be withheld from any child unless there is laboratory evidence of immunity to all three diseases.

The introduction of MMR vaccine in the UK is intended to augment the existing selective vaccination programme and not to replace it. Vaccination of schoolgirls will therefore continue until the present cohort of preschool children given MMR vaccine reaches adolescence. Depending on the uptake of MMR vaccine it may be necessary to keep the schoolgirl programme in place thereafter. In order to eliminate CRS, the high level of immunity that has been achieved in the UK antenatal population must be maintained. Obstetricians and gynaecologists have a key role to play in this by ensuring that no woman under their care enters her next pregnancy still susceptible to rubella. Women who catch rubella in their sixth and seventh pregnancies (Miller *et al.* 1987), or who catch rubella in a first pregnancy after being investigated for 16 years infertility (Communicable Disease Surveillance Centre, unpublished report) will hopefully not be reported again.

## References

Alford C.A., Neva F.A. & Weller T.H. (1964) Virologic and serologic studies on human products of conception after maternal rubella. *New England Journal of Medicine* **271**, 1275–81.

Anon. (1968) Studies on rubella in pregnancy. Report of the Public Health Laboratory Service Working Party on Rubella. *British Medical Journal*, **3**, 203–6.

Assaad F. & Ljungars-Esteves K. (1985) Rubella — world impact. *Reviews of Infectious Disease*, **7**, 29–35.

Balfour H.H., Groth K.E., Edelman C.K., Amren D.P., Best J.M. & Banatvala J.E. (1981) Rubella viraemia and antibody responses after rubella vaccination and reimmunisation. *Lancet*, **i**, 1078–80.

Banatvala J.E. & Best J. (1990) Rubella. In *Topley and Wilson's Principles of Bacteriology, Virology and Immunity*, 8th edn. (Ed. by L. Collier & M. Timbury)

Bart K.J., Orenstein W.A., Preblud S.R., Hinman A.R., Lewis F.L. & Williams N.M. (1985) Elimination of rubella and congenital rubella from the United States. *Pediatric Infectious Disease*, **4**, 14–21.

Brokelmann J., Niesen M., Schneweis K.E., Weitzel H. & Wolff M.H. (1974) Prakonzeptionelle roteln-hinweis auf eine besondere form der pathogenese von rotelnembryopathien. *Geburtshilfe und Frauenheilkunde*, **12**, 1007–11.

Chantler S., Evans C.J., Mortimer P.P., Cradock-Watson J.E. & Ridehalgh M.K.S. (1982) A comparison of antibody capture radio- and enzyme immunoassays with immunofluorescence for detecting IgM antibody in infants with congenital rubella. *Journal of Virological Methods*, **4**, 305–13.

Chu S.Y., Bernier R.H., Stewart J.A., Herrmann K.L., Greenspan J.R., Henderson A.K. & Liang A.P. (1988) Rubella antibody persistence after immunization. *Journal of the American Medical Association*, **259**, 3133–6.

Cooper L.Z. (1975) Congenital rubella in the United States. In *Infections of the Fetus and the Newborn Infant*, (Ed. by S. Krugman & A.A. Gershon), pp. 1–22. Alan R. Liss Inc, New York.

Cooper L.Z. & Krugman S. (1967) Clinical manifestations of postnatal and congenital rubella. *Archives of Ophthalmology*, **77**, 434–49.

Cradock-Watson J.E., Miller E., Ridehalgh M.K.S., Terry G.M. & Ho-Terry L. (1989) Detection of rubella virus in fetal and placental tissues and in the throats of neonates after serologically confirmed rubella in pregnancy. *Prenatal Diagnosis* (in press).

Cradock-Watson J.E., Ridehalgh M.K.S., Anderson M.J. & Pattison J.R. (1981) Outcome of asymptomatic infection with rubella virus in pregnancy. *Journal of Hygiene, Cambridge*, **87**, 147–54.

Cradock-Watson J.E., Ridehalgh M.K.S., Anderson M.J. & Pattison J.R. (1985) Rubella reinfection and the fetus. *Lancet*, **i**, 1039.

Cradock-Watson J.E., Ridehalgh M.K.S., Bourne M.S. & Vandervelde E.M. (1973) Nasal immunoglobulin responses in acute rubella determined by the immunofluorescent technique. *Journal of Hygiene*, **71**, 603–17.

Daffos F., Forestier F., Grangeot-Keros L., Pavlovsky M.C., Lebon P., Chartier M. & Pillot J. (1984) Prenatal diagnosis of congenital rubella. *Lancet*, **ii**, 1–3.

DHSS (1988) *Immunisation Against Infectious Diseases*. Department of Health and Social Security, Welsh Office and Scottish Home and Health Department. HMSO, London.

Enders G. & Jonatha W. (1987) Prenatal diagnosis of intrauterine rubella. *Infection*, **15**, 162–4.

Enders G., Nickerl-Pacher U., Miller E. & Cradock-Watson J.E. (1988) Outcome of confirmed periconceptional maternal rubella. *Lancet*, **i**, 1445–7.

Gregg N.M. (1941) Congenital cataract following German measles in the mother. *Transactions of the Ophthalmological Society Australia*, **3**, 35–46.

Hayes K., Ross L. & Leydon J. (1982) Experience with prenatal diagnosis of fetal rubella infection by amniocentesis. International Symposium on Recent Developments in Perinatal and Childhood Infection, Jerusalem.

Holzel H., Jones G., Smithells R.W. & Sheppard S. (1987) National Congenital Rubella Surveillance Report: Communicable Disease Report 88/15.

Iuorio J.L., Hoskings C.S. & Pyman C. (1984) Retrospective diagnosis of congenital rubella. *British Medical Journal*, **289**, 1566–8.

Just M., Just V., Berger R. Burkhadt F. & Schilt U. (1985) Duration of immunity after rubella vaccination: a longterm study in Switzerland. *Reviews of Infectious Diseases*, **7** (suppl.), 91–4.

Marshall W.C., Sheppard S., Stark O., Milton A & Smithells R.W. (1983) Rash in early pregnancy. *British Medical Journal*, **287**, 609.

Menser M.A., Hudson J.R., Murphy A.M. & Upfold L.J. (1985) Epidemiology of congenital rubella and results of rubella vaccination in Australia. *Reviews of Infectious Disease*, **7**, 37–41.

Miller C.L., Miller E., Sequeira P.J.L., Cradock-Watson J.E., Longson M. & Wiseberg E.C. (1985) Effect of selective vaccination on rubella susceptibility and vaccination in pregnancy. *British Medical Journal*, **291**, 1398–1401.

Miller C.L., Miller E. & Waight P.A. (1987) Rubella susceptibility and the continuing risk of infection in pregnancy. *British Medical Journal*, **294**, 1277–8.

Miller E. (1986) Can congenital rubella be eliminated. In *Public Health Virology*, (Ed. by P.P. Mortimer), pp. 36–49. Public Health Laboratory Service.

Miller E., Cradock-Watson J.E. & Pollock T.M. (1982) Consequences of confirmed maternal rubella at successive stages of pregnancy. *Lancet*, **ii**, 781–4.

Morgan-Capner P. (1986) Does rubella reinfection matter? In *Public Health Virology*, (Ed. by P.P. Mortimer), pp. 50–62. Public Health Laboratory Service.

Morgan-Capner P. Hodgson J., Hambling M.H., Dulake C., Coleman T.J., Boswell P.A., Watkins R.P., Booth J., Stern H., Best J.M. & Banatvala J.E. (1985a) Detection of rubella-specific IgM in subclinical rubella reinfection in pregnancy. *Lancet*, **i**, 244–6.

Morgan-Capner P., Rodeck C.H., Nicolaides K.N. & Cradock-Watson J.E. (1985b) Prenatal detection of rubella-specific IgM in fetal sera. *Prenatal Diagnosis*, **5**, 21–6.

Morgan-Capner P., Wright J., Miller C.L. & Miller E. (1988) Surveillance of antibody to measles, mumps and rubella by age. *British Medical Journal*, **297**, 770–2.

Munro N.D., Sheppard S.S., Smithels R.W., Holzel H. & Jones G. (1987) Temporal relations between maternal rubella and congenital defects. *Lancet*, **ii**, 201–4.

O'Shea S., Best J.M. & Banatvala J.E. (1983) Viraemia, virus excretion, and antibody responses after challenge in volunteers with low levels of antibody to rubella virus. *Journal of Infectious Diseases*, **148**, 639–47.

O'Shea S., Best J.M., Banatvala J.E., Marshall W.C. & Dudgeon J.A. (1984) Persistence of rubella antibody 8–18 years after vaccination. *British Medical Journal*, **288**, 1043–6.

Peckham C.S. (1972) Clinical and laboratory study of children exposed *in utero* to maternal rubella. *Archives of Disease in Childhood*, **47**, 571–7.

Peckham C.S. (1985) Congenital rubella in the United Kingdom before 1970: the prevaccine era. *Reviews of Infectious Disease*, **7**, 11–16.

PHLS (1987) Report of the Working Party on the Laboratory Diagnosis of Rubella. Public Health Laboratory Service.

Plotkin S.A. (1969) Rubella viruses. In *Diagnostic Procedures for Viral and Rickettsial Infections*, 4th edn (Ed. by E.H. Lennette & N.J. Schmidt), pp. 364–413. American Public Health Association, Washington D.C.

Plotkin S.A. (1988) Rubella vaccine. In *Vaccines*, (Ed. by S.A. Plotkin & E.A. Mortimer), pp. 235–62. W.B. Saunders, Philadelphia.

Smithells R.W., Sheppard S., Holzel H. & Dickson A. (1985) National Congenital Rubella Surveillance Programme: 1 July 1971–30 June 1984. *British Medical Journal*, **291**, 40–1.

Terry G.M., Ho-Terry L., Warren R.C., Rodeck C.H., Cohen A. & Rees K.R. (1986) First trimester prenatal diagnosis of congenital rubella: a laboratory investigation. *British Medical Journal*, **292**, 930–3.

Thomas H.I.J. & Morgan-Capner P. (1988) Rubella-specific IgG subclass avidity ELISA and its role in the differentiation between primary rubella and rubella reinfection. *Epidem Inf.*, **101**, 591–8.

Thompson K.S. & Tobin JO'H. (1970) Isolation of rubella virus from abortion material. *British Medical Journal*, **2**, 264–6.

# 14: Human immunodeficiency virus infection in pregnancy and the newborn

FRANK D. JOHNSTONE AND JACQUELINE MOK



## Virology

The acquired immunodeficiency syndrome (AIDS) was first described in 1980, and the aetiological agent soon discovered as the human immunodeficiency virus (HIV). HIV belongs to the oncovirus subfamily of retroviruses which are characterized by the production of reverse transcriptase, an enzyme which converts viral RNA into a complementary DNA copy prior to insertion into the chromosomal DNA of an infected cell. Integration of the viral genome into host genetic material means that infection is lifelong, although the integrated DNA provirus may remain latent until activated. Activation signals which are thought to trigger a latent to an active infection include chronic antigenic stimulation as well as several DNA viruses (herpes simplex virus type 1, varicella-zoster virus).

The main target for HIV is the helper subset of T lymphocytes which express the CD4 antigen on the cell membrane. Other cells which are susceptible include monocyte–macrophages in blood, alveoli and brain, follicular dendritic cells in lymph nodes and neuroglial tissue. Following acute infection and in the period prior to seroconversion, there is marked viraemia which renders the individual highly infectious in the absence of clinical evidence of disease. Thereafter, antibody production occurs and infectivity wanes until the immune system fails and the full-blown syndrome is apparent.

## Epidemiology

Currently, three global patterns of AIDS and HIV infection are described, based on the introduction and spread of the virus in a given population (Piot *et al.* 1988). Countries with pattern I include North America, many western European countries and parts of Latin America where HIV is thought to have spread extensively in the late 1970s amongst homosexual and bisexual males, and urban intravenous drug misusers (IDM) who shared infected needles. The male : female ratio is about 10 : 1, with heterosexual transmission responsible for a small, albeit increasing, percentage of cases.

Heterosexual spread is common in pattern II areas, where the male : female ratio is 1 : 1 and consequent transmission from mother to infant occurs. This pattern prevails in central, eastern and southern Africa, where HIV was introduced in the late 1970s. In pattern III areas (eastern Europe, Middle East, Asia) HIV was introduced in the 1980s, and only small numbers of cases of AIDS have been reported, mainly from individuals with sexual contact from infected persons in pattern I and II areas.

Based on a conservative estimate of about 5 million HIV infected individuals throughout the world, and using observed male : female ratios for each pattern, it is thought that about 1.5 million females are infected with HIV. Of almost 10 000 adult AIDS cases reported to the WHO Collaborating Centre on AIDS (European region) 20 per cent were IDM with about half the female cases in the 20–29 year age group. Between December 1984 and December 1987, a 20-fold increase has occurred in the proportion of heterosexual IDM with AIDS. This has serious implications for the spread of HIV into the wider, non-drug using heterosexual population, and to children through maternofetal transmission.

## HIV transmission

Although HIV has been identified in peripheral blood, cervical secretions, amniotic fluid, semen and saliva, the documented modes of spread are by sexual intercourse, parenteral exposure to infected blood, and transmission from mother to child. Initial emphasis was on receptive anal intercourse amongst homosexual men, but it is now clear that on a global basis, heterosexual vaginal intercourse is the most effective means of transmission of HIV. The risks of heterosexual transmission have not yet been evaluated, and appear to depend upon characteristics of the infected individual and sexual partner. Important co-factors which might contribute to the risk include the coexistence of other sexually transmitted diseases, the clinical state of the infected partner and the practice of anal sex. It is not known if the same rate of transmission occurs from man to woman as from woman to man.

Other modes of transmission have not been well documented, and there is no evidence that casual contact with an HIV infected person carries a risk of infection.

## Transmission from mother to child

A pregnant HIV infected woman could transmit the infection to her child during the antenatal, perinatal or postnatal period. It is likely that antenatal infection occurs, as HIV has been documented from placenta (Hill *et al.* 1987), amniotic fluid (Mundy *et al.* 1987) and from fetal tissues from mid-term abortions (Jovaisas *et al.* 1985; Sprecher *et al.* 1986). The actual timing of infection has not been established, although the description of a dysmorphic syndrome associated with paediatric AIDS suggests that infection occurs early in pregnancy (Marion *et al.* 1986). However, a causal relationship between HIV and dysmorphism has not been proven because it is difficult to separate the effects of concurrent maternal drug or alcohol abuse.

Intrauterine infection can result from physical damage to the placenta allowing passage of free virus particles; from passage of infected maternal lymphocytes to the fetus; or from actual infection of trophoblast tissue leading to secondary infection of the fetus, as occurs with congenital rubella. Preliminary data suggest that placental pathology (chorioamnionitis, vasculopathy) may correlate with HIV infection in the newborn (Nelson *et al.* 1988). The presence of HIV antigen is more difficult to detect, and two groups (Jimenez *et al.* 1988; Peuchmaur *et al.* 1988) were unable to demonstrate HIV antigen consistently from the placentae of HIV seropositive women, even in the presence of chorioamnionitis. Further studies are therefore needed to define the mechanism of maternofetal infection.

The isolation of HIV from cervical secretions (Vogt *et al.* 1986; Wofsy *et al.* 1986) and the uterine cervix (Pomerantz *et al.* 1988), together with the presence of maternal blood at delivery led to the hypothesis that perinatal infection of the fetus could be prevented by Caesarean section. Results from prospective studies (Mok *et al.* 1987; European Collaborative Study 1988) show that the mode of delivery did not influence the infection status of the child.

The infectivity of breast milk is more controversial. HIV has been isolated from the cell-free fraction of breast milk of asymptomatic infected women (Thiry *et al.* 1985), and case reports have described infants who were thought to have been infected as a result of breast feeding (Ziegler *et al.* 1985; Lepage *et al.* 1987; Weinbreck *et al.* 1988). All these infants were born to mothers who were presumed to have been infected by receiving HIV contaminated blood transfusions in the immediate postpartum period. Breast feeding then took place during seroconversion, a time when the mothers were likely to be highly infectious. The same risk may not apply to all HIV infected women. However, more convincing evidence has emerged from experience with other retroviruses, where transmission has been shown to occur through breast feeding (Ando *et al.* 1987). Where a safe alternative to breast feeding exists, it is prudent to advise against breast feeding for HIV infected women. In the developing world, however, breast feeding by the mother continues to be the method of choice irrespective of HIV status, in view of the morbidity and mortality from malnutrition and gastrointestinal infections caused by inappropriate making of bottle feeds. Changes in this method of feeding would also have serious implications on control of family size.

## Risk of maternofetal transmission

Early reports on the risk of HIV transmission from mother to child were pessimistic and probably misleading, as mothers were identified after their child was diagnosed as having AIDS (Scott *et al.* 1985; Minkoff *et al.* 1987). The results were biased by the method of case selection, since these women were presumably more advanced in the disease and hence more likely to pass the virus to their offspring. Prospective studies which have recruited all infants born to HIV seropositive women from birth (European Collaborative Study 1988) are underway, and preliminary reports reveal vertical transmission rates of 20–30 per cent.

There are also problems with the criteria used to define an infected child. HIV antibody results are unreliable in young infants, due to the presence of passively acquired maternal antibody. It was initially thought that maternal antibody would clear during the first year, and studies which reported on infection rates using only antibody testing at six months of age resulted in falsely high figures (Semprini *et al.* 1987). The present estimate is that 70 per cent of infants born to HIV positive mothers will clear maternal antibodies by 15 months of age, although in some circumstances, these can persist until 22 months.

Some infants have been documented to become HIV positive at about 20 months, having been previously HIV negative (Aiuti *et al.* 1987). Clinical manifestations of HIV infection can appear without antibody; while seronegative children can be clinically free of symptoms and have normal tests of immune function, yet have positive results on HIV antigen testing or virus culture. These diagnostic difficulties have led to other markers of infection being studied.

While antigen assays have allowed virus expression to be detected, sometimes before antibody appears, the timing of antigenaemia in perinatal infection has not been evaluated. A single negative antigen result is unhelpful, as antigen may be missed if serial samples of blood are not obtained. Peripheral blood mononuclear cells can be cultured for HIV, its presence being detected by syncytia formation, immunofluorescence, the presence of reverse transcriptase activity or of p24 antigen in the supernatant. A positive virus culture would prove that the infant is infected, but falsely negative results are common due to small sample sizes and insensitive methods. The technique of virus culture is laborious and costly, and therefore not routinely available.

Other tests that might prove useful for early diagnosis include the *in-vitro* production of HIV antibody from lymphocytes; and the polymerase chain reaction technique for amplifying HIV DNA or RNA in small numbers of infected cells (De Rossi *et al.* 1988). These methods require careful evaluation, and the clinical outlook is still unknown for children who test positive by these very sensitive methods.

Using currently available laboratory test results (persistence of HIV antibody over 15 months; HIV antigen and HIV culture) together with clinical criteria the risk of transmission from mother to child is about 30–40 per cent. Although rarely seen at birth, symptoms and signs of HIV infection usually appear within the first year of life with about 30 per cent of those infected developing AIDS or AIDS related conditions by 9 months.

## Testing and screening

While there has been controversy about HIV screening of antenatal populations, both for clinical and disease surveillance purposes, there is general agreement that women who acknowledge risk activities should be offered testing, after full counselling (Royal College of Obstetricians and Gynaecologists 1987). Experience from several centres suggests that in the early phases of an HIV epidemic most affected individuals do give a positive history. However, as the epidemic develops and spreads more widely within the heterosexual, non-drug using population, use of these risk factors becomes increasingly less sensitive. Acknowledgement or recognition of risk factors by the patient may also be incomplete. In a London study only 9 of 1500 antenatal women consented to be tested in a voluntary scheme, although 12 out of 2200 sera tested anonymously were positive (Heath *et al.* 1988). The overall result is that in some centres only a minority of HIV infected pregnant women may be discovered using selective case finding in this way. Despite an aggressive teaching and testing programme in one study in New Jersey for example, only 9 of 26 HIV positive women were identified (Connor *et al.* 1988). Each geographical area therefore needs to define its testing and screening programme in response to surveillance data or, in the absence of this, to perceived risk.

Purely from the point of view of the fetus, there are advantages in knowing the HIV status of the mother. Invasive procedures which could infect the baby, such as fetal blood sampling or applying scalp electrodes, can be avoided; breast feeding, which may also provide an occasional route for infection may be replaced by bottle feeding; and the mother can take care with any possible exposure to her own blood. Knowledge that the infant is infected can be helpful in ensuring that any other infections are treated effectively and promptly, and will also allow antiviral chemotherapy to be started at the optimal time. The case for routinely offering HIV testing to pregnant women has been persuasively argued by Minkoff & Landesman (1988).

## Pregnancy effects on HIV

There appears to be a mild immunosuppression of predominately cell-mediated type in normal pregnancy. Absolute T4 cell counts decrease slightly (Sridama *et al.* 1982; Biggar *et al.* 1988) and lymphocytic responses are decreased (Gehrz *et al.* 1981). In addition, there appears to be greater risk to pregnant women from a number of viral diseases including influenza, poliomyelitis, hepatitis, and varicella infections. The evidence for this is reviewed well by Schoenbaum *et al.* (1988). This knowledge prompted concern that pregnancy might hasten progression to AIDS, and initial studies, based on identification of women whose children had subsequently developed AIDS suggested that this did indeed occur (Scott *et al.* 1985; Minkoff *et al.* 1987). However, this is a biased method of selection, as such women are probably at a more advanced stage of disease during their pregnancy, and more recent prospective studies have not substantiated these early findings. MacCallum *et al.* (1988 and unpublished data) studied HIV infected women, some of whom had had a pregnancy since seroconversion. No adverse clinical, immunological or virological effects were found in those who had been pregnant. Similar results have been reported from other centres (Berrebi *et al.* 1988; Terragna *et al.* 1988).

At present there is no good evidence to show that pregnancy accelerates maternal progression of HIV infection. However, reported series are small, with short follow-up, and predominantly with women in the early years of infection. In addition, we do not know whether a further pregnancy carries a greater risk. This important subject therefore needs to be reassessed as more information becomes available.

## The effect of HIV on pregnancy

It is important to recognize that in most series there are other adverse factors likely to compromise pregnancy outcome. Thus our experience in Edinburgh has largely been with intravenous drug injectors, and these women have tended to be young, heavy smokers, have poor family relationships and come from deprived areas of the city. Regardless of HIV serostatus this group of women tends to have higher rates of preterm delivery, growth retardation, intrauterine death, and sudden infant death syndrome. However, HIV infected women have experienced the same rate of adverse pregnancy outcome as seronegative women tested for the same indications (Johnstone *et al.* 1988 and unpublished data). Similar findings have been reported in other controlled studies from France (Ciraru-Vigneron *et al.* 1988) though Willoughby *et al.* (1988) from New York reported more abnormal pregnancies in HIV infected women.

It seems likely that two major factors affect the relationship between HIV infection and pregnancy outcome: the presence of background risk factors (mainly involvement in the drug scene) and the clinical status of the infected woman. Current evidence from studies controlling for the former factor is not extensive, and not consistent. However, in women who are clinically well, there may be little or no additional adverse affect of being seropositive. It seems inevitable that women who are clinically ill with AIDS will have a higher probability of unfavourable outcome, but information on this is lacking.

## Antenatal supervision

All HIV infected women in pregnancy face major psychosocial problems, and doctors looking after such patients must be prepared to provide both psychological reassurance and information and advice about HIV infection. The subjects which need to be discussed are:

- The nature, course and seriousness of the infection.
- The steps which should be taken to maintain health.
  - Stopping injecting drugs.
  - Good dietary habits.
  - Avoiding other infections.
- The modes of transmission of infection.
- The prevention of transmission.
  - Safer drugs.
  - Safer sex.
  - Other general precautions with blood.
- Hospital confidentiality.
- Precautions which need to be taken to protect staff.
- Testing of sexual or needle sharing partners.
- Risks of pregnancy for the mother.
- Risks of transmission of virus to the baby.
- The infected baby's subsequent risk of AIDS.
- The option of terminating the pregnancy.

This should occur over several sessions, be supplemented by information sheets, and the woman has to know about the support systems available to her. In addition, she should be introduced to an agency geared to offer long-term support and clinical follow-up.

Termination of pregnancy is clearly an option that many women will consider, and in our recent experience 50 per cent of women who know themselves to be seropositive for HIV early in pregnancy do have an abortion. This has been discussed (Johnstone 1988) but is outside our present subject.

Early pregnancy assessment should include general physical examination, and estimates of full blood count, T4 count, HIV antigen and p24 antibody. From this some prediction of the stage of HIV disease is possible. Women who continue their pregnancy should be reassessed immunologically and virologically at intervals and there has to be high awareness of symptoms which could mean progression to clinical illness. Many symptoms are non-specific however and may easily be dismissed as due to pregnancy, as discussed by Minkoff *et al.* (1986) who report three cases of *Pneumocystis carinii* pneumonia in pregnancy with subsequent maternal death. Some of the clinical and laboratory predictors of progression to AIDS are shown in Table 14.1

*Pneumocystis carinii* pneumonia is the most common presentation of AIDS, particularly in drug users. The most typical presentation is with slowly progressive dyspnoea, often with a dry cough, and sometimes mild pleuritic chest pain. Examination of the chest may show little

**Table 14.1** Clinical and laboratory predictors of progression to AIDS

| |
|---|
| *Clinical predictors of progression to AIDS* |
| Persistent oral candidal infections |
| Weight loss |
| Fever |
| Diarrhoea |
| Seborrhoeic dermatitis |
| Hairy cell leukoplakia of the tongue |
| |
| *Laboratory predictors of progression to AIDS* |
| Normochromic anaemia |
| Leukopenia |
| Low platelet count |
| Low T4 lymphocytes |
| Decline in antibody to p24 (core protein) |
| Reappearance of HIV antigenaemia |
| Raised $\beta_2$-microglobulin |

abnormality but there is usually a low grade fever and there may be other stigmata of AIDS such as oral candidasis; a chest X-ray may be negative or show a perihilar haze, progressing to diffuse shadowing of the mid and lower zones (Weber & Pinching 1985). Progress of the disease may be fulminating and the first four cases reported in pregnancy all resulted in death of the mother during the initial infective episode (Jensen *et al.* 1984; Minkoff *et al.* 1986). The standard treatment is parenteral co-trimoxazole in high doses, and for prolonged periods, because of the difficulty of eradicating the organism (Wharton *et al.* 1986). Although there are theoretical concerns about the safety of this drug in pregnancy (trimethoprim is a folate antagonist), published studies have failed to demonstrate an increase in fetal abnormalities or risk (Briggs *et al.* 1983). Sulphonamides compete with bilirubin for binding to plasma albumin, but although hyperbilirubinaemia and kernicterus are well known to occur when sulphonamides are given directly to the newborn, kernicterus in babies has never been reported after *in utero* exposure. In any case the seriousness of the maternal risk with *Pneumocystis carinii* pneumonia makes treatment mandatory regardless of the stage of pregnancy. Pentamidine is a second line drug usually used when treatment with co-trimoxazole is unsuccessful. Little is known about its effect in pregnancy, but it can be given with a nebulizer so that systemic absorption is minimal, and this may be preferable to high dose co-trimoxazole immediately before delivery. HIV infected women who are immunocompromised are also at higher risk of episodes of herpes simplex infection, toxoplasmosis and cytomegalovirus which all have profound implications for the fetus. Treatment of these conditions in the context of HIV infection is well discussed by Feinkind & Minkoff (1988) who recommend that baseline antibody titres to toxoplasmosis and cytomegalovirus should be obtained in early pregnancy to assist in maternal or neonatal diagnosis if there are later symptoms. Azidothymidine (AZT, Retrovir) is of proven value in the treatment of AIDS and is now being given to infected individuals who are asymptomatic but who have unfavourable immunological or virological features. There is currently no information on its use in human pregnancy.

As far as general obstetric care is concerned, HIV infected women, most of whom in our experience have been intravenous drug injectors, may be at greater risk of sexually transmitted disease, and swabs should be taken to exclude, particularly, gonorrhoea and *Chlamydia trachomatis*. Such patients in our experience also have high default rates from clinics, and antenatal care must involve good communication between hospital staff, patient and community services. There often needs to be an intensive social work involvement. In late pregnancy the index of suspicion of intrauterine growth retardation should be high, and antenatal fetal monitoring should be instituted readily.

Continuing drug use is a problem. Narcotics do appear to retard fetal growth, both in women and in experimental studies in animals, and as preterm delivery is also more common, the combined effect is that the rate of low birth weight is around 30 per cent in most large series (Stone *et al.* 1971; Newman *et al.* 1975; Connaughton *et al.* 1979; Ostrea & Chafez 1979). There is also a tendency to fetal asphyxia as suggested by the high incidence of meconium staining of the amniotic fluid, fetal distress in labour, low Apgar scores, and aspiration pneumonia in this group of infants (Ostrea & Chavez 1979). Cocaine use also seems to be associated with adverse pregnancy outcome (Chasnoff *et al.* 1985).

Ideally, the patient should withdraw from all drugs during pregnancy, and some women are willing to attempt this. It is widely believed that sudden cessation of drug use may cause fetal distress or even death (Finnegan 1978). This belief is based on theoretical considerations of the effects of fetal withdrawal, the demonstration of raised noradrenaline levels in the amniotic fluid of a patient being detoxified in the third trimester of pregnancy (Zuspan *et al.* 1975) and several antedotal reports of fetal death (Rementaria & Nunag 1973; Zuspan *et al.* 1975; Finnegan 1978). Though not all authors agree (Hepburn & Forrest 1988), it seems prudent to attempt methadone substitution and gradual reduction as described by Finnegan (1978) rather than acute detoxification, particularly in the second or third trimester. If stopping drugs is unacceptable to the patient, then maintenance with oral methadone linctus is preferable to injecting street drugs, and for the occasional patient who insists on continuing to inject, the risk of other infections and transmission of HIV can be minimized by asking her to stop sharing equipment and supplying her with sterile needles and syringes on an exchange basis.

There is no way at present of knowing whether a baby is infected *in utero*. Management therefore has to minimize risk of infection, and invasive procedures such as chorion villus sampling, cordocentesis, fetal blood sampling or attachment of a scalp electrode should be avoided if at all possible. Theoretically, such procedures could expose the fetus to maternal cells containing virus and thus infect an otherwise non-infected baby. Amniocentesis is likely to pose a much lesser risk, but again should be performed only after balancing the risks involved carefully.

## Delivery

As already discussed, there is at present no good evidence to suggest that elective Caesarean section can reduce the likelihood of the fetus being infected. Nevertheless, this has been suggested (Chiodo *et al.* 1986) and this important subject needs to be reviewed as more information becomes available. Currently, vaginal delivery should be the aim, and indeed most of our patients have delivered quickly and with a minimum of obstetric interference. Management of labour is changed little by HIV serostatus, but premature rupture of the membranes, which may occur more commonly, should probably also be treated more aggressively, antibiotics being used more readily in the immune compromised woman, while scalp electrodes and fetal blood sampling should be avoided.

Finally, maximum caution should be taken by the obstetric and midwifery staff to avoid contact with infected blood. Although even needlestick injury appears to pose only a small statistical risk of infection (less than 1 per cent; Henderson *et al.* 1986), the calamitous consequences of being infected mandate that 'no reasonably avoidable risk is acceptable' (Hudson 1988, who deals well with this important aspect of care). Reports of cases of seroconversion in health workers after exposure of intact skin only emphasize that maximum precautions are warranted (Anon. 1987).

## Future care

Postnatal care is outside the remit of our subject, but careful follow-up of both mother and baby is essential. Where bottle feeding is safe, this method should be advised because of the risk of infecting the baby, as discussed earlier. Discussions about contraception, and advice about prevention of transmission of infection to the new baby should occur.

## References

Aiuti F., Luzi G., Mezzaroma I., Scano G. & Papetti C. (1987) Delayed appearance of HIV infection in children. *Lancet*, **ii**, 858.

Ando Y., Nakano S., Saito K. *et al.* (1987) Transmission of adult T-cell leukaemia retrovirus (HTLVI) from mother to child: comparison of bottle with breastfed babies. *Japanese Journal of Cancer Research*, **78**, 322–4.

Anon. (1987) Update: Human immunodeficiency virus infections in health care workers exposed to blood of infected patients. *Morbidity and Mortality Weekly Report*, **36**, 285–9.

Berrebi A., Puel J., Tricoire J. *et al.* (1988) The influence of pregnancy on the evolution of HIV infection. IV International Conference on AIDS, Abstract no. 4041, Book 1, p. 270.

Biggar R.J., Pahwa S., Landesman S. & Goedert J.J. (1988) Helper and suppressor lymphocytic changes in HIV-infected mothers and their infants. IV International Conference on AIDS, Abstract no. 4031, Book 1, p. 267.

Briggs G.G., Bodendorfer T.W., Freeman R.K. & Yaffe S.J. (1983) *Drugs in Pregnancy and Lactation*, pp. 365–66. Williams and Wilkins, Baltimore.

Brossard Y., Goudeau A., Larsen M. *et al.* (1988) A sero-epidemiological study of HIV in 15465 pregnant women screened in Paris area between Feb. 1987 and Oct. 1987. IV International Conference on AIDS, Abstract no. 4632, Book 2, p. 219.

Chasnoff I.J., Burns W.J., Schnoll S.M. & Burns K.A. (1985) Cocaine use in pregnancy. *New England Journal of Medicine*, **313**, 666–9.

Chiodo F., Ricchi E. & Costigliola P. (1986) Vertical transmission of HTLV III. *Lancet*, **i**, 739.

Ciraru-Vigneron N., Nguyen Tan Lung R., Bercau G. *et al.* (1988) Prospective study for HIV infection among high risk pregnant women. IV International Conference on AIDS, Abstract no. 4627, Book 2, p. 218.

Connaughton J.F., Reeser D. & Finnegan L.P. (1977) Pregnancy complicated by drug addiction. *Perinatal Medicine*,

Connor E., Goode L., Morrison S. *et al.* (1988) Seroprevalence of human immunodeficiency virus (HIV) of parturients at University Hospital, New Jersey, USA. IV International Conference on AIDS, Abstract no. 6085, Book 1, p. 375.

De Rossi A., Amadori A., Chieco-Bianci L. *et al.* (1988) Polymerase chain reaction and *in-vitro* antibody production for early diagnosis of paediatric HIV infection. *Lancet*, **ii**, 278.

European Collaborative Study. (1988) Mother to child transmission of HIV infection. *Lancet*, **ii**, 1039–43.

Feinkind L. & Minkoff H.L. (1988) HIV in pregnancy. *Clinics in Perinatology*, **15**, 189–202.

Finnegan L.P. (1978) Management of pregnant drug-dependent women. *Annals of the New York Academy of Sciences*, **311**, 135–46.

Gehrz R.C., Christianson W.R., Linner K.M. *et al.* (1981) A longtitudinal analysis of lymphocyte proliferative responses to mitogens and antigens during human pregnancy. *American Journal of Obstetrics and Gynecology*, **140**, 665–70.

Heath R.B., Grint P.C.A. & Hardiman A.E. (1988) Anonymous testing of women attending antenatal clinics for evidence of infection with HIV. *Lancet*, **i**, 1394.

Henderson D.K., Saah A.J., Zak B.J. *et al.* (1986) Risk of nosocomial infection with human T-cell lymphotropic virus type III/lymphadenopathy-associated virus in a large cohort of intensively exposed health care workers. *Annals of Internal Medicine*, **104**, 644–7.

Hepburn M. & Forrest C.A. (1988) Does infection with HIV affect the outcome of pregnancy? (letter to Editor). *British Medicial Journal*, **296**, 934.

Hill W.C., Bolton V. & Carlson J.R. (1987) Isolation of acquired immunodeficiency syndrome virus from the placenta. *American Journal of Obstetrics and Gynecology*, **157**, 10–11.

Hudson C.N. (1988) Special precautions in delivery suites and operating theatres for normal labour and delivery and operative delivery including episiotomy. In *AIDS and Obstetrics. Proceedings of the Nineteenth Study Group of the Royal College of Obstetricians and Gynaecologists*, (Ed. by C.N. Hudson & F. Sharp), pp. 189–92. The Peacock Press.

Jensen L.P., O'Sullivan M.J., Gomez-del-Rio M. *et al.* (1984) Acquired immunodeficiency (AIDS) in pregnancy. *American Journal of Obstetrics and Gynecology*, **148**, 1145–6.

Jimenez E., Unger M., Vogel M. *et al.* (1988) Placental morphology in HIV positive pregnancies. IV International Conference on AIDS, Abstract no. 6586, Book 2.

Johnstone F.D. (1988) Termination of pregnancy. In *AIDS and Obstetrics. Proceedings of the Nineteenth Study Group of the College of Obstetricians and Gynaecologists, 1988*, (Ed. by C.N. Hudson & F. Sharp), pp. 151–6. The Peacock Press.

Johnstone F.D., MacCallum L., Brettle R., Inglis J.M. & Peutherer J.F. (1988) Does infection with HIV affect the outcome of pregnancy? *British Medicial Journal*, **296**, 467.

Jovaisas E., Koch M.A., Schafer A., Stauber M. & Lowenthal D. (1985) LAV/HTLVIII in 20 week fetus. *Lancet*, **ii**, 1129.

Lepage P., Van de Perre P., Carael M. *et al.* (1987) Postnatal transmission of HIV from mother to child. *Lancet*, **ii**, 400.

MacCallum L.R., France A.J., Jones M.E. *et al.* (1988) The effects of pregnancy on the progression of HIV infection. IV International Conference on AIDS, Abstract no. 4032, Book 1, p. 267.

Marion R., Wizna A.A., Hutcheon R.G. & Rubinstein A. (1986) Human T-cell lymphotropic virus type III (HTLVIII) embryopathy. *American Journal of Diseases of Children*, **140**, 638–40.

Minkoff H., de Regt. R.H., Landessman S. *et al.* (1986) *Pneumocystis carinii* pneumonia associated with acquired immunodeficiency syndrome in pregnancy: a report of three maternal deaths. *Obstetrics and Gynecology*, **67**, 284–7.

Minkoff M. & Landesman S.H. (1988) The case for routinely offering prenatal testing for human immunodeficiency virus. *American Journal of Obstetrics and Gynecology*, **159**, 793–6.

Minkoff H., Nanda D., Menez R. *et al.* (1987) Pregnancies resulting in infants with acquired immunodeficiency syndrome or AIDS related complex. *Obstetrics and Gynecology*, **69**, 285–7.

Mok J.Q., Giaquinto C., De Rossi A., Grosch-Worner I., Ades A.E. & Peckham C.S. (1987) Infants born to mothers seropositive for human immunodeficiency virus. *Lancet*, **i**, 1164–8.

Mundy D.C., Schinazi R.F., Gerber A.R., Nahmias A.J. & Randall H.W. (1987) Human immunodeficiency virus isolated from amniotic fluid. *Lancet*, **ii**, 459–60.

Nelson A.M., Anderson V., Ryder R. *et al.* (1988) Placental pathology as a predictor of perinatal HIV infection in infants born to HIV seropositive women in Kinshasa, Zaire. IV International Conference on AIDS, Abstract no. 6585, Book 2.

Newman R.G., Bashkow S. & Calko D. (1975) Results of 313 consecutive live births of infants delivered to parents in the New York City Methadone Maintenance Treatment programme. *American Journal of Obstetrics and Gynecology*, **121**, 233–7.

Ostrea E.M. & Chavez C.J. (1979) Perinatal problems (excluding neonatal withdrawal) in maternal drug addiction. A study of 830 cases. *Journal of Pediatrics*, **94**, 292–5.

Peuchmaur M., Pons J.C., Vazeu R., Brossard Y., Papiernik E. & Delfraissy J.F. (1988) Prospective study for immunodetection of HIV viral proteins in 55 placentas. IV International Conference on AIDS, Abstract no. 6587, Book 2.

Piot P., Plummer F.A., Mhalu F.S., Lamboray J.L., Chin J. & Mann J.M. AIDS: An international perspective. *Science*, **239**, 573–9.

Pomerantz R.J., de la Monte S.M., Donegan S.P. *et al.* (1988) Human immunodeficiency virus (HIV) infection of the uterine cervix. *Annals of Internal Medicine*, **108**, 321–7.

Rementeria J.L. & Nunag N.N. (1973) Narcotic withdrawal in pregnancy: stillbirth incidence with a case report. *American Journal of Obstetrics and Gynecology*, **116**, 1152–6.

Royal College of Obstetricians and Gynaecologists (1987) Report of the RCOG Subcommittee on problems associated with AIDS in relation to Obstetrics and Gynaecology.

Schoenbaum E.E., Davenny K. & Selwyn P.A. (1988) The impact of pregnancy on HIV-related disease. In *AIDS and Obstetrics. Proceedings of the Nineteenth Study Group of the Royal College of Obstetricians and Gynaecologists*, (Ed. by C.N. Hudson & F. Sharp) pp. 65–75. The Peacock Press.

Scott G.B., Fischl M.A., Klimas N. *et al.* (1985) Mothers of infants with the acquired immunodeficiency syndrome. *Journal of the American Medical Association*, **253**, 363–6.

Semprini A.E., Vucetich A. Pardi G. & Cossu M.M. (1987) HIV infection and AIDS in newborn babies of mothers positive for HIV antibody. *British Medical Journal*, **294**, 610.

Skinnider L.F. & Laxdal V. (1981) The effect of progesterone, oestrogen, and hydrocortisone on the mitogenic response of lymphocytes to phytohaemagglutinin in pregnant and non-pregnant women. *British Journal of Obstetrics and Gynaecology*, **88**, 1110–14.

Sprecher S., Soumenkoff G., Puissant F. & Degueldre M. (1986) Vertical transmission of HIV in 15 week fetus. *Lancet*, **ii**, 288–9.

Sridama V., Pacini, F., Yang S.L. *et al.* (1982) Decreased levels of helper T cells — a possible cause of immunodeficiency in pregnancy. *New England Journal of Medicine*, **307**, 352–6.

Stone M.L., Salerno L.J., Green M. & Zelson C. (1971) Narcotic addiction in pregnancy. *American Journal of Obstetrics and Gynecology*, **109**, 716–23.

Terragna A., De Maria A., Sampietro F. *et al.* (1988) Perinatal HIV infection: evaluation of the risk for mother and child. IV International Conference on AIDS, Abstract no. 4028, Book 1, p. 266.

Thiry 1, Sprecher-Goldberger S., Jonckheer T. *et al.* (1985) Isolation of AIDS virus from cell-free breast milk of three healthy virus carriers. *Lancet,* **ii**, 891–2.

Vogt M.W., Witt D.J., Craven D.E. *et al.* (1986) Isolation of HTLV III/LAV from cervical secretions of women at risk for AIDS. *Lancet,* **i**, 525–7.

Weber J. & Pinching A. (1985) The clinical management of AIDS and HTLV III infection. In *The Management of AIDS Patients,* (Ed. by J. Miller, J. Weber & J. Green), pp. 1–33. MacMillan Press, London.

Weinbreck P., Loustaud V., Denis F., Vidal B., Mounier M. & DeLumley L. (1988) Breastfeeding in the transmission of HIV infection. *Lancet,* **i**, 482.

Wharton M., Coleman D.L., Fitz G. *et al.* (1986) Trimethoprim–sulphamethiazole or pentamidine for *Pneumocystis carinii* pneumonia in AIDS. *Annals of Internal Medicine,* **105**, 37–44.

Willoughby A., Mendez H., Hittelman J. *et al.* (1988) Epidemiology of the perinatal transmission of Human Immunodeficiency Virus (HIV). IV International Conference on AIDS, Abstract no. 6588, Book 2, p. 293.

Wofsy C.B., Cohen J.B., Hauer L.B. *et al.* (1986) Isolation of AIDS-associated retrovirus from genital secretions of women with antibodies to the virus. *Lancet,* **i**, 527–9.

Ziegler J.B., Cooper D.A., Johnson R.O. & Gold J. (1985) Postnatal transmission of AIDS associated retrovirus from mother to infant. *Lancet,* **i**, 896–9.

Zuspan F.P., Gumpel J.A., Mejia-Zelaya A. *et al.* (1975) Fetal stress from methadone withdrawal. *American Journal of Obstetrics and Gynecology,* **122**, 43–6.

# 15: Chorion villus sampling

RICHARD WARREN



Although it is every parent's wish that their baby be born free from abnormality or handicap, sadly still over 2 per cent of liveborn babies are born with a significant congenital or inherited disorder. Most disorders arise unexpectedly, without a relevant family or obstetric history. However, a small number of parents, an estimated 7 per cent of the population, are at particular risk of fetal abnormality, and as such should be offered the available methods of prenatal diagnosis (Table 15.1).

The development of safe and accurate techniques of prenatal diagnosis (Table 15.2) is one of the most important areas of advance in medicine and the introduction of ultrasound by Donald in the late 1950s is undoubtedly one of the greatest milestones. Ultrasound is the backbone of all forms of prenatal diagnosis, being able to detect fetal structural abnormalities of only a few millimetres in size. It also allows the accurate and safe guidance of invasive techniques such as amniocentesis or biopsy of placental or fetal tissue for those conditions, often without structural defect, which require tissue analysis for diagnosis.

Advances in the field of medical genetics have progressed as rapidly as advances in clinical techniques. Following the use of the amniotic fluid cell's Barr bodies for fetal sexing to detect the risk of X-linked conditions (Serr *et al.* 1955) there has been a relentless progression in scientific and clinical skills. The use of second trimester amniocentesis is well established and is widely available with proven accuracy and safety. The wait to 15 weeks gestation before amniocentesis and the further delay for

**Table 15.1** Prenatal diagnosis: techniques

| |
|---|
| Ultrasound |
| Amniocentesis |
| Fetoscopy |
| Cordocentesis |
| Chorion villus biopsy |

**Table 15.2** Historical landmarks in prenatal diagnosis

| | | |
|---|---|---|
| 1955 | Amniotic cell Barr body determination | (Serr) |
| 1966 | Amniocytes cultured | (Steele) |
| 1967 | Fetal karyotyping by amniocentesis | (Jacobson) |
| 1968 | First attempts at chorion biopsy | (Hahnemann) |
| 1972 | Amniotic fluid AFP and neural tube defects | (Brock) |
| 1972 | Ultrasound diagnosis of anencephaly | (Campbell) |
| 1974 | Fetal blood sampling | (Hobbins) |
| 1976 | DNA prenatal diagnosis of alpha-thalassaemia | (Kan) |
| 1982 | Prenatal diagnosis by chorion biopsy | (Kazy) |

tissue analysis has, however, led to the search for a successful and safe early method of prenatal diagnosis. Recent advances in chorion villus sampling mean that for many congenital disorders there is now an early, first trimester, alternative. For most patients early prenatal diagnosis brings early reassurance but for those unfortunate few with an affected fetus a simpler and safer therapeutic abortion may be offered at a time when the patient is not visibly pregnant and before the mother's perception of fetal movements.

## Embryonic development

After fertilization the zygote develops as an inner and outer cell mass. The embryo develops from the inner cell mass whereas chorionic villi develop from the trophoblast cells of the outer cell mass. Initially, chorionic villi surround the blastocyst but gradually, by 14 weeks of gestation, those at the implantation site develop and proliferate to form the placenta (chorion frondosum) whereas those opposite degenerate to form the smooth chorion (chorion laeve). Placental biopsy, or chorion villus sampling, refers to the biopsy of the developing chorion frondosum and is a means of obtaining tissue which is representative of the genetic makeup of the fetus without biopsy of the developing embryo itself.

Much research has occurred, and is still continuing, into the development and assessment of biopsy techniques and into the analysis of chorionic villi in an attempt to provide reliable and safe early prenatal diagnosis.

## History

Although placental biopsy was first evaluated in 1958 for the rapid diagnosis of hydatidiform mole (Acosta-Sison 1958) it was Hahnemann & Mohr (1968) who first started work on chorionic villus sampling for genetic, prenatal diagnosis reporting a transcervical endoscopic method for fetal membrane biopsy under direct visual control. Subsequently, further series were described using similar techniques, but endoscopic biopsy failed on several counts: it required considerable operator skill, success at achieving chromosome analysis was poor, the risk of complication high and the diameter of the endoscope used often required cervical dilatation and anaesthesia. Following this early experience interest in chorion villus sampling waned as the then new technique of amniocentesis developed rapidly into a widely accepted, reliable and safe method of prenatal diagnosis.

In 1975, following a programme of intensive population control in China allowing fetal sex selection, a report from the Tietung Hospital, Anshan described a transcervical aspiration biopsy technique using a rigid metal cannula blindly inserted through the cervix into the developing placenta without guidance by endoscope or ultrasound. This simple technique was highly successful at fetal sex determination using Barr body identification. The fetal loss rate was low, less than 6 per cent, and the continuing pregnancies were delivered at term without maternal

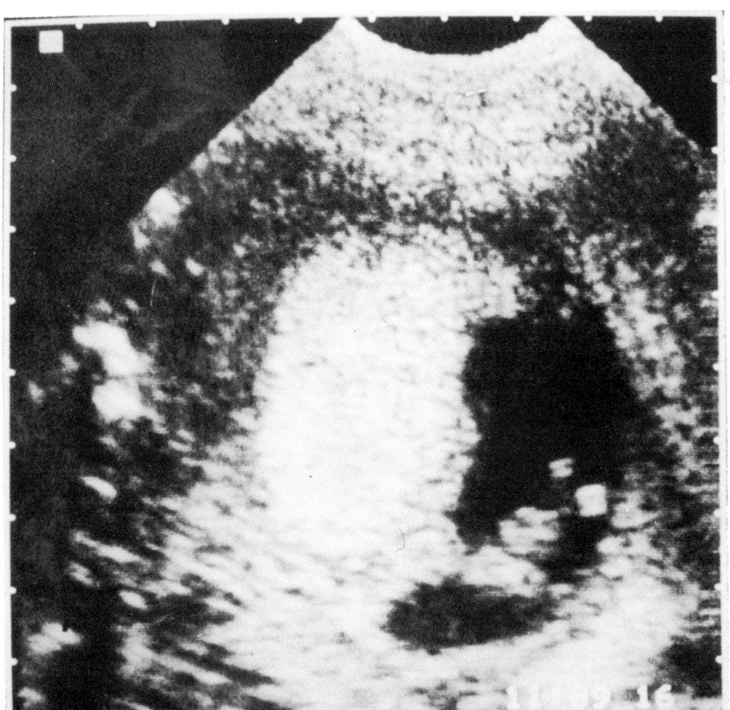

**Fig. 15.1** An ultrasound picture of a pregnancy at 10 weeks gestation. The chorion frondosum is clearly visible and well localized.

or fetal complication. Such success encouraged further research into chorion villus sampling.

It was the use of ultrasound allowing localization of the placenta (Figure 15.1) and accurate biopsy (Kazy *et al.* 1982) which heralded improved success with fewer complications. Subsequently, many different biopsy techniques have been used successfully for prenatal diagnosis (Fraccaro *et al.* 1984). Biopsy may be achieved transabdominally using a needle for aspiration (Smidt-Jensen & Hahnemann 1984) or transcervically using biopsy forceps (Kazy *et al.* 1982) or with an aspiration cannula (Rodeck *et al.* 1983; Ward *et al.* 1983). Whichever method is employed ultrasound guidance has been shown to be essential for successful and safe biopsy.

## Timing

The desire for early prenatal diagnosis led to the assessment of placental biopsy or chorion villus sampling techniques from as early as 7 weeks gestation. Apart from the difficulties of arranging referral so early in pregnancy, at this stage the implantation site is poorly localized and thin, making accurate biopsy very difficult. As well as this major technical reason against early biopsy this is the time of rapid embryonic development and disturbance of the placenta theoretically risks fetal damage.

Early research suggested that biopsy after 12 weeks gestation was associated with increased fetal loss. The reason for this was unclear but it may reflect the technical difficulties of transcervical sampling when the uterus is larger and the placenta more inaccessible. As well as this, it has been suggested that around this time there is a morphological change in the structure of the placenta making biopsy more difficult to achieve. However, further experience with transcervical chorion villus sampling beyond 12 weeks has not been associated with increased fetal loss. Nevertheless, the transabdominal route has advantages and is preferred as gestation advances.

## Methods

### Transcervical

The transcervical technique of placental biopsy was the first method to gain clinical application (Old *et al.* 1982) and has until recently been the most popular mode of chorion villus sampling.

Although transcervical endoscopic guided biopsy and ultrasound guided biopsy using forceps (Figure 15.2) have been used, the greatest experience and most favoured method has been aspiration biopsy using a malleable plastic (Ward *et al.* 1983) or metal cannula (Rodeck *et al.* 1983) (Figure 15.3) guided by ultrasound. This simple out-patient technique requires neither local anaesthesia nor sedation. Careful and detailed

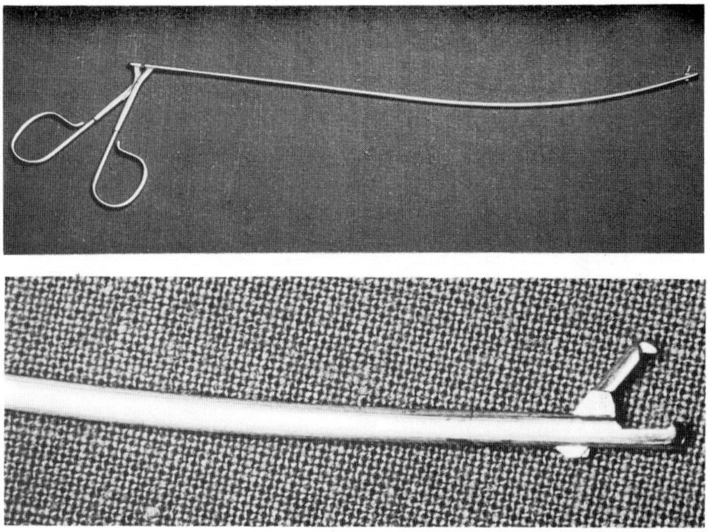

**Fig. 15.2** Transcervical biopsy forceps (RM Surgical Developments).

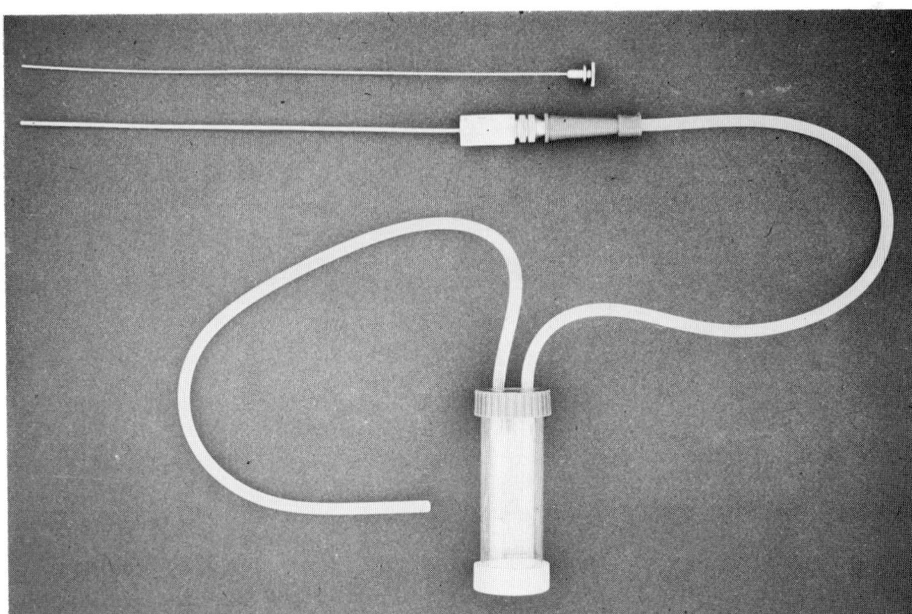

**Fig. 15.3** The King's College Hospital Silver Cannula (Downs plc) for single operator transcervical chorion villus sampling.

ultrasound scanning using a high resolution real-time scanner confirms gestation and viability as well as excluding multiple pregnancies, fibroids, uterine contractions and evidence of placental or membrane separation. The position of the uterus, the implantation site, and its relation to the cervix is confirmed so that the passage of the cannula can be planned. The patient is made comfortable in the lithotomy position on a col-

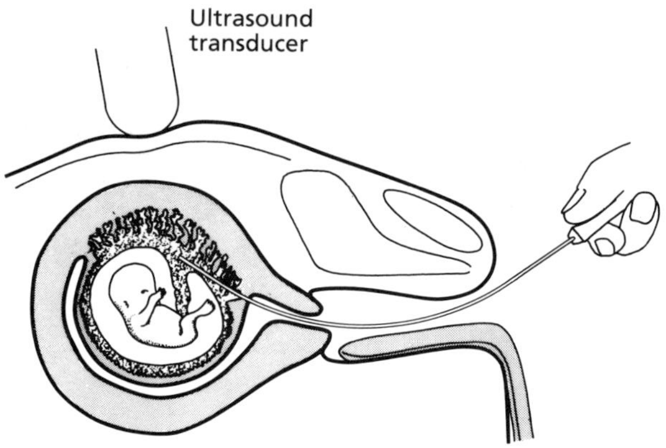


**Fig. 15.4** Ultrasound guided transcervical aspiration chorion villus sampling.

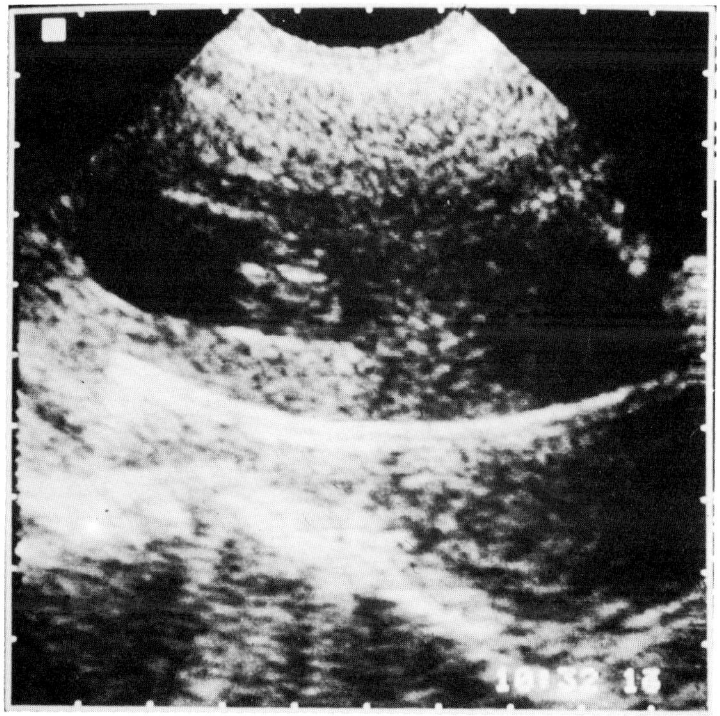

**Fig. 15.5** The King's College Hospital Silver Cannula is highly echogenic and can be seen clearly entering the chorion frondosum.

poscopy couch. Thorough cleansing of the inner thighs, vulva, vagina and cervix is performed to minimize any potential risk of infection. The malleable cannula is bent to the required shape and introduced gently into the cervical canal under ultrasound guidance (Figure 15.4). The cannula is carefully advanced around the gestation sac into the implantation site (Figure 15.5). Aspiration using a syringe or vacuum pump achieves placental biopsy.

## Transabdominal

Transabdominal needle aspiration biopsy (Smidt-Jensen & Hahnemann 1984) has recently been developed as an alternative to the transcervical method and is rapidly gaining in popularity. This route avoids the potential risk of transmitting cervical infection and offers technical advantages as gestation advances.

During the first trimester the rapid growth of the uterus soon brings it into contact with the maternal anterior abdominal wall through which biopsy may be achieved. Although a double or single needle technique may be used with or without a biopsy guide, the freehand double needle technique has advantages. Under local anaesthesia, a 17 gauge needle with stilette is inserted through the abdominal wall and its passage guided by ultrasound through the uterine wall to reach the edge of the placenta (Figure 15.6). The stilette is removed and a smaller, 19 gauge, needle is threaded down inside the first (Figure 15.7) and advanced into

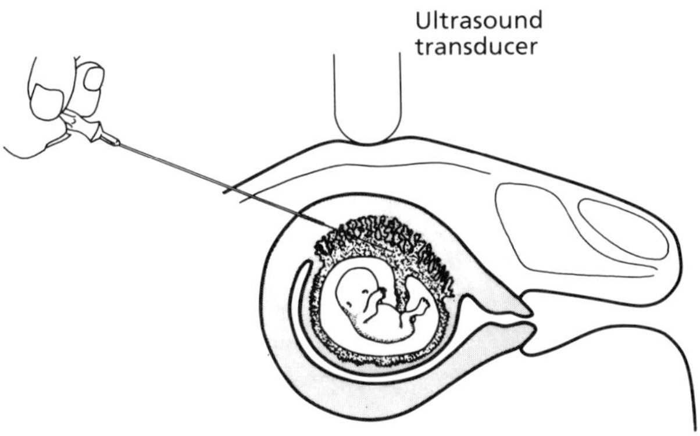


**Fig. 15.6** Transabdominal chorion villus sampling under ultrasound guidance.

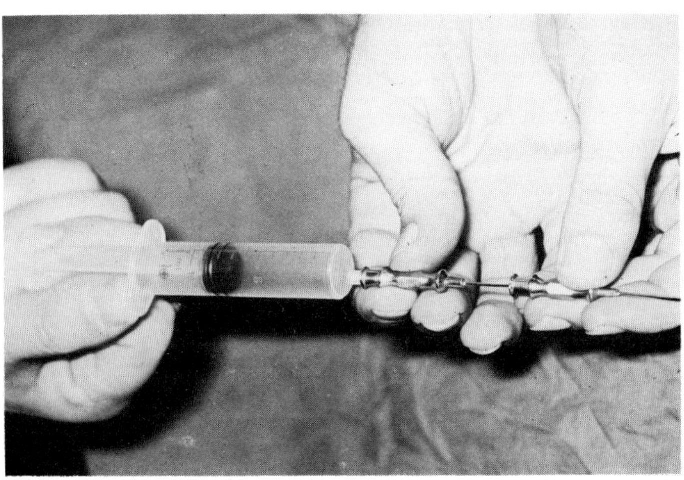

**Fig. 15.7** The 17/19 gauge double needle for transabdominal chorion villus sampling (RM Surgical Developments).

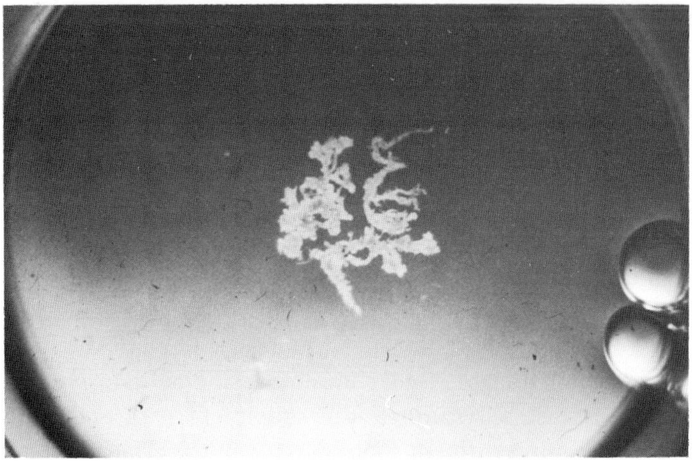

**Fig. 15.8** A typical specimen of chorionic villi in tissue culture medium immediately after biopsy prior to microscopic inspection.

the placental substance parallel to the chorionic plate. A syringe is used to aspirate villi. If further passages of the inner needle are required to achieve a suitable specimen, this can be achieved, without further discomfort to the patient, via the outer needle which remains in position until completion of the sampling.

Whichever method of biopsy is used the tissue obtained (Figure 15.8) is carefully scrutinized under the microscope to confirm the presence of sufficient chorionic villi for prenatal diagnosis and to allow removal of any decidual and maternal blood contamination should it be present.

## Indications

Most of the conditions amenable to diagnosis by amniocentesis may now be diagnosed by chorion villus sampling, viz: (i) karyotyping; (ii) inborn errors of metabolism; and (iii) DNA analysis.

### Karyotyping

Indications include:

**1** Maternal age.

**2** Previous baby with abnormal karyotype.

**3** Abnormal parental chromosomes.

**4** Fetal sexing (X-linked conditions).

The risk of fetal chromosome abnormality associated with advanced maternal age is by far the most frequent indication for prenatal diagnosis and has already become the principal reason for referral for chorion villus sampling.

Cytogenetic analysis of chorionic tissue may be performed directly after biopsy (Simoni *et al.* 1983) or after tissue culture (Heaton *et al.*

1984). The former method examines the spontaneous mitoses in the cytotrophoblast layer of chorionic villi and a result is available within hours of biopsy with little chance of interference by maternal decidua or of culture artefact. However, such preparations are not usually the best and culture techniques offer better quality, more detailed analysis of metaphase spreads, allowing the diagnosis of minor deletions and rearrangements. Most centres now use a modified direct technique (Verlinsky *et al.* 1984) which allows fetal sex to be determined and aneuploidy excluded within 24–48 hours. Cultured examination of cells may then be undertaken for confirmation of the result as well as allowing further, more detailed, analysis. It should be realized, however, that as gestation advances, many abnormal fetuses are lost by natural selection and therefore first trimester chorion villus sampling will reveal more abnormal karyotypes than would be expected either by the incidence in live births or at amniocentesis.

The theoretical risk of discrepancy between the chromosome complement of chorionic villi and the fetus is an infrequent practical problem. Such discordance results if a mosaic occurs early in blastocyst development resulting in an abnormal cell line either within the trophoblast but not within the embryo, or within the fetus but not within the trophoblast. Research suggests that the former occurs in less than 3 per cent of cases and that the latter is extremely rare. Although under such circumstances it may be possible to recognize those cases where the fetus is not at risk, when an unusual or mosaic karyotype is discovered, fetal blood sampling may be required for confirmation of the true fetal karyotype.

## Metabolic disorders

A large number of metabolic disorders may be diagnosed by analysis of chorionic villi either directly after sampling or after cell culture (Crawford 1988).

Most metabolic disorders have an autosomal recessive inheritance and many couples referred for chorion villus sampling have already had an affected baby. Before chorionic villus sampling can be offered, normal, affected and carrier ranges of the relevant enzyme must be established. Thereafter caution is still required as even a small amount of maternal contamination may produce a diagnostic error. Careful selection of villi from the biopsy specimen is essential and for many metabolic disorders amniocentesis is still recommended for confirmation of continuing pregnancies.

## DNA analysis

Advances in the field of molecular genetics have been rapid and have themselves encouraged the further development of chorionic villus sampling.

**Table 15.3** Diseases recognized using DNA technology

| |
|---|
| *Gene specific probes* |
| Sickle cell disease |
| Alpha-thalassaemia |
| Beta-thalassaemia |
| Haemophilia A |
| Haemophilia B |
| Alpha-1 antitrypsin deficiency |
| Phenylketonuria |
| |
| *Gene unknown* |
| Cystic fibrosis |
| Duchenne muscular dystrophy |
| Huntington's chorea |
| |
| *Chromosome-specific probes* |
| e.g. Y chromosome |
| |
| *Viral DNA* |
| e.g. rubella |

DNA technology was first used in conjunction with chorion villus sampling for the prenatal diagnosis of haemoglobinopathies (Old *et al.* 1982) but similar methodology has now been used to diagnose many other conditions (Table 15.3). Such DNA techniques do not rely on the presence or absence of accessible fetal tissue proteins or enzymes but instead upon the direct investigation of genetic material, in some cases permitting diagnosis even when the cause of a disease is unknown, e.g. cystic fibrosis.

Less than 20 mg of chorionic tissue is required to obtain the 20 mcg of DNA necessary for analysis. DNA is extracted and digested into fragments by endonucleases (restriction enzymes). These enzymes recognize and cut DNA at a specific sequence of nucleotides. Each enzyme will cut the DNA into a characteristic and unique range of sizes which may be separated by gel electrophoresis. The DNA fragments are transferred to a stable nitrocellulose filter (Southern blotting). Genetic disease involving a mutation, deletion or insertion of DNA within the gene will be detectable if there is a resulting change in fragment size; this can be detected by hybridization with a complementary DNA probe. The radioactive gene probe recognizes and adheres to a certain sequence of nucleotides and is then read as an autoradiograph. For many conditions, however, direct gene probe analysis is not possible and prenatal diagnosis relies on the presence or absence of endonuclease cutting sites, restriction fragment length polymorphisms, in the DNA between genes. Such analysis requires detailed family studies following the inheritance of detectable restriction fragment length polymorphisms linked to the abnormal gene. These studies are not infallible and are complicated, time consuming and rely on analysis of an affected family member or known carriers. Family investigation should, if possible, always be carried out prior to pregnancy as not all families are informative. An increasing number of conditions are, nevertheless, amenable to such diagnosis and the potential is great. The advent of simple and cheap methodology coupled with further advances will no doubt widen the clinical application of such DNA techniques.

### Other tests

Further methods of analysis may also prove beneficial and widen the scope of first trimester diagnosis. HLA typing and fetal Rhesus group identification are already possible but the promising use of two dimensional electrophoresis and monoclonal and polyclonal antibodies still has to be explored.

## Risks of chorion biopsy

Before chorion villus sampling can be used along with existing methods of prenatal diagnosis, the risks to mother and fetus have to be assessed accurately. To date no prospective controlled series have been reported and we must rely on the International Chorion Villus Sampling Registry (Jackson 1989). This is a voluntary record of the experiences of the majority of centres of the world who are using chorion villus sampling for prenatal diagnosis.

### Fetal losses

The assessment of the risks related to chorion villus sampling is a complex issue. Chorion villus sampling is performed at an early stage in pregnancy (optimal timing 9–11 weeks) when spontaneous fetal loss is not uncommon. This natural background risk has best been assessed by following pregnancies which have a normal appearance on ultrasound; this excludes the majority of subsequent spontaneous losses resulting from anembryonic pregnancies or missed abortions. Such studies show the likelihood of spontaneous abortion increases with maternal age (Christiaens & Stoutenbeek 1984), which is itself the commonest reason for prenatal diagnosis, but decreases with advancing gestational age. The overall risk of spontaneously aborting a pregnancy, shown by ultrasound at 10 weeks to be alive, appears to be less than 2 per cent but this surprisingly low figure rises to as high as 14 per cent once the maternal age reaches 40 years.

The International Registry (Jackson 1989) documents the wide range of post-biopsy losses experienced by the 182 submitting centres; the average fetal loss rate is 3.2 per cent ($n = 65\,747$). Those centres with greatest experience tend, as would be expected, to have the best results with the least number of pregnancy losses. Most experienced centres achieve successful biopsy in over 98 per cent of cases and, if the operator is competent in both transcervical and transabdominal methods of chorion villus sampling, success should approach 100 per cent.

At King's College Hospital, London the last 350 transcervical cases of chorion villus sampling were associated with a pregnancy loss rate of 2.7 per cent, giving an estimated procedure-related loss rate of less than 0.7 per cent. This is comparable to the reported risk of amniocentesis (Tabor *et al.* 1986).

The theoretical advantage of avoiding transcervical spread of infection and the extended use beyond the first trimester has recently encouraged interest in the transabdominal technique of placental biopsy. The combined world experience with this technique is still small ($n$ = 8160) but the average fetal loss rate is already down to 3.07 per cent (International Registry, September 1989). Such early success is very encouraging and further evaluation is eagerly awaited. Until such information is available the skill and experience of the operator appear to be as, if not more, important than the method employed.

## Other risks

Reports of serious maternal infection following transcervical chorion villus sampling have been recorded but are infrequent. In our experience at King's College Hospital, we have had no known cases of infection. Nevertheless, transcervical biopsy should always be avoided in the presence of active local genital tract infection. The transabdominal approach theoretically lessens but does not eradicate the risk of transmitted infection; scrupulous cleanliness is essential for both techniques.

Anxieties that instrumentation may cause membrane rupture have proven to be unfounded. The membranes are resilient and careful biopsy under ultrasound guidance makes membrane rupture highly unlikely even if the cannula tip is advanced and tents the membrane. However, such tenting effectively blocks the end of the cannula tip and prevents successful biopsy.

Revealed vaginal bleeding is frequently seen following transcervical chorionic villus sampling but usually comes from the cervix following the use of a tenaculum and does not indicate placental damage. Research has shown, however, that although fetal cells cannot be detected within the maternal circulation after biopsy (Kleihauer test), a rise in maternal alpha-fetoprotein may occur, suggesting that a small fetomaternal transfusion may accompany biopsy (Warren *et al.* 1985). For this reason anti-D immunoglobulin should be given to all Rhesus negative women. Because of the short half life of alpha-fetoprotein, any rise at chorionic villus sampling will not influence neural tube defect screening at 16 weeks gestation.

The risks of post-biopsy complication in both later pregnancy and childhood still need to be fully evaluated. To date no increase in the incidence of obstetric complications or neonatal mortality or morbidity has been shown (Anguo *et al.* 1985).

As the clinical techniques of chorion villus sampling have improved over the years so has the expertise in tissue analysis. Those laboratories handling trophoblast specimens are now able to process smaller samples successfully with only a small (2 per cent) risk of failure of culture or direct analysis.

## Multiple pregnancy

Despite our experience and other successful reports, prenatal diagnosis of a multiple pregnancy is not without difficulty. Firstly, if possible, clear identification of individual placentae must be made (Figure 15.9) and biopsies taken at widely separate sites close to the individual cord insertions. In the case of a twin pregnancy, at least two invasive procedures will be required and more if either is unsuccessful. Such multiple biopsies have already been shown to be associated with an increased risk of fetal loss. If, on biopsy, the fetuses are found to be of the same sex, DNA techniques may be used to confirm that both have been sampled. Should the result of analysis show discordance, i.e. one fetus abnormal and the other normal, then selective feticide brings further problems. The rapidly and sometimes asymmetric enlargement of the uterus and changing contours associated with uterine contractions may make identification of the abnormal fetus very difficult. Once the abnormal fetus has

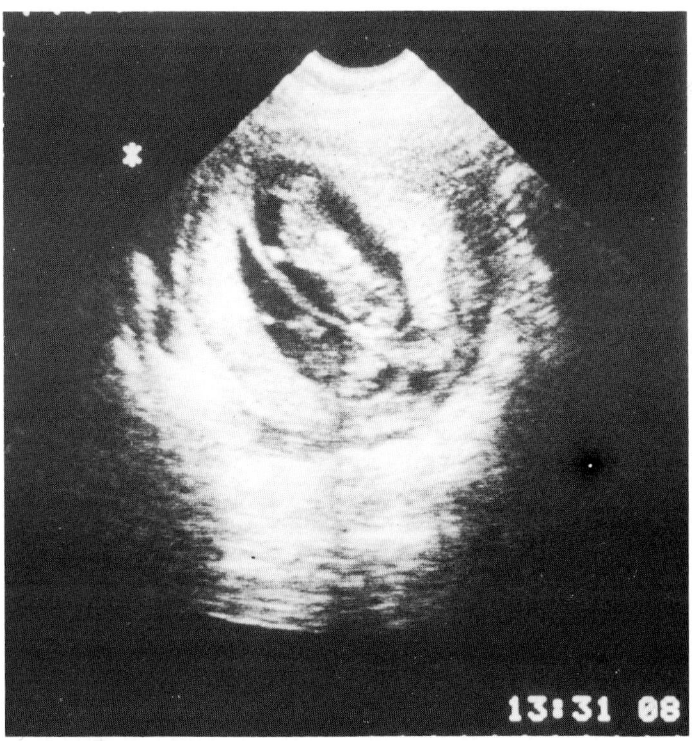


**Fig. 15.9** Ultrasound of a twin pregnancy showing distinctly separate placentae allowing accurate independent biopsy.

been determined, selective feticide must be carried out without damage or loss of the healthy fetus. Even after using extreme care it is still advisable to recheck the surviving fetus to confirm correct selection.

## Ethical considerations

The ability to determine fetal sex so early in pregnancy has been of great benefit to those at risk of X-linked conditions. However, the use of chorionic villus sampling to allow selective abortion if a fetus is normal but not of the perferred sex raises considerable ethical considerations. Similarly, healthy people unaware they are at risk of Huntington's chorea, may be identified as future sufferers by the DNA study of families requesting prenatal diagnosis. Further advances in DNA technology will undoubtedly bring even more complex ethical dilemmas.

The solutions to such problems are not easy and need to be resolved taking into account the interests of the patient, the family and society in general.

## Conclusions

Many patients already feel that chorionic villus sampling has clear advantages over second trimester amniocentesis. The demand for chorionic sampling has been so great that it initially exceeded the number of centres offering chorionic villus sampling, and far exceeded the limited number of laboratories able to analyse the biopsied trophoblast.

Even though amniocentesis is widely available, less than 50 per cent of those patients sufficiently at risk to warrant prenatal diagnosis actually have testing performed. There are many reasons for this poor uptake of amniocentesis: lack of education, late referral, as well as a group of patients who would not consider late diagnosis because of the possibility of a mid-trimester termination of pregnancy. Such patients may well consider first trimester diagnosis. The potential workload of chorionic villus sampling may therefore be even larger than that of amniocentesis. Although widespread chorion villus sampling will require changes in, and possibly additions to, presently available clinical and laboratory facilities, early placental biopsy is, nevertheless, extremely cost effective and compares well with the cost of amniocentesis.

To fully assess chorionic villus sampling, its success, risks and complications, large trials are required. The result of a Medical Research Council prospective multi-centre randomized trial comparing chorionic villus sampling with amniocentesis is expected shortly. In this trial women at low risk of congenital disease through advanced maternal age are randomly allocated either to have chorionic villus sampling or amniocentesis. Subsequent follow-up extending into childhood will be vigilant. Though, for many reasons, criticism is already being levelled at this trial, it is only in this way that the exact role of chorionic villus sampling will be known and its risks fully assessed.

The advantages of first trimester diagnosis have led to enthusiasm by patients and physicians alike. Chorionic villus sampling has already had a major impact on those at risk of congenital disease and has stimulated further advances in the science of prenatal diagnosis. Until the exact risks of chorionic villus sampling are known, initial enthusiasm should be cautioned. Meanwhile, increasing DNA technology and quicker cytology results will mean an ever increasing demand.

As the optimum for biopsy lies between 9 and 12 weeks gestation prepregnancy counselling should be actively encouraged and patients should obtain early confirmation of pregnancy and be quickly referred to a centre performing chorionic villus sampling. Such organization is difficult but essential for early diagnosis.

## References

Acosta-Sison H. (1958) Diagnosis of hydatidiform mole. *Obstetrics and Gynecology*, **12**, 205–8.

Anguo H. Bingru Z. & Hong W. (1985) Longterm follow up results after aspiration of chorionic villi during early pregnancy. In *First Trimester Fetal Diagnosis*, (Ed. by M. Fraccaro, G. Simoni & B. Brambati), pp. 1–6. Springer-Verlag, Berlin.

Anshan Iron & Steel Company, Tietung Hospital (1975) Fetal sex prediction by sex chromatin of chorionic villi cells during early pregnancy. *Chinese Medical Journal*, **1**, 117–26.

Brock D.J.H. & Sutcliffe R.G. (1972) Alpha fetoprotein in the antenatal diagnosis of anencephaly and spina bifida. *Lancet*, **ii**, 197–9.

Campbell S., Johnstone F.D., Holt E.M. & May P. (1972) Anencephaly. Early ultrasonic diagnosis and management. *Lancet*, **i**, 1226–7.

Christiaens G.C.M.L. & Stoutenbeek Ph. (1984) Spontaneous abortion in proven intact pregnancies. *Lancet*, **ii**, 571–2.

Crawford M.d'A. (1988) Prenatal diagnosis of common genetic disorders. *British Medical Journal*, **297**, 502–6.

Fraccaro M., Simoni G. & Brambati B. (Eds) (1984) *First Trimester Fetal Diagnosis*. Springer-Verlag, Berlin.

Hahnemann N. & Mohr J. (1968) Genetic diagnosis in the embryo by means of biopsy from extraembryonic membranes. *Bulletin of the European Society of Human Genetrics*, **2**, 23.

Heaton D.H., Czepulkowski B.H., Horwell D.H. & Coleman D.V. (1984) Chromosome analysis of first trimester chorionic villus biopsies prepared by a maceration technique. *Prenatal Diagnosis*, **4**, 279–87.

Hobbins J.C. & Mahoney M.J. (1974) *In utero* diagnosis of haemoglobinopathies. Technic for obtaining fetal blood. *New England Journal of Medicine*, **290**, 1065–7.

Jackobson C.B. & Barter R.H. (1967) Intrauterine diagnosis and management of genetic defects. *American Journal of Obstetrics and Gynecology*, **99**, 795–805.

Jackson L. (1989) *International CVS Register*. Philadelphia, USA.

Kan Y.W., Golbus M.S. & Dozy A.M. (1976) Prenatal diagnosis of alpha thalassaemia. Clinical application of molecular hybridisation. *New England Journal of Medicine*, **309**, 831–3.

Kazy Z., Rozovsky I.S. & Bakharev V.A. (1982) Chorion biopsy in early pregnancy: A method of early prenatal diagnosis for inherited disorders. *Prenatal Diagnosis*, **2**, 39–45.

Old J.M., Ward R.H.T., Petrou M., Karagozlu F., Modell B. & Weatherall D.J. (1982) First trimester fetal diagnosis for haemoglobinopathies: three cases. *Lancet*, **ii**, 1413–16.

Rodeck C.H., Morsman J.M., Nicolaides K.H., McKenzie F.C., Gosden C.M. & Gosden J.R. (1983) A single operator technique for first trimester chorion biopsy. *Lancet*, **ii**, 1340–1.

Serr D.M., Sachs L. & Danon M. (1955) Diagnosis of sex before birth using cells from the amniotic fluid. *Bulletin of the Research Council of Israel,* **5B**, 137.

Simoni G., Brambati B., Danesino C., Rossella F., Terzoli G., Ferrari M. & Fraccaro M. (1983) Efficient direct chromosome analysis and enzyme determinations from chorionic villi samples in the first trimester of pregnancy. *Human Genetics,* **63**, 349–57.

Smidt-Jensen S. & Hahnemann N. (1984) Transabdominal fine needle biopsy from chorionic villi in the first trimester. *Prenatal Diagnosis,* **4**, 163–9.

Steele M.W. & Breg W.R. Jnr (1966) Chromosome analysis of human amniotic fluid cells. *Lancet,* **i**, 383–5.

Tabor A., Philip J., Madsen M., Bang J., Obel E.B. & Norgaard-Pedersen B. (1986) Randomised controlled trial of genetic amniocentesis in 4606 low risk women. *Lancet,* **ii**, 1287–92.

Verlinsky Y., Chu L. & Pergament E. (1984) Chromosomal preparations of chorionic villi samples (CVS). *Karyogram,* **10**, 1–3.

Ward R.H.T., Modell B., Petrou M., Karagozlu F. & Douratsos E. (1983) A method of chorionic villus sampling in the first trimester of pregnancy under real-time ultrasonic guidance. *British Medical Journal,* **286**, 1542–4.

Warren R.C., Butler J., McKenzie F.C., Morsman J.M. & Rodeck C.H. (1985) Does chorionic villus sampling cause fetomaternal haemorrhage? *Lancet,* **i**, 691.

# 16: Diet and prepregnancy folic acid and vitamin supplementation in the prevention of neural tube defects

K. MICHAEL LAURENCE



The neural tube defects (NTD) are generally considered to include anencephaly, encephalocoele, myelocoele (myelomeningocoele), meningocoele and complicated spina bifida occulta but not isolated hydrocephalus or simple spina bifida occulta, or where an NTD is part of a chromosome abnormality such as trisomy 18 or triploidy, part of a recognized malformation syndrome such as Meckel–Gruber syndrome or part of fetal disruption (amniotic band) syndrome. They are different endproducts of the same general process which is now widely accepted to have a multifactorial aetiology (Carter 1974, Carter *et al.* 1968). A major genetic component which is thought to be polygenic renders the embryo susceptible to interference by intrauterine environmental factors during the fourth week after conception. There are likely to be a number of such factors, perhaps with different ones being of major importance in various populations with a high incidence. As there is very little likelihood of being able to modify the genetic component effectively, primary prevention of the NTD would therefore be dependent on being able to identify the environmental trigger factors so that they can either be removed from the environment or be avoided. However, although NTD can be produced in experimental animals by numerous and very differing environmental insults, intensive epidemiological and clinical studies in man have only recently produced evidence of specific environmental factors which might be of aetiological importance, poor maternal nutrition and more specifically folic acid depletion and folate antagonists. In man a few cases may be precipitated by maternal anticonvulsant therapy with sodium valproate (Oakley 1985; Anon. 1988), poorly controlled maternal diabetes (Soler *et al.* 1976) and hyperthermia caused by virus and other infections (Smith *et al.* 1978).

Poor maternal nutrition has for some time been suspected as an aetiological factor because in the British Isles with its former high incidence, social class IV and V families had a much higher incidence of NTD then those of social classes I and II. (Record & McKeown 1949; Laurence *et al.* 1968a; Nevin 1980). The more deprived regions, such as the Irish Republic, Northern Ireland, South Wales, the north west of England and the south west of Scotland have the highest incidences. There has also been a seasonal variation with a higher incidence amongst conceptions in winter and spring when fresh foods are less plentiful and more expensive (Laurence *et al.* 1968b). In the last two decades or so, not only has the general incidence of NTD fallen dramatically (Bradshaw *et al.* 1980), especially in the previously higher incidence regions (Nevin 1981; Laurence 1983) but also social class differences and seasonal variations have been less pronounced (Laurence *et al.* 1968b). Secular trends have been noted in the past and have usually been difficult to interpret. However, the sharp rise in the incidence of NTD in Boston during the depression years (MacMahon & Yen 1971) has been interpreted as being due to poor maternal nutrition prevailing at the time.

In this connection in China, where in general the incidence of NTD is relatively low (less than 1 per 1000 births), a study of the births in seven townships in the north (Shuniyi area) found an incidence of almost 7 per 1000, as high as that in South Wales three decades ago. It is of special interest that there, winter conceptions are most at risk when the mothers are apparently on a very deficient diet (Ye 1986; Laurence *et al.* 1987).

## Folate deficiency as a possible cause of neural tube defects

Although the effect of poor maternal nutrition on the developing embryo may be due to a number of vitamin deficiencies acting together to interfere with the closure of the neural tube, or to allow some as yet unidentified teratogen to have an influence (Renwick 1982), it seems much more likely based on experimental, embryological, epidemiological as well as clinical evidence, that the main cause in the UK at least, is a lack of folate.

NTD can be induced in the rat by exposing developing embryos to a variety of teratogens, after the 9th day following fertilization (Elwood & Elwood 1980), including anti-folic acid agents. In the rat the neural tube begins to form about the 8th or 9th day, closure being complete towards the middle of the 12th day (F. Beck pers. comm.). This is also the stage when the rat embryo's chorioallantoic placenta begins to develop, the embryonic heart starts to perfuse it and the pace of the development and energy requirement increases significantly (F. Beck pers. comm.). During this time there are also considerable changes in the metabolic processes.

Before the neural tube is formed the rat embryo derives its energy largely from glycolysis and the pentose phosphate shunt, but from that time there is a progressive switch to the Krebs cycle (Shepard *et al.* 1970; Tanimura & Shepard 1970). In the chick embryo it seems to have been shown that neural tube closure is critically dependent on an oxygen gradient in the neural crests (Watt 1977) producing only a narrow band of hypoxic surface cells along the opposing neural crests. Lack of sufficient folate at that stage or a general metabolic disturbance could then intefere with the normal closure process and either the crests do not meet correctly or if they do meet the hypoxic necrosis having progressed too far, they dehisce again.

It may be thought that these findings in rodent or bird embryos bear little relation to the situation in man. However, 'it is an accepted principle of comparative embryology that species differences in form and structure become less striking as earlier embryonic stages are examined and it is an interesting, but largely unstudied possibility that inter-species metabolic differences are also minimal in the early embryo' (Wilson 1973).

Translated to the human embryo, all these processes take place between the 21st and 25th day after fertilization, and there is every reason to suppose that they differ only in detail and in timing from those in the chick and the rat. This is only supposition as it is not possible to investigate the metabolic processes in human embryos at that stage of development. However, research using the technique of New (1978) where explanted rat embryos are grown artificially in various manipulated media up to the 12th day of development has been able to throw some light on the folate requirements for the closure of the neural tube. F. Beck (pers. comm.) grew fetuses removed on the 8th day from folate-depleted rats in serum from similarly folate-depleted rats and obtained in nearly all fetuses defective or non-closure of the neural tube. When either conjugated or non-conjugated folic acid was added to the deficient medium on the 9th day, only about half the fetuses had NTD. When both were added, the fetuses were smaller than normal but with normally closed neural tubes. This suggests that folates play an important part in rat development acting either directly or indirectly and perhaps in early human development also.

Both the serum and the red cell folate levels are low in women who are on an unsatisfactory diet (Table 16.1), and Smithells found similar results in women from social class III, IV and V, both when not pregnant and during the first trimester (Smithells *et al.* 1977) but especially so at the beginning of a pregnancy that ended in an infant with an NTD (Smithells *et al.* 1976). It has recently been shown that women who had previously had one NTD had significantly lower serum and red cell folate levels than matched controls and those who had previously had two or more NTDs had lower levels still (Yates *et al.* 1987). This suggests that there might be an inherited disorder of folic acid metabolism as a predisposing factor. Finally, there is the small human experience with aminopterin in precipitating NTD (Thiersch 1952).

## Studies in South Wales

To elucidate these problems various studies were carried out in South Wales into the nutritional status of women who had had pregnancies with a neural tube defect and a trial of supplementation with folic acid of the diet before and during the first trimester of subsequent pregnancies in these women has been completed.

### First dietary study

In this study women who had had a child with an NTD betwen 1954 and 1974 and were living in the counties of Glamorgan and Gwent were identified. This was a population in which there had been several epidemiologic studies and several registers of patients were available. Those who were still under 35 years of age were visited between 1969 and 1974 (Laurence *et al.* 1980) by two investigators. Both investigators were doctors, one with a long experience of taking dietary histories in diabetic clinics, and the other with wide experience in public health clinics and general practice. One surveyed the western half of the area and the other the eastern area.

Nine hundred and two women were visited in their homes; 442 women who were not pregnant and who had not decided against having any more children were enrolled in the dietary study.

The women were questioned about their usual diet at the time of the survey (the interpregnancy diet). Enquiries about diet in the first trimester of previous pregnancies were also made.

A simple diet sheet was used that provided a general pattern for meals and a check list which included protein-rich foods, dairy products, vegetables and fruits, brown and white bread, confectionery and soft drinks, and was designed to reveal any deficiency in the consumption of foods containing significant amounts of folic acid during an average week.

The diets were classified as good, fair or poor. Good diets were those comprising a large variety of foods including particularly meats, eggs and milk, green vegetables and fruit, and with a relatively low consumption of confectionery and soft drinks. Such a diet would be expected to provide generous intakes of all the nutrients (including folic acid) and dietary fibre. Poor diets were monotonous, restricted in variety, with very low intakes of animal foods, including milk, and of fruits and vegetables, and an over-dependence on convenience foods high in carbohydrate and fat. These diets were often associated with irregular meal patterns, and a high consumption of confectionery, and would provide marginal intakes of vitamins and minerals. The diets judged to be fair were intermediate between these extremes, but in addition were thought to provide low intakes of one or more nutrients. This classification was carried out by an independent research worker after the end of the study who was unaware of the outcome of pregnancies. This assessment was re-examined by one of the investigators but almost no changes to the independent classification were made at this stage.

Blood samples were taken after the interview, but conditions under which they were taken (as to time of month, and day and relationship to meals) could not be standardized. Serum and red cell folic acid concentrations and serum vitamin $B_{12}$ were measured (Hoffbrand *et al.* 1966; Tennant & Withey 1972). Haematocrit was also estimated.

The women in the western area of Glamorgan who were willing to cooperate in the prospective study were counselled to improve their diets and to stop smoking not later than the time when contraceptive precautions were stopped. Those in the eastern area were not specifically counselled. Both groups were instructed to report within 6 weeks of the last menstrual period (LMP) if they missed a period. They were revisited as soon as possible and certainly before the 11th week from the LMP and detailed enquiries were made about the quality of the diet during the pregnancy so far, about illness, nausea and vomiting and medicines used. Another blood sample was taken and the same haematological and biochemical factors measured. They were revisited at least twice more, in mid-pregnancy and immediately after the end of the pregnancy.

There were 442 who were eligible for admission to this study. Of these 26 subsequently proved to have been pregnant at interview and one was on folate treatment leaving 415 subjects in the study. Of these only 65 reported a good interpregnancy diet, 197 a fair diet and 149 a poor diet; four diet histories could not be analysed. The mean serum folate concentration and the red cell folate for these groups are shown in Table 16.1 and the gradient of the measurements suggests that the dietary assessment had some validity. Serum $B_{12}$ concentration did not correlate with this classification of diet.

Of these 415 women, 174 reported within adequate time, 186 subsequently confirmed pregnancies, of whom 12 reported twice. They were all revisited within 11 weeks of their last LMP, a current pregnancy dietary history taken and a blood sample taken. There were 103 from west Glamorgan and 71 from east Glamorgan or Gwent. These 174 were asked about the diet that they remembered to have taken during the first trimester of their previous pregnancies that resulted in an NTD (Index

**Table 16.1** First dietary study. Women with a previous fetal neural tube defect. Quality of interpregnancy diet and mean concentration of serum folate, red blood cell folate and serum $B_{12}$

| Quality of diet | Subjects *n* | Subjects per cent | Mean serum folate μg/l | RBC folate μg/l of red cells | Serum $B_{12}$ μg/l |
|---|---|---|---|---|---|
| Good | 65 | 16 | 8.9 | 295 | 283 |
| Fair | 197 | 47 | 5.4 | 236 | 272 |
| Poor | 149 | 36 | 4.9 | 197 | 285* |
| Not known | 4 | 1 | | | |
| All women | 415 | 100 | 5.9 | 238 | 277 |

* Two sera with concentrations of $B_{12}$ over 1000 μg/l excluded as subjects were likely to have been on $B_{12}$ treatment.

**Table 16.2** First dietary study. Quality of diet during interpregnancy period compared to that during previous pregnancies

| Period of diet | Quality of diet: Good *n* | Good per cent | Fair *n* | Fair per cent | Poor *n* | Poor per cent | All women *n* |
|---|---|---|---|---|---|---|---|
| Interpregnancy | 24 | 14 | 107 | 61 | 43 | 25 | 174 |
| Pregnancy with NTD | 17 | 10 | 65 | 37 | 92 | 53 | 174 |
| Other pregnancy | 23 | 19 | 63 | 51 | 37 | 30 | 123 |

*Note*:
**1** The interpregnancy diet was the diet currently consumed at the time of the first survey.
**2** The pregnancy diets related to the first trimester of previous pregnancies and were obtained by recall.

**Table 16.3** First dietary study. Change in diet in project pregnancy compared to that in index pregnancy

| Instructions on diet | Changes in diet: Improved *n* | Improved per cent | No change *n* | No change per cent | Worse *n* | Worse per cent | All pregnancies *n* |
|---|---|---|---|---|---|---|---|
| Counselled | 78 | 71 | 29 | 27 | 2 | 2 | 109 |
| Not counselled | 9 | 12 | 63 | 82 | 5 | 6 | 77 |
| All diets | 87 | 47 | 92 | 49 | 7 | 4 | 186 |

Six counselled women and 6 non-counselled women had two pregnancies. The project pregnancy diet was recorded at the time of this pregnancy. The index pregnancy diet was taken by recall at the interpregnancy interview.

pregnancies) and in their other pregnancies. Compared with the interpregnancy diet, which was in any case not very good, their diet in early pregnancy deteriorated due to nausea and excessive vomiting, but those that had an abnormal outcome seemed to have deteriorated very much more (Table 16.2).

In previous epidemiological studies no obvious differences in the social and demographic characteristics of the women in the two areas had been found (Laurence *et al.* 1968a,b) and their diets in the interpregnancy period and during the first trimester of previous pregnancies were similar. In the western area where all women had been counselled to improve their diet, the majority had heeded this advice and almost three quarters (71 per cent) had improved their diet in time for their next pregnancy and the reason why many of the remainder did not do so was because of excessive nausea and vomiting (Table 16.3). In the uncounselled area over 80 per cent did not change the pattern of their diet. The outcome of the 109 pregnancies in the western area was 10 miscarriages and three recurrences of NTD; amongst the 77 in the eastern area there

**Table 16.4** First dietary study. Outcome of project pregnancies. By quality of diet in first trimester

| Outcome of pregnancy | Quality of diet: Good *n* | Fair *n* | Poor *n* | All pregnancies *n* |
|---|---|---|---|---|
| Normal child | 53 | 85 | 22 | 160 |
| Recurrent NTD | — | — | 8 | 8 |
| Miscarriage | — | 3 | 15 | 18 |
| All outcomes | 53 | 88 | 45 | 186 |

were eight miscarriages and five recurrences. The ratio of the risk of recurrence in East Glamorgan compared to West Glamorgan was 2.4 although this did not differ statistically significantly from 1.0. All eight recurrences occurred in women whose diets were considered to be poor during the first trimester of that pregnancy, an assessment which was made at the time of the first visit during the pregnancy before any outcome could be known (Table 16.4). There were no recurrences in the pregnancies with a good or fair diet. This distribution was most unlikely to have occurred by chance, ($P < 0.001$). Of the three women with recurrences who had received counselling, one had ignored the advice but two suffered nausea and vomiting during the first month of conception which had continued into hyperemesis gravidarum.

## Second dietary study

A second dietary study was conducted between 1974 and 1979 largely in the western part of South Wales, again with women who had at least one previous pregnancy with NTD, but this time two control groups were also studied; the sisters of the index cases who had only normal babies and a group of University and professional wives (James *et al.* 1980). The dietary investigation was based on a modified form of Burke's dietary history which was more detailed than the one used in the first study (Burke 1947). The diet was again divided into three main categories of good, fair and poor but within the poor diets those subjects whose diet would have been considered to have been fair except that it was unbalanced by excessive amounts of refined carbohydrates and fats were separated.

The 244 index women, visited in their homes, were found to have a dietary pattern very similar to the women in the previous dietary study. One hundred out of 244 (41 per cent) seemed to be on a poor diet. This compared with 32 out of 123 (26 per cent) amongst their sister controls and 3 out of 50 (6 per cent) of the upper class controls (Table 16.5). All the women in this study were given dietary counselling with apparently even greater effect than in the previous study. The 244 index women had 176 further pregnancies by the end of 1979 with only 32 (18 per cent) remaining on a poor diet and with 5 NTD (2.8 per cent), about half the

**Table 16.5** Second dietary study. Interpregnancy diet: cases and controls, number of subjects and row percent

| | Quality of diet | | | | | | | | |
|---|---|---|---|---|---|---|---|---|---|
| | Good | | Fair | | Poor (a) | | Poor (b) | | All cases |
| Group of women | *n* | per cent | *n* | per cent | *n* | per cent | *n* | per cent | *n* |
| Index cases | 34 | 14 | 110 | 45 | 33 | 14 | 67 | 27 | 244 |
| Sister controls | 43 | 35 | 48 | 39 | 23 | 19 | 9 | 7 | 123 |
| Upper class controls | 39 | 78 | 8 | 16 | 3 | 6 | 0 | 0 | 50 |

All diets were current interpregnancy diets. Index cases had had a pregnancy with a fetal NTD. Sisters of index cases had not had an NTD. Upper class controls, university and professional wives had not had an NTD. Poor diets are subdivided into (a) those with an adequate diet but excess refined carbohydrates and fat, and (b) those with a totally inadequate diet.

**Table 16.6** Second dietary study. Diet of index women during first trimester of project pregnancy

| | Quality of diet | | | | | | | | |
|---|---|---|---|---|---|---|---|---|---|
| | Good | | Fair | | Poor(a) | | Poor(b) | | All pregnancies |
| Outcome to fetus | *n* | per cent | *n* | per cent | *n* | per cent | *n* | per cent | *n* |
| Normal | 68 | 40 | 76 | 44 | 15 | 9 | 12 | 7 | 171 |
| NTD | | | | | 3 | 60 | 2 | 40 | 5 |
| All fetuses | 68 | 39 | 76 | 43 | 18 | 10 | 14 | 8 | 176 |

Seven index women had had two previous pregnancies with NTD. 176 index women became pregnant and 5 had an NTD giving a rate of 2.8 per cent. All recurrences had poor diets. All women were counselled to improve their diet.

number of recurrences expected. More important, all five recurrences occurred in the 32 pregnancies with disordered diets, a rate of 16 per cent. This distribution was unlikely to have occurred by chance, ($P <$ 0.01) (Table 16.6).

Quite apart from those who are poorly nourished because of family poverty (now relatively uncommon in the British Isles) and those who live largely on convenience foods or unsatisfactory food materials through ignorance, habit, religious observance, laziness or lack of time, the following distinct groups tend to be on a disordered diet (James *et al.* 1980).

*Pickers* who toy with their food and rarely eat more than a fraction of the helpings on their plate.

*Nibblers* who tend to eat incessantly, especially when viewing television or feeling lonely, bored or anxious. Some of these eat between meals, others never sit down to a proper meal, although they may pick at the dinners prepared for their husband's homecoming.

*Gorgers* who overeat at meals and those who are nibblers also become overweight. This leads to slimming fads and crash diets, interspersed with lapses into compulsive eating. Some of the more figure-conscious then starve themselves for weeks at a time and if this coincided with conception their diet would be markedly deficient in all the essential nutrients during the vital period for the development of the embryo's nervous system.

*Moody women* who also tend to be erratic in their diet and when depressed either go off their food or eat more than usual in an attempt to comfort themselves.

*Food faddists* who have an aversion to one or more foods often including several essentials. A number of these women said they disliked meat, fish, eggs, greens, fruit and salads so they subsisted almost entirely on refined carbohydrates and fats.

*Chip maniacs* was a term often used by their sisters to describe an index mother who ate mounds of chips for one or two meals daily, sometimes with chip sandwiches in between and very little other foods.

## Folic acid supplementation trial

A double-blind randomized controlled trial of folate treatment compared with an inert placebo given before conception and continuing until at least the 12th week of pregnancy was started in South Wales in 1969 and continued until 1974 (Laurence & Campbell 1981; Laurence *et al.* 1981). The subjects were recruited from the same women who at the same time were taking part in the first dietary study. On recruitment to that study, all these women were asked if they would be prepared to take part in a study of the possible causes of NTD, and as part of this they were invited to take tablets at the beginning of their next pregnancy, without any promise of success. Those who agreed to take part were randomized to two treatment groups, either 2 mg twice a day of folic acid in the form of methyl folate in an inert tablet, or the identical tablet of inert filler without folic acid. They were told to advise the investigators as soon as they intended to stop contraceptive precautions; tablets were then sent to them which they were instructed to take until they missed a period when they were to notify the field workers as soon as possible when they were revisited by the field workers. Treatment was continued up to 12 weeks of pregnancy. Women who did not apply for tablets or who received tablets but did not report back that they had become pregnant were not revisited at this stage and were not included in the study.

Neither the doctor not the subject knew the treatment allocated so that this would not influence their willingness to take the tablets, their response to notifying a suspect pregnancy nor the field worker's thoroughness in making the recall visit and taking a history. Once the history had been taken and a blood sample analysed and the pregnancy confirmed, there was no point in maintaining the anonymity of treatment as the outcome could not be subject to any form of subjective bias, although in practice the code was not broken until the end of the study.

All the women who were approached in connection with the first dietary study and folate trial are analysed in Appendix I. There were 415 women who were not pregnant nor on folate therapy in the dietary study. Of these 197 were unwilling to take part in a trial of an unspecified treatment with no assurance of success but were willing to help with the dietary follow-up. The climate of opinion in the aftermath of the Thalidomide disaster was against taking unnecessary medication in pregnancy. Two hundred and eighteen were willing to take part in the trial. Of these, 114 were allocated at random to folate treatment and 104 to placebo. Appendix I gives a complete schedule of the various groups into which the 442 women were analysed.

The criteria for entry to the folate analysis group were more stringent than those for the dietary study. They had to be seen within 11 weeks of last menstrual period, they had to provide pregnancy dietary history, and the serum folate concentration had to be reported by the laboratory. There were 123 pregnancies reported which met these criteria, 60 in the folate group and 63 in the placebo group.

As it is well known that patients and especially pregnant women do not necessarily take medicines prescribed, the serum folate concentration was used as a screening test. When it came to the analyses it was decided that if the folate subjects had a serum level below 10 μg/l they would be considered as non-compliers. There were 15 subjects classified as non-compliers by this criterion. Similar results would have been obtained if red cell folate at a level of 350 μg/l of red cells had been used. The detailed distributions of serum folate and red cell folate are shown in Figure 16.1. No test of compliance in the placebo group was available. The subjects were not asked to confirm that they had taken the tablets in the early years of the study, but in later years it was possible to confirm in some cases that there was non-compliance. While it is reasonable to infer that there was non-compliance from the low folate levels, the possibility that poor absorption may be a cause of low serum folate in some individuals could not be excluded.

We were surprised to find one woman in the folate tablet group with a serum folate level of 212 μg/1 and with a low red cell folate (259 μg/1) but we considered this possibly a laboratory error of estimation and we retained her as a folate complier. She had a miscarriage of an anencephalic fetus at 12 weeks of pregnancy. In 1980 at the time of the publicity following the publication of the paper by Smithells and his colleagues (1980) she came and admitted that she had not taken the tablets during early pregnancy but when she realized that the field

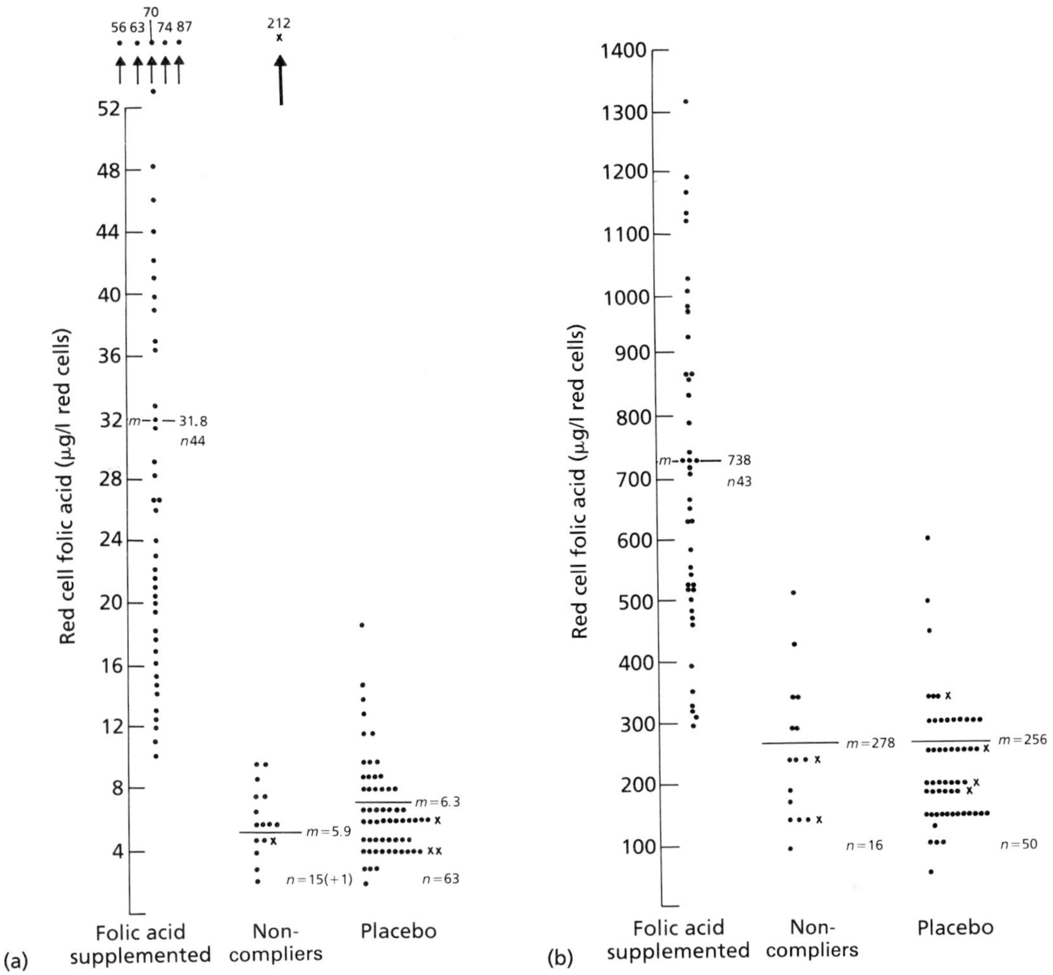


**Fig. 16.1** Serum and red cell folate levels in supplementation study divided into groups according to whether the patients were on folic acid supplementation or placebo, or whether they were non-compliers. All but one of those regarded to have been non-compliers had serum folate levels below 10 μg/l (X denotes patients with a recurrence).

worker would take a blood sample she swallowed a large number on the evening before the visit. A cross-tabulation of serum folate against red cell folate (Figure 16.2) was examined and a reasonable degree of association was found except for this one subject who had a low red cell concentration yet this extraordinarily high serum concentration. Her diet before pregnancy and during pregnancy had been poor, and her $B_{12}$ concentration was consonant with the poor dietary history (112 μg/1). Her story was accepted and she was reclassified as a non-complier.

The outcome of these pregnancies is shown in Tables 16.7, 16.8 and 16.9. There were four recurrences out of 63 (6.4 per cent) in the placebo group and two recurrences out of 60 (3.3 per cent) in the folate prescribed group. Although the relative risk was 2.0 or a possible 50 per cent reduction in recurrences this could not be considered significant statis-

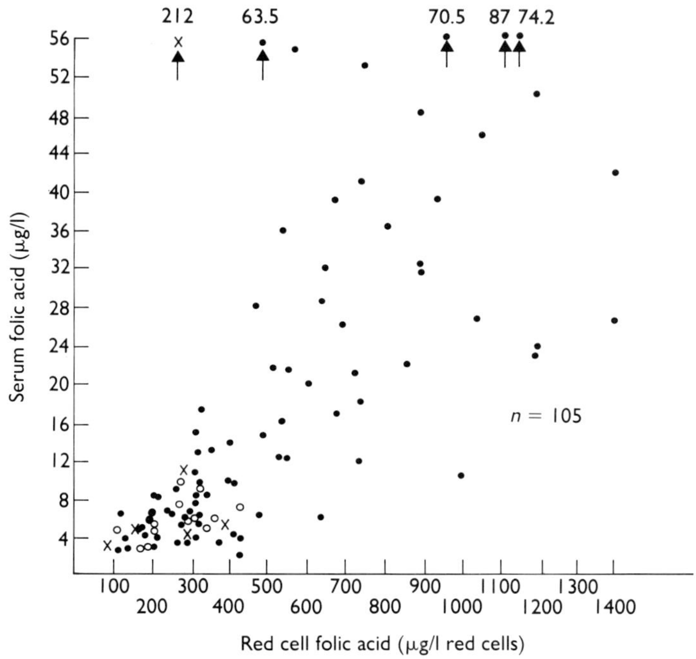


**Fig. 16.2** Relationship between red cell and serum folate levels. All those on folic acid supplementation had greatly elevated serum and red cell folate levels (X = non-compliers; ○ = placebo; ● = folate supplemented).

**Table 16.7** Folic acid supplementation trial. Recurrence of neural tube defects

| | | | | Blood estimations | | | Outcomes | | |
|---|---|---|---|---|---|---|---|---|---|
| Case | Treatment | Diet | Week | Serum folate | Red cell folate | $B_{12}$ | Delivery | Lesion | Gestation (months) |
| A | F.NC | Poor | 7 | 212.0 | 259 | 112 | MC | AN | 3 |
| B | F.NC | Poor | 8 | 4.8 | 155 | 167 | LB | SB | 9 |
| C | PL | Poor | 8 | 3.7 | 228 | 89 | LB | SB | 8 |
| D | PL | Poor | 7 | 11.0 | 275 | 210 | MC | AN | 4 |
| E | PL | Poor | 8 | 5.0 | 380 | 217 | LB | SB | 9 |
| F | PL | Poor | 7 | 2.9 | 76 | 371 | T | AN | 5 |

Estimations in μg/1; F.NC = folate non-complier; PL = placebo; LB = live birth; MC = miscarriage; AN = anencephalic; SB = spina bifida cystica.

*Case A.* Past history: 1 surviving spina bifida, 1 miscarriage. Diet known to be poor, excessive carbohydrate intake. Took no tablets until 7 weeks after LMP. She then took a considerable number 24 hours before blood sample was taken and then continued to take the tablets as instructed. We did not know this until after the end of the whole trial. Outcome, anencephalic miscarriage at 12 weeks.

*Case B.* Past history: 2 normal children, 2 anencephalics and 4 spontaneous abortions. Diet very poor. Started to take tablets 7–10 days after LMP at a time when she was feeling sick, off work with febrile illness. The nausea increased to vomiting and she returned most of the tablets she was taking. Her diet up to 8/52 after LMP was largely milk. Thereafter she felt much better. Outcome, full term spina bifida female, died on first day.

**Table 16.8** Folic acid supplementation trial. Outcome of pregnancy by treatment group

| Outcome of pregnancy | Folate supplement: Compliers | Folate supplement: Non-compliers | Placebo supplement | All cases |
|---|---|---|---|---|
| Normal fetus | 44 | 14 | 59 | 117 |
| Neural tube defect | 0 | 2 | 4 | 6 |
| All outcomes | 44 | 16 | 63 | 123 |

**Table 16.9** Folic acid supplementation trial. Outcome of pregnancy by quality of diet in first trimester; by folate supplementation received

| | Quality of diet | | | | | | All diets | |
|---|---|---|---|---|---|---|---|---|
| | Good | | Fair | | Poor | | | |
| Outcome of pregnancy | F | NF | F | NF | F | NF | F | NF |
| Normal fetus | 18 | 25 | 16 | 32 | 10 | 16 | 44 | 73 |
| Neural tube defect | 0 | 0 | 0 | 0 | 0 | 6 | 0 | 6 |
| All outcomes | 18 | 25 | 16 | 32 | 10 | 22 | 44 | 79 |

F = folate supplemented; NF = folate not supplemented.

tically as the numbers were so small. However, it is important to note that the two recurrent cases in the folate prescribed group were both non-compliers and so six recurrences occurred in 79 unsupplemented pregnancies (7.6 per cent) and none in the 44 supplemented pregnancies (Fisher's exact test $P = 0.04$). Thus the data suggest that there was a biological effect of folate which could be demonstrated even though in practice it was difficult to ensure that women took the tablets and so achieve satisfactory results. The specific effect of taking folate had to be separated from the more general effect of diet. There were no recurrences among 91 pregnancies who received good or fair diet ($P < 0.001$ Fisher's exact test) (Table 16.9). Within this high risk group of women, however, there were no recurrences in the 10 who had taken folate supplementation but six in the 22 who had poor diet and had not taken supplementation ($P = 0.004$ Fisher's exact test). Thus, although there may have been some bias owing to women who were receiving an inadequate diet the preventive effect of supplementation despite an inadequate diet could still be detected.

There were seven further pregnancies which resulted in a fetus with an NTD occurring amongst the women in these studies, which are listed in Appendix II. Four of these pregnancies were excluded because they were not visited within the prescribed 11 weeks from LMP. This was because these women had not requested tablets before conception or notified the pregnancy to us within the 11 weeks. Two patients had been in group O who had refused to take tablets; one had been randomized to the A group (folate) and one to the B group (placebo). Three other pregnancies occurred after the close of the trial, two from the B group and one from the A group. These pregnancies were unsupplemented as no tablets were sent to them.

All seven of these patients had poor pregnancy diets and one of them had had a previous normal pregnancy in the dietary study when she took no tablets but improved her diet. In the subsequent pregnancy outside the study period she relapsed to a poor diet, took no tablets and had a fetus with spina bifida cystica mildly affected who survived.

These further cases confirm our trial conclusions that a poor diet greatly increases the risk of a neural tube defect but offer no evidence either way on the efficiency of folate therapy.

## Conclusions from these trials

What was demonstrated was that in the circumstances of South Wales in 1969–1974, it was very difficult to establish a trial of preventive treatment in pregnancy and there was no assurance that the subjects would actually comply with a protocol, but that if the serum folate level and the red cell folate could be raised above critical thresholds then there were no recurrences of NTD in a high risk group of women.

The two dietary studies were based upon a pragmatic classification of the quality of the diets, but the detailed histories on which they were based were extensive and had been taken by two clinical field workers widely experienced in taking dietary histories from women in these population groups.

They demonstrate first that women who had had a fetal NTD were more likely than others to be taking a poor diet; in the first study there was no control group for comparison purposes but in our second study there were two comparison groups, the sisters of the index cases and the wives of professional families in the same area. The current diets of the index cases were markedly poorer than those of either control group.

They demonstrate secondly, that it is possible to persuade women to change their diet and three-quarters of the counselled group had made considerable improvements compared to only about a tenth of the group not counselled.

They demonstrate thirdly that in the prospective study all the recurrences occurred in the group of women who were shown to have a poor diet from the history taken contemporaneously at the second month of pregnancy.

The supplementation trial demonstrates, firstly, that such trials are very difficult to undertake. No assurances were offered and no pressure was placed on the women to join the trial, publicity was avoided and follow-up of women who did not return voluntarily to the field workers was not carried out. This reduced the possible population by three-quarters. Now that assurances can be given and publicity cannot be avoided the response would be much better.

Secondly, there is a serious problem of how to ensure that any treatment has been taken and how this can be validated. Probably a quarter of the women who did return to us were not taking the medications.

Thirdly, it is essential to distinguish between the effectiveness of an agent which has been used in preventing recurrences and the efficiency of a regime in converting an effective agent into a usable efficient system of treatment. The trial demonstrated that no recurrences occurred to women who took the folate, whether or not they had an adequate diet; similarly no recurrences occurred to women who had an adequate diet whether or not they were supplemented; all the recurrences occurred in the small group who had poor diets and were not supplemented.

The trial, therefore, is persuasive that NTD are the result of deficient diet and that they can be prevented either by an adequate diet or by supplementation with folate. It does not exclude the possibility that there are other deficiencies or some abnormality of folic acid metabolism (Hibbard & Smithells 1965; Yates *et al.* 1987) which can be swamped by an excessive intake of folate.

The supplementation study seems to demonstrate that folic acid unavailability to the embryo during the first 4 weeks of development is an important aetiological factor in NTD in South Wales at least, and probably in the British Isles in general, and that dietary supplementation seems to prevent recurrences (Stone 1980; Smithells *et al.* 1981). It also suggests that the folic acid content of Pregnavite forte F used in the highly successful supplementation trial of Smithells and his colleagues, is the major, if not the only active substance (Nevin 1981). It is not necessary that diets in the first trimester of women who have a fetus with an NTD need always be frankly deficient in foods containing folic acid. Much of the folic acid content of food is often destroyed, first in storage, in processing (e.g. canning), and then in the preparation of the meals. Some women cannot take their usual diets as they suffer from nausea and vomiting almost from the time that they conceive. Analogous to the absorption of dietary zinc (Smithells *et al.* 1976) that of folates may be interfered with by excessive amounts of refined carbohydrates and fats which are so common in the diet of women in South Wales. In others a disordered metabolism of folic acid may also play a part for there seems to be a suggestion that a greater proportion of women who have just had a child with NTD show evidence of impaired folic acid metabolism than do women with a normal outcome (Hibbard & Smithells 1965). Because of the possible folic acid absorption and metabolic problems it was thought that a pharmacological dose of folic acid, i.e. about ten times the daily requirement for a pregnant woman (Mervyn 1984) might swamp any block. Such a dose is thought to be entirely safe and without side effects. Indeed, a recent study where healthy female volunteers took 16 mg of folic acid per day did not seem to cause any untoward symptoms (K.M. Laurence *et al.* pers. comm.).

Contrary to what has been suggested (Edwards 1982), it is not considered that the time has come for supplementation to be used on a population scale or if it were that it would be efficient. A well-controlled study improving on the defects of the previous studies is still required (Chalmers & Sacks 1982). The trial was too small and was confined to a particular group within a particular ethnic group for extrapolation to be made with confidence, and the Pregnavite forte F trial was defective because of the choice of controls (Elwood 1980; Stone 1980; Smithells *et al.* 1981; Seller 1982). Therefore, the large multi-centred randomized controlled trial to prevent recurrence of NTD now being carried out by the Medical Research Council is essential.

## Other supplementation studies

### Periconceptional supplementation with multivitamins (Pregnavite forte F)

Smithells and his colleagues in a careful dietary study of almost 200 first trimester pregnant women found that the dietary intake of those from social class III, IV and V and those under the age of 20 was very much poorer than women from social class I and II (Smithells *et al.* 1977). They also found lower levels of red cell folic acid, leucocyte vitamin C and serum vitamin A, and to a lesser extent of red cell riboflavin in lower class non-pregnant women and more so in those who are pregnant. Because these findings paralleled the population incidence of NTD in Britain they concluded that subclinical deficiencies of these micronutrients probably contributed to their cause. This view was reinforced by their discovery of particularly low levels of these vitamins in the first trimester of pregnancies complicated by a fetus with an NTD (Smithells *et al.* 1976).

Smithells tried to launch a placebo-controlled supplementation trial of the effectiveness of a vitamin cocktail, containing folic acid as well, in the prevention of NTD. He was not able to obtain ethical permission for the use of placebo, so he had to make do with less satisfactory controls. His index patients, recruited mostly from local genetic counselling centres, came from Yorkshire, Lancashire, Cheshire, Northern Ireland and the south-eastern part of England, were volunteer women who had had one or more pregnancies with an NTD and who were planning further pregnancies but were not pregnant at the time. They were asked to take three Pregnavite forte F tablets* per day, not less than 28 days before conception and to continue taking these until the date of the second missed period. Control women were from the same areas but mostly from Northern Ireland, who were already pregnant at the time of recruitment, or who declined to take the tablets. The project was started in 1976 and preliminary reports on the first cohort of fully supplemented women and controls appeared in 1980 (Smithells *et al.* 1980; Smithells *et al* 1981a, b, c). The results from a second cohort were reported in 1983

* Pregnavite Forte F (Bencard). Daily recommended intake (in 3 tablets per day): vitamin A 4000 IU, vitamin $D_2$ 400 IU, vitamin $B_1$ 1.5 mg, vitamin $B_2$ 1.5 mg, vitamin $B_6$ 1 mg, nicotinamide 15 mg, vitamin C 40 mg, dried ferrous sulphate 252 mg, calcium phosphate 480 mg, folic acid 0.36 mg.

**Table 16.10** Outcome of pregnancies supplemented with Pregnavite forte F

| | Supplemented | Unsupplemented |
|---|---|---|
| Number of outcomes* | 459 | 529 |
| Fetuses with NTD | 3 | 24 |
| Miscarriages not examined | 30 | 19 |
| Normal fetuses or infants | 426 | 486 |
| Recurrences | 0.7 per cent | 4.7 per cent |

* Including 15 twin pairs (5 supplemented, 10 unsupplemented) (after Smithells *et al.* 1983, Table 17.6).

giving a total of 454 supplemented mothers and 519 controls from the two cohorts, with 3 and 24 recurrences respectively (Table 16.10), suggesting that the risk of recurrence was reduced from 4.7 per cent down to 0.7 per cent (Smithells 1983). Results of Pregnavite forte F supplementation in the highest incidence area (Northern Ireland) and the lowest (south-east England) in the British Isles suggests that the risks are reduced by over five times and twice respectively (Seller & Nevin 1984). A further review on 1080 fully supplemented pregnancies in high risk women appeared in 1985 with a total of 10 recurrences suggesting an average recurrence risk of just under 1 per cent (Seller 1985). The ability to prescribe this therapy under the Health Service in 1987 was therefore welcome (Anon. 1987; Harris 1988).

There is possibly some doubt whether the folic acid content of Pregnavite forte F (0.12 mg per tablet or 3.6 mg per day) is sufficient to overcome any metabolic block or absorption disorder that might be present. In addition, there is no firm evidence at present that all the substances present in Pregnavite forte F which include two vitamins (A and D), which are at least potentially teratogenic (Anon. 1985; Briggs *et al.* 1986; Martinez-Frias & Salvador 1988) are in any way effective in preventing NTD. Finally, supplementation with Pregnavite forte F is almost 30 times more expensive than with folic acid on its own (BNF 1988), and therefore may eventually not be the best supplementation method.

## Medical Research Council's multi-centre vitamins trial

The results of both the South Wales folic acid supplementation trial (Laurence *et al.* 1983) and the five-centre periconceptional multi-vitamin trial (Smithells *et al.* 1981) appeared to give encouraging results. However, statistical opinion was that the results of neither study were sufficiently clear to justify offering supplementation on a wide scale (Wald 1983; Wald & Polani 1984). In the past, promising results of trials of forms of therapy evaporated on closer scrutiny using stringent unbiased methods. Both the supplementation studies had statistical flaws. The South Wales study, though it was a double-blind randomized placebo-controlled trial was of only a relatively small number of pregnancies and was complicated by a high rate of non-compliance with folate taking (27 per cent). The periconceptional multi-vitamin study though of considerable numbers, lacked proper controls insofar that the non-compliers or the women already pregnant were used as such. There are strong reasons to believe that the index women differ substantially from non-compliers or those who do not enter trials.

Because it was felt that definite data had to be available to identify the possible part that multi-vitamins on the one hand and folic acid on the other play in the prevention of NTD, the Medical Research Council in the UK first considered mounting a randomized placebo-controlled trial at the end of 1981. However, the proposed trial aroused considerable professional and public opposition because of the use of placebo when an apparently effective preventative treatment was already available (Nature, 1982). Eventually the trial started with volunteer women at increased risk being randomized into one of four groups, those in each being asked to take a capsule with a different content. The four arms of the trial are: minerals* plus vitamins†; minerals plus 4 mg of folic acid; minerals plus vitamins plus 4 mg folic acid; and finally minerals only (placebo). The first patient was not recruited until July 1983. The trial was slow to gain momentum and is still on-going. Now there are 29 collaborating centres, 14 in the UK including South Wales, three in Australia and in Canada, two in western Europe, six in Hungary and one in Israel. About one new volunteer is recruited into the trial daily; altogether over 1300 have been recruited, over a 1000 of whom have become pregnant with 717 pregnancies completed (Anon. 1988). So far no clearcut results have been reported, except that non-compliers with the capsule taking assessed by capsule counting and by biochemical methods, seem to have a significantly higher risk of recurrence than the compliers. At the present rate of recruitment it is expected to reach the target number of 2000 in the trial by the end of 1990.

When the study is complete it may be possible to assess the effectiveness of folic acid and vitamins separately and together. Folic acid on its own would cost 1/30th of the price of supplementing with Pregnavite forte F; if it could be shown to be effective on its own in the prevention of NTD then it might be feasible to consider whether folic acid should be added to some staple items of the diet for the automatic primary prevention in the very women who are least likely to comply with any preconceptional supplementation regime and who at the same time tend to be those most at risk of NTD.

## Budapest population supplementation study

With the help of the family planning clinics in Budapest (Hungary) every woman planning a pregnancy regardless of whether she has previously

* Dried ferrous sulphate 120 mg and dicalcium phosphate 240 mg.

† Vitamins A 400 IU, D 400 IU, $B_1$ 1.5 mg, $B_6$ 1.0 mg, C 40 mg; and nicotinamide 15 mg.

had an abnormal child or not, is being invited to join a double-blind supplementation study (Czeizel, pers. comm.). The volunteers are randomized to 0.8 mg per day of folic acid (Elevit, Hoffman la Roche) or to take placebo.



### Dublin high risk supplementation study

Dublin, with its relatively high incidence of NTD (Devals *et al.* 1986), has been the centre for a supplementation trial carried out in the Irish Republic since 1983 with women who have had a pregnancy with an NTD being randomized blindly to taking Pregnavite forte F with its 0.36 mg daily dose of folic acid, Pregnavite forte (vitamins without folic acid) and 0.36 mg of folic acid only (Kirke, pers. comm.). For ethical reasons no placebo group could be included. So far about 370 women, 85 per cent of whom come from Dublin and its environs have enrolled. The study is still on-going and no results have been published yet.

### Folic acid supplementation in South Wales since 1982

Most mothers who have had a pregnancy with NTD in South Wales are referred for genetic counselling. As part of this consultation they are told about the risks of recurrence, the advisability of prenatal diagnostic tests with a view to possible selective termination; they are advised to have a high resolution fetal ultrasound scan and an amniocentesis at about 16 weeks gestation to enable amniotic alpha-fetoprotein to be estimated and isoenzymes of acetylcholinesterase to be looked for, or to have at least blood taken to measure serum alpha-fetoprotein levels. More importantly they are told about primary prevention, given dietary counselling and are advised to have folic acid or multi-vitamin supplementation. It was also suggested that they should allow at least two months between coming off any oral contraception and planning to conceive (Laurence 1989). Those women already pregnant or already on supplementation with folic acid or Pregnavite forte F by their general practitioner or obstetrician, are invited to volunteer for the Medical Research Council's Vitamins Trial; those who decline are advised to have supplementation with 5 mg of folic acid per day for at least one month prior to conception and to be continued until the end of the first trimester.

Since 1982 there have been a total of 192 completed pregnancies with

**Table 16.11** Folic acid supplementation since 1982 in South Wales

| | |
|---|---:|
| Normal outcome | 170 |
| Miscarriage | 15 |
| Recurrence* | 2 |
| Other malformations† | 5 |
| Total completed pregnancies | 192 |

* 1 Spina bifida cystica, 1 encephalocoele.
† 2 Clubfeet, 1 CHD, 1 Klinefelters, 1 extra digit.

preconceptional folic acid supplementation (Table 16.11). Amongst these there have been two recurrences, giving a recurrence risk of 1 in 96 (1.04 per cent). There were, of course, no controls for this further folic acid supplementation series, which is still on-going. The numbers supplemented with folic acid alone in South Wales are quite small compared with those on Pregnavite forte F reported by Sellers (1985) but both have very similar risks of recurrence (1.04 per cent and 0.94 per cent respectively).

## Changes in the incidence of neural tube defects in South Wales

Birth incidence of NTD in South Wales has decreased considerably in the last three decades, as elsewhere in the UK (Bradshaw *et al.* 1980), in The Netherlands (Romijn & Treffers 1983), in Canada (International Clearing House 1982), in Hungary (Czeizel 1983), in Australia (Danks & Halliday 1983) and in the Republic of Ireland (Kirke & Elwood 1984). Most of the fall in the last 14 years in South Wales and elsewhere in the UK can be attributed to prenatal surveillance followed by selective abortion (Laurence 1989). However, the fall before 1973 and the fall in the Irish Republic where there is no early prenatal diagnosis and selective abortion must have other causes.

Mid Glamorgan in the past had been regarded as a high incidence area with 11 NTD births per 1000 in 1957 (Figure 16.3). By 1959 this had dropped to 6.8 where it remained until 1962. For 1964–1966 it had again risen somewhat to 8.7 but since then and latterly with the help of NTD pregnancy screening it has dropped to less than 1 per 1000 births; (the sharp drop for 1976 is probably due to under-reporting following the National Health Service reorganization). Secular changes have been seen previously but never before had there been such a steady and unrelent-

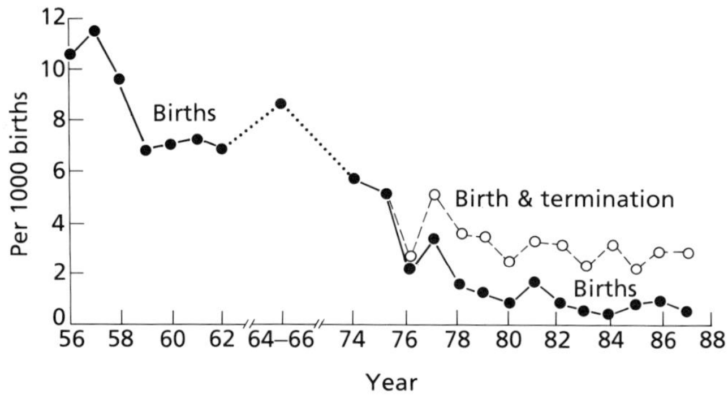


**Fig. 16.3** NTD births from 1956 to 1987 and NTD from 1973 to 1987 in Mid Glamorgan. The chart is based on births reported in two population studies of 1956–1962 births (Laurence *et al.*1968a), of 1964–1966 births (Richards 1971), on OPCS data supplemented with personal data since 1979 and information from the fetal malformation unit for terminations. The dip for reported NTD births in 1976 is due to reporting following the NHS reorganization. No acceptable data is available for 1963 and for 1967–1974.

ing fall in the incidence of NTD lasting several decades. The drop in the number of births since 1973 can very largely be accounted for, first by prenatal diagnosis and selective abortion in high risk pregnancies, and since 1977 by pregnancy screening using serum AFP estimation and more recently by ultrasound. Genetic counselling followed by pregnancy avoidance in high risk women is unlikely to have had much of an impact, not only because genetic clinics did not begin in South Wales until 1967 but also because recurrences in high risk pregnancies accounted for only about 1 in 10 of NTD. Similarly, dietary counselling and preconceptional supplementation given to high risk women available since about 1980 could also not have affected the incidence significantly.

The reason for some of the dramatic fall in the number of births for neural tube defects between 1956 and 1973 and some of the reduction since then may well be attributed to an improvement in maternal nutrition due both to the rise in the standard of living and to improvement of general education and the information available from the media and the women's magazines. The deep freeze revolution of recent years may possibly have been a contributing factor as it often leads to vegetables reaching the dining table with much of the folic acid content intact. Another, and possibly major reason for the reduction in the incidence is the smaller numbers of children being born to the mothers belonging to social class III, IV and V who are well known to have the highest risk and to contribute to the majority of affected pregnancies. There are almost certainly other factors responsible, as yet unidentified.

When the number terminated in the last 15 years are added to those which reached term, there is still a fall in the incidence but this is less dramatic than the number of births alone, and the reduction in the number of affected pregnancies since 1978 has hardly been significant (from 3.2 per 1000 in 1978 to 2.8 in 1987). Parallel to the reduction of the total incidence of affected pregnancies has been a quite dramatic fall in the risk of recurrence. Before 1961 the risk of recurrence estimated from a large family study was 1 in 20 (Carter *et al.* 1968). Between 1974 and 1982 the risk of recurrence in almost 800 high risk women coming to amniocentesis was 1 in 36. Between 1983 and 1985 the risk of recurrence in over 300 such women coming to prenatal diagnosis had fallen to 1 in 50 and between 1986 and 1988 there had been only 1 recurrence in 175. A similar fall has been observed in south eastern England (Seller & Hancock 1985). It is tempting to speculate that the fall in the rate of recurrence may in part be due to preconceptional dietary counselling and supplementation which has become increasingly universal for all high risk women since 1980. Some of the reduction will also relate to the general population incidence (Laurence 1989).

## Conclusions

The effective prevention of NTD will depend on a variety of approaches, including health education which should be part of the school curriculum, preconception and genetic counselling, folic acid supplementation and prenatal diagnosis for women who are recognized to be at increased risk and serum AFP and ultrasound screening for all pregnancies. The ultimate aim must be for primary prevention of NTD as far as possible by improvement in the maternal nutrition and the introduction of supplementation with folic acid before pregnancy is actually embarked upon and where appropriate population supplementation by adding folic acid to some part of the staple diet.

It must not be forgotten that there are almost certainly a number of environmental factors that trigger NTD. Folic acid lack may be an important factor in the UK. Other factors may be relatively more important elsewhere. The search for further triggers must continue.

**Appendix 16.1** Dietary study allocation of subjects with previous NTD

| | |
|---|---|
| Subjects visited on register | 902 |
| | — |
| Subjects accepted for dietary study | 442 |
| Subjects already on folate | 1 |
| Subjects already pregnant | 26 |
| | — |
| Subjects analysed in dietary study | 415 |
| | — |
| Subjects refusing any tablet (O) | 197 |
| Subjects allocated to folate (A) | 114 |
| Subjects allocated to placebo (B) | 104 |
| | — |
| Subjects allocated to treatment groups | 415 |
| | — |
| Subjects on good diet | 65 |
| Subjects on fair diet | 197 |
| Subjects on poor diet | 149 |
| Subjects with inadequate history | 4 |
| | — |
| Subjects to diet groups | 415 |
| | — |
| *Folate intervention trial allocation of pregnancies* | |
| Pregnancies reported | 186 |
| Pregnancies on no tablets (O) | 56 |
| Pregnancies reported too late (A) or (B) | 7 |
| | — |
| Pregnancies admitted to folate trial | 123 |
| | — |
| Pregnancies in folate group > 10 μg/l (A) | 44 |
| Pregnancies in folate group < 10 μg/l (A) (NC) | 16 |
| Pregnancies in placebo group (B) | 63 |
| | — |
| Pregnancies analysed in trial | 123 |
| | — |

## Acknowledgement

A part of this chapter is based on a chapter by K.M. Laurence, H. Campbell and N. James (1983) entitled 'The role of improvement in the maternal diet and preconceptional folic acid supplementation in the prevention of neural tube defects' which appears in *Prevention of Spina*


**Appendix 16.2** All pregnancies with recurrence of neural tube defect in intervention trial

| Patient No. | Diet in this pregnancy | Treatment allocation | Previous obstetric history | Year | Outcome | Reason for exclusion |
|---|---|---|---|---|---|---|
| 86 | P | NC | miss.N.An.N.miss.miss. | 1973 | SBC | — |
| 154 | P | NC | SBC survivor.miss | 1971 | An | — |
| 149 | P | B | An.SBC survivor | 1973 | SBC | — |
| 265 | P | B | An.N. | 1974 | SBC — Exomph | — |
| 288 | P | B | miss.miss.An. | 1973 | An | — |
| 293(i) | P | B | An. | 1974 | An | — |
| *In dietary study only* | | | | | | |
| 99 | P | O | SBC.N.N | 1971 | An | — |
| 108(ii) | P | O | SBC.miss.An | 1973 | An | Incomplete blood chemistry |
| *Excluded from both dietary study and trial* | | | | | | |
| 13 | P | O | An.N(masc) | 1973 | An — Exomph | >3/12 pregnant |
| 91(ii) | P | B | N.SBC.miss | 1973 | SBC) N) twins | >3/12 pregnant |
| 108(i) | P | O | SBC.miss | 1970 | An | >3/12 pregnant |
| 214(ii) | P | A(NC) | miss.miss.miss.SBC.N(A) | 1973 | SBC | >3/12 pregnant |
| 167 | P | B | An.N(G).N(G) | 1977 | SBC | Beyond study period |
| 201(ii) | P | A | N.An.N(A) | 1977 | An | Beyond study period |
| 293(ii) | P | B | An.An | 1976 | An | Beyond study period |

P = Poor diet. G = Good diet. A = Folic acid suppl. B = Placebo. O = No supplementation. NC = Folic acid non-complier. An =Anencephaly. Exomph = Exomphalos. SBC = Spina bifida cystica. miss = Miscarriage. masc = Mascerated. N = Normal outcome.

Note: Subjects 201 and 214 had normal children when taking folate tablets under supervision, but when they became pregnant beyond the supervised period they reverted to an unsupplemented and poor diet and both fetuses had neural tube defects. Subject 167 had two normal pregnancies in the study period when she was on a good supervised diet and treated with the placebo tablet. Outside the study period she reverted to a poor diet and the fetus had a neural tube defect.

*Bifida and other Neural Tube Defects* (Ed. by J. Dobbing) pp. 85–125, Academic Press, London. The permission of both Professor J. Dobbing and of Academic Press is gratefully acknowledged.

## References

Anon. (1985) Vitamin A and teratogenesis (Editorial). *Lancet*, **i**, 319–20.

Anon. (1987) An odd way to license a drug. *Lancet*, **ii**, 376.

Anon. (1988) MRC Vitamin Study. *Lancet*, **ii**, 1322.

Bradshaw J., Weale J. & Weatherall J. (1980) Congenital malformations of the central nervous system. *Population Trends*, **19**, 13–18.

BNF (1988) British National Formulary No.16. British Medical Assoc. and Pharmaceutical Press, London.

Briggs G.G., Freeman R.K. & Yaffee S.J. (1986) *Drugs in Pregnancy and Lactation; a Guide to Fetal and Neonatal Risk*. Williams & Wilkins, Baltimore.

Burke B.S. (1947) The dietary history as a tool in research. *Journal of the American Dietetics Association*, **23**, 1041–6.

Carter C.O. (1974) Clues to the aetiology of neural tube malformations *Developmental Medicine and Child Neurology*. **16** (suppl.) **34**, 3–15.

Carter C.O., David P.A. & Laurence K.M. (1968) A family study of central nervous system malformations in South Wales. *Journal of Medical Genetics*, **5**, 81–100.

Chalmers T.C. & Sacks H. (1982). Vitamin supplements to prevent neural tube defects. *Lancet*, **i**, 748.

Czeizel A. (1983) Spina bifida and anencephaly. *British Medical Journal*, **287**, 429.

Danks D.M. & Halliday J.L. (1983) Incidence of neural tube defects in Victoria, Australia. *Lancet*, **i**, 65.

Editional (1982) Biting off other tongues. *Nature*, **300**, 302.

Edwards J.H. (1982) Vitamin supplementation and neural tube defects. *Lancet*, **i**, 275–6.

Elwood J.H. (1980). Possible prevention of neural tube defects by periconceptional vitamin supplementation. *Lancet*, **i**, 648.

Elwood J.M. & Elwood J.H. (1980) *Epidemiology of Anencephaly and Spina Bifida*, p. 23. Oxford University Press, Oxford.

Harris R (1988) Vitamins and neural tube defects. *British Medical Journal*, **296**, 80–1.

Hibbard E.D. and Smithells R.W. (1965) Folic acid metabolism and human embryopathy. *Lancet*, **i**, 1254.

Hoffbrand A.V., Newcombe B.F.A. & Mollin D.L. (1966) Method of assay of red cell folate activity and the value of the assay as a test for folate deficiency. *Journal of Clinical Pathology*, **19**, 171–81.

International Clearing House for Birth Defects Monitoring Systems (1981) Annual Report. International Clearing House, San Francisco.

James N., Laurence K.M. & Miller M. (1980) Diet as a factor in the aetiology of neural tube malformations. *Zeitschrift für Kinderchirurgie*, **31**, 302–7.

Jongbloet P.H. (1981) Neural tube defects. *Lancet*, **ii**, 1291.

Kirke P.N. & Ellwood J.H. (1984) Anencephaly in the United Kingdom and the Republic of Ireland. *British Medical Journal*, **289**, 1621.

Laurence K.M. (1983) Neural tube defects: a two-pronged approach to primary prevention. *Pediatrics*, **70**, 648–50.

Laurence K.M. (1987). Spina bifida and anencephaly in South Wales. In *Genetic and Population Studies in Wales* (Ed. by P.S. Harper & E. Sunderland). University of Wales Press, Cardiff.

Laurence K.M. (1989) The genetics and prevention of neural tube defects and of uncomplicated hydrocephalus. In *Principles and Practice of Medical Genetics*, 2nd edn (Ed. by A.E.H. Emery & D.L. Rimoin) Churchill Livingstone, Edinburgh (in press).

Laurence K.M. & Campbell H. (1981). Trial of folate treatment to prevent recurrence of neural tube defect. *British Medical Journal*, **282**, 2131.

Laurence K.M., Campbell H. & James N.E. (1983) The role of improvement in the maternal diet and preconceptional folic acid supplementation in the prevention of renal tube defects. In *Prevention of Spina Bificla and other Neural Tube Defects*, (Ed. by J.

Dobbing), pp. 85–106. Academic Press, London.

Laurence K.M., Carter C.O. & David P.A.(1968a) The major central nervous system malformations in South Wales. I. Incidence, local variations and geographical factors. *British Journal of Preventive and Social Medicine* **22**, 146–60.

Laurence K.M., Carter C.O. & David P.A. (1968b) The major central nervous system malformations in South Wales. II. Pregnancy factors, seasonal variations and social class effects. *British Journal of Preventive and Social Medicine*, **22**, 212–22.

Laurence K.M., Harper P.S., Harris R., Nevin N.C. & Roberts D.F. (1987) Report of the Delegation of Clinical Geneticists, Spring 1986. *Biology & Society*, **4**, 61–77.

Laurence K.M., James N. & Campbell H. (1982) Blood folate levels and quality of the maternal diet. *British Medical Journal*, **285**, 216.

Laurence K.M., James N., Miller M. & Campbell H. (1980) Increased risk of recurrence of neural tube defects to mothers on poor diets and the possible benefits of dietary counselling. *British Medical Journal*, **281**, 1542–4.

Laurence K.M., James N., Miller M., Tennant G.P. & Campbell H. (1981) Double-blind randomised controlled trial of folate treatment before conception to prevent recurrences of neural tube defects. *British Medical Journal*, **282**, 1509–11.

MacMahon B. & Yen S. (1971) Unrecognised epidemic of anencephaly and spina bifida. *Lancet*, **ii**, 260–1.

Marking-Frias M.L. & Salvador (1988) Megadose Vitamin A and teralogenricity. *Lancet*, **i**, 236.

Mervyn L. (1984) *Dictionary of Vitamins*, p. 97. Newman Turner, West Byfleet.

Nevin N.C. (1980) Recurrence risk of neural tube defects. *Lancet*, **i**, 1301–2.

Nevin N.C. (1981) Neural tube defects. *Lancet*, **ii**, 1290–1.

New D.A.T. (1978) Whole embryo culture and the study of mammalian embryos during organogenesis. *Biological Reviews*, **53**, 81–122.

Oakley G.P. Jr (1985) Birth defects and surveillance. In *Prevention of Physical and Mental Congenital Defects. Part A*, (Ed. by M. Marois), pp. 71–90. Alan Liss, New York.

Record R.G. & McKeown T. (1949) Congenital malformations of the central nervous system I — survey of 930 cases. *British Journal of Preventive and Social Medicine*, **3** 183–219.

Renwick J.H. (1982) Vitamin supplementation and neural tube defects. *Lancet*, **i**, 748.

Richards I.D.G. (1971) *Incidence of congenital defects is South Wales*. PhD Thesis, University of Wales.

Romijn J.A. & Treffers P.E. (1983) Anencephaly in the Netherlands: a remarkable decline. *Lancet*, **i**, 64–5.

Seller M.J. (1982) Nutritional supplementation and prevention of neural tube defects. In *Clinical Genetics: Problems in Diagnosis and Counselling*, (Ed. by A.M. Willey, T.P. Carter, S. Kelly & I.H. Parker), pp. 1–9. Academic Press, London and New York.

Seller M.J. (1985) Periconceptional vitamin supplementation to prevent recurrence of neural tube defects. *Lancet*, **i**, 1392–3.

Seller M.J. & Hancock P.C. (1985) Is recurrence rate of neural tube defects declining. *Lancet*, **i**, 175.

Seller M.J. & Nevin N.C. (1984) Periconceptional vitamin supplementation and the prevention of neural tube defects in south-east England and Northern Ireland. *Journal of Medical Genetics*, **21**, 325–30.

Shepard T.H., Tanimura T. & Robkin M.A. (1970) Energy metabolism in early mammalian embryos. *Developmental Biology*, **4** (suppl.), 42–58.

Smith D.W., Clarren S.K. & Harvey M.A.S. (1978) Hyperthermia as a possible teratogenic agent. *Journal of Pediatrics*, **92**, 878–83.

Smithells R.W., Ankers C., Carver M.E., Lennon D., Schorah C.J. & Sheppard S. (1977) Maternal nutrition in early pregnancy. *British Journal of Nutrition*, **38**, 497–506.

Smithells R.W., Sheppard S. & Schorah C.J. (1976) Nutritional deficiencies and neural tube defects. *Archives of Disease in Childhood*, **51**, 944–50.

Smithells R.W. (1983) Prevention of neural tube defects by vitamin supplements. In *Prevention of Spina Bifida and other Neural Tube Defects*, (Ed. by J. Dobbing), pp. 53–84. Academic Press, London.

Smithells R.W., Sheppard S., Schorah C.J., Nevin N.C. & Seller M.J. (1981a) Trial of folate therapy to prevent recurrences of neural tube defects. *British Medical Journal*, **282**, 1793.

Smithells R.W., Sheppard S., Schorah C.J., Seller M.J., Nevin N.C., Harris R., Read A.P.

& Fielding D.W. (1980) Possible prevention of neural tube defects by periconceptional vitamin supplementation. *Lancet*, **i**, 339–40.

Smithells R.W., Sheppard S., Schorah C.J., Seller M.J., Nevin N.C., Harris R., Read A.P. & Fielding D.W. (1981b) Apparent prevention of neural tube defects by periconceptional vitamin supplementation. *Archives of Disease in Childhood*, **56**, 911–18.

Smithells R.W., Sheppard S., Schorah C.J., Seller M.J., Nevin N.C., Harris R., Read A.P., Fielding D.W. & Walker S. (1981c) Vitamin supplementation and neural tube defects. *Lancet*, **ii**, 1424–5.

Soler N.G., Walsh C.H. & Malins J.M. (1976) Congenital malformations in infants of diabetic mothers. *Quarterly Journal of Medicine*, **45**, 303–13.

Stone D.H. (1980) Possible prevention of neural tube defects by periconceptional vitamin supplementation. *Lancet*, **i**, 647.

Tanimura T. & Shepard T.H. (1970) Glucose metabolism by rat embryos *in vitro*. *Proceedings of the Society for Experimental Biology and Medicine*, **135**, 51–4.

Tennant G.B. & Withey J.L. (1972) An assessment of work simplified procedures for the microbiological assay of serum vitamin B, and serum folate. *Medical Laboratory Technology*, **29**, 171–81.

Thiersch J.B. (1952) Therapeutic abortions with folic acid antagonist, 4-amino pteroylglutamic acid (4 amino PGA) administered by oral route. *American Journal of Obstetrics and Gynecology*, **63**, 1298–1304.

Tuchmann-Duplessis H. & Mercier-Parot L. (1957) Sur l'action teratogene de l'acid X-methylfolique chez la souris. *Comptes rendues hebdomadaires des seances de l'Academie des Sciences (Paris)*, **245**, 1963–5.

Wald N. (1983) Possible prevention of neural tube defects by vitamin supplementation. In *Prevention of Spina Bifida and other Neural Tube Defects*, (Ed. by J. Dobbing), pp. 231–39. Academic Press, London.

Wald N.J. & Polani P.E. (1984) Neural tube defects and vitamins: the need for a randomised clinical trial. *British Journal of Obstetrics and Gynaecology*, **91**, 516–23.

Watt D.J. (1977) *Mechanism of development of spina bifida in the chick*. PhD thesis, Aberdeen University.

Wilson J.G. (1973) *Environment and Birth Defects*. Academic Press, London and New York.

Yates, J.R.W., Ferguson-Smith M.A., Shenkin R., Gugman-Rodriques M., White M. & Charke B.T. (1987) Is disordered folate metabolism the basis for the genetic predisposition to neural tube defect. *Clinical Genetics*, **31**, 279–87.

Ye H. (1986) The strategy of risk approach in perinatal care in Shuniyi County Beijing. Paper presented in Symposium on Paediatrics in China and Africa, Royal Society of Medicine, London, June 1986.

# 17: The ultrasound diagnosis of neural tube defects

J. MALCOLM PEARCE



Neural tube defects (NTD) account for approximately 50 per cent of the congenital abnormalities diagnosed in the UK and although the prevalence is falling they are still the commonest major abnormality. This chapter considers the problems of whether to screen for NTD and briefly reviews the biochemical methods of screening and diagnosis before discussing the role of real-time ultrasound, both as a screening and diagnostic test.

## Is routine screening for neural tube defects justified?

A half of all cases of NTD are anencephalic; since such infants die shortly after birth it could be argued that screening is not cost effective as they do not produce a long-term drain on finances. However, it is kinder to offer such women a termination of pregnancy rather than to await the natural outcome, especially as induction of labour is not always possible and Caesarean section may become necessary.

Spina bifida presents a different problem because it is a relatively simple surgical matter to close the defect after birth. However, even with optimal care in a specialized centre, the five year survival rate for infants with open spina bifida is only 50 per cent (Althouse & Wald 1980). Furthermore, only 6 per cent of the survivors in this study were free of major handicap, thus strongly suggesting that prenatal screeing should be available. Table 17.1 indicates the recurrence risk of neural tube defects but more than 90 per cent of affected women will not have a relevant

**Table 17.1** The risk of recurrence of neural tube defects

| | Recurrence | |
|---|---|---|
| Family history | Risk | Percentage |
| One affected | 1 in 20 | 5 |
| Two affected | 1 in 10 | 10 |
| Three affected | 1 in 5 | 21 |
| Parent with NTD | 1 in 33 | 3 |
| Parent and child with NTD | 1 in 9 | 13 |

Data from Carter & Roberts (1967) and Carter & Evans (1973) and Laurence (1983).

personal or family history, again reinforcing the need for a screening programme.

## Screening by means of alpha-fetoprotein

Alpha-fetoprotein (AFP) is an oncofetal protein, that is, it is found in embryonic and fetal life and in the presence of some tumours but is not detectable in normal adults. It is produced from the yolk sac in the embryo and from the fetal liver, and its function is as a plasma protein maintaining oncotic pressure. It is transferred to the amniotic fluid via fetal urine or as leaks from neural tissue or exposed bowel. The precise mechanism for its passage to maternal blood is unknown but it is thought to be by diffusion across the placenta.

Figure 17.1 is taken from the UK Collaborative Study (1982) and demonstrates the distribution of maternal serum AFP (MSAFP) in unaffected, singleton pregnancies and in those complicated by NTD. It can be clearly seen that there is no clear separation between the two groups, so some arbitrary cut-off point has to be chosen. The report recommended a level of 2.5 multiples of the median (MoM) and using this

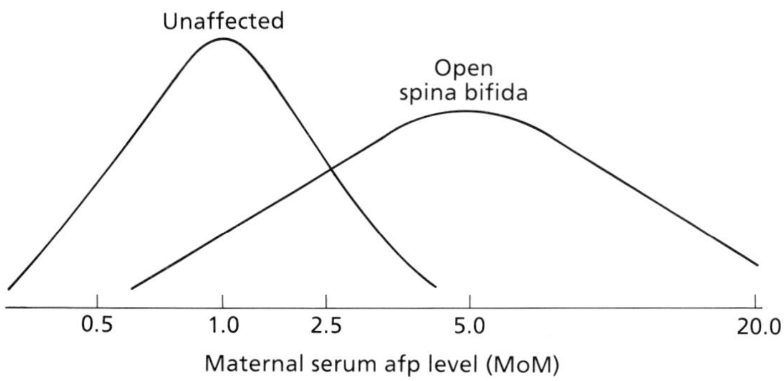


**Fig. 17.1** The distribution of maternal alpha-fetoprotein results in normal patients and in those carrying a fetus with an open spina bifida.

**Table 17.2** The risk of open spina bifida

| | Prevalence per 1000 | | |
|---|---|---|---|
| AFP (MoM) | 0.5 | 1.0 | 1.5 |
| 2.0 | 1 : 1600 | 1 : 800 | 1 : 400 |
| 2.5 | 1 : 560 | 1 : 280 | 1 : 140 |
| 3.0 | 1 : 250 | 1 : 125 | 1 : 65 |
| 3.5 | 1 : 100 | 1 : 50 | 1 : 25 |

level some 79 per cent of cases of open spina bifida should be detected with a false positive rate of about 2 per cent.

However, it must be remembered that a woman's chances of carrying a fetus with an open spina bifida is very dependent upon the prevalence of spina bifida in the area in which the woman lives, as Table 17.2 illustrates.

This means that in areas of low prevalence (less than 1/1000), in order to maintain a high detection rate (sensitivity), it is necessary to lower the cut-off point which in turn increases the number of false positive results. This problem has been demonstrated in actual clinical practice by Standing and colleagues (1981). Using a cut-off point of 2.0 MoM because of their low prevalence of only 2.3 NTD per 1000, they produced the results illustrated in Figure 17.2. Even in areas of high prevalence, such as South Wales, the screening programme has not been entirely successful as illustrated in Figure 17.3. There is a steady decline in the incidence of NTD (Figure 17.4) even when the increased antenatal recognition and subsequent termination of pregnancy is included (Figure 17.5) for reasons which are not clear. This means that the introduction of a new MSAFP screening programme must be carefully questioned and that existing programmes should be subject to regular review.

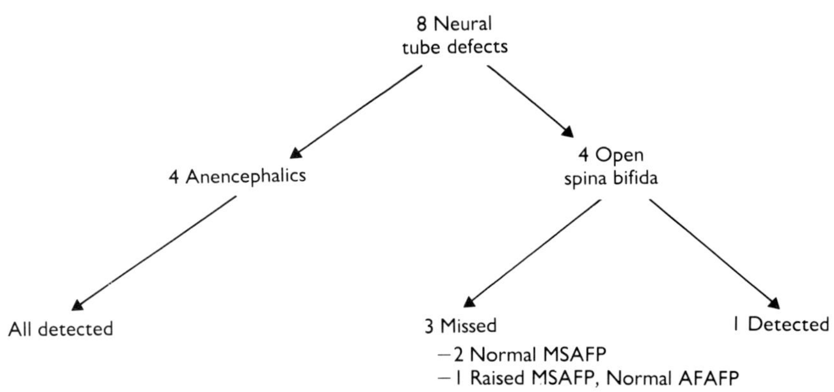


**Fig. 17.2** The outcome of a screening programme in south east England (derived from Standing *et al.* 1981).
MSAFP — maternal serum alpha-fetoprotein.
AFAFP — amniotic fluid alpha-fetoprotein.

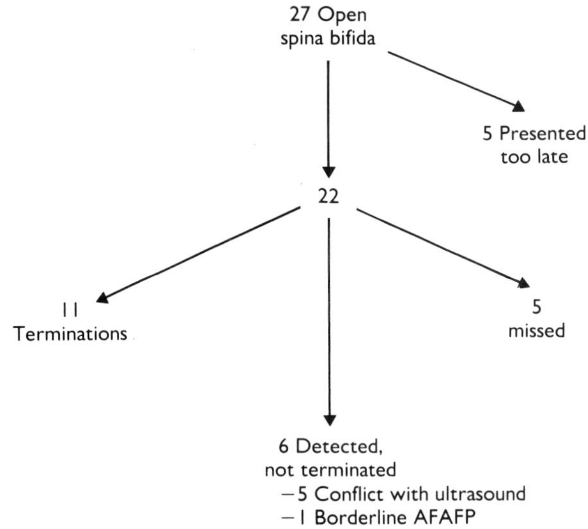


**Fig. 17.3** The South Wales experience of alpha-fetoprotein screening (from Roberts *et al.* 1983).
AFAFP — amniotic fluid alpha-fetoprotein.

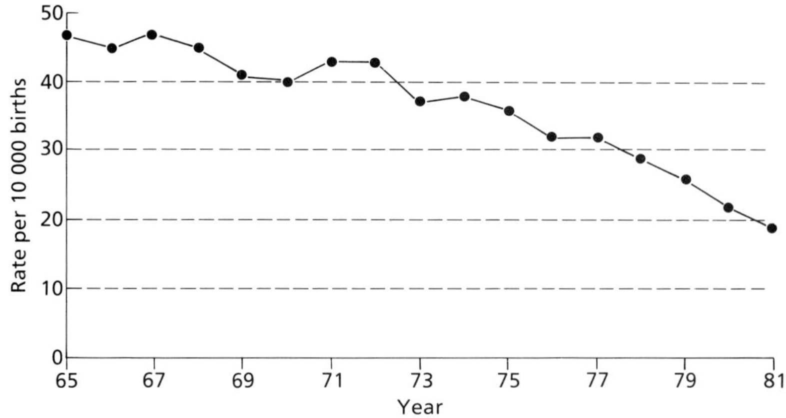


**Fig. 17.4** The decline in the birth prevalence of neural tube defects (data from OPCS).

## Biochemical diagnosis

Prior to the widespread availability of diagnostic ultrasound patients with a raised MSAFP underwent a simple ultrasound examination to exclude the causes of raised MSAFP listed in Table 17.3. The next step was to repeat the MSAFP estimation and if it was still raised an amniocentesis was suggested in order to estimate amniotic fluid AFP (AFAFP) and acetylcholinesterase.

A similar problem arises with the interpretation of AFAFP because

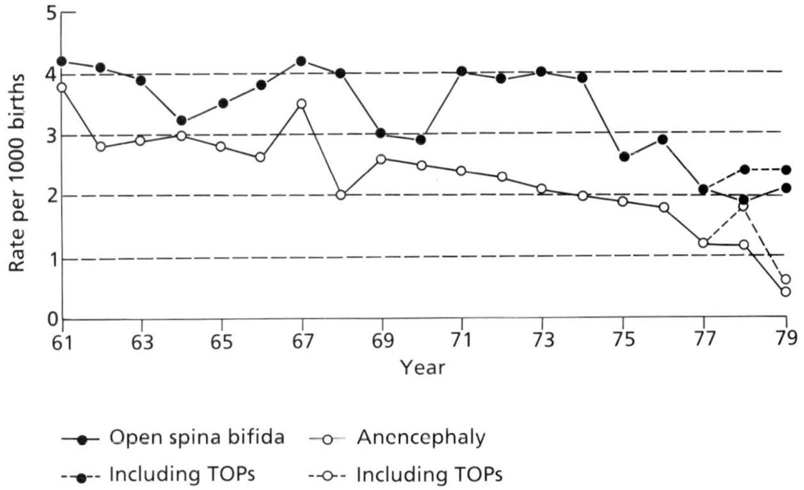


**Fig. 17.5** The decline in the birth prevalence of neural tube defects in the Liverpool and Bootle area, demonstrating that the fall is not due to terminations of antenatally diagnosed cases (from Owens *et al.* 1981).

even at the most favourable time of 16–18 weeks gestation (UK Collaborative Report 1979), there is still an overlap between the levels from unaffected pregnancies and those from cases of open spina bifida. Taking a level of 3.5 MoM this would detect 96 per cent of open cases of spina bifida with a false positive rate of about 0.2 per cent (UK Collaborative Study 1982). The addition of the estimation of acetylcholinesterase (AChE) significantly improves the false positive rate (UK Collaborative Study 1981).

However, AFAFP may be raised in other congenital abnormalities which do not necessarily warrant termination of pregnancy, for example gastroschisis. In addition, diagnosing spina bifida on biochemical grounds does not allow any assessment of the severity of the lesion and therefore it is impossible to determine the prognosis.

Furthermore, as Figure 17.6 demonstrates, hospitals offering a MSAFP screening programme should interpret the results of the tests based upon gestational age, as determined by ultrasonic measurement of the fetal biparietal diameter (BPD). This means that all patients should have an ultrasound examination at the same time as the blood specimen is taken for MSAFP.

**Table 17.3** Causes of raised MSAFP demonstrable on simple ultrasound examination

| |
|---|
| Gestational age more advanced |
| Multiple pregnancy |
| Intrauterine death |
| Hydatidiform mole |
| Anencephaly |

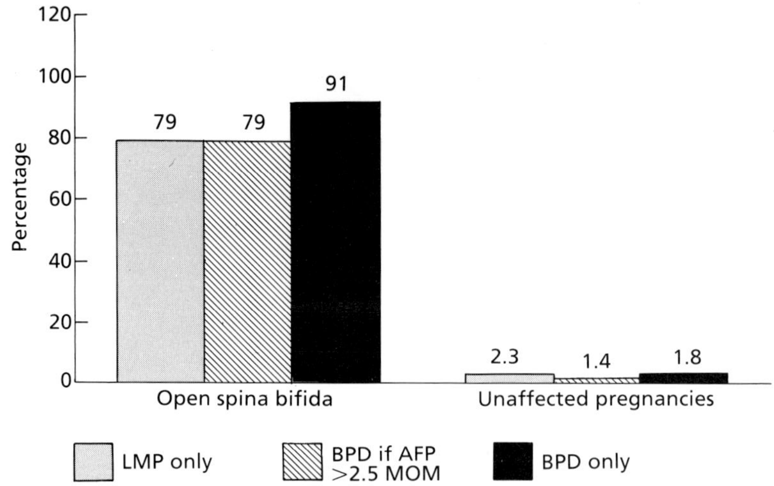


**Fig. 17.6** The sensitivity and false positive rate of maternal serum alpha-fetoprotein based upon the means of establishing gestation (adapted from Wald *et al.* 1982).

## Ultrasound as a screening test

Real-time ultrasound falls into the unique category of being both a screening and a diagnostic test depending upon the skill of the operator. The term high resolution ultrasound examination has frequently appeared in the literature, but modern equipment has excellent resolution so the accuracy of the test is almost entirely operator dependent.

On a screening basis Roberts *et al.* (1983) demonstrated that success is dependent upon experience. In the first half of their study (1977–1980) only 30 per cent of fetuses with spina bifida were detected whereas in the years 1981–1984 the sensitivity rose to 80 per cent. In 1984

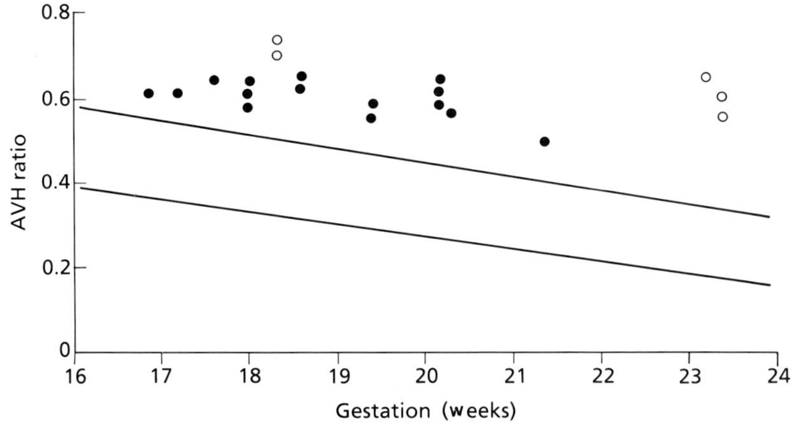


**Fig. 17.7** A.ventricle – hemisphere ratio chart with superimposed cases of ventriculomegaly. The closed circles represent cases associated with spina bifida whilst the open circles represent cases of isolated hydrocephaly.

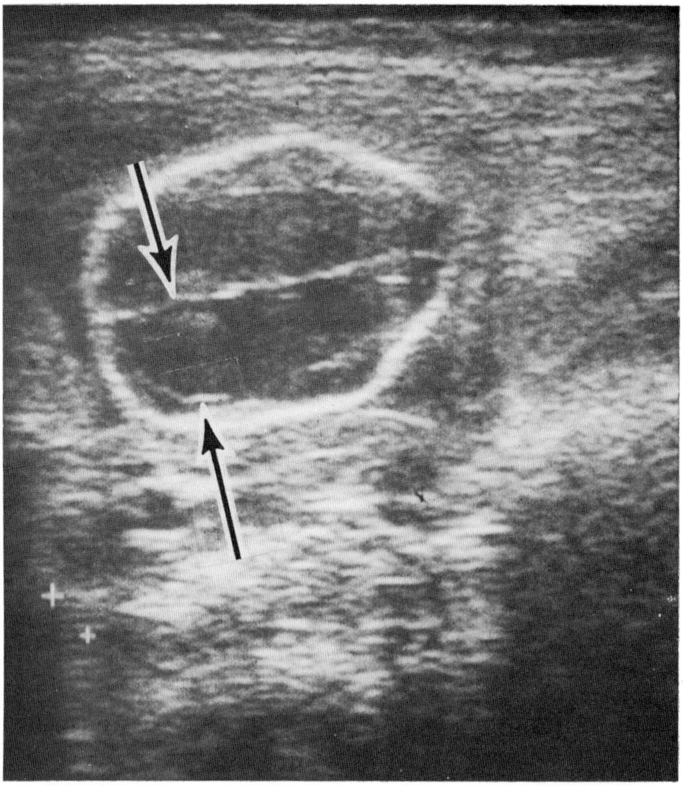

**Fig. 17.8** A transverse section of the fetal head demonstrating the lemon sign (see text). The arrows demonstrate the dilated lateral cerebral verticle.

routine screening by MSAFP was abandoned at St George's Hospital and ultrasound became the only screening modality. All 15 cases of NTD (6 anencephalics and 9 spina bifida) have been detected at the time of the routine ultrasound examination at 18 weeks gestation (St George's Hospital Report 1988). This experience has been confirmed by other workers, for example the group at King's College Hospital, London (Campbell & Pearce 1983).

Screening for anencephaly should be easy and as long as the fetal head is visualized the diagrams should not be missed. The defect of spina bifida is, however, more difficult to visualize but spina bifida is often associated with severe intracranial abnormalities. More than 80 per cent of fetuses with spina bifida at 16–20 weeks gestation will demonstrate dilatation of the lateral cerebral ventricles (Figures 17.7 and 17.8). At this gestation this is correctly called ventriculomegaly as the fetal head does not increase in size (hydrocephaly) until later in pregnancy. Furthermore, the fetal head shape may be unusual (Figure 17.8), producing the lemon sign (Nikolaides *et al.* 1986) and there may also be abnormalities of the cerebellum. This may be absent or may be smaller than expected because of the Arnold–Chiari malformation. A recent small series of 18 cases of spina bifida suggests that one of the above three findings may be present in all cases of spina bifida (Romero *et al.* 1987).

## The ultrasound diagnosis of neural tube defects

### Anencephaly

The first ultrasound diagnosis of a structural abnormality leading to termination of pregnancy was in an anencephalic pregnancy at 17 weeks gestation (Campbell *et al.* 1972). The diagnosis of anencephaly can be made from about 12 weeks gestation onwards as the fetal cranial vault is not visualized and the fetus takes on the appearance of a startled frog (Figure 17.9). The commonest reason for a missed diagnosis is failure to visualize adequately the fetal head. In the setting of a routine ultrasound clinic, gestational age may be confirmed by femur length measurements but unless the patient is brought back a week or so later the opportunity to examine the cranial anatomy will be lost.

### Spina bifida

The method for scanning the fetal spine in order to detect spina bifida was originally described by Campbell *et al.* (1975). Although the technique is based upon static B-scan apparatus it is much quicker and easier

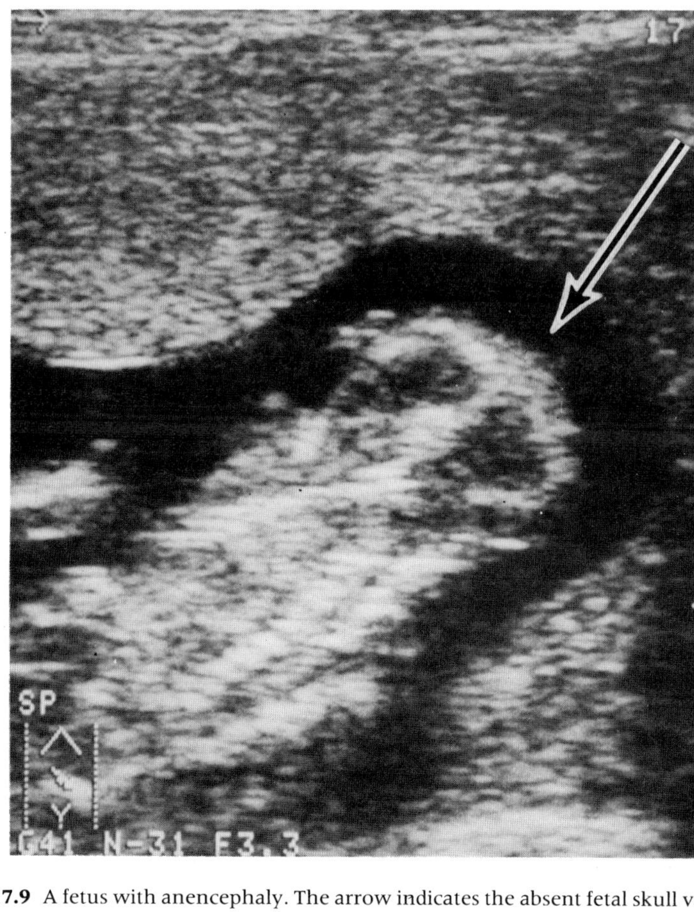


**Fig. 17.9** A fetus with anencephaly. The arrow indicates the absent fetal skull vault.

on modern, real-time apparatus. The entire length of the fetal spine should be viewed in longitudinal section as illustrated in Figure 17.10. The resolution of modern equipment should easily allow the skin covering to be visualized along the entire length of the fetal spine. Figure 17.11 demonstrates an open neural tube defect. In addition to this view each vertebrae should be viewed in transverse section, when the normal, closed neural arch appears as a closed circle, wherese the the incompletely formed arch is saucer-shaped or appears as a V-shaped complex (Figure 17.12).

By careful study the type of defect and an estimation of the number of vertebrae involved can be obtained. The bulge of the sac may be visualized and if strands of nervous tissue can be seen the leison can be diagnosed as a meningomyelocoele rather than a meningocoele, in which the nervous tissue is maintained within the bony confines of the spina bifida. Figure 17.12 shows serial transverse sections of the spinal cord allowing assessment of the length of the defect.

Using the above knowledge, together with the presence or absence of ventriculomegaly, the parents can be given a realistic prognosis, using a modified version of the criteria defined by Lorber & Salfield (1981). Poor prognosis is suggested with extensive meningomyelocoeles associated

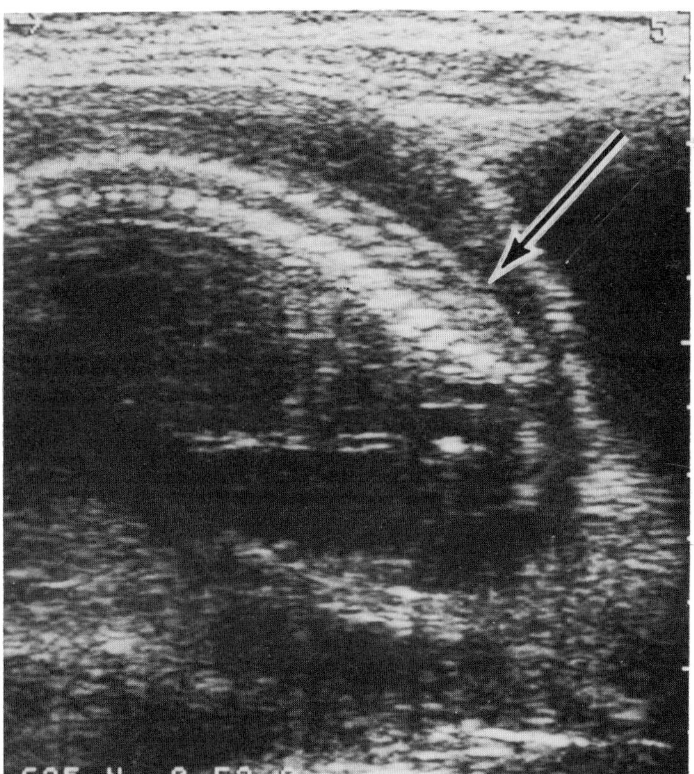


**Fig. 17.10** A longitudinal section of a normal fetal spine demonstrating the skin covering (arrow).

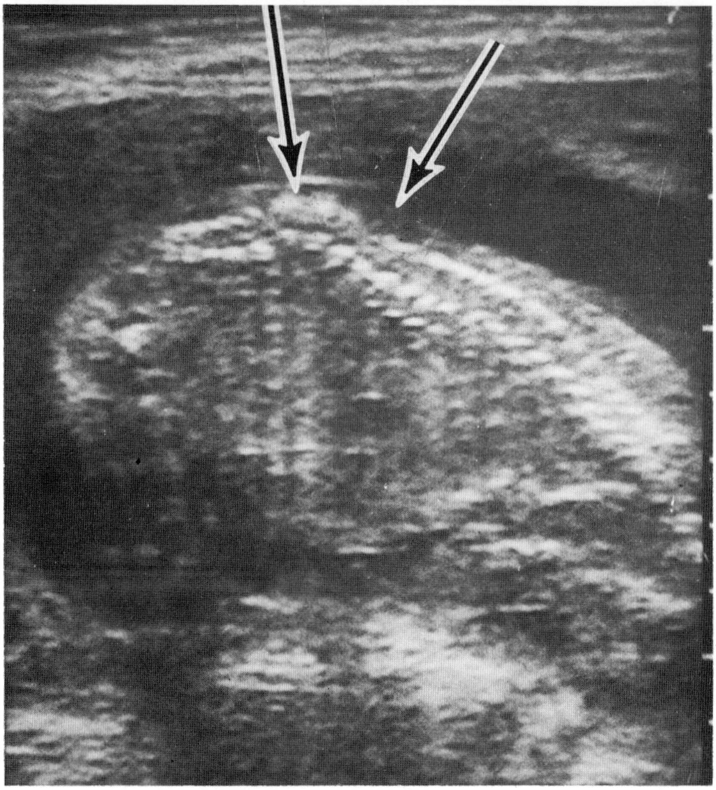

**Fig. 17.11** A longitudinal section of a fetal spine demonstrating spina bifida (arrowed).

(a)

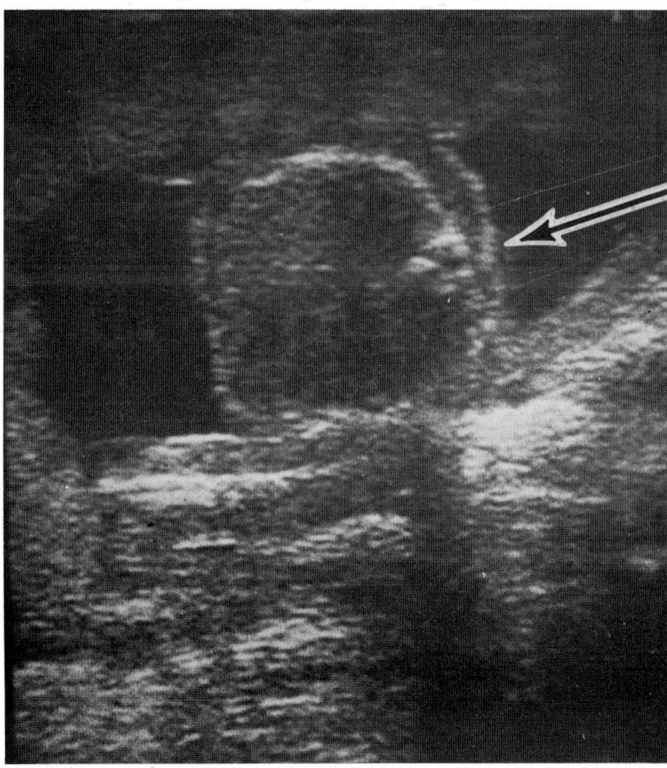

(b)

(c)

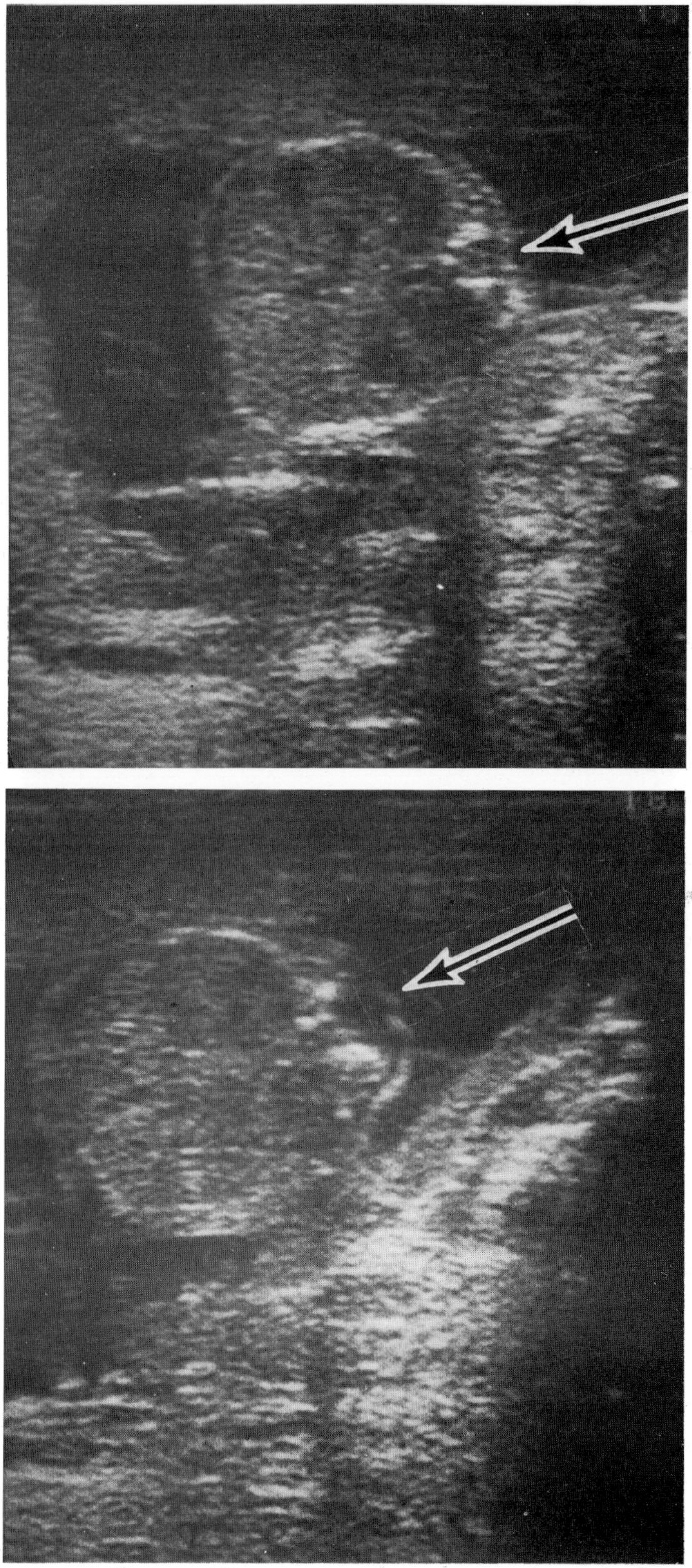

**Fig. 17.12** A series of transverse sections of a fetal spine demonstrating spina bifida. (a) Normal spine. (b) The start of the spina bifida (arrow) with the twelth rib visible. (c) An obvious spina bifida with a sac showing strands on nervous (arrow) at the level of the third sacral vertebrae.

**Table 17.4** The results of 1473 high risk referrals (from Campbell & Pearce 1983)

| Diagnosis | Detected | Not detected | False positives |
|---|---|---|---|
| Anencephaly | 48 | 0 | 0 |
| Spina bifida | 96 | 6 | 2 |
| Encephalocoele | 16 | 1 | 0 |
| Iniencephaly | 3 | 0 | 0 |
| Isolated hydrocephaly | 27 | 1 | 0 |
| Holoprosencephaly | 1 | 0 | 0 |
| Hydranencephaly | 3 | 0 | 0 |
| Microcephaly | 10 | 0 | 0 |
| Other | 17 | 1 | 0 |

with ventriculomegaly, or the presence of a deformed spine, usually the result of a fracture. Coexistent abnormalities are rare with NTD occurring in only 5 per cent of cases. Finally, it must be remembered that if the lesion involves more than two lumbosacral vertebrae there will undoubtedly be associated bladder and anal sphincter problems.

Table 17.4 is taken from Campbell & Pearce (1983) and reports the results of a referral clinic. The overall results for patients referred because they were at risk of a craniospinal defect gave a sensitivity of 96 per cent, a specificity of 99 per cent and the predictive value of a positive test was also 99 per cent.

### Ventriculomegaly

Enlarged cerebral ventricles are easily diagnosed on the same section that ultrasonographers use to measure the biparietal diameter (BPD). Figure 17.13 illustrates this section, whereas Figure 17.14 is a pathological section taken at the same level and demonstrates that the ultrasound image is a good reflection of the anatomy.

Enlargement of the ventricles is expressed by use of the ventricle–hemisphere ratio, and this clearly separates abnormal fetuses (Figure 17.7). Ventricular dilatation does not usually cause an increase in the BPD or measurement of the fetal head circumference in early pregnancy and so should not strictly be called hydrocephaly.

Over 80 per cent of cases of ventriculomegaly diagnosed in the first half of pregnancy will be associated with spina bifida. Isolated hydrocephaly is rarer in the UK and usually is more severe (Figure 17.7). Accurate post-mortem diagnosis is important if the parents accept the option of termination of pregnancy because the recurrence rate of isolated hydrocephaly is 1 in 30 but if due to aqueduct stenosis this is a sex-linked condition.

As equipment has improved, cases of mild dilatation of the posterior, cerebral ventricle have started to pose a problem. In our experience of 22 cases followed to at least one year of postnatal age, 20 have been normal with the growing brain eventually compressing the ventricles to

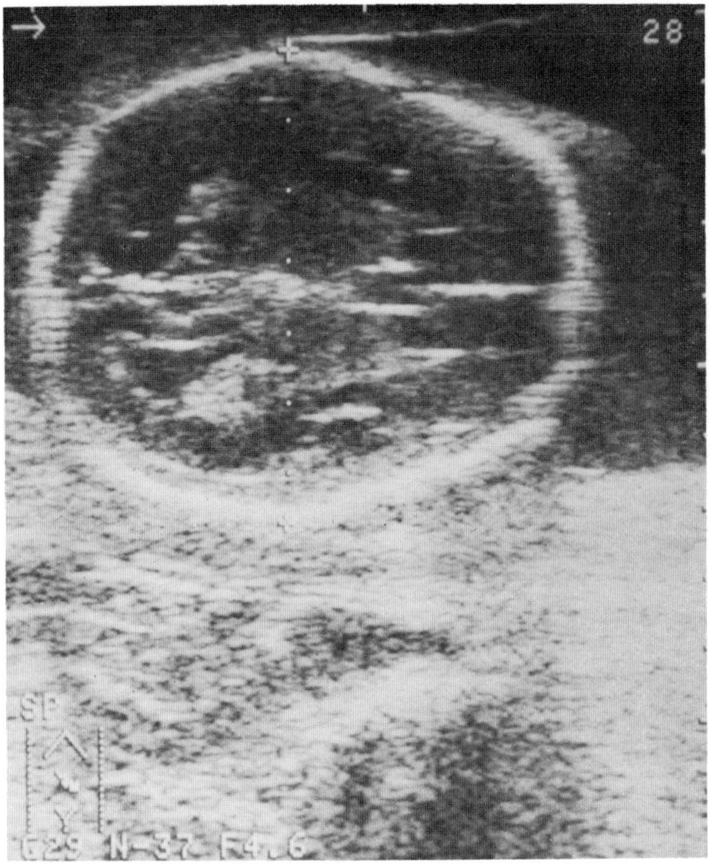

**Fig. 17.13** A transverse section of the fetal head demonstrating the section on which the biparietal diameter is usually measured.

normal size. In two cases, however, we have detected other structural markers suggestive of chromosomal abnormality; rocker bottom feet in one case and Ebstein's cardiac abnormality. Both these pregnancies were terminated following cordocentesis which resulted in the diagnosis of trisomy 18 in the first case and trisomy 21 in the second case.

## Rare abnormalities

Figure 17.15 demonstrates an encephalocoele, a rare form of NTD; these account for less than 1 per cent of all cases. These lesions are easily diagnosed but may be confused with cystic hygromata. Careful search, however, always reveals a defect in the cranial vault (Pearce *et al.* 1985). The defect most commonly is in the occipital region but may be frontal, nasal or parietal. The size of the defect ranges from small, without herniated brain to absence of large parts of the cranial vault with large quantities of brain in the herniated sac (exencephaly). The prognosis depends upon the amount of brain tissue within the sac (Lorber 1967); the more the extruded brain the worse the prognosis.

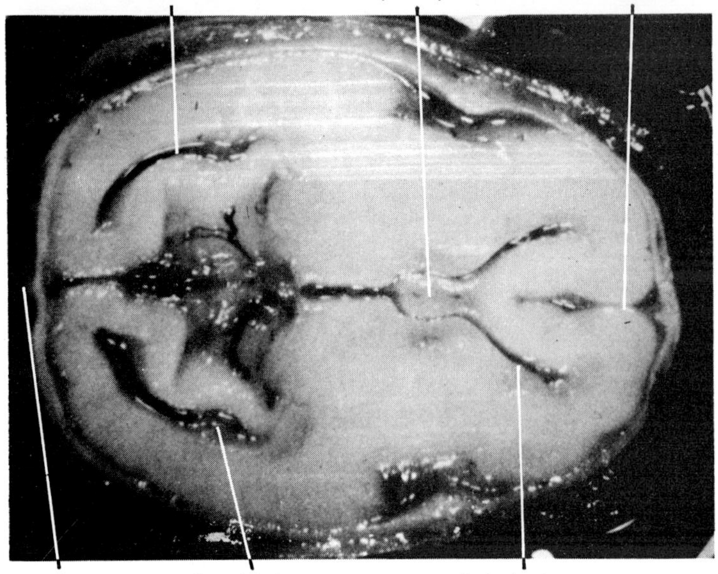


**Fig. 17.14** A pathological section of the fetal head taken at the same section as Figure 17.13.

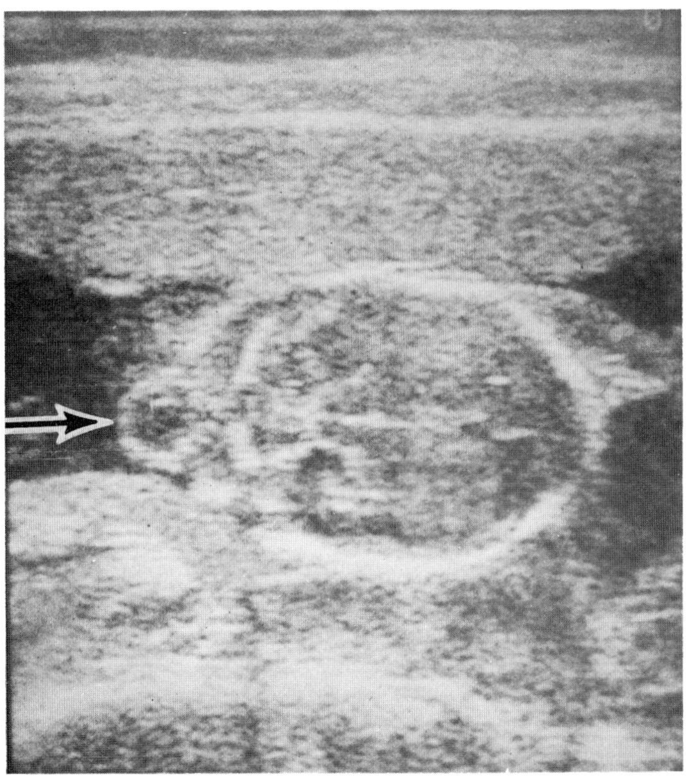

**Fig. 17.15** A section of a fetal head demonstrating an encephalocoele (arrowed).

## A comparison of ultrasound and MSAFP as screening methods

To date there has been no direct comparison of the two tests. Both screening tests should, however, be expected to detect 100 per cent of cases of ancephaly. Given ideal circumstances both modalities should be expected to detect more than 80 per cent of cases of open spina bifida. In the case of ultrasound this value should be obtained if only the cranial signs of spina bifida such as ventriculomegaly, the abnormal cerebellum and the lemon sign are sought. These signs should be apparent to operators after basic training in ultrasound. With increasing experience the sensitivity of ultrasound should be over 95 per cent with only low sacral lesions, unassociated with cranial signs, being overlooked.

A criticism that is frequently levelled at ultrasound as a screening tool is that the test errors have not been evaluated. Intra-batch error with MSAFP is quoted at about 5 per cent whereas inter-batch error is approximately double at about 10 per cent. Figure 17.16 illustrates a study performed by 20 ultrasonographers prior to attending an advanced course in ultrasound. They were each given the same video tape to review and were asked to freeze the tape and measure the anterior ventricle–hemisphere ratio on what they felt was an appropriate section. There were five normal fetuses on the tape and five fetuses who exhibited ventriculomegaly, but this was not revealed to the ultrasonographers. The inter-observer variation was 17 per cent but, as Figure 17.16 demonstrates, in no case would this have resulted in an abnormal result being declared normal or vice versa.

The possibility of combining the tests should be considered strongly as Persson *et al.* (1983) report that all 10 NTD from a screened population of 10 147 were detected using both methods. Interestingly, although ultrasound detected eight of the ten cases, in six cases the diagnosis was not made until after the MSAFP result was known to be elevated. The problem with combining the tests is that the ultrasound examina-

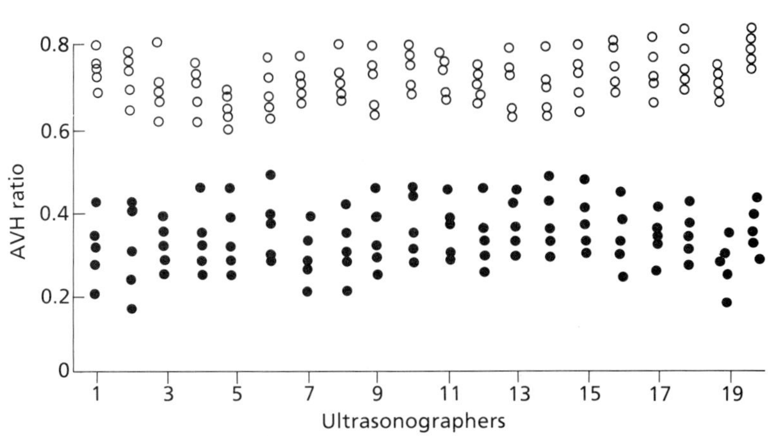


**Fig. 17.16** The inter-observer error of measurement of the anterior ventricle–hemisphere (AVH) ratio. See text for explanation.

tion should be performed simultaneously with the estimation of MSAFP (see Figure 17.6), which means carrying out the ultrasound examination at about 16 weeks gestation. Visualization of fetal anatomy is best performed some 2 weeks later (Chudleigh & Pearce 1983) and the low sensitivity for ultrasound screening reported in several studies may be the result of screening too early in pregnancy.

Of recent interest is the revival of MSAFP estimation together with estimation of human placental lactogen and oestriol as a means of screening for Down's syndrome (see Wald & Cuckle 1989). As more than 60 per cent of infants with Down's syndrome are born to women below 35 years of age, this new approach to screening has a lot of merit. If the tests were performed at the time of routine ultrasound examination at 17–18 weeks gestation we should expect to detect close to 100 per cent of all neural tube defects utilizing both screening methods. If patients who were discovered to be at high risk of Down's syndrome from the combined tests were then submitted to chorionic villus sampling and direct karyotyping, the result would be available at 18–19 weeks gestation which is comparable with the timing of results from amniocentesis for karyotyping.

## Conclusion

There appears to be good evidence for screening for neural tube defects, in that their detection in early pregnancy may allow termination of pregnancy. Both MSAFP and ultrasound have similiar theoretical success rates in screening for NTD in that both methods should detect all cases of anencephaly and more than 80 per cent of cases of open spina bifida; this figure can probably be improved to almost 100 per cent by combining both. However, the declining prevalence of NTD is making screening by means of MSAFP less accurate. This, combined with the fact that successful MSAFP programmes must incorporate an ultrasound estimate of gestation, suggests that if funds are only available for one screening test that ultrasound is the preferred method because of its many other advantages.

The recent suggestion that combining estimation of MSAFP with human placental lactogen and oestriols will improve the screening for Down's syndrome must be seriously considered. Performing these tests together with the routine ultrasound examination at 17–18 weeks gestation would seem to be the best method of screening.

## References

Althouse R. & Wald N. (1980) Survival and handicap of infants with spina bifida. *Archives of Disease in Childhood*, **55**, 854–61.

Campbell S., Johnstone F.D., Holt E.M.T. & May P. (1972) Anencephaly: early ultrasound diagnosis and active management. *Lancet*, **ii**, 1226.

Campbell S. & Pearce J.M.F. (1983) Fetal structural anomalies diagnosed by ultrasound. In *Ultrasound in Obstetrics and Gynaecology: Recent Advances*, (Ed. by S. Campbell), pp. 445–58. Saunders & Co., London.

Campbell S., Pryse-Davies J., Coltart T.M. *et al.* (1975) Ultrasound diagnosis of spina bifida. *Lancet*, **ii**, 1126–7.

Carter C.O. & Evans K. (1973) Children of adult survivors with spina bifida cytica. *Lancet*, **ii**, 924–6.

Carter C.O. & Roberts J.A.F. (1973) The risk of recurrence after two children with central nervous system malformations. *Lancet*, **i**, 306–7.

Chudleigh P. & Pearce J.M.F. (1983) *Obstetric Ultrasound: How, Why and When.* Churchill Livingstone, Edinburgh.

Lorber J. (1967) The prognosis of occipital encephalocoeles. *Developmental Medicine and Child Neurology*, **13** (suppl.), 75–9.

Lorber J. & Salfield S.A.W. (1981) Results of selective treatment of spina bifida cystica. *Archives of Disease in Childhood*, **56**, 822–6.

Nicolaides K.H., Campbell S. & Gabbe S.G. (1986) Ultrasound screening for spina bifida: cranial and cerebellar signs. *Lancet*, **ii**, 272–3.

Ownes J.R., McAllister E., Harris F. & West L. (1981) Year incidence of neural tube defects in an area under constant surveillance. *Lancet*, **ii**, 1032–4.

Pearce J.M.F., Griffin D. & Campbell S. (1985) The differential, prenatal diagnosis of cystic hygromata and encephalocoele by ultrasound examination. *Journal of Clinical Ultrasound*, **13**, 317–20.

Pearce J.M.F. & Chemberlain G.V.P.C. (Eds) (1988) *Report of the Department of Obstetrics & Gynaecology*, St. George's Hospital, London.

Persson P.H., Kullanders S. & Gennser G. (1983) Screening for fetal malformations using ultrasound and measurements of alpha feto protein in maternal serum. *British Medical Journal*, **286**, 747–9.

Roberts C.J., Hibbard B.M. & Roberts E.E. (1983) Diagnostic effectiveness of ultrasound in the detection of neural tube defects. The South Wales experience of 2059 scans in high risk mothers. *Lancet*, **ii**, 1068–70.

Romero R., Pilu G., Jeanty P., Ghidini A. & Hobbins J.C. (1987) *Prenatal Diagnosis of Congenital Abnormalities*, p. 41. Appleton & Lange, Norwalk, Connecticut, USA.

Standing S.J., Brindle M.J., MacDonald A.P. & Lacey R.W. (1981) Maternal alphafetoprotein screening: two year's experience in a low risk district. *British Medical Journal*, **283**, 705–7.

UK Collaborative Study on Acetyl Cholinesterase (1981). Amniotic fluid cholinesterase as a secondary test in the diagnosis of anencephaly and open spina bifida in early pregnancy. *Lancet*, **ii**, 27–33.

UK Collaborative Study on Alphafetoprotein in relation to Neural Tube Defects — Second report (1979) Amniotic fluid alphaprotein measurement in antenatal diagnosis of anencephaly and open spina bifida in early pregnancy. *Lancet*, **ii**, 652–4.

UK Collaborative Study on Alphafetoprotein in relation to Neural Tube Defects — fourth report (1982) Estimating an individuals chance of having an open spina bifida and the value of repeat AFP testing. *Journal of Epidemiology and Community Health*, **36**, 87–92.

Wald N.J. & Cuckle H.S. (1989) Screening for neural tube defects and Down's syndrome by means of serum alphafetoprotein. In *Obstetrics*, (Ed. by A.C. Turnbull & G.V.P. Chamberlain), pp. 269–90. Churchill Livingstone, Edinburgh.

Wald N.J., Cuckle H.S., Boreham J. & Turnbull A.C. (1982) The effect of estimating gestational age by ultrasound cephalometry on the specificity of alphafetoprotein screening for neural tube defects. *British Journal of Obstetrics and Gynaecology*, **89**, 1050–4.

# 18: Detection of congenital abnormalities of the cardiovascular system by ultrasound

GURLEEN SHARLAND AND LINDSEY D. ALLAN



During the past eight years it has been established that normal fetal cardiac anatomy can be defined accurately from eighteen weeks gestation onwards (Allan *et al.* 1980; Lange *et al.* 1980). As a result, it is possible to diagnose structural heart abnormalities (Kleinman *et al.* 1980; Allan *et al.* 1984). Over the years, advances in equipment have enabled a high degree of diagnostic accuracy.

A detailed scan of the fetal heart may be time consuming and requires experienced personnel and high quality equipment. However, by looking for one section of the fetal heart only, the four chamber view, many major cardiac defects may be excluded. Studies from the New England Infant Care Program (Fyler *et al.* 1980) and the Brompton Hospital in this country (Scott *et al.* 1984) imply that about 3/1000 live births present with the most severe forms of congenital heart disease in the first year of life. Of these, 2/1000 can be detected by examining the four chamber view only and will be abnormalities at the severe end of the spectrum of cardiac malformations. Ultrasonographers involved in routine obstetric scanning can readily be taught to obtain, understand and interpret the four chamber view. Thus potentially up to two-thirds of patients normally presenting to paediatric cardiology units are identifiable before birth.

Once this section can be obtained clearly in every patient, the ultrasonographer can attempt to recognize the more difficult arterial views.

## Normal fetal cardiac anatomy

When examining the fetal heart there are six connections that may be sought for, three on either side of the heart. These are at the venous-atrial junction, the atrioventricular junction and the ventriculo-arterial junction.

On the right side of the heart, the inferior and superior vena cavae drain to the right atrium. This then connects via the tricuspid valve to the right ventricle. The pulmonary artery arises from the right ventricle. Similarly, on the left side of the heart, the left atrium receives the pulmonary veins. The left atrium then connects through the mitral valve to the left ventricle, which then gives rise to the aorta.

Heart defects which do not involve a connection abnormality can also be detected antenatally. These are usually more minor and of a type that may be correctable. However, it is mainly the more severe forms of heart disease that are important to diagnose in fetal life, as many carry a very poor prognosis for survival in childhood.

The normality of many of the above connections may be seen on the four chamber view. This is the easiest view to obtain and should be the view with which to start examination of the fetal heart.

## The four chamber view

The four chamber view is achieved by cutting straight across the fetal thorax above the level of the diaphragm between the views normally sought to measure the abdominal circumference and the biparietal dia-

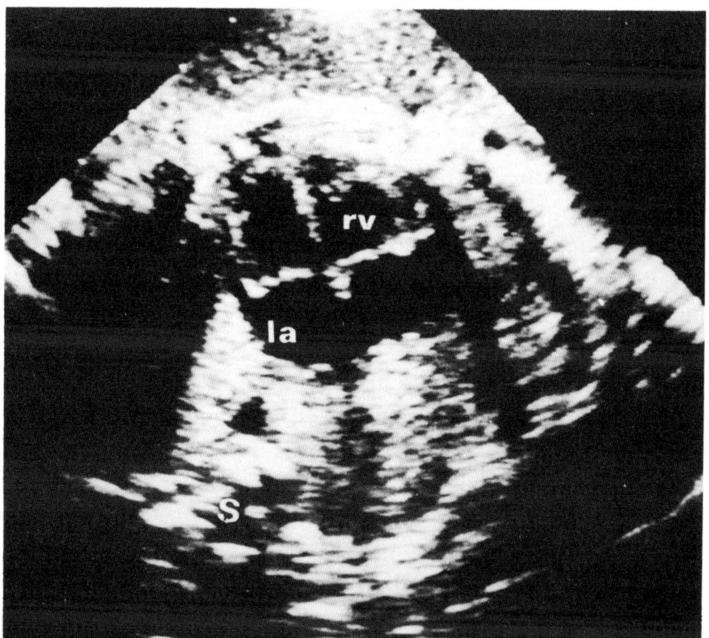


**Fig. 18.1** The four chamber view of the fetal heart is seen with the apex directed towards the transducer. The right ventricle (rv) lies under the anterior chest wall opposite the spine (S). The descending aorta is seen as a circular structure anterior to the spine. The left atrium (la) lies anterior to this. The remaining chambers of the heart, the left ventricle and right atrium can then be identified.

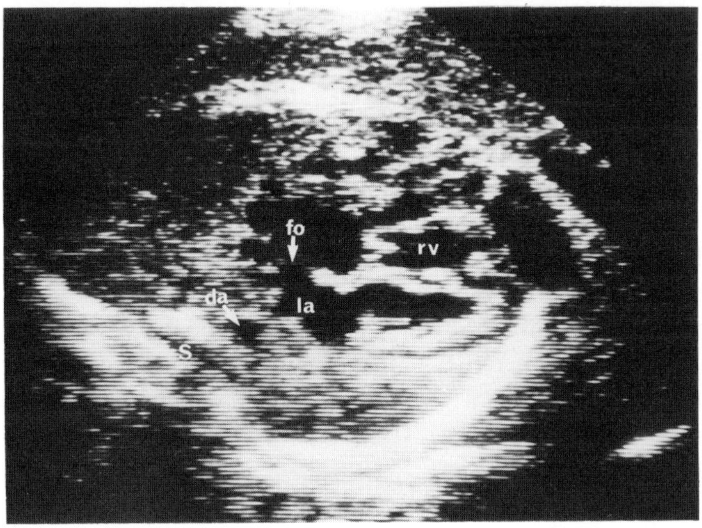


**Fig. 18.2** The four chamber view is seen with the ultrasound beam perpendicular to the line of the septum. The foramen ovale (fo) can be identified. The method of orientation described allows the cardiac chambers to be identified.

meter. The heart lies mainly in the left chest with the apex pointing out of the left anterior chest wall (Figure 18.1). The normal position of the heart within the thorax and in relation to the spine should always be noted.

The appearance of the four chambers will vary depending on the position of the fetus relative to the ultrasound beam (Figures 18.1 and 18.2). Regardless of the fetal lie, however, the method of orientation to identify cardiac chambers is always the same. The spine is located first. Opposite the spine is the anterior chest wall or sternum. Below the sternum lies the right ventricle. Returning to the spine, the descending aorta is seen as a circle in the mediastinum lying anterior to the spine. The left atrium can be identified lying anterior to the descending aorta. The remaining intracardiac chambers, the right atrium and left ventricle can then be identified. The following normal features should always be sought when examining the four chamber view:

**1** The heart occupies about a third of the thorax.

**2** There are two atria of approximately equal size.

**3** There are two ventricles of approximately equal size and thickness.

**4** The atrial and ventricular septa meet the two atrioventricular valves at the crux of the heart in an offset cross.

**5** The foramen ovale defect is seen in the atrial septum.

**6** The ventricular septum appears intact.

After 30 weeks gestation the right ventricle may look slightly larger than the left in the normal fetus. The septal leaflet of the tricuspid valve inserts slightly lower in the ventricular septum than the mitral valve, and this produces the offset cross appearance at the crux of the heart.

The pulmonary veins can be seen connecting to the left atrium in the four chamber view but the ultrasound beam needs to be swept up and down at the back of the left atrium to find the veins.

## The arterial connections

Once the four chamber view is familiar, the arterial connections can be sought Maintaining a horizontal section of the thorax but moving cranially, the origin of the aorta can be found at the crux of the heart arising from the left (posterior) ventricle. Twisting the transducer in this plane will open out the aorta in the long axis view of the left ventricle (Figure 18.3). Moving further cranially, the pulmonary artery can be seen arising close to the anterior chest wall and directed straight back towards the spine. Tilting the transducer cranially will produce the image in Figure 18.4.

The arterial connections may be visualized in many projections and these are described elsewhere (Allan 1986). However, there are certain features to note regarding the great arteries whatever the projection may be:

**1** Two arterial valves can always be seen.

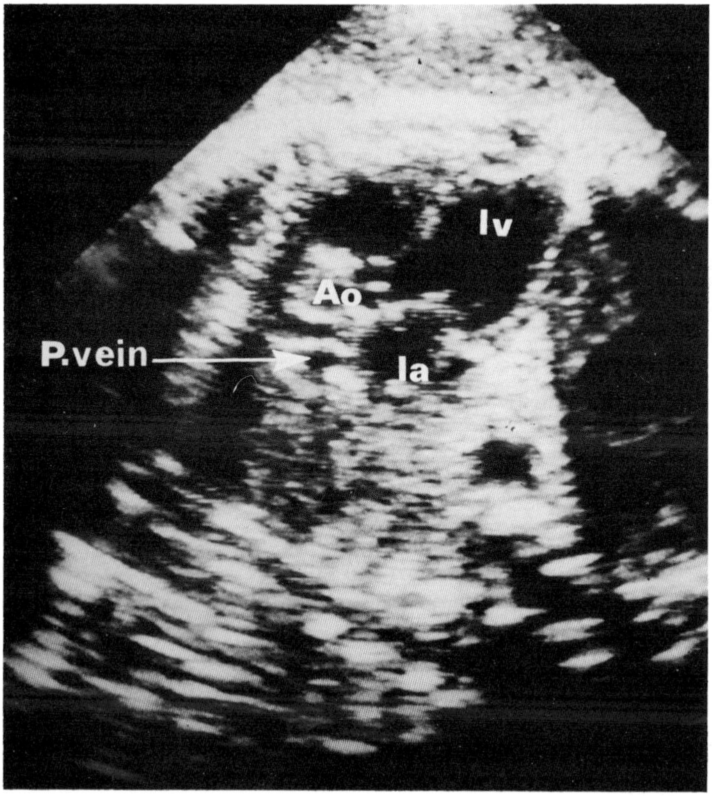


**Fig. 18.3** The aorta (Ao) can be seen arising from the left ventricle (lv). It can be seen that the aorta is totally committed to the left ventricle. In this view a pulmonary vein (P.vein) is seen draining into the left artium (la).

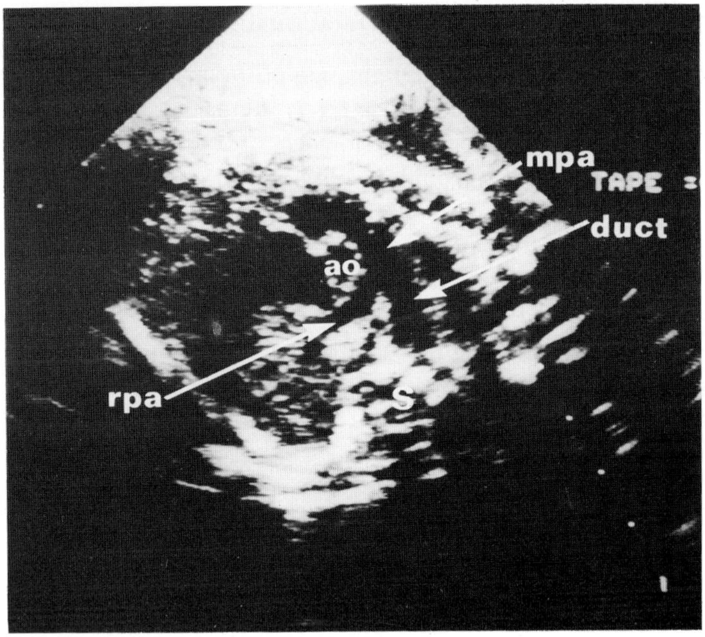


**Fig. 18.4** The pulmonary artery arises from the front of the chest and is directed posteriorly towards the spine. The main pulmonary artery (mpa) is seen branching into the right pulmonary artery (rpa) and ductus arteriosus. The duct joins the descending aorta just anterior to the spine (S). The ascending aorta (ao) is seen in cross section.

**2** The pulmonary artery is slightly larger than the aorta in size.
**3** The aorta arises wholly from the posterior ventricle and gives rise to the aortic arch. The head and neck vessels can be seen to arise from here.
**4** The pulmonary artery arises from the anterior ventricle and branches into the ductus and pulmonary arteries.
**5** The two great arteries cross each other at right angles to each other at their origin.

## Cardiac malformations

Structural abnormalities of the fetal heart are more easily detected if the examination is approached in a systematic manner. The diagnosis may be made by a non-cardiologist but it is important that a paediatric cardiologist is involved to confirm the diagnosis and to counsel the patient accurately with the appropriate prognosis.

### Connection abnormalities

These can occur at the venous-atrial, the atrioventricular or the ventricular-arterial junction. Any of the connections may be missing, displaced or inappropriate. In addition to connection abnormalities there may be valvular stenosis, ventricular septal defects, aortic arch defects and cardiac tumours. The abnormalities seen in practice are discussed below.

## ABNORMALITIES AT THE VENOUS ATRIAL JUNCTION

The venous connection on the right side of the heart, the inferior vena cava, is not usually sought as it is rarely abnormal and as an isolated finding it would be unimportant. However, if it is associated with complex heart disease there would be other features that would alert the examiner to the presence of an anomaly.

Abnormality of the pulmonary venous connection is an important, but difficult, condition to recognize prenatally. It tends to be an isolated anomaly with a good prognosis for corrective surgery if the infant is in good condition at operation. It would therefore benefit from prenatal diagnosis and immediate postnatal therapy. The prenatal features include right ventricular dilatation and failure to identify the normal insertion of the pulmonary veins.

## ABNORMALITIES AT THE ATRIOVENTRICULAR JUNCTION

There may be an absent or atretic connection of either atrioventricular valve, i.e. mitral atresia or tricuspid atresia. In either case, there is no patent valve seen in the normal position between the appropriate atrium and ventricle. The ventricular chamber of the affected side appears small as a consequence of the lack of flow through the related ventricle. An example of mitral atresia is shown in Figure 18.5.

Ebstein's anomaly is a malformation of the tricuspid valve where the septal leaflet of this valve is displaced into the cavity of the right ventricle

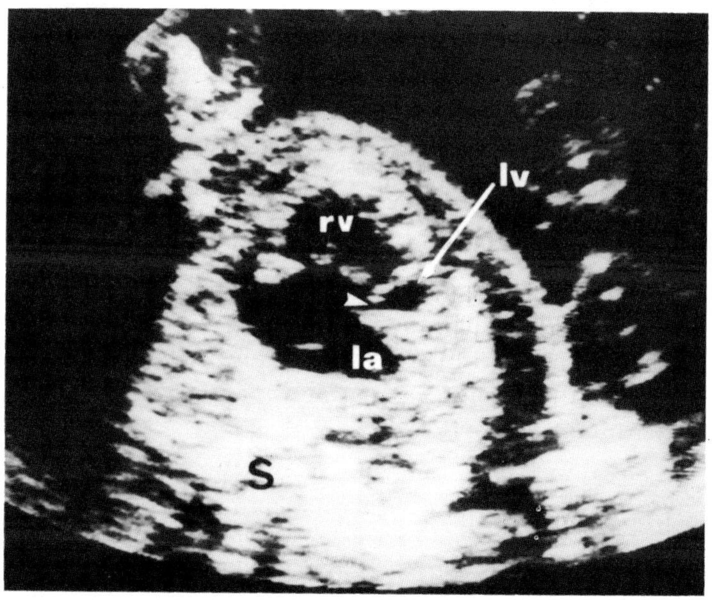


**Fig. 18.5** The heart is seen in the four chamber view but the left ventricle (lv) is much smaller than the right (rv). There is no direct connection between the floor of the left atrium (la) and the left ventricle. A small ventricular septal defect is seen (arrow). This is an example of mitral atresia.

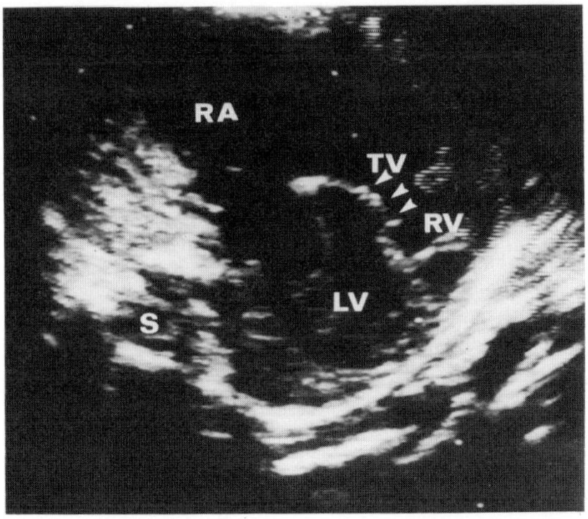


**Fig. 18.6** The septal leaflet of the tricuspid valve (TV) is tethered to the ventricular septum. The tricuspid valve was incompetent resulting in right atrial (RA) dilatation.

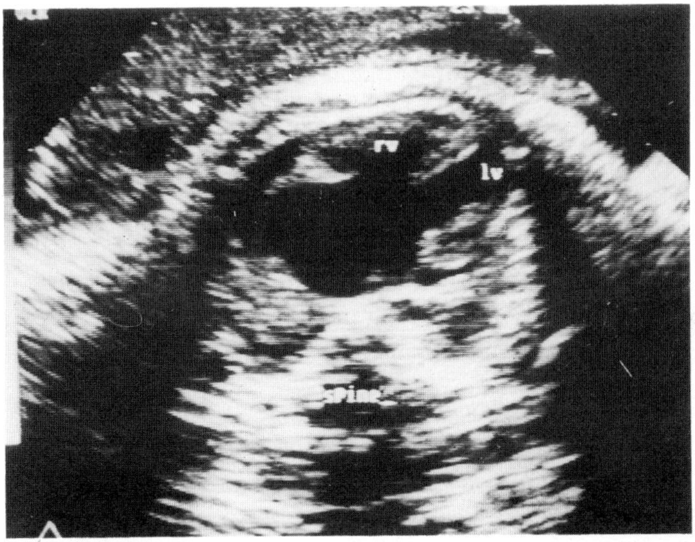


**Fig. 18.7** The heart is seen in a four chamber view. There is a common atrioventricular valve. In diastole, as shown here, the common valve is open and there is a large defect seen at the crux of the heart. This is due to a defect in both the atrial and ventricular septa.

altering the normal appearance of the crux of the heart (Figure 18.6). The valve is usually incompetent, a finding that accounts for the right atrial dilatation associated with this condition. The enlarged heart can cause secondary pulmonary hypoplasia and consequently the prognosis is poor postnatally.

Figure 18.7 shows an example of a complete atrioventricular septal defect. There is a defect in both the atrial and ventricular septa at the point at which the two septa meet the two atrioventricular valves at the centre of the heart. The echocardiographic appearance is of the single valve opening astride the crest of the ventricular septum. It is one of the commonest forms of heart disease seen in prenatal life (Machado *et al.* 1988). This type of defect detected prenatally is found commonly in two situations: associated with complex cardiac anomalies or associated with trisomy 21. It is therefore important to exclude the coexistence of Down's syndrome as this affects the prognosis and must be taken into account when counselling the parents.

Double inlet connection is an unusual defect where both atrioventricular valves drain to one ventricle. The appearance is that of absence of the interventricular septum. This is a rare type of congenital heart disease.

## ABNORMALITIES AT THE VENTRICULO-ARTERIAL JUNCTION

Connection abnormalities at the atrioventricular junction may involve either of the two arterial valves. The valves may be atretic or absent as in pulmonary or aortic atresia. The great arteries may arise inappropriately as in transposition or double outlet right ventricle. The other abnormality to consider is an overriding great artery.

In pulmonary atresia, the pulmonary root will not be found in its usual position or it will be very tiny in relation to the aorta. A secondary finding will be that the right ventricle is small and hypertrophied (Figure 18.8). However, in some cases of pulmonary atresia there is gross right atrial and ventricular dilatation due to severe tricuspid regurgitation. On routine scanning the heart will occupy more than a third of the fetal thorax and the right side will appear larger than the left. This is an unusual form of pulmonary atresia in postnatal practice but seen more commonly in prenatal life (Allan *et al.* 1986). The prenatal cardiac en-

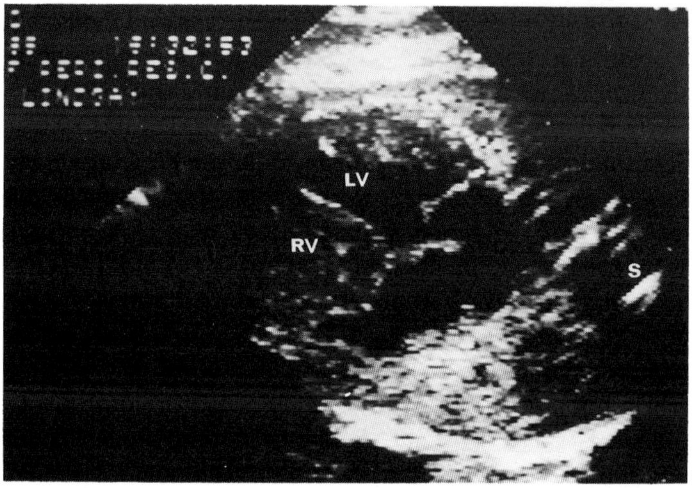


**Fig. 18.8** The heart is seen in the four chamber view. The cavity of the right ventricle (RV) is almost completely obliterated by ventricular hypertrophy. In this case this was due to pulmonary atresia.

largement compresses the lung tissue and causes pulmonary hypoplasia such that difficulties arise in ventilating the newborn. This condition is often not recognized as being primarily a cardiac problem and may explain why it is less commonly seen in postnatal practise.

In aortic atresia, the aorta will be tiny and the left ventricle small. This may occur with mitral atresia to form the hypoplastic left heart syndrome (Figure 18.9).

In transposition of the great arteries, the aorta arises from the right ventricle and lies anterior to the pulmonary artery. The great arteries will arise in parallel orientation to each other instead of arising at right angles to each other at their origin. Figure 18.10 shows the appearance of the aortic arch in this condition. The aortic arch makes a wider sweep than normal and arises close to the anterior chest from the right ventricle. This can be a difficult diagnosis to make but is important to recognize prenatally as it has a relatively good prognosis if early corrective surgery takes place.

In some forms of heart disease, the aorta is displaced anteriorly and arises astride the ventricular septum with a subaortic ventricular septal defect (Figure 18.11). There are three conditions to consider when this finding is seen: Fallot's tetralogy, pulmonary atresia with a ventricular septal defect and common arterial trunk. These three conditions are differentiated by examination of the pulmonary outflow tract. The distinction is important as each carries a very different prognosis for corrective surgery. In the tetralogy, the pulmonary outflow is obstructed but patent. It is completely obstructed in pulmonary atresia and arises from the aorta in common arterial trunk.

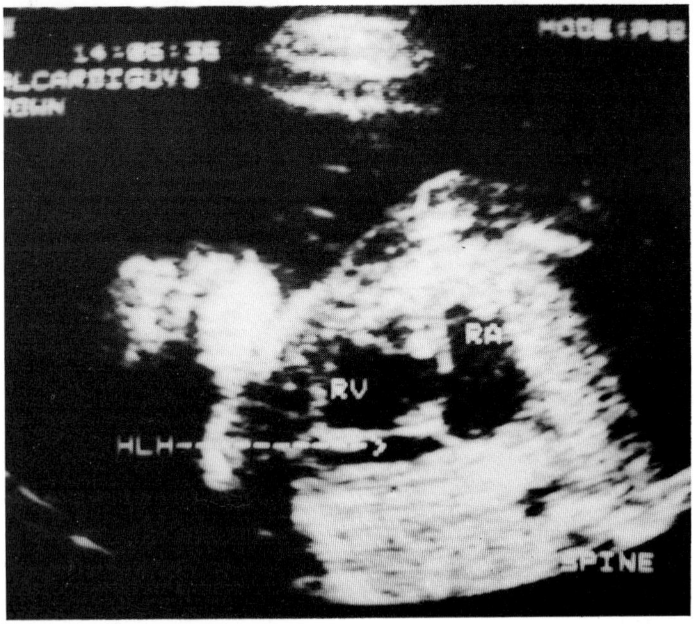


**Fig. 18.9** The heart is seen in four chambers. The small hypoplastic left ventricle is indicated (HLH). This was associated with mitral and aortic atresia.

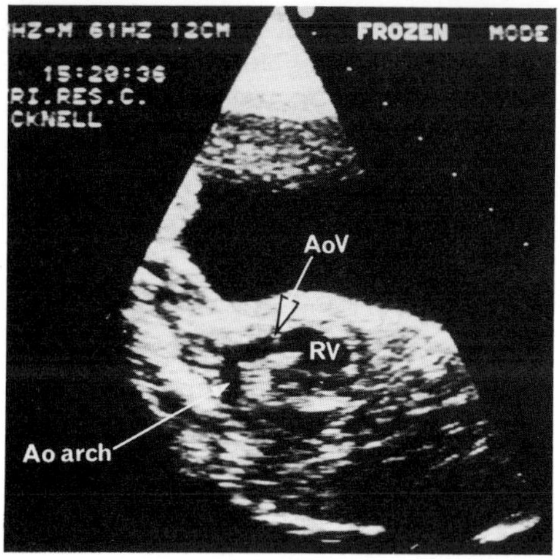


**Fig. 18.10** The aortic arch was seen rising close to the anterior chest wall from the right ventricle (RV). The pulmonary artery in this case was found to rise from the left ventricle. This is an example of transposition of the great arteries.

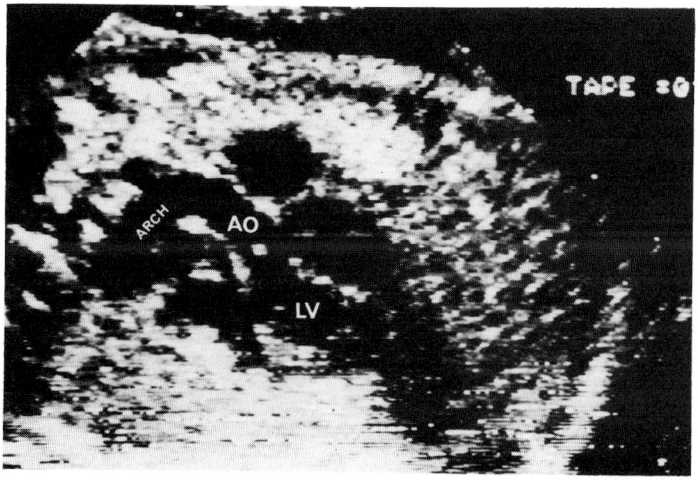


**Fig. 18.11** The aorta is seen to arise astride the crest of the ventricular setpum. The arch and head and neck vessels are seen. There is a ventricular septal defect present.

In double outlet right ventricle, both great arteries arise from the right ventricle anterior to the ventricular septum (Figure 18.12). The position of the great arteries relative to each other can vary but again the great arteries will arise in parallel and do not cross over in the normal way.

## Other abnormalities

### VALVE STENOSIS

Any intracardiac valve can be stenosed or partially obstructed but in practice this mainly occurs at the aortic or pulmonary valve. The re-

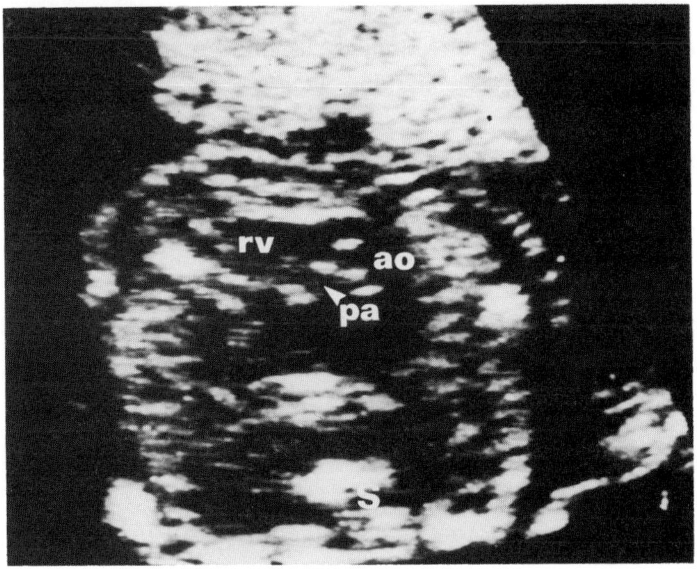


**Fig. 18.12** The two great arteries are seen rising in parallel anterior to the ventricular septum from the right ventricle (rv). The aorta (ao) is anterior to, and larger than, the pulmonary artery (pa). This is an example of double outlet right ventricle.

spective ventricular chamber may appear thickened due to hypertrophy secondary to the obstruction. The valve itself may also appear thick and dysplastic. The affected artery will often be disproportionately small in size relative to the other artery. The Doppler sample volume placed in the stenosed artery sometimes will show a velocity of blood flow above the normal range (Allan *et al.* 1987), and may be helpful in diagnosis.

### VENTRICULAR SEPTAL DEFECTS (VSD)

These can be present in various sizes and positions or be part of more complex anomalies. These factors will influence the prognosis. The majority of isolated VSD close spontaneously postnatally. An example of a ventricular septal defect associated with another cardiac abnormality is seen in Figure 18.5.

### CARDIAC TUMOURS

These are not infrequently seen in prenatal life. They carry a high risk of blood flow obstruction, fetal hydrops and intrauterine death. Rhabdomyomas which are associated with tuberose sclerosis can be detected *in utero* and this may be helpful where there is a positive family history.

### COARCTATION OF THE AORTA

This is a difficult diagnosis to make antenatally (Allan *et al.* 1988). The clue to this diagnosis in prenatal life is relative ventricular disproportion, so that the right-sided structures appear relatively dilated. There is often hypoplasia of the distal aortic arch, although the coarctation shelf itself cannot be seen in early pregnancy. The outlook for successful surgery will depend on the precise anatomy.

## High risk groups

There are certain high risk pregnancies that are recognized to be associated with an increased risk of congenital heart disease (CHD).
These include those with:

**1** A family history of CHD. If one previous child has had CHD the recurrence risk is 1 in 50. If there have been two affected children the risk increases to 1 in 10. When a parent is affected the risk to the next generation is of the order of 1 in 10.

**2** Maternal diabetes is associated with an increased risk of congenital abnormalities and the statistical risk of cardiac malformation of about 1 in 50. It is thought that good diabetic control in early pregnancy probably diminishes this risk.

**3** Exposure to teratogens in early pregnancy such as lithium, phenytoin or steroids is reported to be associated with a 1 in 50 risk of heart malformation.

**4** Extracardiac fetal anomalies may be associated with congenital heart disease and so evidence of heart anomalies should be sought in every case.

**5** Some fetal arrhythmias are associated with structural heart disease, especially complete heart block.

**6** Non-immune fetal hydrops can be due to congenital heart disease and a fetal echocardiogram should be an essential part of the investigation of these patients. Fetal hydrops will have a cardiac cause in up to 25 per cent of cases.

**7** The most important group, however, in which congenital heart disease has been detected in the last two years in our centre is in normal pregnancies where the obstetrician notices an abnormality of the four chamber view on a routine scan. Over the last two years more than 80 per cent of the anomalies seen in our department have been referred because of the suspicion of CHD from examination of the four chamber view. This emphasizes the importance of the four chamber view being included in the routine obstetric scan.

## Screening for congenital heart disease

At the present time over 90 per cent of pregnant women in Britain have a routine obstetric scan for dating and abnormality detection. It is possible to teach ultrasonographers to include examination of the four chamber view on the routine scan. Such a study has already been performed in France (Fermont *et al.* 1985) and confirms the prediction that 2/1000 cases of congenital heart disease can be detected antenatally by examining the four chamber view only.

Widespread prenatal cardiac screening would have profound implications for the practice and organization of paediatric cardiology in the future. Ideally, ultrasonographers performing a high standard of fetal obstetric ultrasound working in with collaboration with a centre specializing in paediatric echocardiography should produce the optimum service and accuracy in fetal cardiac diagnosis. The paediatric specialist must be included in order to counsel the parents correctly on the prognosis for the child. Some forms of defect will benefit from early diagnosis by preparing medical staff for early neonatal intervention.

## Spectrum of congenital heart disease seen antenatally

During an eight year period over 5000 high risk pregnancies have been examined in the department at Guy's Hospital and over 300 anomalies have been detected accurately. In no patient has it proved impossible to visualize the atrioventricular connections and the two great arteries. Some minor defects, such as small ventricular septal defects, secundum atrial septal defects, and valve stenosis have been overlooked. No false positive predictions have been made.

It is apparent from consideration of the forms of CHD seen prenatally that a different spectrum of disease is seen in prenatal life from those who survive to infancy (Allan *et al.* 1985). Malformations detected tend to be the most severe forms of heart disease and defects which are not commonly seen postnatally are frequently recognized, such as tricuspid dysplasia and cardiac tumours. Many of these fetuses do not survive intrauterine life which accounts partly for this discrepancy between prenatal and postnatal data. Up to 25 per cent of continuing pregnancies with CHD result in spontaneous fetal loss. Figure 18.13 shows the outcome of the abnormalities detected to date. A high proportion of parents,

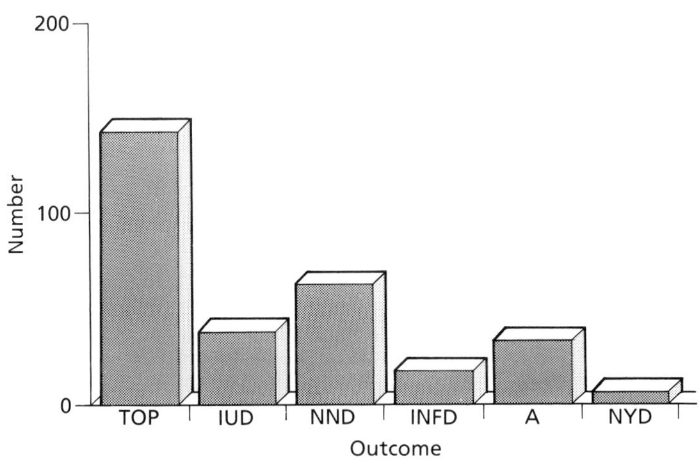


**Fig. 18.13** The outcome of 306 cases of congenital heart disease diagnosed antenatally is shown. TOP = termination of pregnancy, IUD = intrauterine death, NND = neonatal death, INFD = infant death, A = alive, NYD = not yet delivered.

up to 75 per cent where the diagnosis is made in time, will elect termination of pregnancy. A significant proportion (25 per cent) of our detected abnormalities have had associated chromosome defects. This is an important factor in counselling and partially accounts for the high mortality seen *in utero*.

## Conclusions

Fetal echocardiography can accurately detect structural heart disease from an early stage in pregnancy. Almost all forms of congenital heart disease have been recognized prenatally. There is potential for widespread screening for cardiac malformations by the inclusion of the four chamber view on all routine obstetric scans. Once this is familiar the arterial connections can also be sought in every patient. Deviations from the normal appearance or failure to find the standard views will indicate the need for specialist help from the paediatric echocardiographer.

## References

Allan L.D. (1986) *Manual of Fetal Echocardiography*. MTP Press, Lancaster.

Allan L.D., Chita S.K., Anderson R.H., Fagg N., Crawford D.C. & Tynan M.J. (1988) Coarctation of the aorta in prenatal life: an echocardiographic, anatomical and functional study. *British Heart Journal*, **59**, 356–60.

Allan L.D., Chita S.K., Al Ghazali W., Crawford D.C. & Tynan M.J. (1987) Doppler echocardiographic evaluation of the normal human fetal heart. *British Heart Journal*, **57**, 528–33.

Allan L.D., Crawford D.C., Anderson R.J. & Tynan M.J. (1984) Echocardiographic and anatomical correlates in fetal congenital heart disease. *British Heart Journal*, **52**, 542–8.

Allan L.D., Crawford D.C., Anderson R.H. & Tynan M.J. (1985) Spectrum of congenital heart disease seen in prenatal life. *British Heart Journal*, **54**, 523–6.

Allan L.D., Crawford D.C. & Tynan M.J. (1986) Pulmonary atresia in prenatal life. *Journal of the American College of Cardiology*, **8**, 1331–6.

Allan L.D., Tynan M.J., Campbell S., Wilkinson J.L. & Anderson R.H. (1980) Echocardiographic and anatomical correlates in the fetus. *British Heart Journal*, **44**, 444–51.

Fermont L., De Geeter B., Aubry M.C., Kachaner J. & Sidi D. (1985) A close collaboration between obstetricians and cardiologists allows antenatal detection of severe cardiac malformation by 2D echocardiography (abstract). 2nd World Congress of Paediatric Cardiology, New York.

Fyler D.C., Buckley L.P., Hellenbrand W.E. & Cohn H.E. (1980) Report of the New England Regional Infant Cardiac Care Programme. *Pediatrics*, **65**, 375–461.

Kleinman C.S., Hobbins J.C., Jaffe C.C., Lynch D.C. & Talner N.S. (1980) Echocardiographic stuides of the human fetus: prenatal diagnosis of congenital heart disease and cardiac dysrhythmias. *Pediatrics*, **65**, 1059–66.

Lange L.W., Sahn D.J., Allen H.D., Goldberg S.J., Anderson C. & Giles H. (1980) Qualitative real-time cross-sectional echocardiographic imaging of the human fetus during the second half of pregnancy. *Circulation*, **62**, 799–806.

Machado M.V.L., Crawford D.C., Anderson R.H. & Allan L.D. (1988) Atrioventricular septal defect in prenatal life. *British Heart Journal*, **59**, 352–5.

Scott D.J., Rigby M.L., Miller G.A.H. & Shinebourne E.A. (1984) The presentation of symptomatic heart disease in infancy based on 10 years experience (1973–1982). Implications for the provision of services. *British Heart Journal*, **52**, 248–57.

# 19: Detection of congenital abnormalities of the renal and urinary tract by ultrasound

NICHOLAS M. FISK AND CHARLES H. RODECK



Disorders of the renal and urinary tract account for 20–30 per cent of all congenital abnormalities detected by ultrasound (Gauderer *et al.* 1984; Grisoni *et al.* 1986). Compared with anomalies in other organ systems, their presence is relatively easy to detect, largely because obstructive lesions manifest as easily seen cystic spaces, while those with poor urine output are characterized by oligohydramnios. Indeed renal and urinary tract anomalies were amongst the first congenital abnormalities diagnosed by ultrasound (Garrett *et al.* 1970; Garrett *et al.* 1975). They are found in 0.1–0.3 per cent of pregnancies (Kullendorf *et al.* 1984; Arger *et al.* 1985; Helin & Persson 1986), depending on the indication for scanning and the gestation at which performed. Most major abnormalities such as renal agenesis and low obstructive uropathy will be detected by a detailed mid-trimester anomaly scan, provided that this can be delayed until 18–19 weeks, when urinary output begins to make a major contribution to amniotic fluid volume. However, the majority of diagnoses have been made in the third trimester on indicated scans, even in those previously screened and found to be normal at 16–20 weeks (Gunn *et al.* 1988; Watson *et al.* 1988). Thus the later in pregnancy that ultrasound is performed, the more likely it becomes that a renal or urinary abnormality will be detected and that such abnormality will be minor.

## Sonographic anatomy and physiology

The kidneys are recognized in the transverse plane as hypoechoic structures either side of the fetal spine. They are most easily visualized in the third trimester with the fetus in the spine anterior position, when the well delineated cortex gives them the appearance of *pince-nez*. In longitudinal section they appear as bean-shaped structures in a paraspinous locaton. As in the adult, the right is often slightly lower than the left. Over the last 5 years, the earliest gestation at which kidneys can be routinely visualized has decreased markedly. Although it has been known for some time that the fetal kidneys can be seen from as early as 12 weeks, and reliably from 15 weeks (Grannum *et al.* 1980), a safe working rule has been that it is not until 18–20 weeks that almost all kidneys will be apparent on routine sonography using standard equipment (Duval *et al.* 1985a). Advances in high resolution and computed sonography have enabled their demostration from as early as 9 weeks, and it has been recently claimed that 98 per cent can be seen by 11 weeks (Green & Hobbins 1988), when they appear more echogenic than in the second trimester. The clinical significance of this observation is unclear, and indeed a recent detailed transvaginal ultrasound study of first trimester anatomy made no mention of fetal renal and urinary tract structures (Timor-Tritsch *et al.* 1988). The visualization of intrarenal structures such as pyramids and arcuate arteries that is possible in the third trimester is of little diagnostic significance.

Renal length, width and thickness increase linearly with gestation in most studies (Grannum *et al.* 1980; Jeanty *et al.* 1982; Duval *et al.* 1985a; Sagi *et al.* 1987) although Bertagnoli *et al.* (1983) found a quadratic relationship for both length and thickness. Nomograms exist for these measurements, but are of little diagnostic importance, as renal enlargement, when unilateral, may be gauged by comparison with the contralateral kidney, and when bilateral, is usually so gross that reference to normal values is unnecessary. If measurements are required, the simple ratio of kidney circumference to abdominal circumference has the advantage of not varying significantly with gestation (mean = 0.27–0.30, upper limit of normal = 0.32–0.36) (Grannum *et al.* 1980; Jeanty *et al.* 1982).

The renal pelves are identified as central hypoechoic areas whose outlines become defined with increasing gestation as bright specular reflectors. Major calyces may be seen in the third trimester, although normal ureters are not visible. Minor pelvicalyceal dilatation may be physiological (Duval *et al.* 1985b) as discussed later.

Visualization of the fetal bladder depends on both renal function and the state of bladder filling. The fetal bladder is not usually seen until 13 weeks, although it can be demonstrated in some cases as early as 10–11 weeks (Green & Hobbins 1988). Failure to demonstrate a fetal bladder in the presence of normal amniotic fluid volume, suggests that it has just emptied. In the presence of oligohydramnios, the scan should be continued for, or repeated within, 30 min to confirm bladder filling.

Campbell *et al.* (1973) devised an elegant method for estimating fetal urine output based on changes in bladder volume, using the formula for an ovoid, observed over a 15–30 min interval in the third trimester. Using this technique normal values have since been described from 20 weeks until term (Kurjak *et al.* 1981). The supposition on which this methodology is based is that complete voiding occurs at defined intervals. However, observation of fetal bladder dynamics on real-time ultrasound, and the voiding pattern of very preterm babies, would suggest that frequent partial voiding is more likely, at least in early and mid-gestation. Certainly, many fetuses with idiopathic polyhydramnios have chronically full bladders which on prolonged scanning do not appear to empty (unpublished observations). This technique has also been used to show evidence of fetal diuresis following diuretic administration to the mother (Wladimiroff & Campbell 1975; Kurjak *et al.* 1981), an event which is now considered unlikely (Chamberlain *et al.* 1984). In addition, doubt has been cast on the accuracy of measuring hourly fetal urine production rates by the demonstration of wide standard deviations and large interobserver variability in bladder measurements (Chamberlain *et al.* 1985).

Assessment of amniotic fluid volume provides an indirect index of fetal urine output. Although several semiquantitative schemes for measuring amniotic fluid volume have been proposed (Crowley 1980; Manning *et al.* 1981), none makes any reference to gestation with which amniotic fluid volume varies considerably, and all are characterized by poor reproducibility (Patterson *et al.* 1987). Thus subjective assessments of amniotic fluid volume as normal or reduced are in widespread usage. Nevertheless, some gradation of severity of oligohydramnios is of clinical benefit, and we would advocate either simple measurement of the deepest vertical pool devoid of umbilical cord and fetal parts, or the more accurate amniotic fluid index which comprises the sum of the same measurement from each of four abdominal quadrants (Rutherford *et al.* 1987).

## Renal anomalies

### Renal agenesis

Bilateral renal agenesis occurs in approximately 1 in every 4000 births (Potter 1965) and is fatal soon after delivery. Most cases are sporadic, although rarely some occur as part of wider chromosomal and autosomal syndromes as reviewed by Romero *et al.* (1988). An autosomal dominant mode of inheritance has been observed in some families (Morse *et al.* 1987). Agenesis is the result of either failure of development of the ureteric bud or its failure to grow into the metanephric mass of mesoderm and thereby induce tubule formation. Absence of renal function causes no metabolic problem *in utero* due to the excretory function of the placenta, but does lead to virtual absence of amniotic fluid from 15–20 weeks onwards. This produces in the fetus the classical compressed facies and postural deformities due to fixation within the uterus (Potter 1965) and pulmonary hypoplasia, although the exact mechanism by which oligohydramnios produces the latter is still not understood (Nicolini *et al.* 1989a).

Bilateral renal agenesis should only be diagnosed when each of the following three features is demonstrated: bilateral absence of renal tissue, non-visualization of the fetal bladder, and severe oligohydramnios. The kidneys should be sought in both transverse and longitudinal planes and care taken to distinguish the adrenals, which in the absence of the compressive effect of the kidneys assume a discoid shape in the renal fossae (Dubbins *et al.* 1981). An adrenal may be distinguished by its thick central hyperechoic line and absence of a renal pelvis. A fetal bladder should not be seen when sought on serial views at 20 min intervals over 1 hour. This diagnosis should not be made before 16 weeks when amniotic fluid is predominantly non-renal in origin. The recent suggestion that renal agenesis can be reliably diagnosed in the first trimester (Green & Hobbins 1988) may prove applicable in a few centres of excellence, but would seem particularly unwise in the district hospital setting.

The diagnosis of bilateral renal agenesis is made difficult by poor visualization secondary to lack of amniotic fluid. Occasional false positive and negative diagnoses have been reported (Romero *et al.* 1985), and accordingly confirmatory measures are advised. If the fetal abdomen is within the lower half of the uterus, transvaginal ultrasound may provide superior views both because higher frequency sound is used, and because the probe may be manipulated within the vaginal fornix nearer to the fetal renal fossa (Figure 19.1). Unless the diagnosis is clear, invasive confirmation is then indicated. Amnioinfusion of a warmed sterile isotonic solution recreates the acoustic window absent in oligohydramnios. Gembruch & Hansmann (1988) found this improved visualization in 11 fetuses with renal agenesis, while Reuss *et al.* (1987) considered this technique necessary in 5 of 16 fetuses with bilateral renal agenesis before a definitive diagnosis could be made. Amniorrhexis complicated 12 percent of amnioinfusions in one series (Gembruch & Hansmann 1988), and

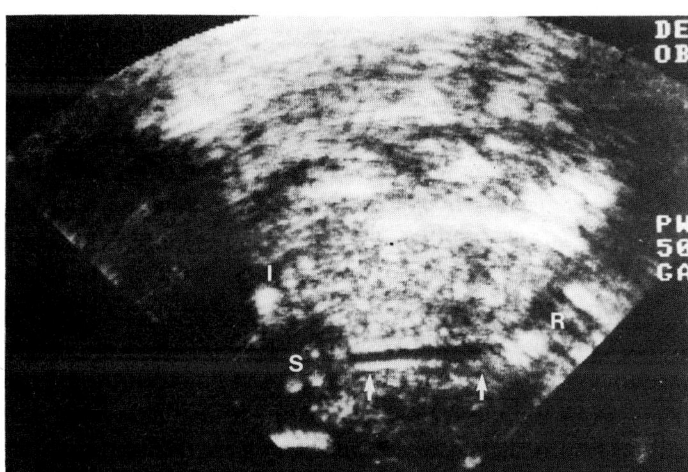


**Fig. 19.1** Transvaginal scan of bilateral renal agenesis. No renal tissue is identified on either side of the fetal aorta (arrows). I = fetal iliac crests, S = fetal spine, R = ribs.

(a)

(b)

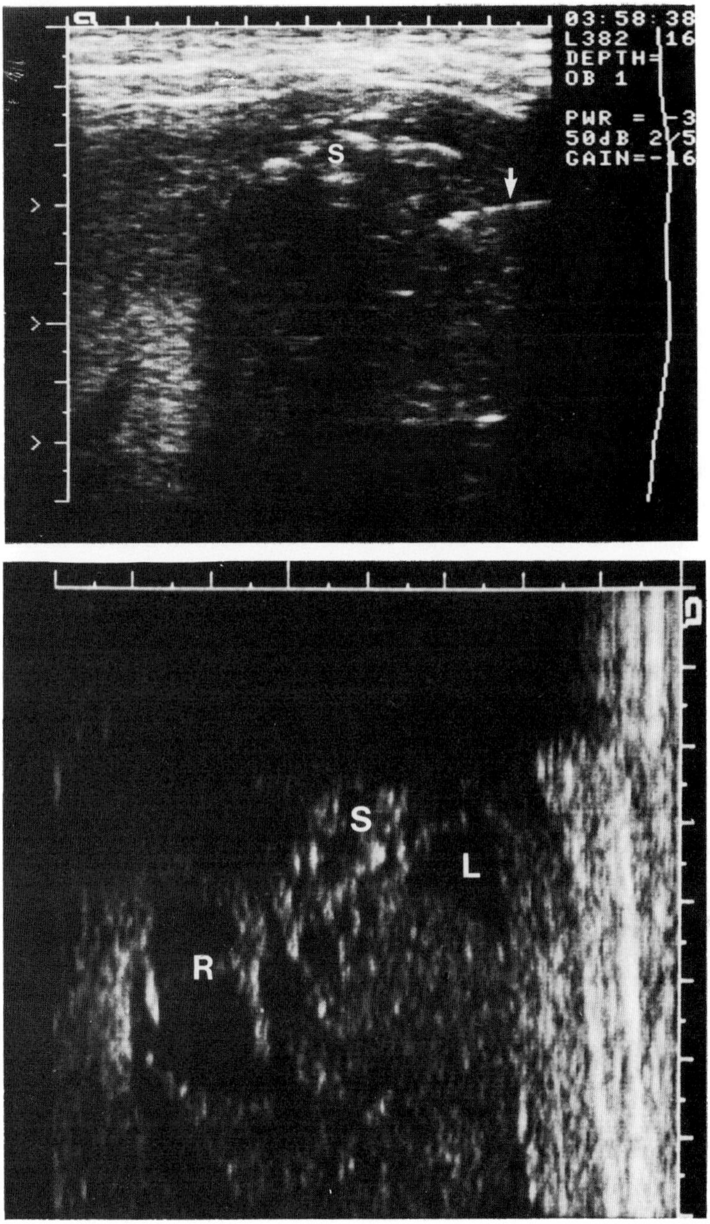


**Fig. 19.2** (a) Ultrasound demonstrating oligohydramnios and the fetal abdomen in cross section. No kidney tissue is seen on either side of the fetal spine (S). The arrow indicates the needle inserted for intraperitoneal infusion of saline. (b) After the saline infusion, the lack of a left kidney (L) is evident as is the liver and a right multicystic kidney (R) (from Nicolini *et al.* 1989c reproduced with permission of J. Wiley).

may be related to the volume infused. More than 200 ml is seldom necessary and we have not experienced this complication in 25 cases since the introduction of pressure monitoring (Nicolini *et al.* 1989b). Alternately, infusion of saline into the fetal peritoneal cavity (Figure 19.2) also improves visualization of retroperitoneal structures (Nicolini *et al.* 1989c) and requires less fluid. The procedure appears safe as it is known from intraperitoneal transfusion data that fetal heart rate changes occur only when large volumes are infused and intraperitoneal pressure rises by >15 mmHg (Nicolini *et al.* 1989d).

Although the prognosis associated with mid-trimester oligohydramnios from whatever cause is poor (Mercer & Brown 1986), confirmation of bilateral renal agenesis permits a definitive recommendation for termination. The main differential diagnosis is severe growth retardation producing fetal oliguria and oligohydramnios (Steele *et al.* 1988). In this regard, maternal administration of frusemide has been used for many years in an attempt to provoke fetal diuresis in the presence of a structurally normal renal tract (Wladimiroff 1975; Kurjak *et al.* 1981; Barrett *et al.* 1983). However, numerous false negative diagnoses have been reported (Goldenberg *et al.* 1984; Harman 1984; Romero *et al.* 1985), and it is now known that maternally administered frusemide in the chronic sheep model neither produces a fetal diuresis nor indeed crosses the placenta (Chamberlain *et al.* 1985). In the same animals, direct administration of diuretic into the fetal circulation produced a fetal diuresis in some but not all, only when high doses were used. It is not known in humans whether the fetal and indeed very preterm neonatal kidney is capable of an immediate diuretic response to frusemide (Yeh *et al.* 1985). We have not observed bladder filling following injection into the umbilical vein of frusemide (3 mg/kg estimated fetoplacental weight) in 6 fetuses with anhydramnios, one of whom was shown to have normal kidneys and bladder at autopsy (unpublished observations).

Unilateral renal agenesis is more common and of less clinical significance, being associated with an excellent prognosis. Absence of one kidney may be missed on ultrasound, as the bladder and amniotic fluid will be normal, and one kidney is often not seen due to shadowing beneath the fetal spine. A pelvic kidney is another possibility (Hill & Peterson 1987).

## Multicystic kidney

Multicystic kidney is a form of renal dysplasia characterized by grape-like clusters of cysts corresponding to dilated collecting tubules, separated by thick fibrous septa. Its pathogenesis is not understood. One theory suggests that failure of induction of nephron development by the ureteric bud produces tubule formation which does not connect to the collecting system (Bernstein 1971). Multicystic kidneys are associated with either pelvi-infundibular atresia or an atretic or absent ureter and therefore do not function (Glassberg *et al.* 1987). Most are sporadic, although rarely some occur in association with recessive syndromes (Romero *et al.* 1988). Multicystic kidneys, of which 20 per cent are bilateral (Kleiner *et al.* 1986), account for 10 per cent of fetal uropathies (Avni *et al.* 1985).

Their ultrasound appearance is typical: multiple peripheral cysts of variable size around a central hyperechoic stroma (Figures 19.3 and 19.4).

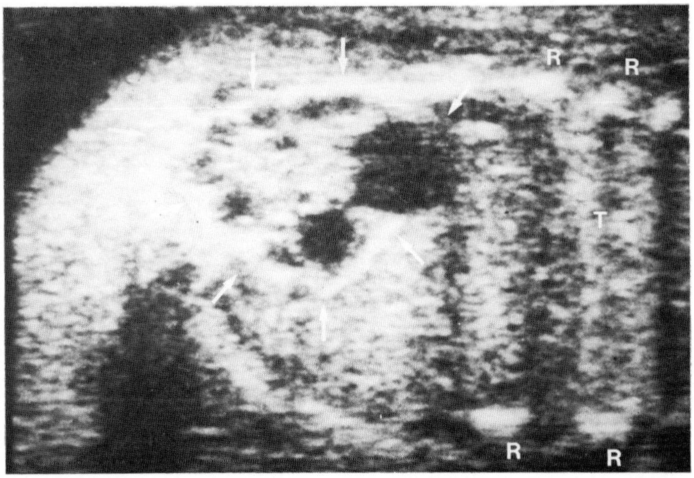


**Fig. 19.3** A predominantly solid multicystic kidney is outlined by arrows. Note the multiple peripheral cysts of variable size situated around the more central hyperechoic stroma. T = fetal thorax, R = ribs.

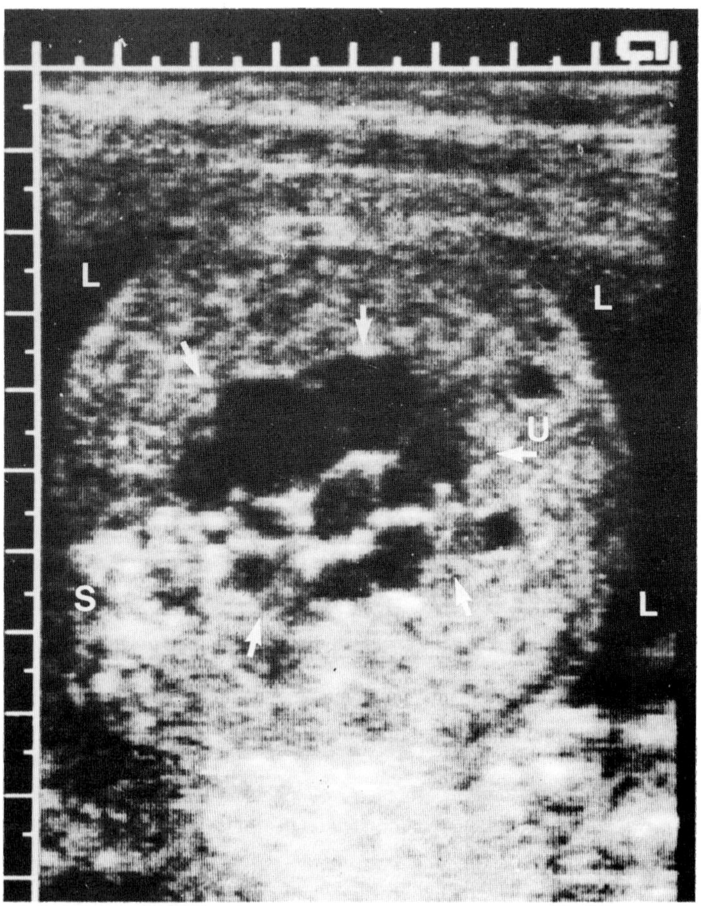


**Fig. 19.4** In contrast to Figure 19.3, the multicystic kidney seen in this cross-sectional view of the fetal abdomen is larger, predominantly cystic with little stroma, and extends anteriorly. S = spine, U = intrahepatic vein, L = amniotic fluid.

The kidney is usually moderately enlarged and retains its reniform shape, but may be huge, crossing the midline (Figure 19.4) and even produce polyhydramnios secondary to compression on the gastrointestinal tract (Henderson *et al.* 1980). Bilateral multicystic kidney is similar to bilateral renal agenesis in that absence of renal function leads to bladder non-visualization and anhydramnios. The approach to diagnosis and management is similar, except that amnioinfusion is usually only required to confirm that the characteristic multicystic appearance arises from both rather than just one kidney.

Unilateral multicystic kidney, like unilateral agenesis, is usually found with a normal bladder and amniotic fluid. Although the appearance alone is normally diagnostic, difficulty may occasionally exist in differentiating these from hydronephrotic kidneys, especially if the cystic spaces are very large (Beretsky *et al.* 1984; Rizzo *et al.* 1987). Ultrasound guided needle aspiration may prove helpful in this situation, as the electrolytes in the multicystic fluid are similar to serum, whereas those from the dilated renal pelvis are more like urine (Nicolini *et al.* 1989b), depending on the degree of obstructive renal damage. Furthermore, there also exists a rare hydronephrotic form of multicystic kidney (Felson & Cussen 1975) with components of both pathologies. An increased frequency of chromosomal and other congenital anomalies is found in unilateral multicystic kidney, and antenatal management should be directed towards their exclusion. Rizzo *et al.* (1987) found serious structural abnormalities in 6 of 16 and abnormal karyotypes in 2 of 7 fetuses with multicystic kidneys, while 3 of 25 unilateral multicystic kidneys in another series were associated with contralateral renal agenesis (Kleiner *et al.* 1986). Pyeloureteric junction obstruction, the most common of the contralateral renal anomalies (Griscom *et al.* 1975), may develop subsequently and therefore follow-up scans are advised. The appearance of a multicystic kidney can change markedly during the pregnancy, either gaining in size or showing evidence of regression (Avni *et al.* 1987) There is increasing evidence that many multicystic kidneys regress or involute in infancy (Avni *et al.* 1987). Previously nephrectomy was standard postnatal practice in view of perceived risks of malignant change and hypertension, but as these are now known to be small (Hartmann *et al.* 1986), conservative management is increasingly employed (Stanisic 1986).

## Polycystic kidneys

The infantile form of polycystic kidney is autosomal recessive and is found in 1:50 000 infants (Potter 1972). Some occur in association with an encephalocoele and polydactyly as the Meckel–Gruber syndrome. Both kidneys contain numerous cylinders 1–2 mm in diameter, arising from the proximal collecting tubules and extending to the cortex. Both nephrons and collecting ducts are normal, and therefore the pathogenetic mechanism is unlikely to be obstruction or a defective blastema. One theory postulates them to be related to secondary hyperplasia of

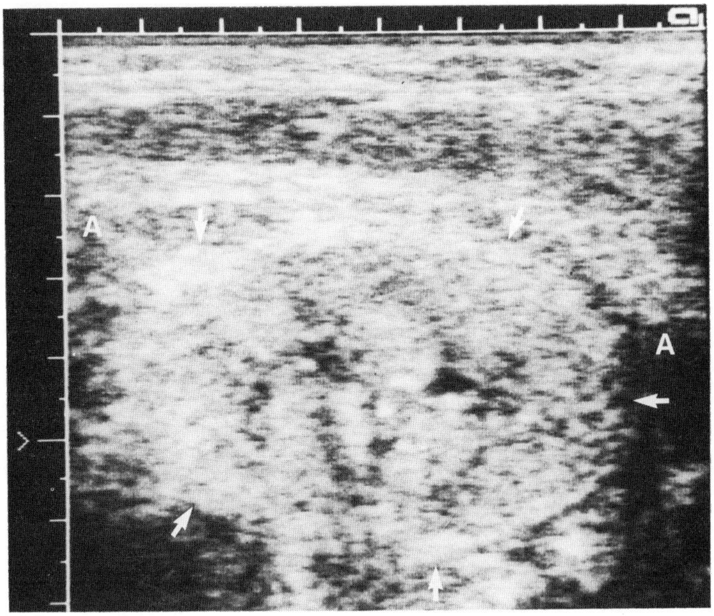


**Fig. 19.5** Enlarged hyperechogenic polycystic kidney (outlined by arrows). Note the poorly defined pelvicalyceal system and the anhydramnios. A = fetal abdominal wall.

cellular elements in the collecting tubules (Potter 1972). Ultrasonically, the kidneys are massively enlarged and may occupy the entire abdomen. Cyst size is usually below ultrasound resolution, so that the lesion appears solid and hyperechoic (Figure 19.5) Nephromegaly often is apparent by 24 weeks (Romero *et al.* 1984; Zerres *et al.* 1988), but need not be, even in the third trimester (Romero *et al.* 1984). As with bilateral renal agenesis, the bladder is not usually seen and there is anhydramnios (Hobbins *et al.* 1979; Romero *et al.* 1984; Luthy & Hirsh 1985), although occasionally liquor volume may remain normal into late pregnancy (Simpson *et al.* 1982; Romero *et al.* 1984; Zerres *et al.* 1988). In the most common, the perinatal form, the kidneys do not function, with death occurring in the neonatal period, whereas in less severe forms, milder renal and hepatic involvement may allow survival into childhood (Blyth & Ockenden 1971). In 10 fetuses with proven infantile polycystic kidneys, Romero *et al.* (1984) reported one false negative diagnosis, due to a milder form of the disease. Prenatal diagnosis may therefore only be possible in severe cases of the perinatal form (Zerres *et al.* 1988). In at-risk women, i.e. those with a previously affected child, the first scan should be performed at 18–20 weeks. If negative, serial scans should be performed at 4 weekly intervals as several cases have been reported of normal ultrasound findings at 16–23 weeks, with a subsequently severely affected baby (Reilly *et al.* 1979; Simpson *et al.* 1982; Luthy & Hirsch 1985).

The adult form of polycystic kidney disease is more common, with 1:1000 people carrying the dominant gene on chromosome 16. It has almost complete penetrance by age 70, but with variable expressivity. Affected individuals usually remain asymptomatic into the third and fourth decade, eventually progressing to chronic renal failure. On the other hand, adult polycystic disease can rarely manifest in childhood, and prenatal diagnoses by third trimester ultrasound have been made in a few cases (Sedman *et al.* 1987; Smedley & Bailey 1987). Pretorius *et al.* (1987) reported 5 and reviewed 8 cases of perinatal ultrasound diagnosis to reveal that 85 per cent showed renal enlargement and 90 per cent had increased echogenicity. Although all had an affected parent, only 5 of 13 were aware of their own diagnosis. Despite cysts being more often seen in the adult than infantile form (Pretorius *et al.* 1987), the ultrasound features may be impossible to distinguish. Family ultrasound screening and the use of a polymorphic gene probe on chorion villi (Reeders *et al.* 1986) may help in distinguishing the adult form. The prognosis of the adult form when detected *in utero* is not known, but would appear reasonably good (Pretorius *et al.* 1987).

### Other renal anomalies

Congenital mesoblastic nephroma is the most common renal tumour in the newborn and is benign. Several cases of ultrasonic visualization in the third trimester fetus have been reported (Ehman *et al.* 1983; Walter & McGahan 1985; Apuzzio *et al.* 1986), and the principle features are a solid unilateral mass arising from the renal fossa. Differential diagnosis is difficult and includes congenital adrenal neuroblastoma, which has a mixed cystic and solid appearance (Giulan *et al.* 1986), teratomas, and Wilm's tumour, the prenatal diagnosis of which has not yet been reported. Recently renal vein thrombosis has been observed on ultrasound in several fetuses, the features being renal enlargement with hyperechoic foci in the parenchyma, thrombosis protruding into the inferior vena cava and fetal ascites (Furness *et al.* 1988; Patel & Connors 1988).

## Upper tract uropathies

### Pyeloureteric junction obstruction

Hydronephrosis is the commonest uropathy detected both in fetuses and children. Obstruction at the pyeloureteric junction (PUJ) is the most common finding (Grignon *et al.* 1986a; Nicolini *et al.* 1987a; Guys *et al.* 1988; Reuss *et al.* 1988a), and in a few, anatomical causes such as adhesions, mucosal folds or polyps have been found (Hanna *et al.* 1976). However most PUJ obstructions appear to be partial, consistent with histological studies of junctional smooth musculature suggesting a functional basis for this disorder (Antonakopoulos *et al.* 1985). The chief ultrasonic feature, dilatation of the renal pelvis, varies greatly in appearance depending on the severity. In mild hydronephrosis, oblong dilatation of the renal pelvis is the sole abnormal finding (Figure 19.6), whereas

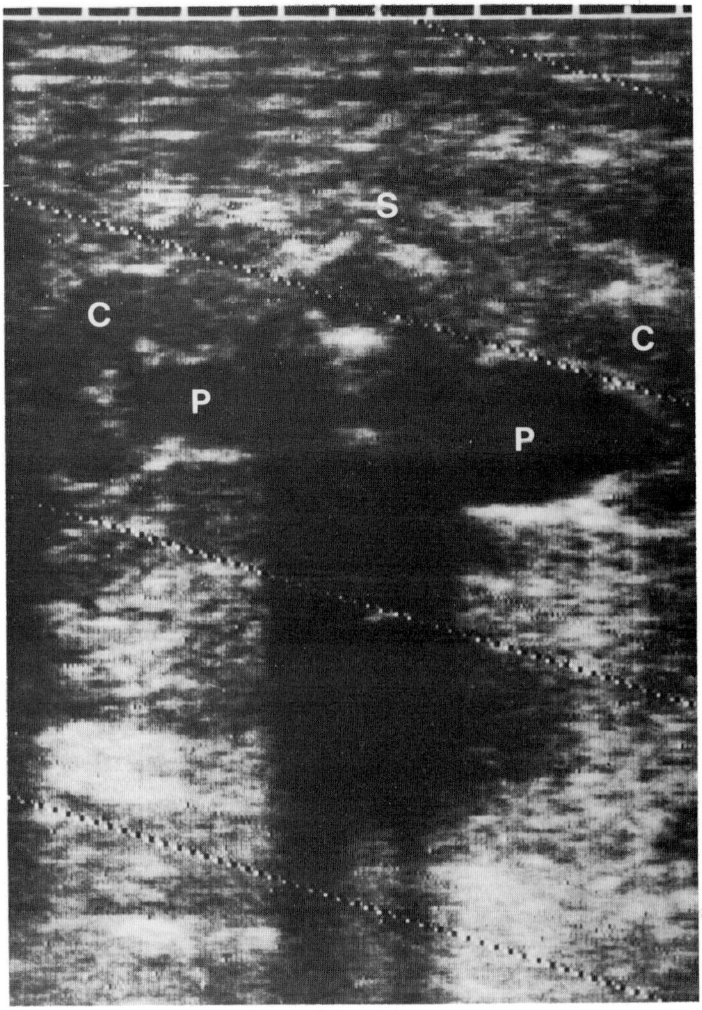


**Fig. 19.6** Mild bilateral hydronephrosis is seen in this transverse plane of the fetal abdomen in the spine anterior position (S). Note the asymmetry of renal pelvic dilatation (P) between the two sides, and the normal echogenicity of the renal cortex (C).

when moderate, the dilated renal pelvis communicates with dilated major calyces (Figure 19.7). In severe hydronephrosis, the kidney enlarges, the renal pelvis loses its normal anatomic configuration and appears as multiple circular anechoic areas, and the renal parenchyma looks thin and hyperechoic (Figure 19.8). Although several classification systems have been proposed, none are uniformly accepted, and qualitative descriptions of mild, moderate and severe hydronephrosis loosely based on the features described above, are in widespread usage. Duval *et al.* (1985b) use an ultrasound classification of four grades similar to that used in postnatal urography, based on renal pelvis diameter, calyceal shape and parenchymal thickness. The usual measurement of the renal pelvis is an anteroposterior diameter taken in the transverse plane. Grignon *et al.* (1986a) have proposed another system, of five grades but based on similar

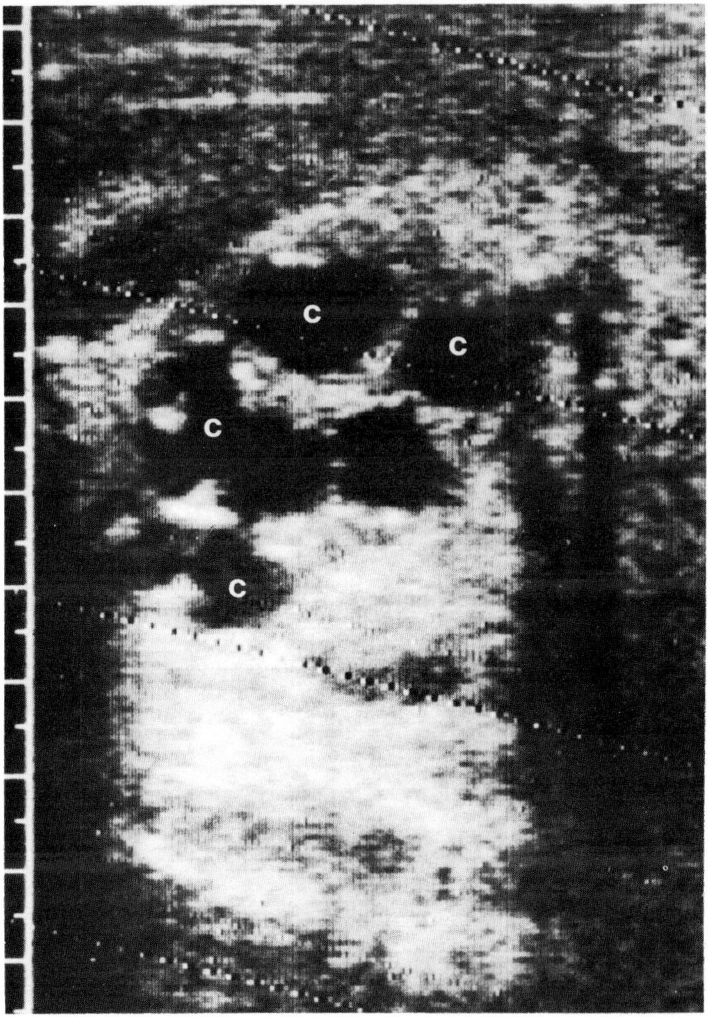


**Fig. 19.7** Moderate unilateral hydronephrosis with dilatation of major calyces (C).

parameters, in which they categorize Grade I pyeloureteric dilatation (renal pelvis ≤10 mm) as physiological. This distinction of mild hydronephrosis from physiological renal pelvic dilatation remains an area of controversy. Whereas one recent paper categorized as hydronephrotic any kidney with fluid visible in its collecting system (Gunn *et al.* 1988), others have been able to measure renal pelvic thickness in most pregnancies after 16 weeks (Duval *et al.* 1985a). Renal pelvic thickness >10 mm appears at present to the best definition currently available of hydronephrosis. In one study, 28 of 29 fetuses with pyelectasis <10 mm were shown not to have hydronephrosis postnatally (Grignon *et al.* 1986a). Problems with definition may also explain some reports of hydronephrosis resolving *in utero* (Harrison *et al.* 1982a; Sanders & Graham 1982; Blane *et al.* 1983; Nicolini *et al.* 1987a). Duval *et al.* (1985b) suggest that 9–12 mm dilatation is a grey zone which may indicate either physiological dilatation or pathological obstruction. None of these measurements are

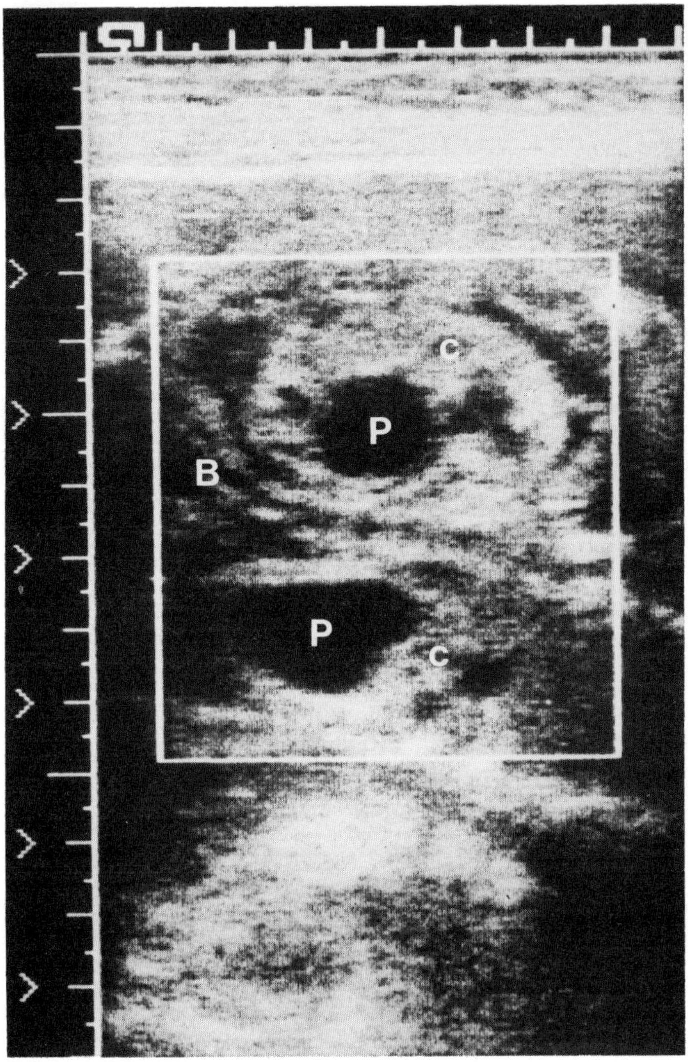


**Fig. 19.8** Severe bilateral hydronephrosis. The enclosed area shows two kidneys in coronal section either side of the fetal aorta. Note the asymmetry of cortical thinning (C) and pelvic dilatation (P). Residual renal tissue is hyperechoic in comparison with surrounding tissue. B = aortic bifurcation.

referenced to gestation, and therefore Arger *et al.* (1985) include in their definition of hydronephrosis a kidney in which the ratio of pelvic to renal thickness exceeds 0.5. This definition on the other hand seems too stringent as the ratio can still be <0.5 and pyeloplasty be required postnatally (Kleiner *et al.* 1987). Although maternal hydration is well recognized in adults as leading to minimal dilatation of the collecting system (Morin & Baker 1979), Hoddick *et al.* (1985) were able to decrease signs of minimal pyelectasis in only 4 of 17 fetuses following maternal fluid restriction, supporting animal work suggesting that the state of maternal hydration has little effect on fetal urine output (Hurley *et al.* 1977).

As with many ultrasound detected anomalies, the discovery of unilateral hydronephrosis should prompt a diligent search for congenital abnormalities in other organ systems, which are found in approximately 20 per cent (Lebowitz & Griscom 1977). A wide range of abnormalities may also be present in the remainder of the urinary tract, with a frequency of 27 per cent in one series (Drake *et al.* 1978). Unilateral hydronephrosis is more commonly left sided (Johnston *et al.* 1977; Drake *et al.* 1978), and associated with normal amniotic fluid volume, although as discussed earlier, large renal masses may produce polyhydramnios (Henderson *et al.* 1980; Kleiner *et al.* 1987; Reuss *et al.* 1988a). In 30 per cent, hydronephrosis will be bilateral, usually with asymmetrical involvement of the kidneys. Amniotic fluid volume will be normal in most of these, consistent with the partial nature of the obstruction at the PUJ. There is general agreement that *in utero* drainage is not warranted for bilateral hydronephrosis with normal amniotic fluid volume (Hellstrom *et al.* 1984; Seeds & Mandell 1986). Even when significant progression of dilatation is observed *in utero*, an uncommon event (Kleiner *et al.* 1987), there would not appear to be a role for preterm delivery and early surgical correction, as the severity of renal damage postnatally correlates poorly with either the degree of antenatal dilatation (Kleiner *et al.* 1987) or the interval from prenatal diagnosis (Nicolini *et al.* 1987a). There may be a role for intervention in bilateral hydronephrosis with oligohydramnios and a persistently empty bladder, but such cases are exceedingly rare.

Differential diagnosis includes multicystic kidney, perinephric urinoma, vesico-ureteric reflux and obstructive megaureter. Multicystic kidneys can be difficult to distinguish from severe hydronephrosis, especially late in gestation (Beretsky *et al.* 1984; Nicolini *et al.* 1987a), and attention should be directed to the latter's more uniform cyst size, their communication with both each other and the renal pelvis, and the overlying renal parenchyma. A pseudocyst or urinoma refers to an elliptical collection of urine located in the perinephric space posterolateral to the kidney (Figure 19.9) (Callen *et al.* 1983), and is usually associated with severe ipsilateral obstruction (Kleiner *et al.* 1987). Occasionally a connection can be demonstrated histologically between the urinoma and a calyx, suggesting that urinomas result from calyceal rupture, which decompresses a high pressure obstructed system (Callen *et al.* 1983; Adzick *et al.* 1985a).

After birth confirmatory neonatal ultrasound is best delayed for 24–48 hours, as the comparative dehydration and low glomerular filtration rate of the newborn may produce a normal appearance of kidneys which both antenatally and later in the first week are shown to have hydronephrosis (Laing *et al.* 1984). Antenatal ultrasound identifies and allows early postnatal confirmation of PUJ obstructions that may have otherwise remain unidentified for many years into childhood (dell'Agnola *et al.* 1983; Grignon *et al.* 1986b). The critical period for recovery of renal function is the first 6 months of life (McCrory *et al.* 1971); some authors have claimed that better renal functon can be attained in those under-

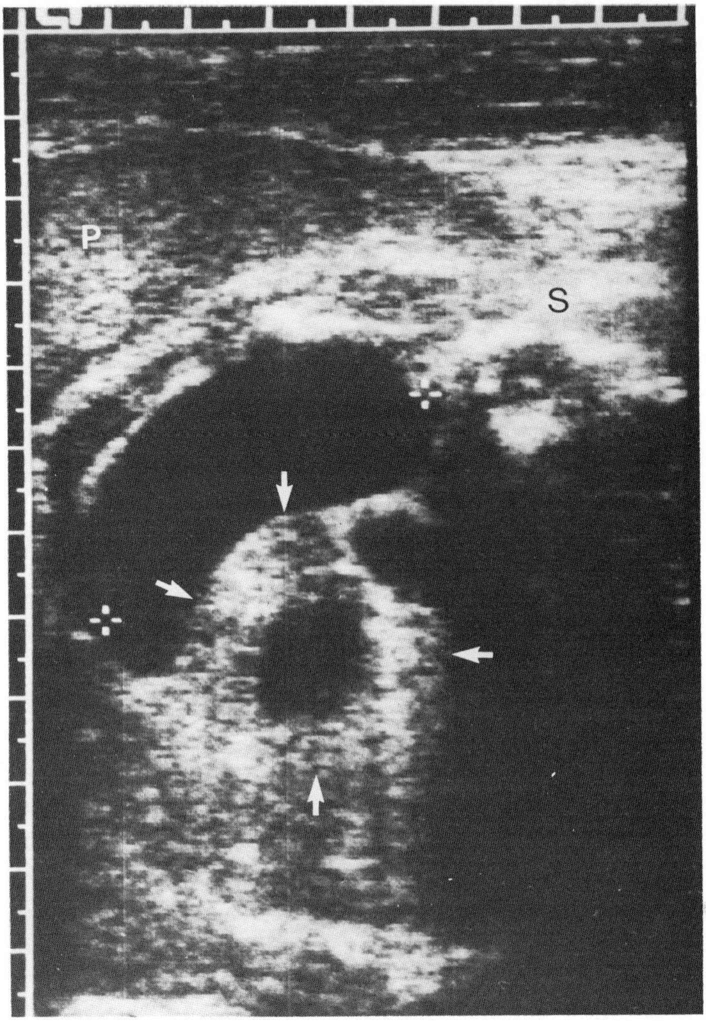


**Fig. 19.9** A large ellipsoid urinoma is seen (between the crosses) displacing a hydronephrotic kidney (arrows) anteriorly. Note the hyperechoic renal cortex. S = spine, P = placenta.

going pyeloplasty in infancy rather than later in childhood (Mayor *et al.* 1975; King *et al.* 1984), but this remains controversial (Thorup *et al.* 1985). It has thus been suggested that earlier postnatal intervention in those first detected by antenatal ultrasound, may improve long-term results (Koyle & Ehrlich 1988). Nevertheless, many infants may still be managed conservatively, postnatal surgery being reserved for those with both severe obstruction and significant impairment of renal function on isotope scans (Koyle & Ehrlich 1988).

## Megaureter

Dilatation of the ureter may occur with or without dilatation of the renal pelvis. The majority of megaureters are secondary to distal pathology, most commonly low urinary tract obstruction in which they occur as part of generalized dilatation of the renal tract. The markedly dilated ureter appears elongated and folds back on itself to give a sinous appearance (Figure); when gross, its margins may be difficult to delineate from concomitant severe pyelectasis.

Primary megaureters result from anatomical obstruction at the vesico-ureteric junction. Like PUJ obstruction, their pathogenesis is debated, with localized stenosis and muscular abnormalities implicated in the failure of transmission of normal peristaltic waves along the distal ureter (Pitts & Muecke 1974; Juskiewenski *et al.* 1984). Ultrasound features noted in the few reported cases of antenatal diagnosis of primary megaureter include dilatation of the proximal but not distal ureter and absence of both significant calyceal dilatation and renal cortical atrophy, although pyelectasis may be present (Deter *et al.* 1980; Dunn & Glasier 1985).

Megaureter also occurs in association with vesico-ureteric (VU) reflux. The International Classification subdivides these into primary abnormalities at the VU junction and those secondary to low urinary tract obstruction, neuropathic bladder, ureteral ectopia, ureterocele etc. (Smith *et al.* 1977). A specific antenatal diagnosis of primary refluxing megaureter (primary VU reflux) is difficult and has not been reported. Scott (1987) in describing 7 infants with VU reflux on postnatal investigation, all of whom showed evidence of renal tract dilatation antenatally, postulated that fetal VU reflux had been present *in utero*. Several fetuses with false positive diagnoses of posterior urethral valves, have been found postnatally to have VU reflux (Philipson *et al.* 1984; Reuter & Lebowitz 1985; Laxova

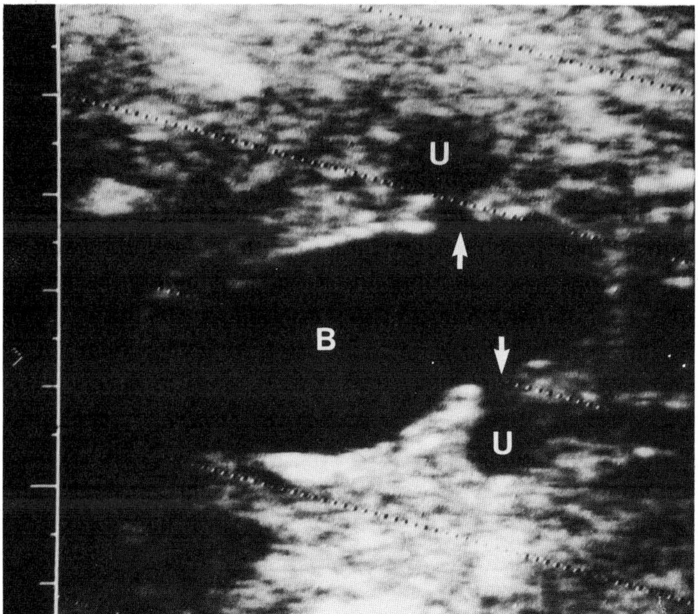


**Fig. 19.10** Bilateral gaping vesico-ureteric valves (arrows) in a fetus with reflux. B = bladder, U = distal ureter.

*et al.* 1987). The antenatal characteristics of VU reflux consist of a slightly enlarged or constantly full bladder, which may or may not be thick walled, and absence of oligohydramnios (Philipson *et al.* 1984; Reuter & Lebowitz 1985). Just as postnatally gaping ureteric orifices may be observed at cystoscopy, antenatally chronic pouting of the VU orifices can also be observed in gross cases on ultrasound (Figure 19.10). We have inferred the presence of significant reflux in several fetuses with low obstructive uropathy due to immediate refilling post aspiration of the upper tract from an emptying bladder. Antenatal radiological studies following contrast injection into the fetal renal tract have been reported in a few cases (Gore *et al.* 1982; Weiner *et al.* 1986), and with the advent of ultrasonic contrast agents, dynamic fetal urographic studies may make it possible to diagnose VU reflux with greater accuracy, along the lines of postnatal investigation (MRC 1979).

## Lower tract uropathies

### Posterior urethral valves

The most frequent cause of lower urinary tract obstruction is posterior valves (PUV) (Lebowitz & Griscom 1977), a heterogeneous group of disorders characterized by membranous or mucosal folds in the prostatic urethra, probably due to abnormal insertion of the distal Wolffian ducts. PUV are found exclusively in males, and thus the detection of lower tract obstruction in a female suggests other diagnoses such as a prolapsing ectopic ureterocele in a duplex system, a urogenital sinus, urethral atresia, primary VU reflex or the megacystis–microcolon–intestinal hypoperistalsis syndrome. In severe cases enlargement of the bladder may occur as early as 11 weeks (Bulic *et al.* 1987) although in general megacystis is not apparent before 16–18 weeks. Thickening of the bladder wall is seen on ultrasound only after decompression, usually by ultrasound guided needle aspiration (Figures 19.11 and 19.12), while urachal dilatation may occasionally be observed at its superior pole when the bladder has partially refilled. Although the valves themselves are too small to be seen, to diagnose PUV with any certainty, it is important to visualize a dilated upper urethra (Gore *et al.* 1982; Hobbins *et al.* 1984; Sholder *et al.* 1988). A variable degree of upper tract dilatation will also be present, and it seems likely that the marked asymmetry commonly seen in the degree of hydronephrosis is related to reflux, which accompanies most gross obstructions. Amniotic fluid volume ranges from normal to markedly reduced. Initial assessment should be directed towards identification of the 1/3 associated with extraurinary anomalies (Lebowitz & Griscom 1977; Glick *et al.* 1985; Reuss *et al.* 1988a) and the 6–24 per cent with chromosomal abnormalities (Nicolaides *et al.* 1986; Reuss *et al.* 1988a).

In fetuses with PUV unassociated with other anomalies, the two main factors determining perinatal outcome are pulmonary hypoplasia and renal dysplasia (Tsingoglou & Dickson 1972; Harrison *et al.* 1982a;

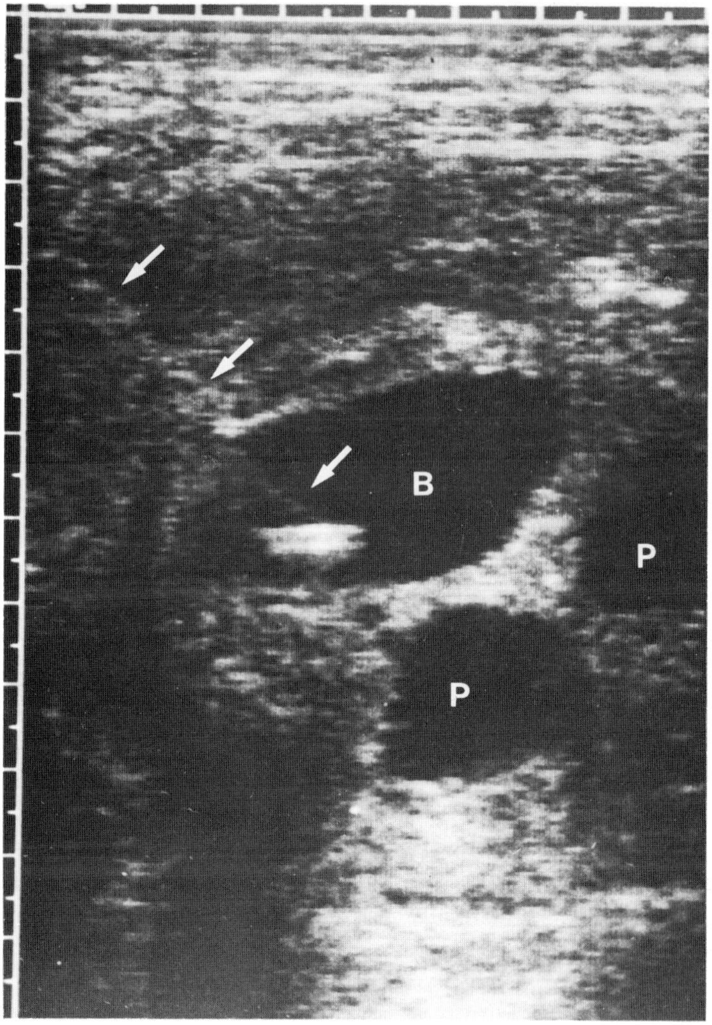


**Fig. 19.11** Dilated renal pelves (P) and bladder (B) in an obstructive uropathy; note the tip of the needle inserted for urine aspiration. Very little amniotic fluid is observed outside the fetal abdomen in this cross-sectional view.

Nakayama *et al.* 1986), which seem related to the duration and severity of obstruction. Lack of a urinary contribution to amniotic fluid in the mid-trimester leads to pulmonary hypoplasia. Although its pathogenesis is not understood, as reviewed by Nicolini *et al.* (1989a) there is general agreement from numerous animal and human studies that lung hypoplasia is related to oligohydramnios. Urethral obstruction has also been considered responsible for associated changes in the proximal renal tract such as renal dysplasia, presumably mediated by increased urinary pressure (Harrison *et al.* 1981; Kurth *et al.* 1981). Spontaneous urinary extravasations in cases of PUV which can be seen on ultrasound as urinomas or ascites support this concept of a raised pressure system (Parker 1974; Kay *et al.* 1980; Adzick *et al.* 1985a). However, in 7 fetuses with low obstructive uropathies, we have recorded intravesical pressures of only

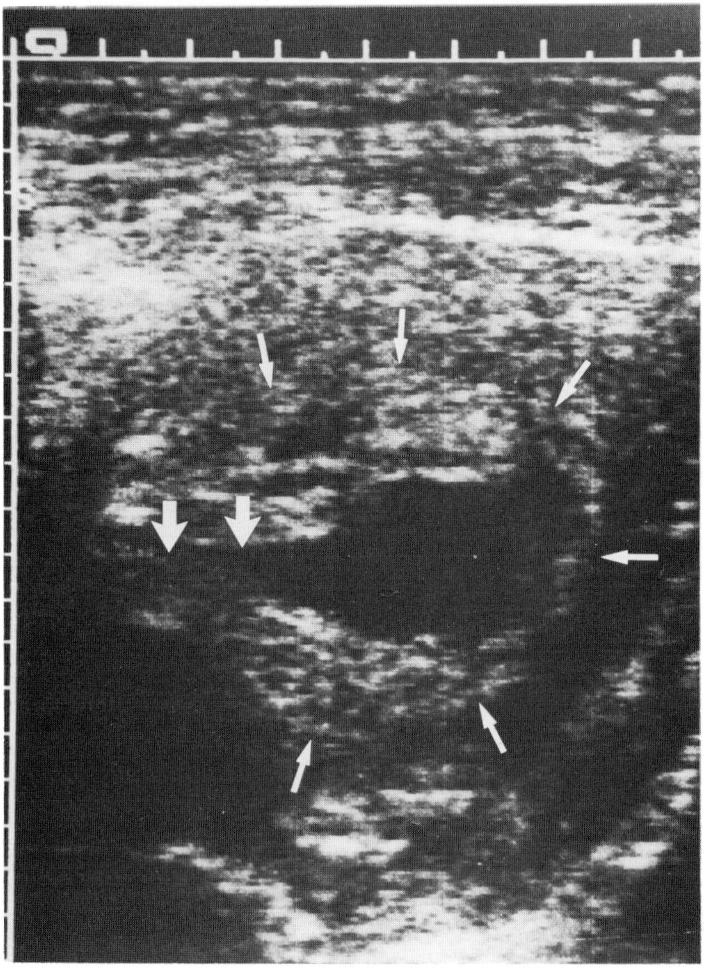

**Fig. 19.12** Thick walled bladder (thin arrows) and dilated upper urethra (thick arrows) in a case of posterior urethral valves.

2–10 mmHg (Nicolini *et al.* 1989b). An alternate embryological theory suggests that renal dysplasia is not secondary to PUV, but results from the same insult: abnormally lateral origin of the ureteric bud from the Wolffian duct (Stephens 1983).

As the surgical correction of PUV on their own is a relatively simple technical procedure, a hypothesis has emerged that bypassing the obstruction *in utero* would not only minimize renal dysplasia but also restore amniotic fluid and thus prevent pulmonary hypoplasia (Harrison *et al.* 1981). The basis for such therapeutic intervention has been rigorously studied in animal models. Essentially, in experimental fetal lambs, urinary obstruction produced both renal dysplasia and lung hypoplasia (Glick *et al.* 1983; Harrison *et al.* 1983), whereas early decompression prevented these sequelae (Harrison *et al.* 1982b; Glick *et al.* 1984).

The presence of a relatively normal quantity of amniotic fluid implies that lung hypoplasia will not occur, that the obstruction is incomplete, and that the fetal kidneys are producing adequate amounts of urine. Any benefit from bypass procedures would therefore be restricted to those fetuses with severe oligohydramnios, in which irreversible renal damage has not yet developed. Vesico-amniotic shunting of a fetus with severe renal dysplasia would not only fail to prevent eventual perinatal death from renal failure, but would also fail to prevent pulmonary hypoplasia if the kidneys *in utero* were incapable of restoring amniotic fluid volume. Accordingly, several parameters have been evaluated for their predictive value for both renal dysplasia and perinatal outcome. Although renal cysts are visualized in only 44 per cent of dysplastic kidneys, their presence strongly suggests dysplasia (Mahoney *et al.* 1984). Hyperechogenicity of the renal parenchyma predicts dysplasia with a sensitivity of 73 per cent and specificity of 80 per cent (Mahoney *et al.* 1984). In view of the inaccuracy of ultrasound features in predicting renal function, biochemistry on fetal urine has become the accepted predictive parameter. This is aspirated from either the fetal bladder (Glick *et al.* 1985) or the renal pelvis (Nicolini *et al.* 1987b). Glick *et al.* (1985) found in a retrospective analysis of 20 fetuses with low obstructive uropathy that urinary $Na^+ > 100$ mEq/l, $Cl^- > 90$ mEq/l and osmolality >210 mOsm/l were indicative of irreversible renal damage. These cut-offs, however, take no account of normal changes in renal function with gestation (Rodeck & Nicolini 1988). Furthermore, Wilkins *et al.* (1987) have recently drawn attention to the considerable disparity between renal function and urinary electrolytes in 9 fetuses with obstructive uropathy, only 1 of which could be accounted for by differences in gestational age. Other biochemical indices of tubular function currently under evalution include amino acids (Lenz *et al.* 1985) and microglobulins (Dumez, pers. comm.). Observation of refilling post aspiration suggests continued urine production, but may be misleading due to either polyuric renal failure or passive filling from a dilated upper tract (Harrison *et al.* 1982a; McFadyen *et al.* 1983). An endogenous fetal creatinine clearance test in which maternal creatinine is used to reflect the fetal level, has been shown to correlate well with GFR in animals (Adzick *et al.* 1985b), but is not in clinical usage due to the need for fetal bladder catheterization to the exterior to determine urine output.

The standard method of vesico-amniotic shunting is by ultrasound guided insertion of an indwelling plastic double pigtail catheter (Harrison *et al.* 1982a; Manning *et al.* 1986). As some shunts are prone to blockage or displacement (Golbus *et al.* 1982; Manning *et al.* 1983), one group currently advocates hysterotomy and open decompression (Harrison *et al.* 1982c; Harrison *et al.* 1987), although experience is extremely limited with this major procedure. External shunts (Shalev *et al.* 1984) and serial aspirations (Weinstein *et al.* 1982) have not been popular due to the risk of infection. The results of 73 cases of shunting procedures for low obstructive uropathy reported to the International Registry (Manning *et al.* 1986) are not encouraging with only a 41 per cent perinatal survival rate.

Although it has been questioned whether such procedures are of benefit (Elder *et al.* 1987; Reuss *et al.* 1988b), the available data is far from conclusive as in many of these cases, the aetiology of apparent obstruction was not stated nor was the degree of oligohydramnios. Until the value of shunting procedures is established, selection criteria should be rigorously applied to restrict shunting to those few fetuses in whom it may be of benefit, i.e. otherwise normal male fetuses of normal karyotype with low obstructive uropathy, dilatation of the upper urethra, severe oligohydramnios and biochemical evidence of adequate renal function.

## Prune-belly syndrome

The prune-belly or triad syndrome (PBS) refers to the association of congenital dilatation of the urinary tract, undescended tests and agenesis or hypoplasia of anterior abdominal wall musculature (Nunn & Stevens 1961). Specific antenatal diagnosis of PBS has only been reported in a few severe cases in the third trimester, in which gross ureteric and bladder distension was noted in association with a bulging and misshapen anterior abdominal wall (Christopher *et al.* 1982; Miezner *et al.* 1985). In the majority of PBS fetuses, the ultrasound features are indistinguishable from those of low obstructive uropathy (Anderson *et al.* 1979; Fitzsimmons *et al.* 1985).

The aetiology of PBS is unknown. One theory postulates a primary mesodermal defect affecting the musculature of both the abdominal wall and urinary tract (Nunn & Stevens 1961). However, abdominal wall changes seem non-specific and may follow distension from a variety of causes (Pagon *et al.* 1979; Nakayama *et al.* 1984). There is now increasing evidence that some form of urethral obstruction is implicated in the majority of cases (Pagon *et al.* 1979; Adzick *et al.* 1985a). The major flaw in the latter theory is that most affected babies have no evidence of urethral obstruction at birth (Woodhouse *et al.* 1982). Transient obstruction *in utero* has been documented in PBS (Anderson *et al.* 1979; Fitzsimmons *et al.* 1985; Fisk *et al.* 1989), and it has recently been suggested that an obstruction between 10–20 weeks which subsequently resolves, would account for all the ultrasound features of PBS (Hutson & Beasley 1987). Dilatation of the anterior as well as the prostatic urethra has been documented radiographically in children with PBS, implicating in its pathogenesis a failure of the penile urethra to remain open in the coronal sulcus until the glandular urethra forms and fuses with it (Beasley *et al.* 1988).

Megalourethra is a rare condition of diffuse elongation and expansion of the penile urethral lumen, and most occur in association with PBS (Appel *et al.* 1986). The antenatal diagnosis of megalourethra has recently been reported, and its visualization antenatally in association with non-specific urinary tract dilatation allows a specific diagnosis of PBS to be made (Fisk *et al.* 1989).

## Conclusion

Antenatal sonography has shown itself good in detecting the presence of significant fetal uropathies (Smith *et al.* 1987; Madarikan *et al.* 1988). Its accuracy in arriving at specific diagnoses, on the other hand, has been comparatively bad (Colodny 1987; Grupe 1987), several series reporting incorrect diagnoses in as many as 20–40 per cent when prenatal findings were compared with pathological or paediatric diagnoses (Turnock & Shawls 1984; Broyer *et al.* 1985). This deficiency is currently being corrected, at least in part, by improvements in machine resolution together with a greater understanding of the pathophysiology of congenital renal and urinary abnormalities. In addition to gross uropathies with a poor perinatal prognosis, increasingly minor lesions are being detected, thereby reducing paediatric morbidity from delayed diagnosis (Dell'Agnola *et al.* 1983).

## References

Adzick N.S., Harrison M.R., Flake A.W. & deLorimier A.A. (1985a) Urinary extravasation in the fetus with obstructive uropathy. *Journal of Pediatric Surgery*, **20**, 608–15.

Adzick N.S., Harrison M.R., Flake A.W. & Laberge J. (1985b) Development of a fetal renal function test using endogenous creatinine clearance. *Journal of Pediatric Surgery*, **20**, 602–7.

Anderson J.C., Faulder K.C. & Moir J.E. (1979) 'Prune belly' syndrome. *Medical Journal of Australia*, **1**, 313–4.

Antonakopoulos G.N., Fuggle W.J., Newman J., Considine J. & O'Brien J.M. (1985) Idiopathic hydronephrosis: light microscopic features and pathogenesis. *Archives of Pathology and Laboratory Medicine*, **109**, 1097–101.

Appel R.A., Kaplan G.W., Brock W.A. & Streit D. (1986) Megalourethra. *Journal of Urology*, **135**, 747–51.

Apuzzio J.J., Unwin W., Adhate A. & Nichols R. (1986) Prenatal diagnosis of fetal renal mesoblastic nephroma. *American Journal of Obstetrics and Gynecology*, **154**, 636–7.

Arger P.H., Coleman B.G., Muntz M.C., Snyder H.P., Camardese T., Arenson R.L., Gabbe S.G. & Aquino L. (1985) Routine fetal genitourinary tract screening. *Radiology*, **156**, 485–9.

Avni E.F., Rodesch F. & Schulman C.C. (1985) Fetal uropathies: diagnostic pitfalls and management. *Journal of Urology*, **134**, 921–5.

Avni E.F., Thoua Y., Lalmand B., Didier F., Droulle P. & Schulman C.C. (1987) Multicystic dysplastic kidney: natural history from *in utero* diagnosis and postnatal follow up. *Journal of Urology*, **138**, 1420–4.

Barrett R.J., Rayburn W.F. & Barr M. (1983) Furosemide (Lasix) challenge test in assessing bilateral fetal hydronephrosis. *American Journal of Obstetrics and Gynecology*, **147**, 846–7.

Beasley S.W., Bettenay F. & Hutson J.M. (1988) The anterior urethra provides clues to the aetiology of prune belly syndrome. *Pediatric Surgery International*, **3**, 169–72.

Beretsky I., Lankin D.H., Rusoff J.H. & Phelan L. (1984) Sonographic differentiation between the multicystic dysplastic kidney and the ureteropelvic junction obstruction *in utero* using high resolution real-time scanners employing digital detection. *Journal of Clinical Ultrasound*, **12**, 429–33.

Bernstein J. (1971) Heritable cystic disorders of the kidney: the mythology of polycystic disease. *Pediatric Clinics of North America*, **18**, 435–44.

Bertagnoli L., Lalatta F., Gallicchio R., Fantuzzi M., Rusca M., Zorzolli A. & Deter R.L. (1983) Quantitative characterization of the growth of the fetal kidney. *Journal of Clinical Ultrasound*, **11**, 349–56.

Blane C.E., Koff S.A., Bowerman R.A. & Barr J.M. (1983) Nonobstructive fetal hydronephrosis: sonographic recognition and therapeutic implications. *Radiology*, **147**, 95–9.

Blyth H. & Ockenden B.G. (1971) Polycystic kidney disease of kidneys and liver presenting in childhood. *Journal of Medical Genetics*, **8**, 257–84.

Broyer M., Guest G., Lestage F. & Gacoin F.B. (1984) Prenatal diagnosis of urinary tract malformations. *Advances in Nephrology*, **14**, 21–38.

Bulic M., Podobnik M., Korenic B. & Bistricki J. (1987) First-trimester diagnosis of low obstructive uropathy: an indicator of initial renal function in the fetus. *Journal of Clinical Ultrasound*, **15**, 537–41.

Callen P.W., Bolding D., Filly R.A. & Harrison M.A. (1983) Ultrasonographic evaluation of fetal paranephric pseudocysts. *Journal of Ultrasound in Medicine*, **2**, 309–12.

Campbell S., Wladimiroff J.W. & Dewhurst C.J. (1973) The antenatal measurement of fetal urine production. *Journal of Obstetrics and Gynaecology of the British Commonwealth*, **80**, 680–6.

Chamberlain P.F., Cumming M., Torchia M.G., Biehl D. & Manning F.A. (1985) Ovine fetal urine production following maternal intravenous furosemide administration. *American Journal of Obstetrics and Gynecology*, **151**, 815–19.

Chamberlain P.F., Manning F.A., Morrison I. & Lange I.R. (1984) Circadian rhythym in bladder volumes in the term human fetus. *Obstetrics and Gynecology*, **64**, 657–60.

Christopher C.R., Spinelli A. & Severt D. (1982) Ultrasonic diagnosis of prune-belly syndrome. *Obstetrics and Gynecology*, **59**, 391–4.

Colodny A.H. (1987) Antenatal diagnosis and management of urinary abnormalities. *Pediatric Clinics of North America*, **34**, 1365–81.

Crowley P. (1980) Non-quantitative estimation of amniotic fluid volume in suspected prolonged pregnancy. *Journal of Perinatal Medicine*, **8**, 249–51.

Dell'Agnola C.A., Tomaselli V., Ferrazzi E., Kustermann A. & Nicolini U. (1983) Perinatal ultrasound monitoring: early detection and treatment of congenital uropathy. *British Journal of Urology*, **55**, 469–72.

Deter R.L., Hadlock F.P., Gonzles E.T. & Wait R.B. (1980) Prenatal detection of primary megaureter using dynamic image ultrasonography. *Obstetrics and Gynecology*, **56**, 759–62.

Drake D.P., Stevens P.S. & Eckstein H.B. (1978) Hydronephrosis secondary to ureteropelvic junction obstruction in children: A review of 14 years experience. *Journal of Urology*, **119**, 649–51.

Dubbins P.A., Kurtz A.B., Wapner R.J. & Goldberg B.B. (1981) Renal agenesis: spectrum of *in utero* findings. *Journal of Clinical Ultrasound*, **9**, 189–93.

Dunn V. & Glasier C. (1985) Ultrasonographic antenatal demonstration of primary megaureters. *Journal of Ultrasound in Medicine*, **4**, 101–3.

Duval J.M., Milon J., Coadou Y., Blouet J.M., Langella B., Bourgin T., Nicolas J.C., Fremond B., Duval J.C. & Jouan H. (1985b) Ultrasonographic anatomy and diagnosis of fetal uropathies affecting the upper urinary tract: I Obstructive uropathies. *Anatomia Clinica*, **7**, 301–32.

Duval J.M., Milon J., Langella B., Blouet J.M., Coadou Y., Le Marec B. & Vialard J. (1985a) Ultrasonographic anatomy and physiology of the fetal kidney. *Anatomia Clinica*, **7**, 107–23.

Ehman R.L., Nicholson S.F. & Machin G.A. (1983) Prenatal sonographic detection of congenital mesoblastic nephroma in a monozygotic twin pregnancy. *Journal of Ultrasound in Medicine*, **2**, 555–7.

Elder J.S., Duckett J.W. & Snyder H.M. (1987) Intervention for fetal obstructive uropathy: has it been effective? *Lancet*, **ii**, 1007–10.

Felson B. & Cussen L.J. (1975) The hydronephrotic type of unilateral congenital multicystic disease of the kidney. *Seminars in Roentgenology*, **10**, 113–23.

Fisk N.M., Dhillon H.K., Ellis C.E., Nicolini U., Tannirandorn Y. & Rodeck C.H. (1989) Antenatal diagnosis of megalourethra in a fetus with the prune belly syndrome. *Journal of Clinical Ultrasound*, (In press).

Fitzsimmons R.B., Keohane C. & Galvern J. (1985) Prune belly syndrome with ultrasound demonstration of reduction of megacystis *in utero*. *British Journal of Radiology*, **58**, 374–6.

Furness M.E., Rajadurai S., Haslam R.R., Weckert R.C. & O'Loughlin J.A. (1988) Fetal renal vein thrombosis. *Australian and New Zealand Journal of Obstetrics and Gynaecology*, **28**, 193–6.

Garrett W.J., Grunwald G. & Robinson D.E. (1970) Prenatal diagnosis of fetal polycystic kidney by ultrasound. *Australian and New Zealand Journal of Obstetrics and Gynaecology*, **10**, 7–9.

Garrett W.J., Kossof G. & Osborn R.A. (1975) The dagnosis of fetal hydronephrosis, megaureter, and urethral obstruction by ultrasonic echography. *British Journal of Obstetrics and Gynaecology*, **82**, 115–20.

Gauderer M.W.L., Jassani M.N. & Izant R.J. (1984) Ultrasonographic antenatal diagnosis: will it change the spectrum of neonatal surgery? *Journal of Pediatric Surgery*, **19**, 404–7.

Gembruch U. & Hansmann M. (1988) Artificial instillation of amniotic fluid as a new technique for the diagnostic evaluation of cases of oligohydramnios. *Prenatal Diagnosis*, **8**, 33–45.

Giulan B.B., Chang C.C.N. & Yoss B.S. (1986) Prenatal ultrasonographic diagnosis of fetal adrenal neuroblastoma. *Journal of Clinical Ultrasound*, **14**, 225–7.

Glassberg K.I., Stephens F.D., Lebowtz R.L., Braren V., Duckett J.W., Jacobs E.C., King L.R. & Perlmutter A.D. (1987) Renal dysgenesis and cystic disease of the kidney: A report of the committee on terminology, nomenclature and classification, Section on Urology, American Academy of Pediatrics. *Journal of Urology*, **138**, 1085–92.

Glick P.L., Harrison M.R., Adzick N.S., Noall R.A. & Villa R.L. (1984) Correction of congenital hydronephrosis *in utero*. IV: *In utero* decompression prevents renal dysplasia. *Journal of Pediatric Surgery*, **19**, 649–57.

Glick P.L., Harrison M.R., Golbus M.S., Adzick N.S., Filly R.A., Callen P.W., Mahony B.S., Anderson R.L. & de Lorimier A.A. (1985) Management of the fetus with congenital hydronephrosis. II. Prognostic criteria and selection for treatment. *Journal of Pediatric Surgery*, **20**, 376–87.

Glick P.L., Harrison M.R., Noall R.A. & Villa R.L. (1983) Correction of congenital hydronephrosis *in utero*. III: early mid trimester ureteral obstruction produces renal dysplasia. *Journal of Pediatric Surgery*, **18**, 681–7.

Golbus M.S., Harrison M.R., Filly R.A., Callen P.W. & Katz M. (1982) *In utero* treatment of urinary tract obstruction. *American Journal of Obstetrics and Gynecology*, **142**, 383–8.

Goldenberg R.L., Davis R.O. & Brumfield C.G. (1984) Transient fetal anuria of unknown etiology: a case report. *American Journal of Obstetrics and Gynecology*, **149**, 87.

Gore R.M., Callen P.W., Filly R.A., Harrison M.R. & Golbus M.S. (1982) Prenatal percutaneous antegrade pyelography in posterior urethral valves: songographic guidance. *American Journal of Roentgenology*, **139**, 994–6.

Grannum P., Bracken M., Silverman R. & Hobbins J.C. (1980) Assessment of fetal kidney size in normal gestation by comparison of ratio of kidney circumference to abdominal circumference. *American Journal of Obstetrics and Gynecology*, **136**, 249–54.

Green J.J. & Hobbins J.C. (1988) Abdominal ultrasound of the first-trimester fetus. *American Journal of Obstetrics and Gynecology*, **159**, 165–75.

Grignon A., Filiatrault D., Homsy Y., Robitaille P., Filion R., Boutin H. & Leblond R., (1986b) Ureteropelvic junction stenosis: antenatal ultrasonographic diagnosis, postnatal investigation and follow up. *Radiology*, **160**, 649–51.

Grignon A., Filion R., Filiatrault D., Robitaille P., Homsy Y., Boutin H. & Leblond R. (1986a) Urinary tract dilatation *in utero:* classification and clinical applications. *Radiology*, **160**, 645–7.

Griscom N.T., Vawter G.F. & Fellers F.X. (1975) Pelvoinfundibular atresia: the usual form of mylticystic kidney: 44 unilateral and 2 bilateral cases. *Seminars in Roentgenology*, **10**, 125–31.

Grisoni E.R., Gauderer M.W., Wolfson R.N. & Izant R.J. (1986) Antenatal ultrasonography: the experience in a high risk perinatal centre. *Journal of Pediatric Surgery*, **21**, 358–61.

Grupe W. (1987) The dilemma of intrauterine diagnosis of congenital renal disease. *Pediatric Clinics of North America*, **34**, 629–38.

Gunn T.R., Mora J.D. & Pease P. (1988) Outcome after antenatal diagnosis of upper urinary tract dilatation by ultrasonography. *Archives of Disease in Childhood*, **63**, 1240–3.

Guys J.M., Borella F. & Monfort G. (1988) Ureteropelvic junction obstructions: Prenatal diagnosis and surgery in 47 cases. *Journal of Pediatric Surgery*, **23**, 156–8.

Hanna M.K., Jeffs R.D., Sturgess J.M., *et al.* (1976) Ureteral structure and ultrastructure. Part II. Congenital ureteropelvic junction obstruction and primary obstructive megaureter. *Journal of Urology*, **116**, 725–30.

Harman C.R. (1984) Maternal furosemide may not provoke urine production in the compromised fetus. *American Journal of Obstetrics and Gynecology*, **150**, 322–3.

Harrison M.R., Filly R.A., Parer J.T., Faer M.J., Jacobson J.B. & de Lorimier A.A. (1981) Management of the fetus with a urinary tract malformation. *Journal of the American Medical Associaton*, **246**, 635–9.

Harrison M.R., Golbus M.S., Filly R.A., Anderson R.L., Flake A.W., Rosen M. & Huff R.W. (1987) Fetal hydronephrosis: selection and surgical repair. *Journal of Pediatric Surgery*, **22**, 556–8.

Harrison M.R., Golbus M.S., Filly R.A., Callen P.W., Katz M., de Lorimier A.A., Rosen M. & Jonsen A.R. (1982c) Fetal surgery for congenital hydronephrosis. *New England Journal of Medicine*, **306**, 591–3.

Harrison M.R., Golbus M.S., Filly R.A., Nakayama D.K., Callen P.W., de Lorimier A.A. & Hricak H. (1982a) Management of the fetus with congenital hydronephrosis. *Journal of Pediatric Surgery*, **17**, 728–42.

Harrison M.R., Nakayama D.K., Noall R. & de Lorimier A.A. (1982b) Correction of congenital hydronephrosis *in utero*. II. Decompression reverses the effects of obstruction on the fetal lung and urinary tract. *Journal of Pediatric Surgery*, **17**, 965–74.

Harrison M.R., Ross N.A., Noall R., & de Lorimier A.A. (1983) Correction of congenital hydronephrosis *in utero*. I. The model: fetal urethral obstruction produces hydronephrosis and pulmonary hypoplasia in fetal lambs. *Journal of Pediatric Surgery*, **18**, 247–56.

Hartman G.E., Smolik L.M. & Shochat S.J. (1986) The dilemma of multicystic dysplastic kidney. *American Journal of Diseases of Children*, **140**, 925–8.

Helin I. & Persson P.H. (1986) Prenatal diagnosis of urinary tract abnormalities by ultrasound. *Pediatrics*, **78**, 879–83.

Hellstrom W.J., Kogan B.A., Jeffrey R.B. & McAninch J.W. (1984) The natural history of prenatal hydronephrosis with normal amounts of amniotic fluid. *Journal of Urology*, **132**, 947–50.

Henderson S.C., Van Kolken R.J. & Rahatzad M. (1980) Multicystic kidney with hydramnios. *Journal of Clinical Ultrasound*, **8**, 249–50.

Hill L.M. & Peterson C.S. (1987) Antenatal diagnosis of fetal pelvic kidneys. *Journal of Ultrasound in Medicine*, **6**, 393–6.

Hobbins J.C., Grannum P.A.T., Berkowitz R.L., Silverman R. & Mahoney M.J. (1979) Ultrasound in the diagnosis of congenital anomalies. *American Journal of Obstetrics and Gynecology*, **134**, 331–45.

Hobbins J.C., Romero R., Grannum P., Berkowitz R.L., Cullen M. & Mahoney M. (1984) Antenatal diagnosis of renal anomalies with ultrasound. I. Obstructive uropathy. *American Journal of Obstetrics and Gynecology*, **148**, 868–77.

Hoddick W.K., Filly R.A., Mahony B.S. & Callen P.W. (1985) Minimal fetal renal pyelectasis. *Journal of Ultrasound in Medicine*, **4**, 85–9.

Hurley J.K., Kirkpatrick S.E., Pitlick P.T., *et al.* (1977) Renal response of the fetal lamb to fetal or maternal volume expansion. *Circulation Research*, **40**, 557–60.

Hutson J.M. & Beasley S.W. (1987) Aetiology of the prune belly syndrome. *Australian Journal of Paediatrics*, **23**, 309–10.

Jeanty P. & Dramaix-Wilmet M., Elkhazen N., Hubinont C. & van Regemister N. (1982) Measurement of fetal kidney growth on ultrasound. *Radiology*, **144**, 159–62.

Johnston J.H., Evans J.P., Glassberg K.I. & Shapiro S.R. (1977) Pelvic hydronephrosis in children: A review of 219 personal cases. *Journal of Urology*, **117**, 97–101.

Juskiewenski S., Vaysse P., Moscovici J., De Graeve P. & Guitard J. (1984) The ureterovesical junction. *Anatomia Clinica*, **5**, 251–9.

Kay R., Brereton R.J. & Johnston J.H. (1980) Urinary ascities in the newborn. *British Journal of Urology*, **52**, 451–4.

King L.R., Coughlin P.W., Bloch E.C., Bowie J.D., Ansong K. & Hanna M.K. (1984) The case for immediate pyeloplasty in the neonate with ureteropelvic junction obstruction. *Journal of Urology*, **132**, 725–8.

Kleiner B., Callen P.W. & Filly R.A. (1987) Sonographic analysis of the fetus with ureteropelvic junction obstruction. *American Journal of Roentgenology*, **148**, 359–63.

Kleiner B., Filly R.A., Mack L. & Callen P.W. (1986) Multicystic dysplastic kidney:

observations of contralateral disease in the fetal population. *Radiology*, **161**, 27–9.

Koyle M.A. & Ehrlich R.M. (1988) Management of ureteropelvic junction obstruction in neonate. *Urology*, **31**, 496–8.

Kullendorf C.M., Larsson L.T., & Jorgensen C. (1984) The advantage of antenatal diagnosis of intestinal and urinary tract malformations. *British Journal of Obstetrics and Gynaecology*, **91**, 144–7.

Kurjak A., Kirkinen P., Latin V. & Ivankovic D. (1981) Ultrasonic assessment of fetal kidney function in normal and complicated pregnancies. *American Journal of Obstetrics and Gynecology*, **141**, 266–70.

Kurth K.H., Alleman E.R. & Schroeder F.H. (1981) Major and minor complications of posterior urethral valves. *Journal of Urology*, **126**, 517–19.

Laing F.C., Burke V.D., Wing V.W., Jeffrey R.B. & Hashimoto B. (1984) Postpartum evaluation of fetal hydronephrosis: optimal timing for follow-up sonography. *Radiology*, **152**, 423–4.

Laxova R., Biesecker L.E., Friday R.O., Snyder G., Olson R.W., Krassikoff N. & Gilbert E.F. (1987) Management of the fetus with urinary tract dilatation. *Birth Defects*, **23**, 385–99.

Lebowitz R.L. & Griscom N.T. (1977) Neonatal hydronephrosis: 146 cases. *Radiological Clinics of North America*, **15**, 49–59.

Lenz S., Lund-Hansen T., Bang J. & Christensen E. (1985) A possible prenatal evaluation of renal function by amino acid analysis on fetal urine. *Prenatal Diagnosis*, **5**, 259–67.

Luthy D.A. & Hirsch J.H. (1985) Infantile polycystic kidney disease: observations from attempts at prenatal diagnosis. *American Journal of Medical Genetics*, **20**, 505–17.

McCrory W.W., Shibuya M., Leamann E. & Karp R. (1971) Studies of renal function in children with chronic hydronephrosis. *Pediatric Clinics of North America*, **18**, 445–65.

McFadyen I.R., Wigglesworth J.S. & Dillon M.J. (1983) Fetal urinary tract obstruction: is active intervention before delivery indicated? *British Journal of Obstetrics and Gynaecology*, **90**, 342–9.

Madarikan B.A., Hayward C., Roberts G.M. & Lari J. (1988) Clinical outcome of fetal uropathy. *Archives of Disease in Childhood*, **63**, 961–3.

Mahoney B.S., Filly R.A., Callen P.W., Hricak H., Golbus M.S. & Harrison M.R. (1984) Fetal renal dysplasia: sonographic evaluation. *Radiology*, **152**, 143–6.

Manning F.A., Harman C.R., Lange I.R., Brown R., Decter A. & MacDonald N. (1983) Antepartum chronic fetal vvesicoamniotic shunts for obstructive uropathy: a report of two cases. *American Journal of Obstetrics and Gynecology*, **145**, 819–22.

Manning F.A., Harrison M.R., Rodeck C.H. & Members of The International Fetal Medicine & Surgery Society (1986) Catheter shunts for fetal hydronephrosis and hydrocephalus. *New England Journal of Medicine*, **315**, 336–40.

Manning F.A., Hill L.M. & Platt L.D. (1981) Qualitative amniotic fluid volume determination by ultrasound: antepartum detection of intrauterine growth retardation. *American Journal of Obstetrics and Gynecology*, **139**, 254–8.

Mayor G., Genton M., Torrado A. & Guignard J.P. (1975) Renal function in obstructive nephropathy: long term effect of reconstructive surgery. *Pediatrics*, **56**, 740–7.

Medical Research Council-Bacteruria Committee (1979) Recommended terminology of urinary tract infection. *British Medical Journal*, **2**, 717–19.

Meizner I., Bar-Ziv J. & Katz M. (1985) Prenatal ultrasonic diagnosis of the extreme form of prune belly syndrome. *Journal of Clinical Ultrasound*, **13**, 581–3.

Mercer L.J. & Brown L.G. (1986) Fetal outcome with oligohydramnios in second trimester. *Obstetrics and Gynecology*, **67**, 840–2.

Morin M.E. & Baker D.A. (1979) The influence of hydration and bladder distension on the sonographic diagnosis of hydronephrosis. *Journal of Clinical Ultrasound*, **7**, 192–4.

Morse R.P., Rawnsley E., Crowe H.C., Marinpadilla M. & Graham J.M. (1987) Bilateral renal agenesis in three consecutive siblings. *Prenatal Diagnosis*, **7**, 573–9.

Nakayama D.K., Harrison M.R., Chinn D.H. & de Lorimier A.A. (1984) The pathogenesis of prune belly. *American Journal of Diseases of Children*, **138**, 834–6.

Nakayama D.K., Harrison M.R. & de Lorimier A.A. (1986) Prognosis of posterior urethral valves presenting at birth. *Journal of Pediatric Surgery*, **21**, 43–5.

Nicolaides K.H., Rodeck C.H. & Gosden C.M. (1986) Rapid karyotyping in non-lethal fetal malformations. *Lancet*, **i**, 283–7.

Nicolini U., Ferrazzi E., Kustermann A., Ravizza M., Belotti M., Pardi G., dell'Agnola A., Tomaselli V. & Carmassi L. (1987a) Perinatal management of fetal hydronephrosis with normal bladder. *Journal of Perinatal Medicine*, **15**, 53–60.

Nicolini U., Fisk N.M., Rodeck C.H., Talbert D.G. & Wigglesworth J.S. (1989a) Low amniotic pressure in oligohydramnios: Is this the cause of pulmonary hypoplasia. *American Journal of Obstetrics and Gynecology* (in press).

Nicolini U., Fisk N.M., Talbert D.G., Rodeck C.H., Kochenour N.K., Greco P., Hubinont C. & Santolaya J. (1989b) Intrauterine manometry: technique and application to fetal pathology. *Prenatal Diagnosis*, **9**, 243–54.

Nicolini U., Rodeck C.H. & Fisk N.M. (1987b) Shunt treatment for fetal obstructive uropathy. *Lancet*, **ii**, 1338–9.

Nicolini U., Santolaya J., Hubinont C., Fisk N.M., Maxwell D. & Rodeck C.H. (1989c) Visualization of fetal intrabdominal organs in second trimester severe oligohydramnios by intraperitoneal infusion. *Prenatal Diagnosis*, **9**, 191–94.

Nicolini U., Talbert D.G., Fisk N.M. & Rodeck C.H. (1989d) Pathophysiology of pressure changes during intrauterine transfusion. *American Journal of Obstetrics and Gynecology*, **160**, 1139–45.

Nunn I.N. & Stevens F.D. (1961) The triad syndrome: a composite anomaly of the abdominal wall, urinary system and testes. *Journal of Urology*, **86**, 782–94.

Pagon R.A., Smith D.W. & Shephard T.H. (1979) Urethral obstruction malformation complex: a cause of abdominal muscle deficiency and the 'prune belly'. *Journal of Pediatrics*, **94**, 900–6.

Parker R.M. (1974) Neonatal urinary ascites: a potentially favourable sign in bladder outlet obstruction. *Urology*, **3**, 589–93.

Patel R.B. & Connors J.J. (1988) *In utero* sonographic findings in fetal renal vein thrombosis with calcifications. *Journal of Ultrasound in Medicine*, **7**, 349–52.

Patterson R.M., Prihoda T.J. & Pouliot M.R. (1987) Sonographic amniotic fluid measurement and fetal growth retardation: A reappraisal. *American Journal of Obstetrics and Gynecology*, **157**, 1406–10.

Philipson E.H., Wolfson R.N. & Kedia K.R. (1984) Fetal hydronephrosis and polyhydramnios associated with vesicoureteral reflux. *Journal of Clinical Ultrasound*, **12**, 585–7.

Pitts W.R. & Muecke E.C. (1974) Congenital megaloureter: a review of 80 patients. *Journal of Urology*, **3**, 468–73.

Potter E.L. (1965) Bilateral absence of ureters and kidneys: a report of 50 cases. *Obstetrics and Gynecology*, **25**, 3–12.

Potter E.L. (1972) *Normal and Abnormal Development of the Kidney*, pp. 141–53. Year Book Medical Publishers, Chicago.

Pretorius D.H., Lee M.E., Manco-Johnson M.L., Weingast G.R., Sedman A.B. & Gabow P.A. (1987) Diagnosis of autosomal dominant polycystic kidney disease *in utero* and in the young infant. *Journal of Ultrasound in Medicine*, **6**, 249–55.

Reeders S.T., Zerres K., Gal A., Hogenkamp T., Propping T., Schmidt W., Waldherr R., Dolata M.M., Davies K.E. & Weatherall D.J. (1986) Prenatal diagnosis of autosomal dominant polycystic kidney disease with a DNA probe. *Lancet*, **ii**, 6–8.

Reilly K.B., Rubin S.P., Blanke B.G. & Yeh M.N. (1979) Infantile polycystic kidney disease: a difficult antenatal diagnosis. *American Journal of Obstetrics and Gynecology*, **133**, 580–2.

Reuss A., Wladimiroff J.W., Scholtmeijer R.J., Stewart P.A., Sauer P.J.J. & Niermeijer M.F. (1988a) Prenatal evaluation and outcome of fetal obstruction uropathies. *Prenatal Diagnosis*, **8**, 93–102.

Reuss A., Wladimiroff J.W., Stewart P.A. & Scholtmeijer R.J. (1988b) Non-invasive management of fetal obstructive uropathy. *Lancet*, **ii**, 949–51.

Reuss A., Wladimiroff J.W., Wijngaard J.A., Pijpers L. & Stewart P.A. (1987) Fetal renal anomalies, a diagnostic dilemma in the presence of intrauterine growth retardation and oligohydramnios. *Ultrasound in Medicine and Biology*, **10**, 619–24.

Reuter K.L. & Lebowitz R.L. (1985) Massive vesicoureteral reflux mimicking posterior urethral valves in a fetus. *Journal of Clinical Ultrasound*, **13**, 584–7.

Rizzo N., Gabrielli S., Pilu G., Perolo A., Cacciari A., Domini R. & Bovicelli L. (1987) Prenatal diagnosis and obstetrical management of multicystic dysplastic kidney disease. *Prenatal Diagnosis*, **7**, 109–18.

Rodeck C.H. & Nicolini U. (1988) Physiology of the mid-trimester fetus. *British Medical*

*Bulletin*, **44**, 826–49.

Romero R., Cullen M., Grannum P., Jeanty P., Reece E.A., Venus I. & Hobbins J.C. (1985) Antenatal diagnosis of renal anomalies with ultrasound: III. Bilateral renal agenesis. *American Journal of Obstetrics and Gynecology*, **151**, 38–43.

Romero R., Cullen M., Jeanty P., Grannum P., Reece E.A., Venus I. & Hobbins J.C. (1984) The diagnosis of congenital renal anomalies with ultrasound: II. Infantile polycystic kidney disease. *American Journal of Obstetrics and Gynecology*, **150**, 259–62.

Romero R., Pilu G., Jeanty P., Ghidini A. & Hobbins J.C. (1988) *Prenatal Diagnosis of Congenital Anomalies*, 1st edn, pp. 255–99. Appleton & Lange, Connecticut.

Rutherford S.E., Phelan J.P., Smith C.V. & Jacobs N. (1987) The four quadrant assessment of amniotic fluid volume: An adjunct to antepartum fetal heart rate testing. *Obstetrics and Gynecology*, **70**, 353–6.

Sagi J., Vagman I., David M.P., Van Dongen E., Goudie E., Butterworth A. & Jacobson M.J. (1987) Fetal kidney size related to gestational age. *Gynecological and Obstetrical Investigation*, **23**, 1–4.

Sanders R. & Graham D. (1982) Twelve cases of hydronephrosis *in utero* diagnosed by ultrasonography. *Journal of Ultrasound in Medicine*, **1**, 341–8.

Scott E.S. (1987) Fetal ureteric reflux. *British Journal of Urology*, **59**, 291–6.

Sedman A., Bell P., Manco-Johnson M., Schrier R., Warady B.A., Heard E.O., Butler-Simon N. & Gabow P. (1987) Autosomal dominant polycystic kidney disease in childhood: a longitudinal study. *Kidney International*, **31**, 1000–5.

Seeds J.W. & Mandell J. (1986) Congenital obstructive uropathies. Prenatal and postnatal treatment. *Urological Clinics of North America*, **13**, 155–65.

Shalev E., Weiner E., Feldman E., Sudarsky M., Shilowitz L. & Zuckerman H. (1984) External bladder–amniotic fluid shunt for fetal urinary tract obstruction. *Obstetrics and Gynecology*, **63**, 31S–34S.

Sholder A.J., Maizels M., Depp R., Firlit C.F., Sabbagha R., Deddish R. & Reedy N. (1988) Caution in antenatal intervention. *Journal of Urology*, **139**, 1026–9.

Simpson J.L., Sabbhaga R.E., Elias S., Talbot C. & Tamura R.K. (1982) Failure to detect polycystic kidneys by second trimester ultrasonography. *Human Genetics*, **60**, 295.

Smedley M.G. & Bailey R.R. (1987) Autosomal dominant polycystic kidney disease diagnosed *in utero* using ultrasonography. *New Zealand Medical Journal*, **100**, 606.

Smith D., Egginton J.A. & Brookfield D.K.S. (1987) Detection of abnormality of fetal urinary tract as a predictor of renal tract disease. *British Medical Journal*, **294**, 27–8.

Smith E.D., Cussen L.J., Glenn J., Hendren W.H., Jeffs R.D., Johnston J.H., Perlmutter A.D., Stephens F.D., Whitaker R.H. & Woodward J. (1977) Report of working party to establish an international nomenclature for large ureter. *Birth Defects*, **13**, 3–8.

Stanisic T.H. (1986) Editorial. *American Journal of Diseases of Children*, **140**, 865.

Steele B.T., Paes B., Towell M.E. & Hunter J.S. (1988) Fetal renal failure associated with intrauterine growth retardation. *American Journal of Obstetrics and Gynecology*, **159**, 1200–2.

Stephens F.D. (1983) *Congenital Malformations of the Urinary Tract*, 1st edn, pp. 433–62. Praeger, New York.

Thorup J., Mortensen T., Diemer H., Johnson A. & Nielson O.H. (1985) The prognosis of surgically treated congenital hydronephrosis after diagnosis *in utero*. *Journal of Urology*, **134**, 914–17.

Timor-Tritsch I.E., Farine D. & Rosen M.G. (1988) A close look at early development with the high frequency transvaginal transducer. *American Journal of Obstetrics and Gynecology*, **159**, 676–81.

Tsingoglou S. & Dickson J.A.S. (1972) Lower urinary obstruction in infancy. A review of lesions and symptoms in 165 cases. *Archives of Disease in Childhood*, **47**, 215–17.

Turnock R.R. & Shawls R. (1984) Management of fetal urinary tract anomalies detected by prenatal ultrasonography. *Archives of Disease in Childhood*, **59**, 962–5.

Walter J.P. & McGahan J.P. (1985) Mesoblastic nephroma: prenatal sonographic detection. *Journal of Clinical Ultrasound*, **13**, 686–9.

Watson A.R., Readett D., Nelson C.S., Kapila L. & Mayell M.J. (1988) Dilemmas associated with antenatally detected urinary tract abnormalities. *Archives of Disease in Childhood*, **63**, 719–22.

Weiner C., Williamson R., Bonsib S.M., Erenberg A., Pringle K., Smith W. & Abu-Yousef M. (1986) *In utero* bladder diversion — problems with patient selection. *Fetal Therapy*, **1**, 196–202.

Weinstein L., Anderson C.F., Finley P.R. & Lichti P.A. (1982) The *in utero* management of urinary outflow tract obstruction. *Journal of Clinical Ultrasound*, **10**, 465–8.

Wilkins I.A., Chitkara, U., Lynch L., Goldberg J.D., Mehalek K.E. & Berkowtiz R.L. (1987) The nonpredictive value of fetal urinary electrolytes: Preliminary report of outcomes and correlations with pathological diagnosis. *American Journal of Obstetrics and Gynecology*, **157**, 694–8.

Wladimiroff J.W. (1975) Effect of frusemide on fetal urine production. *British Journal of Obstetrics and Gynecology*, **82**, 221–4.

Wladimiroff J.W. & Campbell S. (1974) Fetal urine production rates in normal and complicated pregnancy. *Lancet*, **i**, 151–4.

Woodhouse C.R.J., Ransley P.G. & Innes-Williams D. (1982) Prune belly syndrome — report of 47 cases. *Archives of Disease in Childhood*, **57**, 856–9.

Yeh T.F., Raval D., John E. & Pilder R.S. (1985) Renal response to frusemide in preterm infants with respiratory distress syndrome during the first three postnatal days. *Archives of Disease in Childhood*, **60**, 621–6.

Zerres K., Hansmann M., Mallmann R. & Gembruch U. (1988) Autosomal recessive polycystic kidney disease. Problems of prenatal diagnosis. *Prenatal Diagnosis*, **8**, 215–19.

# 20: Detection of congenital abnormalities of the limbs and face by ultrasound

DAVID R. GRIFFIN



Accurate measurement of the fetal long bones during ultrasound examination remained difficult until the advent of real-time ultrasound. The technique of following movement and accurate alignment and measurement of a long bone is quickly mastered by anyone familiar with real-time ultrasonography. Over the past ten years there have been numerous nomograms constructed for limb lengths and many reports of the use of limb measurement in the assessment of gestational age and the diagnosis of fetal skeletal abnormalities. The higher resolution afforded by dynamic focusing has also enabled more detailed examination of the soft tissue structures of the fetal face.

The aims of this chapter will be to describe the technique of accurate fetal long bone measurement, to describe its application to the diagnosis of fetal limb reduction deformities and to give a brief outline of the features of some of the commoner dysmorphic syndromes that the ultrasonologist might encounter. The examination of the fetal face will be described and some abnormalities discussed.

## Routine measurement

### Machines

The later generations of multifocus real-time scanners are appropriate for limb length measurements. In the author's opinion the linear array scanners are less prone to distortion of long bone images than sector scanners. Optimally, the equipment should switch instantly from freeze-frame to real-time imaging so that moving limbs may be more easily tracked and frozen. The calliper system should be accurate to 1 mm and omnidirectional. A 3.0–3.5 MHz probe is generally sufficient. A 5 MHz facility will greatly enhance image quality and the definition of bone ends in the near to medium field and is a useful addition for those engaged in level three scanning. I would recommend that all those engaged in a regular obstetric scanning commitment have access to a high resolution video tape recorder as this is invaluable for case review and audit of diagnostic performance.

## Why measure bone length?

Why is it important to measure bone length and to examine limb morphology? Firstly, femur length has been shown to be as accurate an indicator of fetal gestational age as biparietal diameter (O'Brien *et al.* 1981; Hadlock *et al.* 1982; Quinlan *et al.* 1982) and serves as a useful alternative in dating a pregnancy when the head is in a difficult position for measurement. Furthermore, when checked against other fetal measurements, pathologies such as limb reductions or microcephaly should be detected. Fetal limb reductions or deformities are a feature of many lethal or crippling congenital disorders (trisomy 18, the chondrodysplasias, arthrogryposis multiplex congenita, TAR syndrome, etc.) most of which should be detected in the second trimester by diligent mid-trimester ultrasound screening.

## When to do these measurements

At least one long bone should be measured (femur or humerus) at every screening ultrasound scan, be this at 16, 18 or 20 weeks. At the same time all the other long bones should be inspected for normal morphology and appropriate length relative to the bone measured. Some of the severe skeletal dysplasias may be apparent from very early in the second trimester but correct distinction between the normal and shortened or deformed bone will be more likely if the first examination is deferred until 16 to 18 weeks. In other chondrodysplasias (achondroplasia, Jeune thoracic dystrophy) long bone shortening may not be apparent until much later (22–24 weeks).

## How to scan limbs

The femur is best located initially by scanning the fetus across the trunk in the axial plane and running down the fetal axis until the pelvic bones are identified. The proximal ends of one or both femurs will then be seen. Keeping the femur in the image, the transducer is then rotated about the axis of the scanning plane until the whole of the ossified diaphysis (shaft) of the bone is in view (Figure 20.1). The transducer is then rocked so that the bone is as parallel with and perpendicular to the ultrasound beam

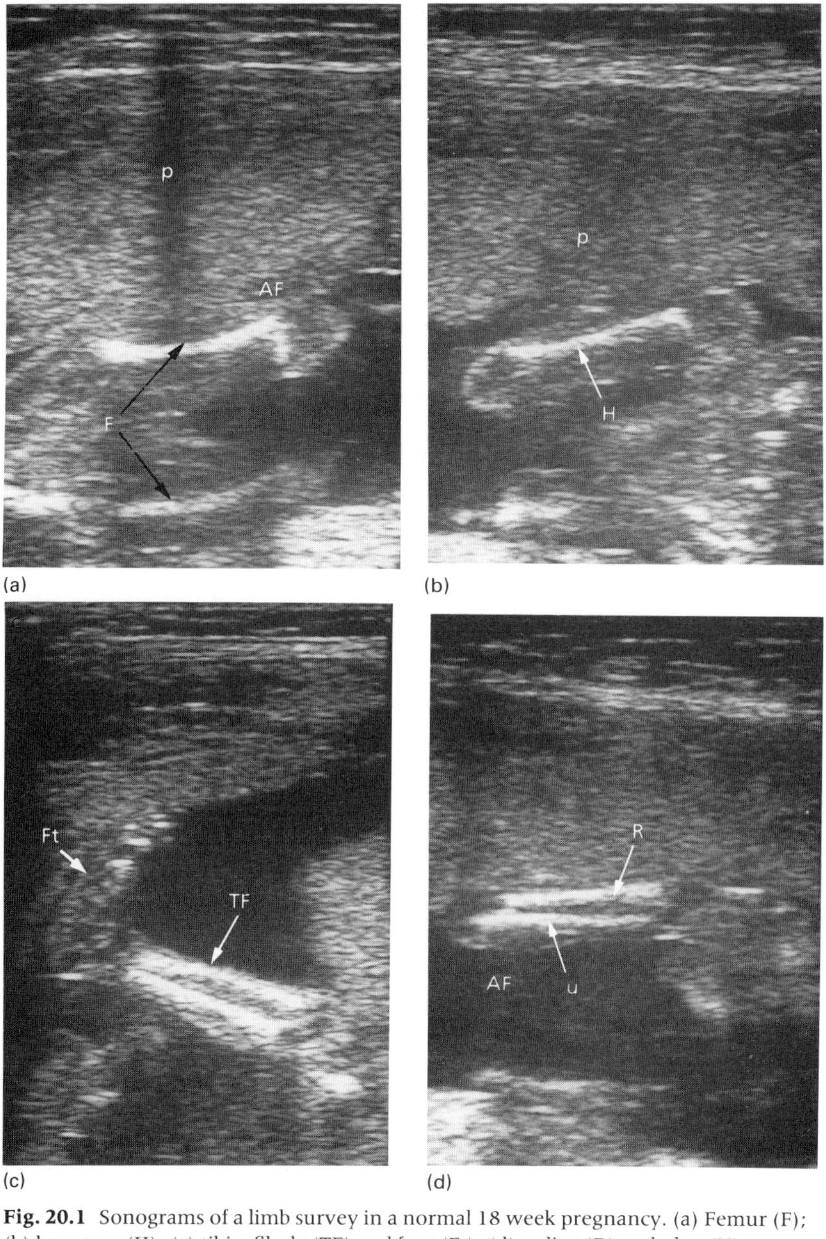


(a) (b) (c) (d)

**Fig. 20.1** Sonograms of a limb survey in a normal 18 week pregnancy. (a) Femur (F); (b) humerus (H); (c) tibia, fibula (TF) and foot (Ft); (d) radius (R) and ulna (U). P = placenta, AF = amniotic fluid.

as possible. At this stage slight lateral shift of the scanning plane should cause the whole bone to disappear from view. If this manoeuvre causes apparent shortening or lateral shift of the bone in the image then the full length of the bone is not covered by the ultrasound beam and further rotational adjustment of the transducer is necessary. Inclusion of the limb extremities (knee and buttocks, elbow and shoulder, etc.) in the image will help in correct alignment. Finally, ensure that the diaphysis to be measured is not overshadowed by other bony structures and that adjacent bones are not included in the measurement. For greatest accuracy several measurements of the bone should be taken until they are consistent.

The technique for humerus measurement is similar to that for the femur. With older machines it may sometimes be difficult to differentiate the humeral extremities from their adjacent articulations (scapula or clavicle and olecranon process of ulna) but with modern focused equipment this should not be a problem. Humerus length is a useful alternative measure of normal limb development or fetal age if the femur is obscured as may occur in a breech presentation.

The distal long bones are identified by following on from the proximal. One forearm is often obscured behind the fetal head or body but will usually move into view eventually. The radius and ulna should be visualized independently in all cases and measured separately in high risk examinations as radial hypoplasia or aplasia is a feature of many important syndromes. The tibia and fibula are of such similar lengths that they need not be measured independently but should be individually identified.

Measurements should be checked against each other, against other somatic measurements (BPD, head and abdomen circumference) and against post-menstrual age. Some excellent limb length nomograms have been published (O'Brien *et al.* 1981; Hadlock *et al.* 1982; Wladimiroff *et al.* 1984) but for general use throughout pregnancy in a Caucasian population those of Jeanty *et al.* (1981, 1982a) are recommended. These are reproduced in texts by Hansmann *et al.* (1985) and Romero *et al.* (1988). Discussion of the appropriate use of cross-sectional or longi-

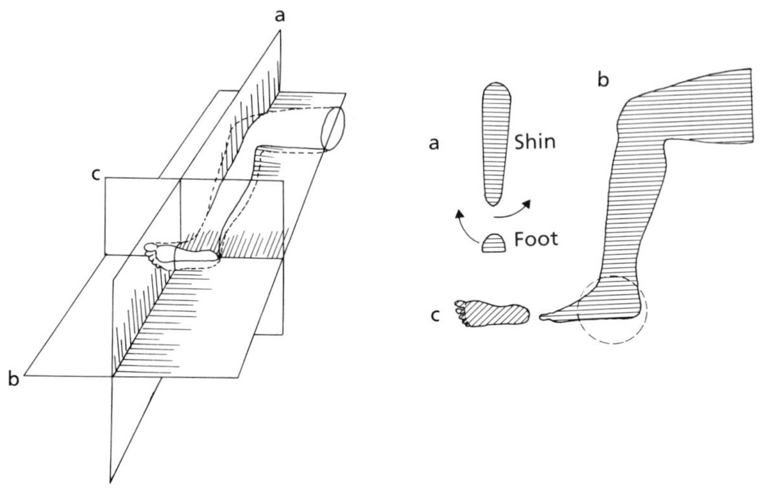


**Fig. 20.2** A diagrammatic representation of the scanning planes used to demonstrate the anatomy of the fetal leg. (a) Longitudinal coronal plane. The sole of the foot and the line of toes should be perpendicular to the foreleg. Internal rotation (↻) is indicative of talipes. (b) Longitudinal sagittal plane. This gives an anteroposterior view of the leg and foot (Figure 20.16b). Rocker-bottom feet (Figure 20.24c) may be recognized and talipes should be suspected if the full plantar view of the foot (c) is seen in this plane (Figure 20.17a). (c) Axial plane giving full plantar view of foot. This is the best view for foot length measurement and counting toes (Figure 20.16a).

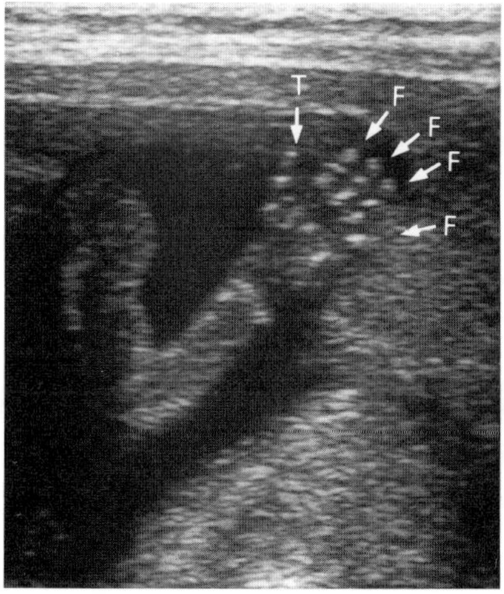


**Fig. 20.3** Sonogram of fetal arm at 17 weeks demonstrating full-fanned hand, thumb (T) and fingers (F).

tudinal data is also fully covered in these texts. It is likely that certain Asian fetal populations do not conform to these growth patterns. Appropriate alternatives should be found or constructed if possible.

The feet may be viewed in three major planes (Figure 20.2) to identify deformities such as talipes, rocker-bottom feet, polydactyly or syndactyly, etc. Foot length (heel to great toe) and femur length should be approximately equal in the second trimester. Hands should be examined so as to reveal four fingers and a normal thumb (Figure 20.3). Hip, knee, ankle, elbow, wrist, and finger joints should be studied for normal position and movement.

Finally examination of the remainder of the skeletal system (spine, thoracic cage, clavicle, mandible and skull) and internal organs completes the survey.

## High risk scanning

### Patient selection for detailed skeletal survey

#### FAMILY HISTORY OF DEFORMITY

Most of the syndromes described here are single gene disorders of autosomal dominant (AD) or autosomal recessive (AR) inheritance. Nonlethal dominant conditions may either be sporadic or show a typical family history with approximately 50 per cent of members affected. All affected members may not be affected to the same extent as a result of variable expression of the gene. Examples of conditions showing dominant inheritance are cleidocranial dysostosis, achondroplasia, Holt–Oram syndrome, etc. and some polydactylies. Lethal dominant conditions will obviously not occur in other generations and are usually new mutations unlikely to recur in the family. Lethal conditions with recessive inheritance, on the other hand, will only occur in the homozygous offspring of heterozygous, unaffected parents. In general the condition will not have presented in that family before. Following the first affected child those parents run a 25 per cent risk of having another and a 50 per cent risk of passing the gene on to their other children. Happily, the gene frequency of these conditions is very low and the chance of two carriers meeting is extremely remote. However, if members of the same family (particularly first cousins) marry, the likelihood of two carriers of the same recessive gene meeting is considerably increased. Such consanguineous marriages are commoner amongst Asian Moslems who should be considered at high risk for recessive syndromes. Many of the lethal and crippling deformities described are recessive.

#### DRUGS IN EARLY PREGNANCY

It is as well to perform a skeletal survey on any patient who has taken significant quantities of medication in the first trimester during this critical time of organogenesis. All are familiar with the devastating effects of the tranquillizer thalidomide. Other drugs that have been specifically implicated in skeletal dysmorphism are warfarin, which may produce a syndrome identical to chondrodysplasia punctata, phenytoin (digital hypoplasia), alcohol, known teratogens such as methotrexate and aminopterin and some anaesthetic agents. A comprehensive list of drug associated malformations has been published by Koren *et al.* (1987).

#### DIABETICS

Poorly controlled diabetics, particularly those with an elevated HbA1c at the time of conception, run a ten-fold risk of fetal malformation, particularly congenital heart disease, renal anomalies and skeletal anomalies (caudal regression syndrome).

#### THE FINDING OF ANY FETAL ANOMALY DURING SCANNING

The abnormalities particularly associated with skeletal malformations are:

polyhydramnios
oligohydramnios
fetal hydrops
small thorax
short femur during routine examination
facial clefting.

### Aids to diagnosis of skeletal dysplasias

The skeletal dysplasias are a heterogeneous group of over 100 rare disorders, many of which have only subtle differences. It is therefore helpful for those particularly interested in the differential diagnosis of these conditions to have access to a comprehensive reference either of fetal and neonatal pathology (Winter *et al.* 1988) or of ultrasound diagnostic features (Romero *et al.* 1988). It is also helpful to cultivate a good working relationship with the local geneticists who may have access to a dysmorphology computerized database.

Before scanning a patient at known risk of a skeletal dysplasia request as much information on the affected members of the family (proband) as possible. This may include photographs, X-rays, detailed pathology reports and reports of any genetic consultations.

## Skeletal malformations

### OSTEOCHONDRODYSPLASIAS

These bone dysplasias are rare with incidences ranging from 1 : 30 000 to a few reported cases (Table 20.1). The list of syndromes and subgroups grows steadily. The degree of limb shortening (Figure 20.4) and deformity is variable between (and sometimes within) syndromes.

The diagnosis or exclusion of recurrence of a limb reduction syndrome in a family known to be at risk is an easy matter as the diagnostician is primed in his search by knowledge of the previous malformations. Accurate diagnosis of an unexpected case discovered at routine scanning is a challenge which demands expert knowledge and diligent attention to detail. Some of the features to note before making a diagnosis are described here.

*Long bones.* Note the degree of shortening in relation to nomograms. Is the shortening greater in the proximal (rhizomelic) femur and humerus or distal (mesomelic) radius and ulna and tibia and fibula or equal in all? Do the bones appear straight, bowed or crumpled?

*Joints.* Note attitude and movement of joints with particular attention to lower limbs and talipes equinovarus.

*Spine.* Examine the spine for deformities, normal ossification of the vertebral bodies and platyspondyly (flattened vertebrae).

**Table 20.1** Incidence of the commoner lethal bone dysplasias

| | |
|---|---|
| Thanatophoric dysplasia | 1 in 30 000 |
| Osteogenesis imperfecta (type 2) | 1 in 55 000 |
| Achondrogenesis (all types) | 1 in 75 000 |
| Chondrodysplasia punctata | 1 in 85 000 |
| Hypophosphatasia (severe form) | 1 in 110 000 |
| Campomelic dysplasia | 1 in 150 000 |

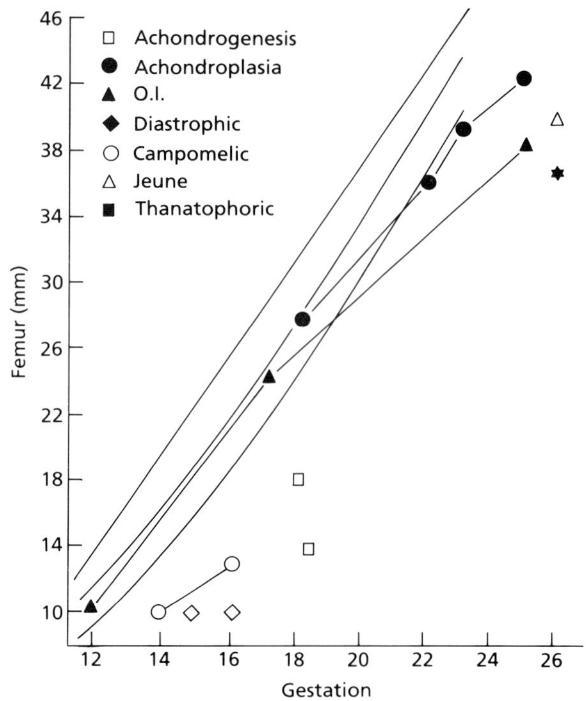


**Fig. 20.4** Nomogram of fetal femur length (O'Brien *et al.* 1981) showing measurements of femur length in fetuses confirmed as having achondrogenesis type 2, achondroplasia, osteogenesis imperfecta type 2a (OI), diastrophic dysplasia, campomelic dysplasia, Jeune thoracic dystrophy and thanatophoric dysplasia. Note the late deviation from normal growth in two fetuses with achondroplasia and one with Jeune thoracic dystrophy.

*Ribs and thorax.* The heart should normally fill about one-third of the thoracic cavity. If the ribs are short the thorax will be small, narrow and bell-shaped and the abdomen protruberant (champagne cork appearance). The ribs may appear beaded in osteogenesis imperfecta type 2 or 3.

*Skull.* A poorly ossified skull will be anechoic or only weekly echoic casting little or no acoustic shadow. The intracranial contents will be more than usually clear and the cerebral hemispheres anechoic (pseudohydrocephaly). In later pregnancy the skull will deform easily if pressed. Note any brachycephaly, cloverleaf deformity or other abnormality.

*Hands and feet.* Count fingers to exclude polydactyly. Extra fingers are usually found next to the fifth finger (post-axial) but thumbs or great toes may be split or duplicated (pre-axial). Note the position of wrists and fingers and the length of the fingers.

*Limb girdles.* There is little data on normal fetal limb girdle dimensions but some osteochondrodystrophies are characterized by short clavicles and hypoplastic ilia and scapulae.

*Face.* A facial profile (sagittal plane) may show a depressed nasal bridge or prominent forehead (frontal bossing) or a receding chin. Micrognathia may be checked by measuring the mandible from the temporomandibular joint to the mental prominence. A full facial view in the coronal plane (see Figure 20.18) will show cleft lip.

*Non-skeletal features.* A full examination of the rest of the fetus including the heart, kidneys, cerebral ventricles and amniotic fluid may uncover further anomalies to narrow down the differential diagnosis.

Table 20.2 shows syndromes associated with specific malformations. Table 20.3 is a rapid diagnostic guide to some of the commoner osteochondrodystrophies.

### *Lethal osteochondrodystrophies*

*Achondrogenesis* types 1 and 2 are of autosomal recessive inheritance occurring with an incidence of approximately 1 : 75 000. Both types may be complicated by polyhydramnios.

**Table 20.2** Clues to the differential ultrasound diagnosis of bone dysplasias

| | |
|---|---|
| Polyhydramnios | Achondrogenesis type 1 or 2<br>Thanatophoric dysplasia<br>Short rib–polydactyly (SRP) syndrome |
| Fetal hydrops | Achondrogenesis type 1<br>SRP syndromes |
| Hypomineralized skull | Osteogenesis imperfecta (IIa)<br>Achondrogenesis type 1<br>Hypophosphatasia |
| Cloverleaf skull | Thanatophoric dysplasia |
| Small thorax | Achondrogenesis<br>Hypochondrogenesis<br>Thanatophoric dysplasia<br>SRP syndromes<br>Chondroectodermal dysplasia<br>Campomelic dysplasia |
| Marked femoral bowing | Campomelic dysplasia<br>Osteogenesis imperfecta<br>Hypophosphatasia |
| Talipes equinovarus | Campomelic dysplasia<br>Diastrophic dysplasia |
| Polydactyly | Chondroectodermal dysplasia<br>SRP syndromes<br>Grebe syndrome<br>? Jeune thoracic dystrophy |
| Short clavicles | Campomelic dysplasia<br>Cleidocranial dysostosis<br>Kniest syndrome |

**Table 20.3** Table showing the chief distinguishing features of the commoner osteochondrodysplasias

| Type | Inheritance | Long bones | Spine | Ribs | Other features | Prognosis | References |
|---|---|---|---|---|---|---|---|
| Achondrogenesis type 1 | (AR) | Extreme micromelia | Poorly mineralized<br>Short | Short | Polyhydramnios, hydrops, very poor cranial ossification | Lethal | Golbus *et al.* (1977)<br>Smith *et al.* (1981)<br>Glen & Teng (1985)<br>Muller *et al.* (1985a)<br>Donnenfeld & Mennuti (1987) |
| Achondrogenesis type 2 | (AR) | Severe micromelia | Unossified spine and sacrum | Short | Polyhydramnios<br>Micrognathia | Lethal | Griffin *et al.* (1985) |
| Thanatophoric dysplasia | (Sporadic) | Severe micromelia<br>Thick diaphysis<br>+/− bowing | Flat vertebral bodies | Short | Polyhydramnios<br>Megalocephaly<br>Ventriculomegaly<br>+/− cloverleaf skull<br>Renal and cardiac anomalies<br>Trident hand | Lethal | Chervenak *et al.* (1983)<br>Beetham & Reeves (1984)<br>Burrows *et al.* (1984)<br>Camera *et al.* (1984)<br>Elejalde *et al.* (1985)<br>Weiner *et al.* (1986) |
| Hypochondrogenesis | (?AR) (Mainly sporadic) | Moderate shortening<br>Flared metaphyses | Flat vertebral bodies | Short | Poor ossification of cervical and sacral spine | Lethal | Stoll *et al.* (1985) |
| Kniest syndrome (Severe neonatal form) | (?AR) | Moderately short<br>Dumb-bell shaped | Lumbar kyphoscoliosis | Normal | Cleft palate<br>Short clavicles | Normal IQ | — |
| Jeune thoracic dystrophy | (AR) | Variable or moderate (especially mesomelic) shortening. | Normal | Short thin | +/− Post-axial polydactyly<br>Hypoplastic lungs<br>Renal dysplasia | 70 per cent lethal<br>Renal problems later | Little (1984)<br>Elejalde *et al.* (1985) |

| | | | | | | | |
|---|---|---|---|---|---|---|---|
| Short rib–polydactyly syndromes Saldino–Noonan (type 1) | (AR) | Moderate shortening<br>Spikey metaphyses | Normal | Very short | Post-axial polydactyly<br>Hydrops, anal atresia<br>Median cleft lip | Lethal | Wladimiroff *et al.* (1984)<br>Meizner & Bar-Ziv (1985) |
| Majewski (type 2) | | Tibia hypoplastic | | | Cardiac and renal anomalies | | Gembruch *et al.* (1985) |
| Ellis–van Crefeld syndrome (chondroectodermal dysplasia) | (AR) | Variable shortening<br>Hypoplastic tibia | Normal | Short | Post-axial polydactyly<br>50 per cent cardiac anomaly (ASD) | 50 per cent lethal<br>Normal IQ | Mahoney & Hobbins (1977)<br>Filly & Golbus (1982)<br>Muller *et al.* (1985a) |
| Campomelic dysplasia | (AR) | Moderate shortening<br>Bowed femur/tibia<br>Hypo/aplastic fibula | Flat vertebrae | Short | Short clavicles, micrognathia<br>Talipes eq. varus<br>Sex reversal | Usually lethal | Fryns *et al.* (1981)<br>Hobbins *et al.* (1982)<br>Redon *et al.* (1984)<br>Winter *et al.* (1985)<br>Griffin (see text) |
| Diastrophic dysplasia | (AR) | Moderate or severe shortening<br>Flexion deformities | Normal | Normal | Talipes eq. varus<br>Proximal hitch-hiker thumbs | 25 per cent lethal | O'Brien *et al.* (1980)<br>Mantagos *et al.* (1982)<br>Kaitila *et al.* (1983)<br>Wladimiroff *et al.* (1984)<br>Gembruch *et al.* (1988) |
| Chondrodysplasia punctata (severe rhizomelic form) | (AR) | Proximal shortening<br>Splayed metaphyses<br>Stippled epiphyses | Coronal clefts | Normal | Joint contractures<br>Microcephaly | Usually lethal<br>Low IQ | Griffin *et al.* (1989) |
| Grebe syndrome | (AR) | Severe mesomelia and acromelia<br>Legs very short | Normal | Normal | Microdactyly<br>Polydactyly | Often lethal<br>Normal IQ | — |
| Achondroplasia | (AD) | Late shortening by 22+ weeks | Normal | Normal | Megalocephaly<br>Frontal bossing<br>Occasional ventriculomegaly | Normal IQ | Campbell *et al.* (1981)<br>Filly *et al.* (1981)<br>Filly & Golbus (1982)<br>Kurtz & Wapner (1983) |

*Achondrogenesis type 1* is characterized by extreme micromelia (very short limbs), a short poorly mineralized spine, short ribs and almost absent ossification of the calvarium. Glenn & Teng (1985) noted femur lengths of 10 mm at 19 weeks. As a result of poor skull mineralization details of the brain structure will be unusually clear. The skull is soft so that the head may be deformed by depressing the transducer.

*Achondrogenesis type 2* shows micromelia to a lesser degree than in type 1. The characteristic feature is absent mineralization of the vertebral bodies. In a personal diagnosis of a new presentation the femur lengths were 18 mm and 19 mm and the radius and ulna combination 19 mm and 20 mm at 18+ post-menstrual weeks. The correct diagnosis was made on finding an anechoic column extending from the sacrum to the base of the skull (Figure 20.5) which represented the unossified vertebral bodies (Figure 20.6). The skull appeared normal.

*Thanatophoric dysplasia* is the commonest of the lethal dysplasias. Its occurrence is sporadic. There is severe micromelia, the diaphyses of the long bones being thick and bowed (Figure 20.7). The ribs are very short and thick and the thoracic cavity constricted. The combination of small chest and normal abdominal size gives the torso a champagne cork appearance in a longitudinal anteroposterior view (Figure 20.8) Vertebrae are flat (platyspondyly) making the spine short. The skull tends towards brachycephaly and in some cases may show cloverleaf deformity (Elejalde & de Elejalde 1985; Weiner *et al.* 1986). There may be associated megalencephaly and cerebral ventriculomegaly. Polyhydramnios

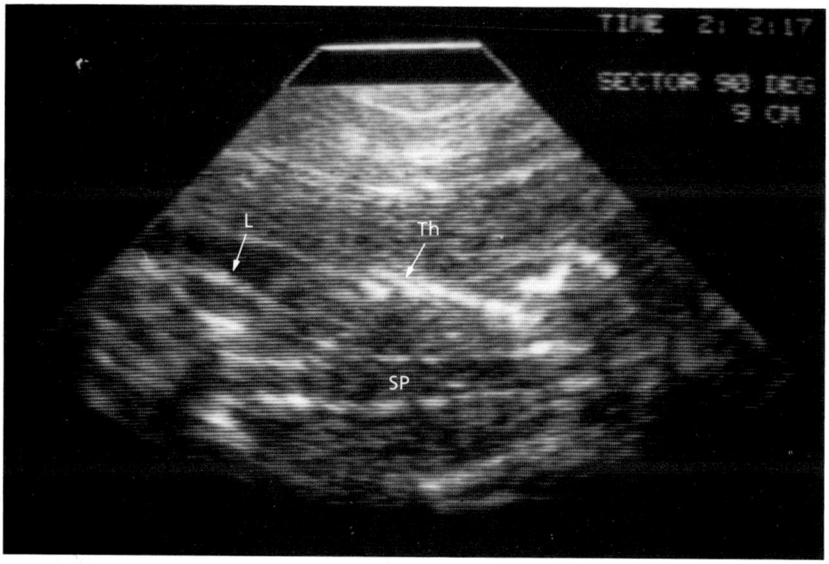


**Fig. 20.5** Longitudinal coronal section of the fetal trunk at 18 weeks in a case of achondrogenesis type 2. Note the anechoic space replacing the vertebral bodies in the spine (Sp). Thorax = Th, Leg = L.

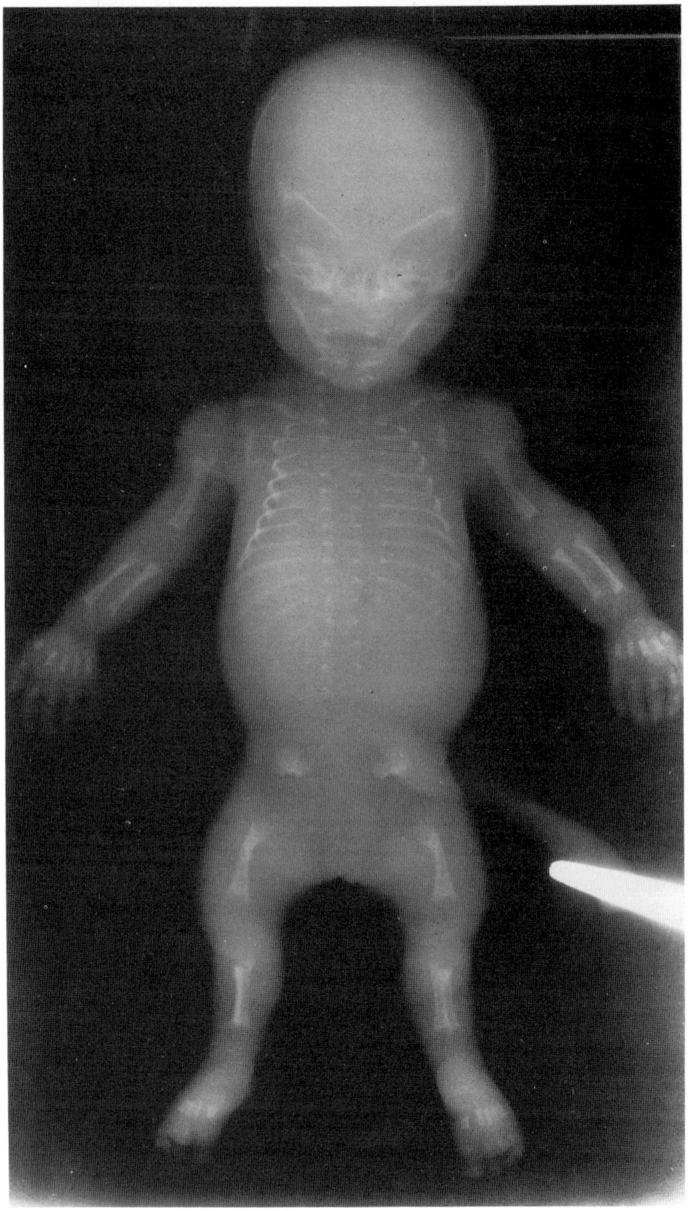

**Fig. 20.6** Radiograph of the fetus in Figure 20.5 showing unossified vertebral bodies and severe micromelia.

is a common presenting sign in the late second or early third trimester.

In a personal case diagnosed at 18 weeks the femur length was 14 mm. Other authors have reported femur lengths of between 18 mm and 21 mm at 19–20 weeks, 23 mm at 22 weeks and only 26–27 mm at 32 weeks. It is thus apparent that very little growth of the long bones occurs from the middle of the second trimester onwards. The condition may be associated with cardiac and renal anomalies. In later pregnancy other dysmorphic features of the condition such as frontal bossing and

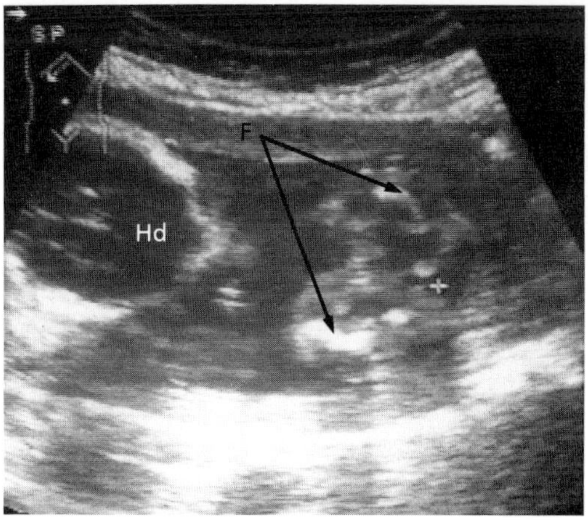


(a)

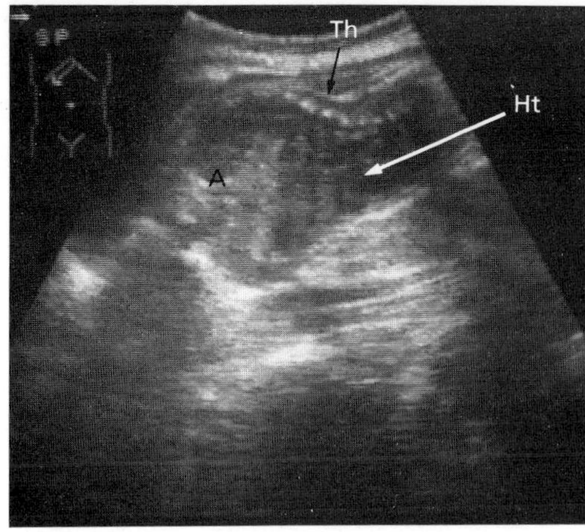


(b)

**Fig. 20.7** Sonograms of a 19 week fetus showing features of thanatophoric dysplasia. (a) Short, bowed femurs (F) and large head (H). (b) The heart (Ht) fills a small, bell-shaped thorax (Th). The ribs are short, thick and splayed at the lower costal margin. (A = abdomen.)

depressed nasal bridge, short splayed fingers (trident hand) and excessive skin folds may be evident (see Figure 20.8).

*Hypochondrogenesis* is of mainly sporadic occurrence but recessive inheritance may occur. A case referred to Watford General Hospital at 31 weeks was diagnosed as Jeune thoracic dystrophy because of moderately short, straight long bones (femur length 42 mm) with thickened metaphyses and short ribs. The diagnosis was revised to hypochondrogenesis after expert examination of neonatal radiographs. Radiologically the condition is characterized by flared metaphyses and poor mineralization of the cervical and sacral vertebral bodies.

*Dys-segmental dysplasia* has been diagnosed by antenatal ultrasonography at 18 weeks (Kim *et al.* 1986). The diagnosis was based on marked shortening of the extremities and a deformed, hypomineralized spine. The condition is lethal and inheritance is autosomal recessive.

*Short rib–polydactyly syndromes (SRPS)* are characterized by moderate micromelia, very short ribs and narrow thorax and post-axial polydactyly (although there have been reports of cases with similar dysmorphic features without polydactyly). They have a recessive pattern of inheritance. Associated anomalies may include anal atresia and renal, cardiac and intestinal deformities. Ambiguous genitalia may give a false impression of a preponderance of females with the condition (see also campomelic dysplasia). *Saldino–Noonan (SRPS type 1)* typically has shortened long bones with pointed metaphyses. *Majewski (SRPS type 2)* may be distinguished from SRPS type 1 by finding median cleft lip or palate and disproportionately short and ovoid tibiae.

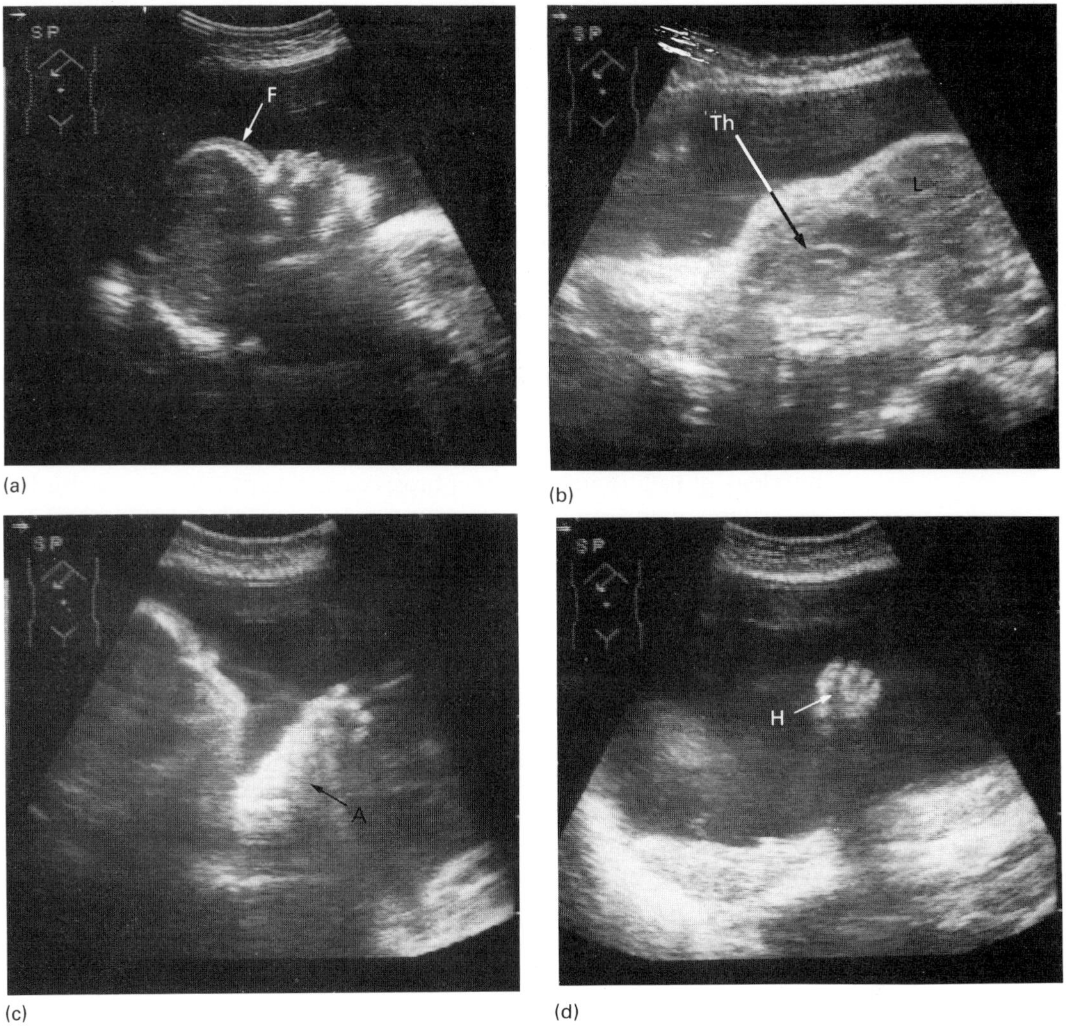


**Fig. 20.8** Thanatophoric dysplasia at 31 weeks showing the features demonstrable in later pregnancy. (a) Facial profile showing frontal bossing (F) and depressed nasal bridge. (b) Small thorax and normal liver giving champagne-cork appearance. (c) Redundant fold of skin on the arm (A). (d) Short, stubby fingers of trident hand (H).

*Frequently lethal dysplasias*

*Ellis–van Crefeld syndrome (chondroectodermal dysplasia)* is recessively inherited, being particularly prevalent amongst the inbred Amish community in Pennsylvania. Affected fetuses may show variable degrees of shortening of long bones which is more pronounced in the forearm and lower leg (mesomelic). There is post-axial polydactyly of hands and feet. The ribs are short and horizontal causing a reduced thoracic cavity and lethal pulmonary hypoplasia in about half of affected infants. Fifty per cent of cases have congenital heart disease (ASD).

*Jeune (asphyxiating) thoracic dystrophy* is another short-ribbed limb reduction syndrome showing minimal to moderate diaphysial shortening. Bone measurements may not fall below normal ranges until late in the second trimester, if at all. There may be severe rib shortening and thoracic reduction. There is high (70 per cent) perinatal and infant mortality from respiratory failure and infection. Associated renal, liver and pancreatic dysplasia often complicate later life in survivors.

*Campomelic dysplasia.* This syndrome is typified by variable shortening and bowing of the femur and tibia. The femurs show angulation in the mid shaft (telephone receiver femur). Shortening or deformity in the upper limbs are less marked or absent. Associated skeletal deformities include macrocephaly (often with associated ventriculomegaly), micrognathia, short clavicles, talipes and small scapulae and ilia. Most of these features should be detectable on careful ultrasonic survey. The ribs are usually short and the thorax small. Congenital heart disease (VSD, ASD, tetralogy of Fallot) and hydronephrosis each occur in about one-third of cases. Phenotypic sex reversal of XY fetuses is common. In about 95 per cent of cases the condition is lethal in the first year of life.

At Watford General Hospital the condition was correctly diagnosed ultrasonically in a low risk pregnancy at 15 weeks on the basis of the appearance of the bent femur (Figure 20.9), severely shortened and deformed tibia and the relative absence of deformity in the upper limbs (Figure 20.10). Review of the video tapes shows evidence of other features of the syndrome not recognized at the time of the examination. The pregnancy was terminated and the diagnosis confirmed radiographically (Figure 20.10).

*Diastrophic dysplasia* is characterized by rhizomelic micromelia, flexion deformities of the arms and legs, talipes equinovarus and proximal displacement of the thumbs (hitch-hiker thumbs). Reports of prenatal

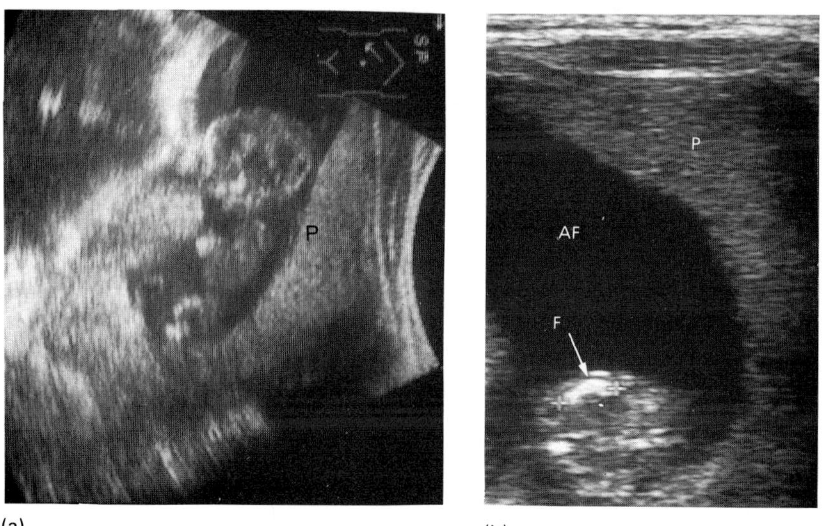


**Fig. 20.9** Sonograms of a 15 week fetus with confirmed campomelic dysplasia. (a) Full sagittal scan of fetus showing short legs (P = placenta). (b) Short femur (F) bowed in the middle. (AF = amniotic fluid.)

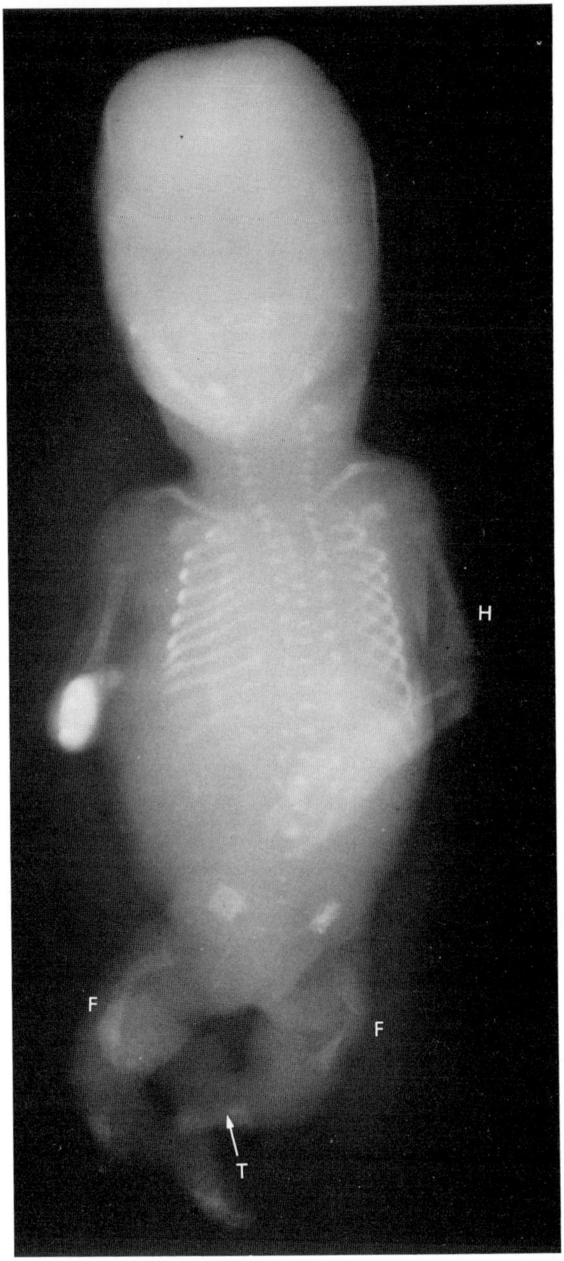


**Fig. 20.10** Post-abortion radiograph of fetus (16+ weeks) in Figure 20.9. Note the telephone receiver femurs (F), hypoplastic tibia (T) and less shortened humerus (H).

diagnosis are mainly in high risk pregnancies and are based on short flexed limbs. Hitch-hiker thumbs have been recognized on ultrasound by Mantagos *et al.* (1982) at 20 weeks and Gembruch *et al.* (1988) at 31 weeks.

*Chondrodysplasia punctata (rhizomelic type)* is a condition characterized by rhizomelic shortening, particularly of the humerus. A recent case occuring *de novo* in a primigravid mother showed short fetal humeri and femora at routine 18 week scan. More detailed examination revealed the typical splayed metaphyses and disorganized echoes around the epiphyses (stippled epiphyses). The limbs were flexed and showed severe limitation of movement. Fetal radiography gave little useful additional information. The pregnancy was terminated on the basis of the very poor prognosis associated with this condition. Infant death within the first two years of life is usual.

*Generally non-lethal dysplasias*

*Heterozygous achondroplasia* has been diagnosed by ultrasound mensuration of the long bones in the second trimester of pregnancy. Considerable caution should be exercised in the delivery of a definitive diagnosis before the 24th week of pregnancy and clinicians should resist pressure from patients to do so. It can be seen from Figure 20.4 that limb measurements in this condition may not deviate from the normal range until 24 weeks or so. This experience is confirmed by other reports of radiographic (Golbus & Hall 1974) and ultrasonic diagnosis (Filly *et al.* 1981; Kurtz & Wapner, 1983). The condition is associated with good survival and normal intelligence although orthopaedic problems are common. Inheritance is dominant.

There has only been one report of *homozygous achondroplasia* (Filly & Golbus 1982) in which there was severe micromelia and small thorax. The condition was lethal.

Many other milder forms of dysplasias may not show sufficient limb shortening for second trimester diagnosis. Malformation of the spine because of hemivertebrae (Benacerraf *et al.* 1986) may give a clue to diagnosis in high risk pregnancies. *Cleidocranial dysplasia* is characterized by shortened or absent clavicles and skull hypomineralization. These and other features of the condition are variable in expression. In a high risk pregnancy the condition was diagnosed in the second trimester at King's College Hospital (London) on finding unilateral clavicular hypoplasia.

The reader is referred for further reading to the excellent coverage of these conditions by Romero *et al.* (1988).

*Dysplasias characterized by hypomineralization*

Achondrogenesis (types 1 and 2) have already been described.

*Osteogenesis imperfecta* is subdivided into four types. Types 1 and 4 are manifest in childhood and are probably rarely amenable to antenatal

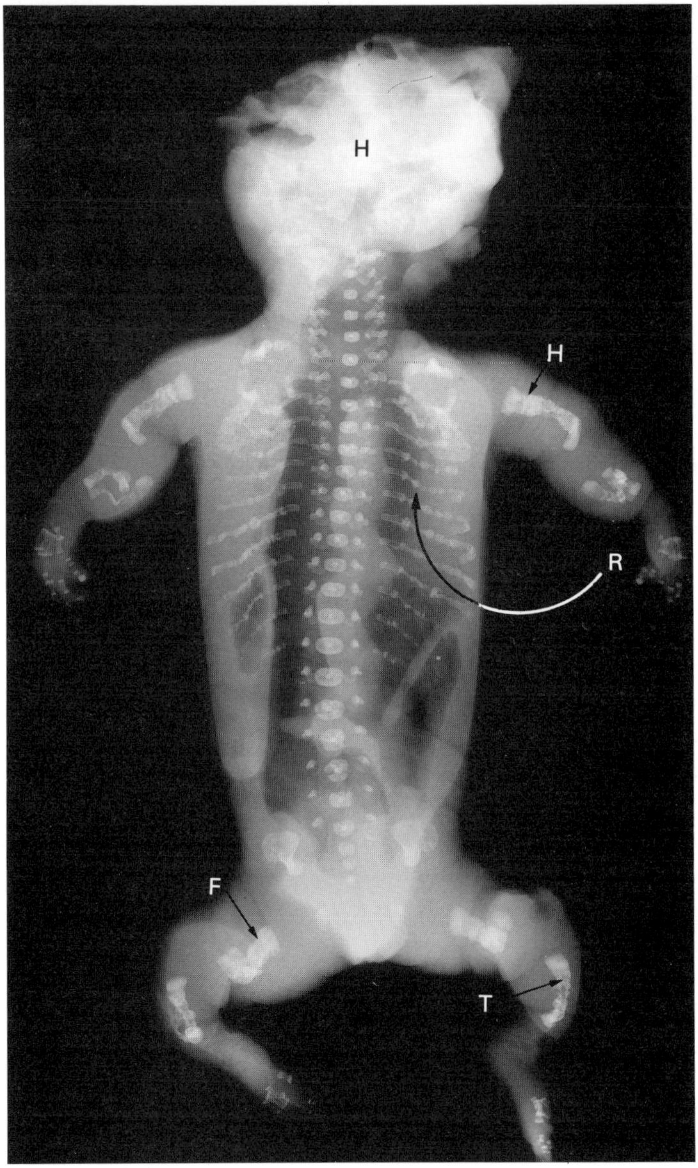


**Fig. 20.11** Xeroradiograph of a 20 week fetus with OI type 2a. The cranium was displaced during delivery. The diaphyses are crumpled and bowed by multiple intrauterine fractures. The ribs are the thin and beaded. F = femur, H = humerus, T = tibia, H = head.

diagnosis. Individuals affected by osteogenesis imperfecta type 3 are usually born with fractures and there is progressive deformity in childhood. Diagnosis *in utero* at 19 weeks has been reported (van der Harten *et al.* 1988). The lethal *type 2* has been the subject of many reports of early antenatal diagnosis with ultrasound (Dinno *et al.* 1982; Hobbins *et al.* 1982; Milsom *et al.* 1982; Shapiro *et al.* 1982; Elejalde & de Elejalde 1983; Brons *et al.* 1988a). The author has personal experience of the correct diagnosis of three cases of osteogenesis imperfecta type 2 in the mid-second trimester and one in the third trimester, all in low risk pregnancies.

The long bones are short, deformed and crumpled by multiple intrauterine fractures (Figure 20.11) (the positional appearance of the lower limbs may be similar to that in campomelic dysplasia and diastrophic dysplasia). Fetal movement is reduced. The ribs appear thin, short and beaded and the thorax may be small. All reported cases and those seen by the author have shown marked hypomineralization of the skull (Figure 20.12). In later pregnancy the gyri may be seen clearly and the skull can easily be distorted by the pressure of the ultrasound transducer. The appearance of the spine is usually normal. There may be associated polyhydramnios.

The outlook is almost invariably fatal, usually due to pulmonary hypoplasia. It is believed that the majority are of sporadic occurrence but occasional autosomal recessive inheritance may be apparent. The approximate recurrence risk is 5 per cent unless a family history suggests recessive inheritance (Thompson *et al.* 1986).

*Hypophosphatasia* presents four clinical pictures depending upon the age of presentation of the condition. It is the severe lethal form which is the main concern of the prenatal diagnostic ultrasonologist. Although its occurrence (1 : 100 000) is said to be about half that of osteogenesis imperfecta type 2, reports in the literature of ultrasound diagnosis are few (Kurtz & Wapner 1983; Wladimiroff *et al.* 1985). Measurement of amniotic fluid alkaline phosphatase is unreliable (Mulivor *et al.* 1978) There are reports of successful diagnosis from the measurement of cellular alkaline phosphatase from amniocytes or chorionic cells (Warren *et al.* 1985). The gene locus for this condition has now been identified and a gene probe is available.

The ultrasonographic appearance is of a hypomineralized skull, similar to that of osteogenesis imperfecta, and short, bowed long bone diaphyses. In the case reported by Wladimiroff *et al.* (1985) the femur length (14 mm) was below the fifth centile at 16 weeks. There was also displacement of the long bones at the elbows and knees. A recent case reviewed by the author showed moderate demineralization of the skull, long bone shortening and marked angulation of the femur.

Inheritance is autosomal recessive. The severe neonatal form of hypophosphatasia is invariably lethal.

## LIMB REDUCTION DEFORMITIES

This group of deformities is characterized by absence or reduction of limbs or segments of limbs. In general, this is a heterogeneous group of disorders many of which are not of genetic origin. The deformity may involve absence of all limbs (amelia) or reduction (phocomelia) of one, more or all (tetraphocomelia) limbs. There may also be reduction of a

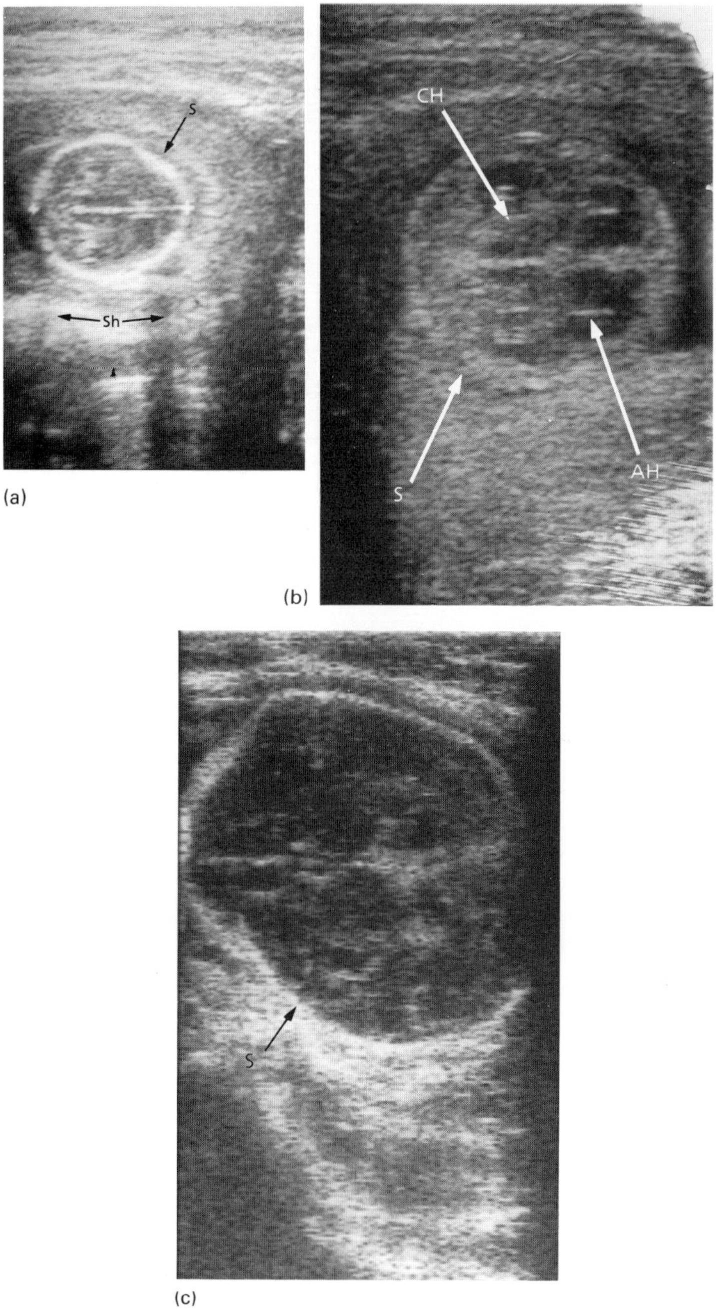


(a) (b) (c)

**Fig. 20.12** Osteogenesis imperfecta (OI) type 2a. (a) Sonogram of a normal fetal head at 17 weeks. Note the high echogenicity of the skull (S) and the accoustic shadow (Sh) cast by it. (b) Head of a 19 week fetus with OI. The skull is poorly echoic and casts no accoustic shadow. The cerebral hemispheres (CH) are anechoic. The lateral borders of the anterior horns (AH) of the lateral ventricle are evident. (c) Skull in a case of OI at 31 weeks showing poor ossification and deformation.

longitudinal segment of a limb (hemimelia) such as the radius. In the absence of associated abnormalities prognosis is generally good as technological advances in limb prostheses are such that excellent functional

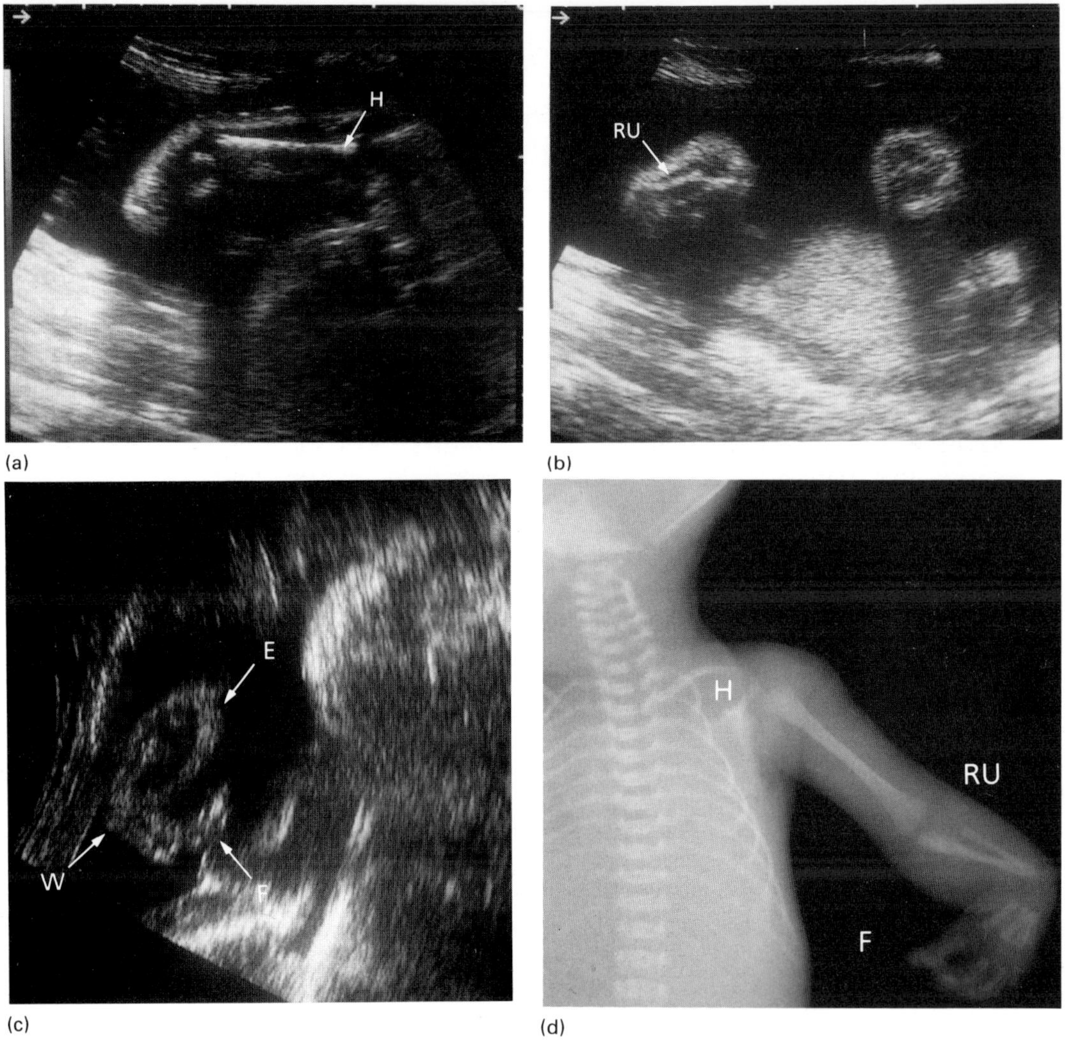


**Fig. 20.13** Sonograms and radiograph of forearm and wrist malformations in a fetus with trisomy 18. H = humerus, RU = radius and ulna, E = elbow, F = fingers.

and cosmetic results can be obtained, even in apparently severe reductions. However, a detailed general examination of the fetus is indicated as a limb reduction deformity may be part of a spectrum of abnormalities which will increase the risk of an underlying chromosomal defect (Figure 20.13) or genetic syndrome.

*Amniotic band syndrome (ABS).* This group of disorders shows great variation in severity from minor digital constriction rings or amputations to major structural disruption of the head (encephalocele) and face, trunk (ventral wall defects) and limbs (deformity and amputations). The lesions are asymmetrical. Careful ultrasonic examination may reveal bands of amnion attatched to and immobilizing deformed fetal parts (Mahony *et al.* 1985).

If multiple asymmetrical abnormalities are found ABS should be considered and bands sought. A fetal karyotype should be obtained to exclude a chromosomal anomaly. Bands or ridges in the amnion may be seen in normal pregnancies. If these are not attached to the fetus and a careful search reveals no deformity they should be regarded as harmless.

Whether amniotic band syndrome is of genetic origin or occurs as a result of early amnion rupture or vascular occlusion during embryonic or fetal development is a continuing debate that remains unresolved.

### *Genetic syndromes associated with limb reduction*

*Roberts syndrome* is a recessive syndrome characterized by severe tetraphocomelia and median facial clefting associated with marked growth deficiency. Other features of the syndrome are syndactyly, talipes and microcephaly. Many are stillborn or die in infancy. Mental retardation is a common complication in the few survivors. An affected individual presents features similar to those associated with the teratogenic effects of the drug thalidomide. The syndrome has been diagnosed prenatally in a high risk family (Hobbins *et al.* 1982).

*Thrombocytopenia–absent radius (TAR) syndrome.* The defects are usually bilateral radial aplasia or variable hypoplasia. The thumbs are usually present. Ulnar or humeral reductions are seen in some cases. These deformities are diagnostic markers for the underlying haemopoietic defect of hypomegakaryocytic thrombocytopenia which may be recognized on fetal blood sampling. In one-third of cases there is coexistent congenital heart disease (Fallot's tetralogy, VSD). Successful ultrasonographic diagnosis in the second trimester has been reported (Luthy *et al.* 1981; Hobbins *et al.* 1982; Filkins *et al.* 1984).

In the 60 per cent that survive infancy the thrombocytopenia tends to improve with age and support with platelet transfusions (Smith 1982). Inheritance is autosomal recessive.

*Fanconi pancytopenia syndrome* is an autosomal recessive syndrome associated with bone marrow failure and severe anaemia. Nearly 80 per cent of affected individuals have aplasia or hypoplasia of the thumb which may be unilateral. Anaemia tends to be progressive, usually presenting in the later part of the first decade of life. Prenatal diagnosis of this syndrome has not been reported but there is potential for diagnosis in high risk families.

*Holt–Oram syndrome* is an autosomal dominant syndrome of upper limb or limb girdle deformity and congenital heart disease of very variable expression. The limb reductions are commoner on the left side and vary in severity. They may involve any part of the upper limb and shoulder girdle. Thumbs may be absent, hypoplastic or triphalangeal (finger-like) or associated with syndactyly. ASD and VSD are the commoner cardiac abnormalities. Successful diagnosis in the second and third trimesters of high risk pregnancies has been based on the ultrasonographic demonstration of both limb and cardiac deformities (Muller *et al.* 1985b; Brons *et al.* 1988b).

### POLYSYNDACTYLY

Abnormalities of the fingers are best seen in a fully fanned hand (Figure 20.3). The fetus is not always obliging enough to give this view and a section across the clenched hand in the axial plane will suffice to detect extra (or a deficiency of) bones. A full plantar view of the foot should display polydactyly.

Polydactyly (Figure 20.14) may be pre-axial (duplicate or bifid thumbs or big toes) or post-axial (on the ulnar side of the index finger or lateral aspect of the foot). Syndactyly denotes fusion of either the bones (osseous syndactyly) or soft tissues (cutaneous syndactyly) of the fingers or toes.

There are many syndromes with these abnormalities as a feature. The commoner ones are listed in Table 20.4. For a more detailed list and description of the various syndromes the reader is referred to Smith (1982). As the syndromes have differing prognostic significance it behoves the ultrasonologist to make a detailed search for other fetal abnormalities before coming to a diagnosis. Fetal karyotyping should also

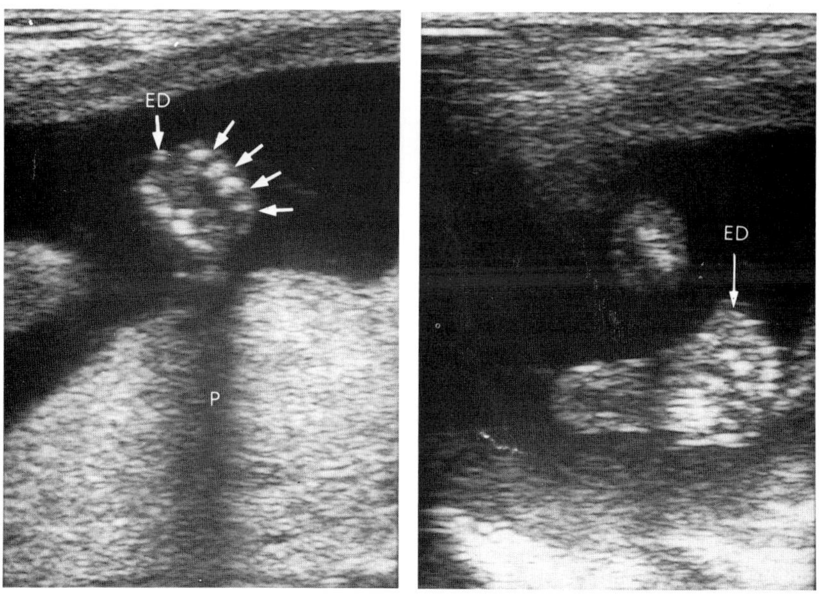


(a) (b)

**Fig. 20.14** Sonograms showing polydactyly of hands and feet of a fetus with a family history of Greig cephalopolysyndactyly syndrome. (a) Clenched hand showing four fingers (↓) and post-axial extra digit (ED). (b) Plantar view of fetal right foot showing pre-axial duplication of the great toe. P = placenta.

**Table 20.4** Some syndromes associated with polysyndactyly

| Polydactyly | Syndactyly |
|---|---|
| Polysyndactyly | Polysyndactyly |
| Meckel–Gruber | Apert |
| Ellis–van Crefeld | De Lange |
| Grebe | Multiple pterygium |
| Oral facial digital | Holt–Oram |
| Towne | Oral facial digital |
| Trisomy 13 | Roberts |

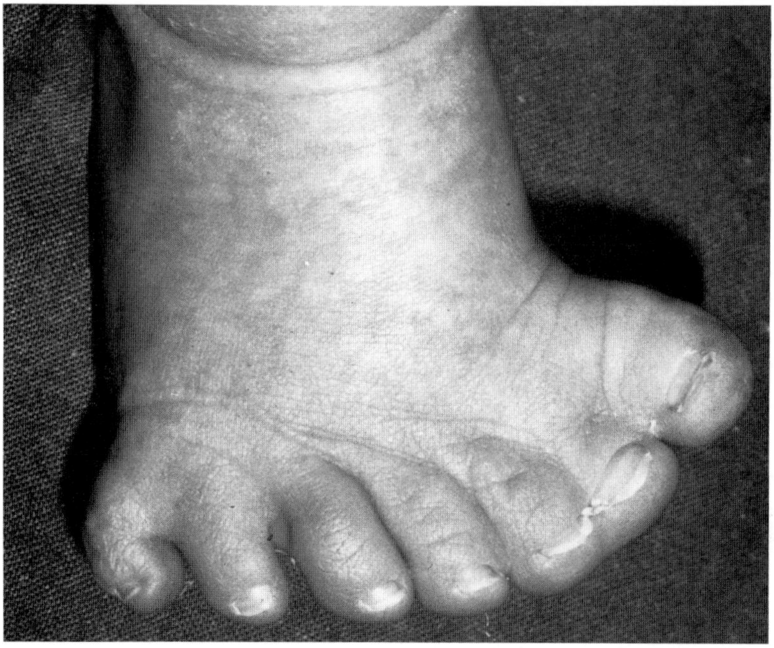

**Fig. 20.15** Photograph of the foot of infant with cephalopolysyndactyly after birth.

be considered. Isolated polysyndactyly occurs as an autosomal dominant condition in some families.

POSITIONAL DEFORMITIES

*Talipes (club foot).* In this condition the foot is plantar-flexed and internally rotated. The condition can be detected on ultrasound examination by observing the relationship between the shaft of the tibia and the axis of the toes or plantar surface of the foot. The views of the leg employed to detect abnormalities are shown in Figures 20.2 and 20.16. Talipes may occur as an isolated malformation, as a response to asymmetrical intrauterine environmental pressures (oligohydramnios, amniotic bands or

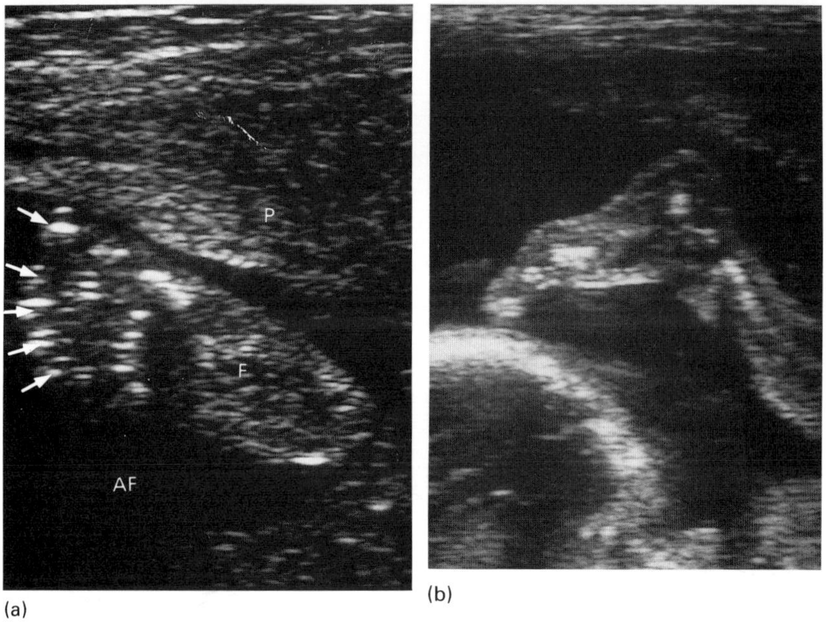


**Fig. 20.16** Sonograms of fetal foot. (a) Axial plane showing plantar view (see Figure 20.2c) of the foot and toes. (b) Sagittal scan (see Figure 20.2b) showing contour of heel and the plantar arch.

intrauterine tumours) or as an integral part of a multitude of genetic syndromes (Smith 1982).

*Rocker-bottom feet* are a feature of trisomy 18 (Edwards syndrome), 18q syndrome and Pena–Shokeir type 2 syndrome. The deformity is characterized by a prominent heel, and replacement of the normal concavity of the plantar arch by convexity. The finding of this deformity should be a stimulus to detailed fetal examination for other defects (see Figure 20.24) and fetal karyotyping.

*Multiple congenital contractures (arthrogryposis multiplex congenita).* This is a heterogeneous group of disorders thought mainly to be of neuromuscular origin. Reduction in joint mobility at a critical stage in early development leads to severe contractures, joint dislocations and deformity. Hageman *et al.* (1988) have reviewed 75 newborns with multiple congenital contractures and found abnormalities in the CNS (55 per cent), the peripheral neuromuscular system (8 per cent) and connective tissues and skin (11 per cent). Seven per cent were associated with oligohydramnios and the remaining 19 per cent were miscellaneous.

These conditions should be recognized on ultrasound examination in the second trimester on seeing fixed, immobile limbs in bizarre positions. Polyhydramnios and fetal hydrops are frequent accompanying features. Specific syndromes of *Pena–Shokeir syndrome type 1* (Pena & Shokeir 1976; Hall 1986), *lethal multiple pterygium syndrome* (Hall *et al.* 1984) and *congenital muscular dystrophy* have been described but it appears uncertain whether they are separate entities or different manifestations of the same pathological process. These syndromes are mainly autosomal recessive. Kirkinen *et al.* (1987) describe ultrasonic observation of six high risk pregnancies from the first trimester. Although apparently normal at between 8 and 12 weeks, all six fetuses showed severe generalized subcutaneous oedema with restricted fetal movement by the 16th week. In two there was ascites or hydrothorax which are common accompaniments to these syndromes (Shenker *et al.* 1985).

The author has personal experience of the diagnosis of three cases of fetal multiple contractures. One was in a high risk family where a previous neonatal death had occurred diagnosed as congenital muscular dystrophy. In the following pregnancy ultrasound examination at the 18th week showed a fetus of appropriate size for dates, a small chest and bilateral talipes (Figure 20.17a). Two were in low risk pregnancies where at routine second trimester scan, positional deformity was noticed in one and small cystic hygromata in the other. Detailed further examination of the latter fetus revealed restricted fetal movement and multiple pterygia at the joint flexures (Figure 20.17b). In none of the three was there noted to be fetal hydrops. All pregnancies were terminated and the contractures confirmed in two. The third has been lost to follow-up. Further antenatal diagnoses have been made by Chen *et al.* (1984), Jeanty *et al.* (1985), MacMillan *et al.* (1985), Shenker *et al.* (1985), Muller & de Jong (1986), Goldberg *et al.* (1986) and Zeitune *et al.* (1988).

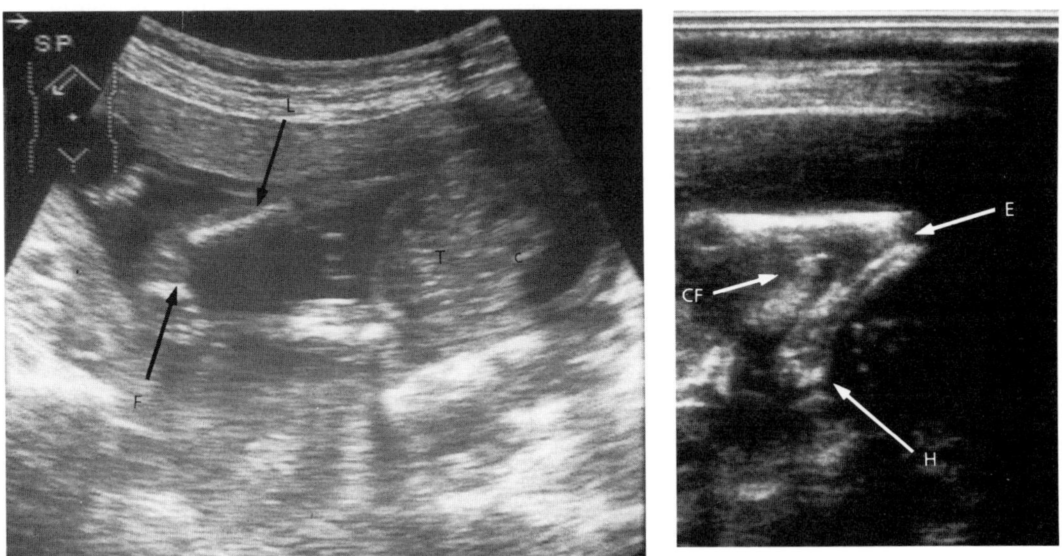


(a) (b)

**Fig. 20.17** Sonograms showing multiple congenital contractures. (a) Fetus with family history of congenital muscular dystrophy demonstrating severe talipes (plantar view of the foot seen in the sagittal plane). (b) The arm of a fetus with lethal multiple pterygium syndrome. Note webbing (pterygium) of the antecubital fossa (CF). F = foot, L = leg, T = trunk, H = hand, E = elbow.

*The distal arthrogryposes* (Hall *et al.* 1982) are a group of milder conditions affecting peripheral joints such as hands, feet and the jaw. The deformities may be corrected with surgery. Life expectancy and neurological function are normal. These conditions are autosomal dominant. Prenatal ultrasound diagnosis at 18 weeks in an affected family has been described on the detection of flexed fingers and extended wrists (Baty *et al.* 1988).

### Counselling and follow-up

Some of the characteristic features of a wide spectrum of skeletal and postural deformities have been described. Diagnostic accuracy will be improved if time is spent examining the fetus in detail. A handy reference may be very helpful in coming to an accurate diagnosis of many of the lethal dysplasias. In cases where the diagnosis or prognosis are in doubt it may be prudent to consult a geneticist or paediatrician before finally counselling a couple who may themselves wish a further specialist consultation before they come to a final decision on management.

On delivery of the affected fetus professional anteroposterior and lateral photographs and detailed X-ray or xeroradiograph should be taken. If the fetus is dead but fresh ask that fetal blood or skin be sent for cytogenetic studies and fetal spleen be rapidly frozen and stored for future DNA analysis. It is also important, where appropriate, that postmortem examination is done by a pathologist interested in skeletal dysplasias. Only when all this information has been gathered should the definitive diagnosis be made and the couple finally counselled by a geneticist as to risks of recurrence in future pregnancies and the implications for other family members. Copies of all investigations and reports should be requested and stored for the purposes of ultrasonographic diagnostic audit.

## The fetal face

### Examination and normal anatomy

Coarse fetal facial features begin to become apparent on ultrasound examination in the late first trimester. By about the 14th post-menstrual week nose, lips, ears, etc. are evident and by the time of a routine 18 week scan a detailed picture of the face may be constructed. Although a standard 3.5 MHz transducer will suffice the added resolution afforded by a 5 MHz transducer is a great help in defining finer structures such as the ears or lips. In order to build up a full three dimensional mental image of the head and face three basic views are employed (Figure 20.18).

The *axial* plane is that used to measure a biparietal diameter. The same plane shifted caudally reveals the orbits (Figure 20.19). The inter-

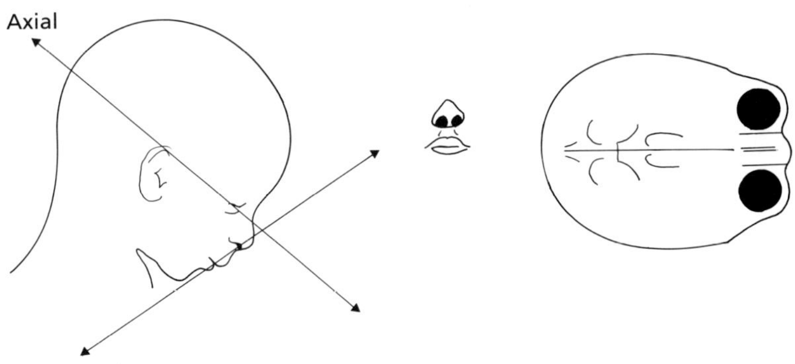


**Fig. 20.18** Diagrammatic representation of the views of the fetal face in sagittal, axial and coronal planes.

nal and external orbital diameters may be measured and checked against published nomograms (Jeanty *et al.* 1982b; Mayden *et al.* 1982). A further caudal shift reveals the hard palate. In the author's opinion this is the best view to detect cleft palate. The tongue may be seen, often moving within the mouth. On a slightly lower plane and with slight rotation of the transducer the mandible can be visualized and measured in its full length from the temporomandibular joint to the mental prominence.

The *sagittal* plane shows the fetal profile. The contours of the fetal forehead, nasal bridge, nose, upper and lower lips and chin can be assessed (Figure 20.19). Laterally in the same plane the ears can be seen if they are not compressed against the amnion.

The soft tissue features of the face are best visualized in the *coronal* plane. This shows the full frontal fetal face including upper and lower lips, external nares, cheeks, eye lids and eyes. Slight adjustments of the plane are necessary to see all these features but the technique can be mastered with a little perseverance. In this view mouthing, sucking and yawning movements are evident.

## Abnormalities

### THE ORBITS AND NOSE

Abnormalities of the eyes and orbits are rare. Hypertelorism (wide spaced eyes) is associated with numerous syndromes and malformations including Down's syndrome (Smith 1982). The efficacy of ultrasound in detecting hypertelorism in fetal life has not been fully evaluated but measurement of internal orbital diameter has not met with success in screening for Down's syndrome. Microphthalmia (Figure 20.20), anophthalmia and cyclopia have a strong association with Patau syndrome (trisomy 13) and other syndromes (Romero *et al.* 1988). The association of ophthalmic abnormality, midline facial defects, holoprosencephaly

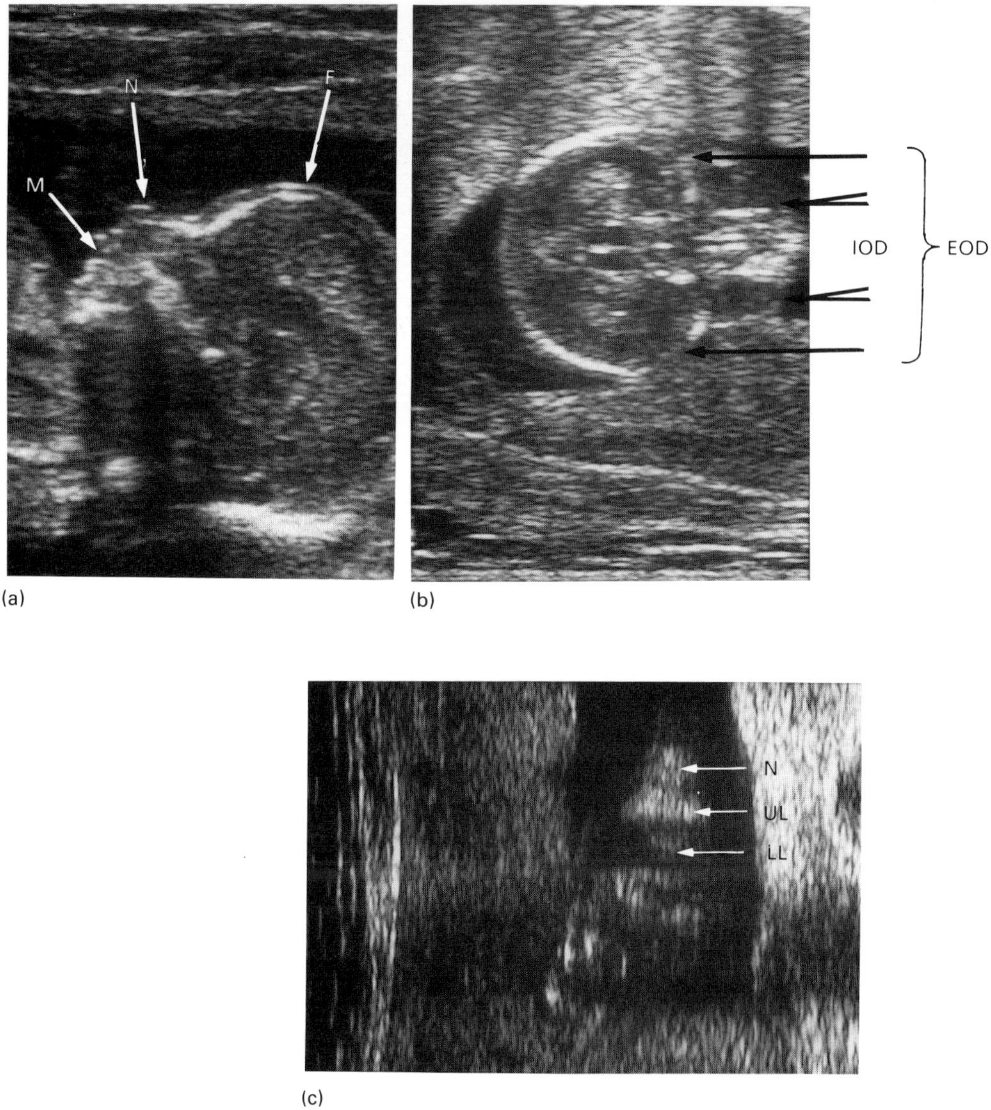


**Fig. 20.19** Sonograms showing views of the fetal face at 18 weeks. (a) Sagittal view of fetal mouth (M), nose (N) and forehead (F) in profile. (b) Axial plane showing orbits and nasal septum, internal (IOD) and external (EOD) orbital diameters. (c) Coronal plane with upper lip (UL), lower lip (LL), nose (N) and nostrils.

(single cerebral ventricle) and polydactyly is strongly indicative of Patau syndrome.

Nasal abnormalities include absence (anosmia), displacement of a proboscis above the orbit (ethmocephaly) in association with cyclopia and single nasal cavity (cebocephaly) (Figures 20.21 and 20.22). These abnormalities are usually found with ophthalmic defects and holoprosencephaly. A bifid nose occurs as part of the frontonasal dysplasia syndrome (see later).

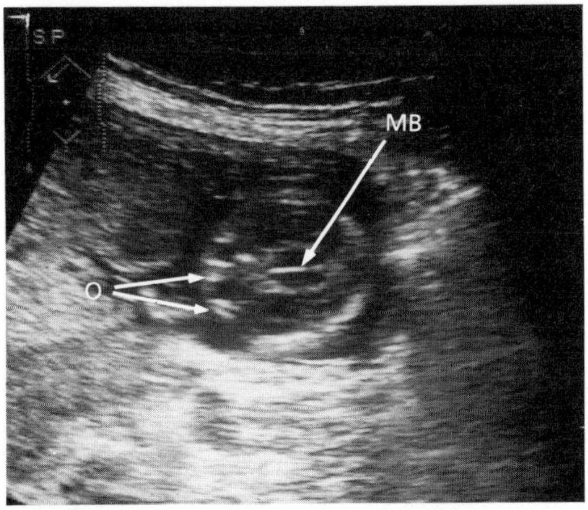


**Fig. 20.20** Axial sonograms of the fetal head at 17 weeks showing microphthalmia and the typically prominent midbrain and malformed lateral ventricles of holoprosencephaly. Karyotype trisomy 13. (O = orbits, MB = midbrain.)

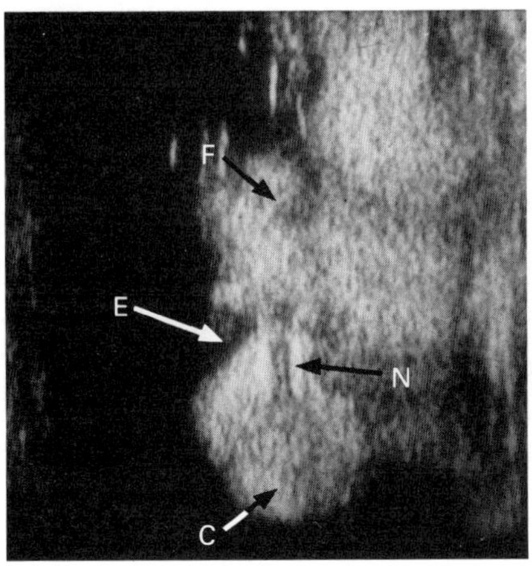


**Fig. 20.21** Coronal scan of fetal face demonstrating single nasal cavity (cebocephaly).

## LIPS AND PALATE

Paramedian cleft lip (CL) or palate (CP) occurs in about 1/1000 of all births. Nine per cent of cases of CL or CP are stillbirths and 12 per cent neonatal deaths. However, in the absence of other associated fetal anomalies the mortality is less than 1 per cent. Half of affected fetuses have both cleft lip and palate (CL–CP), one-quarter have CL alone and one-quarter have only CP. CL or CP may occur as an isolated defect or as part of a spectrum of abnormalities making up a genetic or non-genetic syndrome or chromosomal anomaly. In cases of isolated CL or CP recurrence risks are between 2 and 20 per cent depending upon the number and sex of affected members of the family. In cases where CL or CP

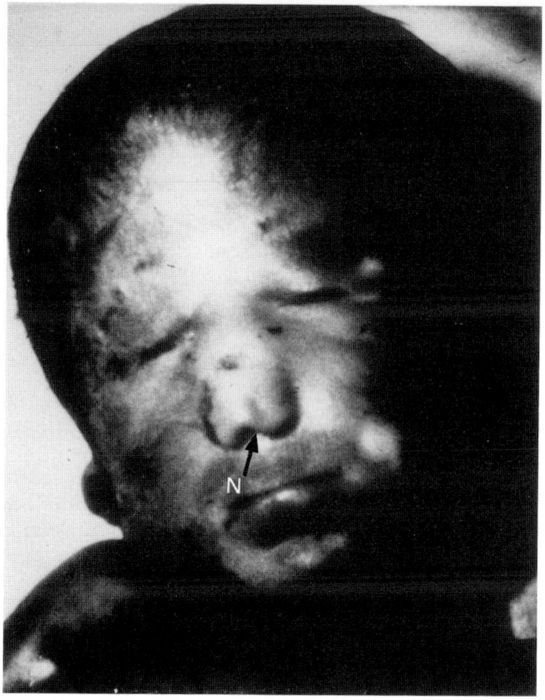


**Fig. 20.22** Photograph of the same fetus after termination of pregnancy. Karyotype trisomy 13.

presents as part of a syndrome the recurrence risk will be that accorded to the syndrome. Some of the syndromes in which ultrasound diagnosis may be possible are listed in Table 20.5 Common non-genetic associations are with talipes (isolated CL or CP), polydactyly (CP–CL) and congenital heart disease. For a more detailed account and more comprehensive list of over 70 associations the reader is referred to Romero *et al.* (1988).

The defect may range from a simple cleft of the lip or soft palate to more extensive lesions involving facial bones, nares or the hard palate. Clefting is bilateral in 20–25 per cent of cases, some of whom are severely disfigured.

An examination of the face and palate should be part of any routine mid-second trimester scan. It is not difficult and may be rewarded by the detection of a facial cleft, the second most common congenital defect and the marker for some lethal conditions. Special attention should be paid to the lips and palate if other defects have been found or if polyhydramnios is evident. The diagnosis of clefting of the facial soft tissues is best accomplished in the full facial (coronal) plane (Figure 20.23). In the author's opinion the best view to diagnose CP is in the axial plane where the defect will be seen as a dark rift between the rather densely echoic lateral processes. With increasing mineralization of the maxillae the defect becomes more difficult to visualize as pregnancy progresses. A diligent

**Table 20.5** Some conditions associated with cleft lip or cleft palate



| |
|---|
| Early amnion rupture |
| EEC (Ectrodactyly–Ectodermal dysplasia–Clefting) syndrome |
| Oral facial digital syndrome |
| Kniest syndrome |
| Miller syndrome |
| Roberts syndrome |
| |
| Trisomy 18 |
| Trisomy 13 |
| |
| *Drugs* |
| Barbiturates |
| Busulfan |
| Carbamazepine |
| Cortisone |
| Diazepam |
| Diphenhydramine |
| Ethanol |
| Ethosuccimide |
| Fluphenazine |
| Imipramine |
| Phenytoin |
| Sodium valproate |
| |
| *Cleft palate alone* |
| Meckel–Gruber syndrome |
| Robin sequence |
| Treacher Collins syndrome |

search for other fetal anomalies must be made to exclude syndromes that will adversely affect the prognosis. If other defects are found then a fetal karyotype should be obtained (Figure 20.24). It is debatable whether a karyotype should be advised for isolated CL or CP as the risks of chromosomal abnormality are low but there is always the risk that other abnormalities present, such as minor congenital heart disease or rocker-bottom feet, may be difficult to detect.

Median cleft lip and palate account for less than 1 per cent of all CL or CP. There is a strong association with other midline defects of the face including, anosmia, cebocephaly, ethmocephaly, microphthalmia, cyclopia, etc. There is usually concomitant defective cleavage of the prosencephalon (holoprosencephaly). These defects are seen in trisomies 13, 18, and 13/15 and are generally lethal. With these associations hypotelorism is the rule.

Rarely, midline clefts of the lip, palate or nose may occur with hypertelorism (frontonasal dysplasia sequence). In these cases the brain and intelligence are generally normal and the prognosis good with cosmetic surgery. The distinction between these two groups with widely differing prognoses may be made by checking internal and external orbital diameters against the appropriate nomograms and by careful examination of intracerebral anatomy.

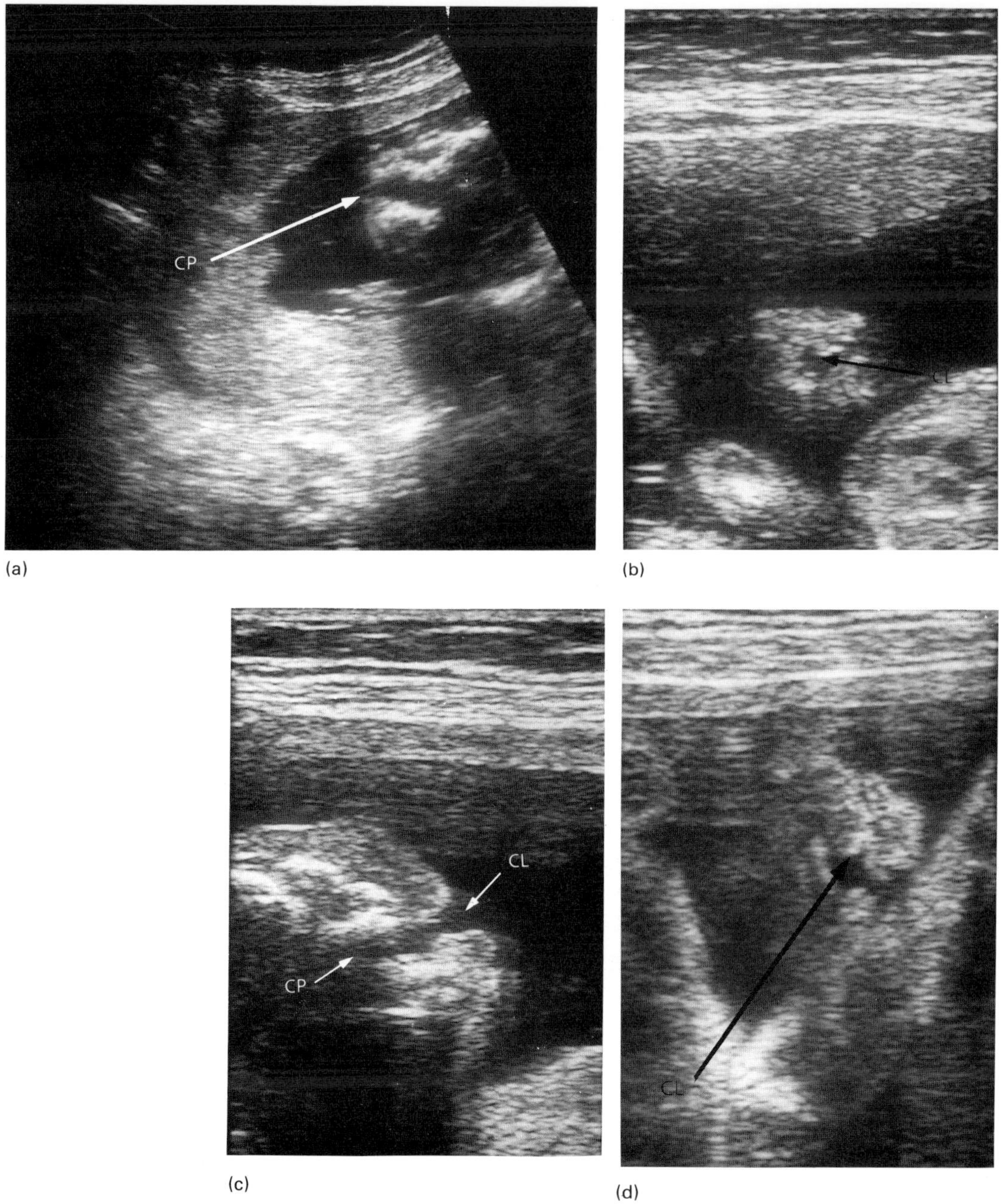


**Fig. 20.23** Sonograms of a fetus at 18 weeks (a and b) and 22 weeks (c and d) with isolated CL–CP. The CP is clearer at 18 weeks and the CL at 22 weeks. (a and c) Axial scans, (b and d) coronal scans. These defects were repaired after birth of the child.

Abnormalities of fusion between the maxillary and mandibular divisions of the first branchial arch may produce horizontal clefts, macrostomia, preauricular pits or accessory auricles and inner ear anomalies causing deafness. Treacher Collins syndrome demonstrates these features. Mandibular hypoplasia and micrognathia are features of the Robin

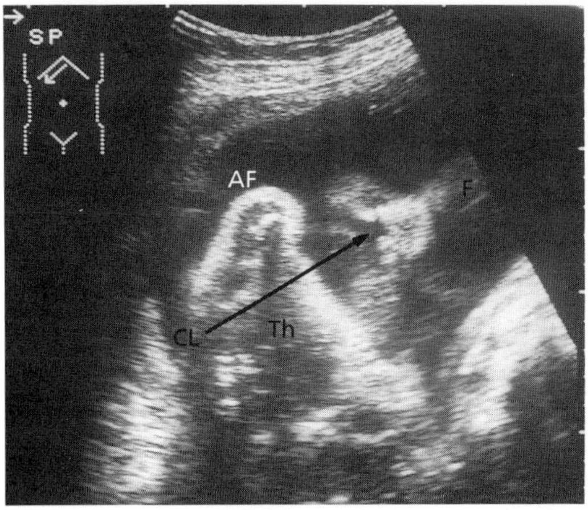


(a)

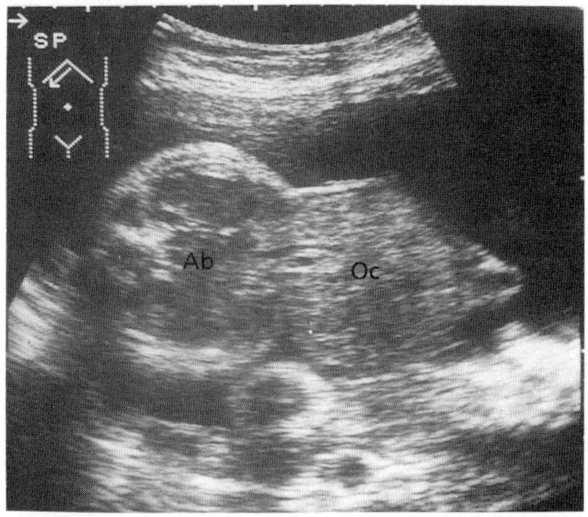


(b)

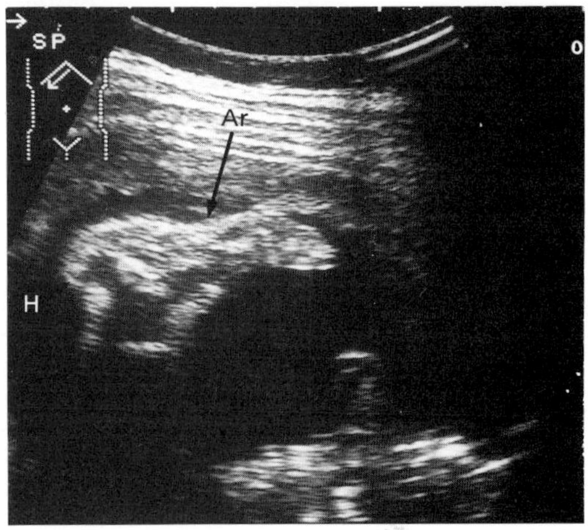


(c)

**Fig. 20.24** Sonograms of a fetus at 30 weeks with features of trisomy 18. (a) Coronal view of the fetal face showing part of the forehead (F), the upper thorax (Th) and paramedian cleft of the upper lip (CL). (b) Axial section of the abdomen (Ab) showing omphalocele (Oc). (c) Sagittal section of the foot with prominent heel (H) and loss of the plantar arch (Ar) (rocker-bottom foot).

sequence of malformations which include cleft palate, ear and ophthalmic abnormalities.

## Counselling and follow-up

When fetal facial clefts are found as an isolated malformation parents should be counselled with optimism. Plastic surgery for cleft lip is now generally performed early. Infants with cleft palate may have difficulties with feeding. Parents usually find it valuable to talk with a paediatric plastic surgeon during the pregnancy as this may allay many of their fears.

The offer of termination of pregnancy should be considered if there are multiple fetal abnormalities and particularly if the karyotype is abnormal. A reference such as Smith (1982) may again be useful. Following birth or termination of pregnancy professional photographs and X-rays should be obtained where appropriate and fetal blood or tissue for karyotyping or DNA analysis sent to the local cytogenetics laboratory. Ideally a geneticist should be informed at the time of birth. In the event of termination of pregnancy, or perinatal death parents should be encouraged to consent to a full post-mortem. A follow-up consultation between the parents and an obstetrician, paediatrician or geneticist will enable full discussion of the malformations and their genetic implications.

For a couple to be told that their baby has an abnormality is a great and lasting emotional trauma, even if the prognosis is good. Sensitivity is required in initial counselling and patients will welcome continued support throughout the pregnancy and thereafter. In the event of termination of pregnancy parents should be encouraged to see the child. These parents in particular suffer not only the concern that they have created an abnormal child but also the emotional distress, and sometimes the guilt, of terminating a wanted pregnancy. Active domiciliary support and reassurance from medical, nursing and ancillary services with free availability of information and advice will help them through the crisis which may be prolonged.

## Acknowledgements

My thanks to Dr L.S. Chitty for genetic advice and her invaluable help with the manuscript.

## References

Baty B.J., Cubberley D., Morris C. & Cary J. (1988) Prenatal diagnosis of distal arthrogryposis. *American Journal of Medical Genetics*, **29**, 501–10.

Beetham F.G.T. & Reeves J.S. (1984) Early ultrasound diagnosis of thanatophoric dwarfism. *Journal of Clinical Ultrasound*, **12**, 43–4.

Benacerraf B.R., Greene M.F. & Barss V.A. (1986) Prenatal sonographic diagnosis of congenital hemivertebra. *Journal of Ultrasound in Medicine*, **5**, 257–9.

Brons J.T.J., van der Harten J.J., Wladimiroff J.W., van Geijn H.P., Dijkstra P.F., Exalto N.E., Reuss A., Niermeijer M.F., Meijer C.J.L.M. & Th. Arts N.F. (1988a) Prenatal ultrasonographic diagnosis of osteogenesis imperfecta. *American Journal of Obstetrics and Gynecology*, **159**, 176–81.

Brons J.T.J., Van Geijn H.P., Wladimiroff J.W., Van Der Harten J.J., Kwee M.L., Sobotka-Plojhar M. & Th.Arts N.F. (1988b) Prenatal ultrasound diagnosis of the Holt–Oram syndrome. *Prenatal Diagnosis*, **8**, 175–81.

Burrows P.E., Stannard M.W., Pearrow J., Sutterfield S. & Baker M.L. (1984) Early antenatal sonographic recognition of thanatophoric dysplasia with cloverleaf skull deformity. *American Journal of Radiology*, **143**, 841–3.

Camera, G., Dodero D. & De Pascale S. (1984) Prenatal diagnosis of thanatophoric dysplasia at 24 weeks. *American Journal of Medical Genetics*, **18**, 39–43.

Campbell S., Griffin D., Roberts A., & Little D. (1981) Early prenatal diagnosis of abnormalities of the fetal head, spine, limbs and abdominal organs. In *Recent Advances in Prenatal Diagnosis*, (Ed. by P. Orlandi, P. Polani & L. Bovicelli), pp. 41–59. John Wiley & Sons.

Chen H., Immken L., Lachman R., Yang S., Rimoin D., Rightmire D., Eteson D., Stewart F., Beemer F., Optiz J., Gilbert E., Langer L., Shapiro L. & Duncan P. (1984) Syndrome of multiple pterygia, camptodactyly, facial anomalies, hypoplastic lungs and heart, cystic hygroma and skeletal anomalies: Delineation of a new entity and review of lethal forms of multiple pterygium syndrome. *American Journal of Medical Genetics*, **17**, 809–23.

Chervenak F.A., Blakemore K.J., Isaacson G., Mayden K. & Hobbins J.C. (1983) Antenatal sonographic findings of thanatophoric dysplasia with cloverleaf skull.

*American Journal of Obstetrics and Gynecology*, **146**, 984–5.

Chervenak F.A., Romero R., Berkowikz R.L., Mahoney M.J., Tortora M., Mayden K. & Hobbins J.C. (1982) Antenatal sonographic findings of osteogenesis imperfecta. *American Journal of Obstetrics and Gynecology*, **143**, 228–30.

Dinno N.D., Yacuob U.S., Kadlec J.F. & Garver K.L. (1982) Midtrimester diagnosis of osteogenesis imperfecta, type II. *Birth Defects*, **18**, 125–32.

Donnenfeld A.E. & Mennuti M.T. (1987) Second trimester diagnosis of fetal skeletal dysplasias. *Obstetrical and Gynecological Survey*, **42**, 199–217.

Elejalde B.R. & de Elejalde M.M. (1983) Prenatal diagnosis of perinatally lethal osteogenesis imperfecta. *American Journal of Medical Genetics*, **14**, 353–9.

Elejalde B.R. & de Elejalde M.M. (1985) Thanatophoric dysplasia: fetal manifestations and prenatal diagnosis. *American Journal of Medical Genetics*, **22**, 669–83.

Elejalde B.R., de Elejalde M.M. & Pansch D. (1985) Prenatal diagnosis of Jeune Syndrome. *American Journal of Medical Genetics*, **21**, 433–8.

Filkins K., Russo J. & Bilinki I (1984) Prenatal diagnosis of thrombocytopenia absent radius syndrome using ultrasound and fetoscopy. *Prenatal Diagnosis*, **4**, 139.

Filly R.A. & Golbus M.S. (1982) Ultrasonography of the normal and pathologic fetal skeleton. *Radiologic Clinics of North America*, **20**, 311–23.

Filly R.A., Golbus M.S., Cary J.C. & Hall J.G. (1981) Short limbed dwarfism: ultrasonographic diagnosis by mensuration of fetal femoral length. *Radiology*, **138**, 653–6.

Fryns J.P., van den Berghe K., van Assche A. & van den Berghe H. (1981) Prenatal diagnosis of campomelic dwarfism. *Clinical Genetics*, **19**, 199–201.

Gallop T.R. & Eigier A. (1987) Brief clinical report: prenatal ultrasound diagnosis of diastrophic dysplasia at 16 weeks. *American Journal of Medical Genetics*, **27**, 321–4.

Gembruch U., Hansmann M. & Frodisch H.J. (1985) Early prenatal diagnosis of short rib–polydactyly (SRP) syndrome type 1 (Majewski) by ultrasound in a case at risk. *Prenatal Diagnosis*, **5**, 357–62.

Gembruch U., Niesen M., Kehrberg H. & Hansmann M. (1988) Diastrophic dysplasia: A specific prenatal diagnosis by ultrasound. *Prenatal Diagnosis*, **8**, 539–45.

Golbus M.S., Hall B.D., Filly R.A. & Poskanzer L.B. (1977) Prenatal diagnosis of achondrogenesis. *Journal of Pediatrics*, **91**, 464.

Goldberg J.D., Chervenak F.A., Lipman R.A. & Berkowitz R.L. (1986) Antenatal sonographic diagnosis of arthrogryposis multiplex congenita. *Prenatal Diagnosis*, **6**, 45–9.

Glenn L.W. & Teng S.S.K. (1985) *In utero* sonographic diagnosis of achondrogenesis. *Journal of Clinical Ultrasound*, **13**, 195–8.

Griffin D., Campbell S., Allan L., Roberts A. & Little D. (1985) Fetal anomalies. In *Clinical Diagnostic Ultrasound*, (Ed. by E. Barnet & P. Morley), pp. 559–80. Blackwell Scientific Publications, Oxford.

Hadlock F.P., Harris R.B., Deter R.L. & Park S.K. (1982) Fetal femur length as a predictor of menstrual age: sonographically measured. *American Journal of Radiology*, **138**, 875–8.

Hageman G., Ippel E.P.F., Beemer F.A., de Pater J.M., Lindhout D. & Willemse J. (1988) The diagnostic management of newborns with congenital contractures: A nosologic study of 75 cases. *American Journal of Medical Genetics*, **30**, 883–904.

Hall J.G. (1984) The lethal multiple pterygium syndromes. *American Journal of Medical Genetics*, **17**, 803–7.

Hall J.G., Reed S.D. & Green G. (1982) The distal arthrogryposes: Delineation of new entities — review and nosological discussion. *American Journal of Medical Genetics*, **11**, 185–239.

Hansmann M., Hackeloer B-J., & Staudach A. (1985) *Ultrasound Diagnosis in Obstetrics and Gynecology*. Springer-Verlag, Berlin.

Hobbins J.C., Bracken M.B. & Mahoney M.J. (1982) Diagnosis of fetal dysplasias with ultrasound. *American Journal of Obstetrics and Gynecology*, **142**, 306–12.

Jeanty P., Dramaix-Wilmet M., Van Gansbeke D., van Regemorter N. & Rodesch F. (1982b) Fetal ocular biometry by ultrasound. *Radiology*, **143**, 513–16.

Jeanty P., Dramaix-Wilmet M., Van Kerkem J., Petroons P. & Schwers J. (1982a) Ultrasonic evaluation of fetal limb growth. Part 2. *Radiology*, **143**, 751–4.

Jeanty P., Kirkpatrick C., Dramaix-Wilmet M. & Struyven J. (1981) Ultrasonic evaluation of fetal limb growth (part 1). *Radiology*, **140**, 165–8.

Jeanty P., Romero R., d'Alton M., Venus I. & Hobbins J. (1985) *In utero* sonographic detection of hand of foot deformities. *Journal of Ultrasound in Medicine*, **4**, 595–601.

Kaitila I., Ammala P., Karjalainen O., Liukkonen S. & Rapola J. (1983) Early prenatal detection of diastrophic dysplasia. *Prenatal Diagnosis*, **3**, 237–44.

Kim H.J., Costales F., Bouzouki M. & Wallach R.C. (1986) Prenatal diagnosis of dysegmental dwarfism. *Prenatal Diagnosis*, **6**, 143–50.

Kirkinen P., Herva R. & Leisti J. (1987) Early prenatal diagnosis of a lethal syndrome of multiple congenital contractures. *Prenatal Diagnosis*, **7**, 189–96.

Koren G., Edwards M.B. & Miskin M. (1987) Antenatal sonography of fetal malformations associated with drugs and chemicals: A guide. *American Journal of Obstetrics and Gynecology*, **176**, 79.

Kurtz A.B. & Wapner R.J. (1983) Ultrasonographic diagnosis of second trimester skeletal dysplasias: a prospective analysis in a high risk population. *Journal of Ultrasound in Medicine*, **2**, 99–106.

Little D. (1984) Prenatal diagnosis of skeletal dysplasias. In *Prenatal Diagnosis*, (Ed. by C.H. Rodeck & K.H. Nicolaides), pp. 301–6. Royal College of Obstetricians and Gynaecologists, London.

Luthy D.A., Mack L., Hirsch J. & Cheng E. (1981) Prenatal diagnosis of thrombocytopenia with absent radii. *American Journal of Obstetrics and Gynecology*, **141**, 350–1.

MacMillan R., Harbart G., Davis W. & Kelly T. (1985) Prenatal diagnosis of Pena–Shokeir syndrome type 1. *American Journal of Medical Genetics*, **21**, 279–84.

Mahony B.S., Filly R.A., Callen P.W. & Golbus M.S. (1985) Amniotic band syndrome: Antenatal sonographic diagnosis and potential pitfalls. *American Journal of Obstetrics and Gynecology*, **152**, 63–8.

Mahoney M.J. & Hobbins J.C. (1977) Prenatal diagnosis of chondroectodermal dysplasia (Ellis–van Creveld Syndrome) with fetoscopy and ultrasound. *New England Journal of Medicine*, **297**, 258–60.

Mantagos S., Weiss R.W., Mahoney M. & Hobbins J.C. (1981) Prenatal diagnosis of diastrophic dwarfism. *American Journal of Obstetrics and Gynecology*, **139**, 111–13.

Mayden K.L., Tortora M., Berkowitz R.L., Braken M. & Hobbins J.C. (1982) Orbital diameters: A new parameter for prenatal diagnosis and dating. *American Journal of Obstetrics and Gynecology*, **144**, 289–97.

Meizner I. & Bar-Ziv J. (1985) Prenatal ultrasonic diagnosis of short-rib polydactyly syndrome (SRPS) type 3: A case report and a proposed approach to the diagnosis of SRPS and related conditions. *Journal of Clinical Ultrasound*, **13**, 284–7.

Milsom I., Mattsson L-A. & Dahlen-Nilsson I. (1982) Antenatal diagnosis of osteogenesis imperfecta by real-time ultrasound: Two case reports. *British Journal of Radiology*, **55**, 310–12.

Mulivor R.A, Mennuti M., Zackai E.H. & Harris H. (1978) Prenatal diagnosis of hypophosphatasia: Genetic, biochemical and clinical studies. *American Journal of Human Genetics*, **30**, 271–82.

Muller L.M. & Cremin B.J. (1985) Ultrasonic demonstration of fetal skeletal dysplasia. *South African Medical Journal*, **65**, 222–6.

Muller L.M. & de Jong G. (1986) Prenatal ultrasonic features of the Pena–Shokeir 1 syndrome and the trisomy 18 syndrome. *American Journal of Medical Genetics*, **25**, 119–29.

Muller L.M., de Jong G. & van Heerden K.M.K. (1985) The antenatal ultrasonographic detection of the Holt–Oram syndrome. *South African Medical Journal*, **68**, 313–15.

O'Brien G.D. & Queenan J.T. (1981) Growth of the ultrasound femur length during normal pregnancy, Part 1. *American Journal of Obstetrics and Gynecology*, **141**, 833–7.

O'Brien G.D., Queenan J.T. & Campbell S. (1981) Assessment of gestational age in the second trimester by real-time ultrasound measurement of the femur length. *American Journal of Obstetrics and Gynecology*, **139**, 540–5.

O'Brien G.D., Rodeck C. & Queenan J.T. (1980) Early prenatal diagnosis of diastrophic dwarfism by ultrasound. *British Medical Journal*, **280**, 1300.

Orioli I.M., Castilla E.E. & Barbosa-Neto J.G. (1986) The birth prevalence rates for the skeletal dysplasias. *Journal of Medical Genetics*, **23**, 328–32.

Quinlan R.W., Brumfield C., Martin M. & Cruz A.C. (1982) Ultrasonic measurement of femur length as a predictor of fetal gestational age. *Journal of Reproductive Medicine*, **27**, 392–4.

Redon J.Y., Le Grevellec J.Y., Marie F., Le Coq E. & Le Guern H. (1984) Un diagnostic antenatal de dysplasie campomelique. *Journal de Gynecologie Obstetrique et Biologie de la Reproduction,* **13**, 437–41.

Romero R., Pilu G., Jeanty P., Ghidini A. & Hobbins J.C. (1988) Skeletal dysplasias. In *Prenatal Diagnosis of Congenital Anomalies,* pp. 311–84. Appleton and Lange, Connecticut/California.

Shaff M.I., Fleischer A.C., Battino R., Herbert C. & Boehm F.H. (1980) Antenatal sonographic diagnosis of thanatophoric dysplasia. *Journal of Clinical Ultrasound,* **8**, 363–5.

Shapiro J.E., Phillips J.A., Byers P.H., Sanders R., Holbrook K.A., Levin L.S., Dorst J., Barsh G.S., Peterson K.E. & Goldstein P. (1982) Prenatal diagnosis of lethal osteogenesis imperfecta (OI type II). *Journal of Pediatrics,* **100**, 127–33.

Shenker L., Reed K., Anderson C., Hauck L. & Spark R. (1985) Syndrome of camptodactyly, anklyoses, facial anomalies and pulmonary hypoplasia (Pena–Shokeir syndrome): Obstetric and ultrasound aspects. *American Journal of Obstetrics and Gynecology,* **152**, 303–7.

Smith D.W. (1982) *Recognizable Patterns of Human Malformations: Genetic, Embryologic and Clinical Aspects.* WB Saunders & Co., Philadelphia.

Smith W.L., Breitweiser T.D. & Dinno M. (1981) *In utero* diagnosis of achondrogenesis type 1. *Clinical Genetics,* **19**, 51.

Socol M., Sabbagha R., Elias S., Tamura R., Simpson J., Dooley S. & Depp R. (1985) Prenatal diagnosis of congenital muscular dystrophy producing arthrogryposis. *New England Journal of Medicine,* **313**, 1230.

Stoll C., Manini P., Bloch J. & Roth M-P. (1985) Prenatal diagnosis of hypochondroplasia. *Prenatal Diagnosis,* **5**, 423–6.

van der Harten J.J., Brons J.T.J., Dijkstra P.F., Niermeijer M.F., Meijer C.J.L.M., Van Geijn H.P. & Th. Arts N.F. (1988) Prenatal lethal osteogenesis imperfecta: radiologic and pathologic evaluation of seven prenatally diagnosed cases. *Pediatric Pathology,* **8**, 233–52.

Warren R.C., McKenzie C.F., Rodeck C.H., Moscoso G., Brock D.J. & Barron L (1985) First trimester diagnosis of hypophosphatasias with a monoclonal antibody to the liver/bone/kidney isoenzyme of alkaline phosphatase. *Lancet,* **ii**, 856.

Weiner C.P., Williamson R.A. & Bonsib S.M. (1986) Sonographic diagnosis of cloverleaf skull and thanatophoric dysplasia in the second trimester. *Journal of Clinical Ultrasound,* **14**, 463–5.

Winter R., Rosenkranz W., Hofmann H, Zierler H., Becker H. & Borkenstein M. (1985) Prenatal diagnosis of campomelic dysplasia by ultrasonography. *Prenatal Diagnosis,* **5**, 1–8.

Winter R.M., Knowles S.A.S., Bieber F.R. & Baraitser M. (1988) *The Malformed Fetus and Stillbirth; a Diagnostic Approach,* pp. 166–201. John Wiley and Sons.

Wladimiroff J.W., Niermeijer M.F., Laar J., Jahoda M. & Stewart P.A. (1984) Prenatal diagnosis of skeletal dysplasia by real-time ultrasound. *Obstetrics and Gynecology,* **63**, 360–4.

Wladimiroff J.W., Niermeijer M.F., Van der Harten J.J., Stewart F.G.A., Bloms W. & Huijmans J.G.M. (1985) Early prenatal diagnosis of congenital hypophosphatasia: case report. *Prenatal Diagnosis,* **5**, 47–52.

Zeitune M., Fejgin M.D., Abramowicz, J., B- Aderet N. & Goodman R. (1988) Prenatal diagnosis of the pterygium syndrome. *Prenatal Diagnosis,* **8**, 145–9.

# Index